Mathog's
Atlas of
Craniofacial Trauma

2nd edition

Mathog's Atlas of Craniofacial Trauma

2nd edition

Editor

Robert H. Mathog, MD
Professor and Chairman
Residency Program Director
Department of Otolaryngology – Head and Neck Surgery
Wayne State University
School of Medicine
Chief of Otolaryngology Karmanos Cancer Hospital
Detroit, Michigan

Associate Editors

Michael A. Carron, MD
Assistant Professor
Chief-Division of Facial Plastic and Reconstructive Surgery
Department of Otolaryngology-Head and Neck Surgery
Wayne State University
School of Medicine
Detroit, Michigan

Terry Y. Shibuya, MD, FACS
Assistant Clinical Professor
Department of Otolaryngology/Head and Neck Surgery
University of California Irvine School of Medicine
Co-Director Anterior Skull Base Surgery Center of Excellence
Co-Director SCPMG Head & Neck Regional Tumor Board
Department of Head and Neck Surgery
Southern California Permanente Medical Group
Orange County, California

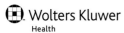 Wolters Kluwer | Lippincott Williams & Wilkins
Health
Philadelphia · Baltimore · New York · London
Buenos Aires · Hong Kong · Sydney · Tokyo

Acquisitions Editor: Robert A. Hurley
Developmental Editor: Franny Murphy
Product Manager: Dave Murphy
Marketing Manager: Lisa Lawrence
Manufacturing Manager: Ben Rivera
Design Manager: Steven Druding
Compositor: SPi Global

Copyright © 2012 Wolters Kluwer Health | Lippincott Williams & Wilkins.

Printed in China

Library of Congress Cataloging-in-Publication Data
Mathog's atlas of craniofacial trauma / editor, Robert H Mathog ; associate editors, Michael A. Carron, Terry Y. Shibuya. — 2nd. ed.
    p. ; cm.
  Atlas of craniofacial trauma
  Rev. ed. of: Atlas of craniofacial trauma. c1992.
  Includes bibliographical references and index.
  ISBN 978-1-60913-700-7 (alk. paper)
 I. Mathog, Robert H., 1939- II. Carron, Michael A. III. Shibuya, Terry Y. IV. Title: Atlas of craniofacial trauma.
  [DNLM: 1. Maxillofacial Injuries—Atlases. 2. Skull—injuries—Atlases. WU 17]
  LC classification not assigned
  617.1'56—dc23

2011045418

LWW.com

9 8 7 6 5 4 3 2 1

This Atlas is dedicated to our wives, Deena, Gretchen and Joyce, whom we love very much. We want to thank them for their patience and support that made this publication possible.

CONSULTANTS

Chenicheri Balakrishnan, MD
Associate Professor
Department of Surgery, Division of Plastic Surgery
Wayne State University School of Medicine
Chief of Hand & Plastic Surgery, John Dingell VAMC
Chief of Plastic Surgery, Detroit Receiving Hospital
Detroit, Michigan

Dennis I Bojrab, MD
Clinical Professor of Otolaryngology and
    Neurosurgery
Wayne State University School of Medicine
Detroit, Michigan
CEO and Director of Research
Michigan Ear Institute
Farmington Hills, Michigan

Lewis Clayman, DMD, MD
Associate Clinical Professor
Department of Otolaryngology-Head and Neck
    Surgery
Wayne State University School of Medicine
Former Chairman of Department of Dentistry/Oral
    and Maxillofacial Surgery
Grace Sinai Hospital
Detroit, Michigan

James M. Coticchia MD, FACS
Associate Professor and Vice Chairman
Director of Pediatric Otolaryngology
Department of Otolaryngology Head and Neck Surgery
Wayne State University School of Medicine
Detroit, Michigan

John J. Fath, MD, MPH, FACS, FCCM
Medical Director of Trauma Services
Oakwood Hospital and Medical Center
Dearborn, Michigan

Adam J. Folbe MD, MS
Assistant Professor
Department of Otolaryngology-Head and Neck
    surgery
Wayne State University School of Medicine
Director, Rhinology, Allergy and Endoscopic Skull
    Base Surgery
Detroit, Michigan

Jerry V. Glowniak, MD, MS
Associate Professor, Department of Radiology
Wayne State University School of Medicine
Chief, Department of Radiology
Detroit Receiving Hospital
Detroit, Michigan

Robert S. Hong, MD, PhD
Fellow in Otology/Neurotology and Skull Base
    Surgery
Michigan Ear Institute
Farmington Hills, Michigan

Mark Hornyak, MD
Assistant Professor
Department of Neurosurgery
Wayne State University School of Medicine
Detroit, Michigan

Michael J. LaRouere, MD
Clinical Associate Professor
Department of Otolaryngology-Head and Neck
    Surgery
Wayne State University School of Medicine
Detroit, Michigan
Attending Neurotologist, Michigan Ear Institute
Farmington Hills, Michigan
Chief, Section of Neurotology Providence Hospital
Southfield, Michigan

Mark Marunick, DDS, MS
Professor
Department of Otolaryngology-Head and Neck
    Surgery
Wayne State University School of Medicine
Chief of Dentistry
Director of Maxillofacial Prosthetics
Detroit, Michigan

Lynne M. Moseley, DDS
Director of Oral Oncology
Karmanos Cancer Center
Detroit, Michigan

Ilka Charlotte Naumann, MD
Fellow in Otology/Neurotology and Skull Base
   Surgery
Michigan Ear Institute
Farmington Hills, Michigan

Jeffrey R. Rubin, MD, FACS
Professor of Surgery
Chief of Vascular Surgery
Wayne State University School of Medicine
And
Detroit Medical Center
Detroit, Michigan

George Yoo, MD, FACS
Professor
Department of Otolaryngology-Head and Neck Surgery
Wayne State University School of Medicine/
   Karmanos Cancer Institute
Chief Medical Officer, Karmanos Cancer Center
Detroit, Michigan

Giancarlo F. Zuliani MD
Assistant Professor
Department of Otolaryngology-Head and Neck Surgery
Division of Facial Plastic and Reconstructive Surgery
Wayne State University School of Medicine
Detroit, Michigan

PREFACE

The diagnosis and treatment of craniofacial trauma are ongoing processes that require periodic documentation of progress and results. The previous Atlas of Craniofacial Trauma was published in 1992, and since then, there have been many developments that need consideration. A charge was thus given to generally respected consultants to serve as authors to update and report on their specialty areas according to their knowledge and expertise. All procedures discussed in this atlas are therefore time-tested and approved by the authors.

This second edition provides a comprehensive approach to injuries of the head, face, and neck areas with the objective of defining what is important for the reader to be a successful practitioner. This atlas is intended to provide information that is easy to read and illustrations that document a stepwise approach to carry out the procedure[s]. To adequately cover the field, there are now discussions of emergency measures, imaging, materials and equipment, and the management of soft tissue, complex fractures, temporal bone, and pediatric injuries. A section on fibula free flaps has been added to deal with the avulsion injury of the mandible. Advances in the use of endoscopic techniques found useful in the reduction and fixation of a variety of facial fractures have been added. Appropriate chapters have been updated to reflect the popularity of rigid fixation.

One of the major objectives of this publication is to develop clearly understood protocols and algorithms. Each subject matter is introduced with the anatomy of the area and pathophysiology of the injury. The procedures are then discussed according to indications, techniques, complications, and pitfalls. Alternative methods that are recognized as being useful are added to the presentation.

PREFACE FROM THE FIRST EDITION

There is much interest in craniofacial trauma. Many people drive or ride in automobiles and play sports, and these activities often lead to accidents and injury to the head and neck region. New textbooks and articles have been published carefully documenting the exciting advances in diagnostic and treatment modalities. Cost-effective treatment methods and ways to prevent these injuries are foci of research activity.

At present, there are many methods to analyze and treat patients with head and neck injuries.

Imaging studies such as computed tomographic (CT) and magnetic resonance scans clearly define skeletal and soft tissue abnormalities. Electrodiagnostic techniques help determine temporary or permanent neurologic deficits. The surgeon has many new approaches and methods available to reinforce or repair damaged tissues. Nonreactive alloplastic implants, free vascularized grafts, and tissue expanders are all recent additions to the surgical armamentarium. Wire fixation is no longer the only method of stabilization, and there are a number of reliable fixation plates of different size and composition.

This atlas is an attempt to provide a series of selected time-proven methods that, in the hands of the author, have been successful in the treatment of craniofacial injury. Each section reviews the pathophysiology of the injury and indications for surgery. The usual format is to illustrate a "typical" injury and then describe what is considered to be an appropriate technique. Modifications, options, and alternatives are provided to give some breadth to the management protocol. Methods to make the procedures easier and ways to prevent and treat complications are also included. The atlas is not intended to be comprehensive, but it does highlight common injuries and one or several chosen methods that will work for that specific situation.

One of the guidelines of this atlas is to provide simple, expedient methodology. With the advent of new techniques, it is tempting to try new approaches and apply new procedures, but these should only be used if they will truly help the patient. A technique should not cause additional morbidity. There is no excuse for a prolonged operative time, unless the surgeon can be assured that the result that can be achieved, in terms of form and function, is an improvement over that which can be achieved by a simpler approach. Overoperation must be avoided.

It should also be noted that this atlas uses consultants to discuss several associated injuries. Although there are many practitioners who can cross specialties, for the most part, the specialists provide an advantage in the management of complex multisystem injuries that often affect the head and neck region. Dentists, orthodontists, oral surgeons, and prosthodontists add invaluable expertise with regard to dental health, tooth stabilization, and occlusal status. For patients with cranial injury, the neurosurgeon plays an important part of the treatment program. Ophthalmologic consultation is essential when there is eye involvement. Laryngologists and otologists are important for evaluation and treatment of laryngeal and temporal bone trauma. The vascular surgeon is also invaluable when the injury involves one of the great vessels of the neck. Craniofacial trauma demands a multidisciplinary approach, and for this reason, we have used consultants liberally to describe their role in the treatment of the patient.

This atlas is written to provide management protocols for the head and neck trauma patient. The methods should help in the training of students, residents, and fellows, and hopefully, the alternative and modified techniques will be of interest to the active practitioner. A base of information is thereby established, setting up future challenges for improvements in patient care.

ACKNOWLEDGMENTS

This surgical atlas is a compilation of surgical techniques that have been developed and taught to many physicians over many lifetimes. It is almost impossible to determine who is responsible for a particular procedure or modification which is often considered an improvement in patient care. The authors appreciate these contributions and want to thank all of those individuals who had a part in development of this expertise. An extensive bibliography toward the end of the book should recognize these contributions.

The authors also want to acknowledge the accurate artistic rendering of surgical procedures performed by professional illustrators William Loechel and Bernie Kida. These illustrations demonstrate their surgical knowledge of the head and neck anatomy and their ability to portray steps a surgeon must use to obtain satisfactory results. Without their contributions, the objectives of this book could not have been obtained.

Finally, the authors would like to recognize those other individuals who have had a place in the development of this atlas. Associate editors, Michael Carron, MD, and Terry Shibuya, MD, were very important in authoring some of the new chapters and in editing the first and last third of the atlas, respectively. Lori Lemonnier, MD, Ilka Naumann, MD, and Robert Hong, MD, PhD, helped several of the senior authors in the writing and editing of text. Also, to be commended is Rita Florkey, executive assistant in the Department of Otolaryngology-Head and Neck Surgery at Wayne State University, who helped in the coordination and communications of this project.

CONTENTS

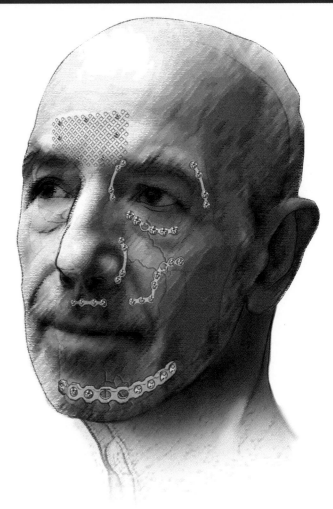

PART ONE

Technical and General Considerations

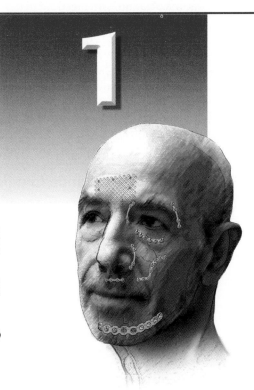

CHAPTER

Imaging of Craniofacial Trauma

In Consultation With Jerry Glowniak, MD

Different imaging methods are available to evaluate the location, severity, and extent of a craniofacial injury. Plain x-rays, which are useful for rapid evaluation at the onset of injury, have largely been replaced by digital scanning and magnetic resonance. Panorex (orthopantograms) and a complete mandible series are, however, helpful for dental and mandible fractures. Computed tomography (CT) scans are commonly employed for most facial fractures, whereas CT angiography (CTA), magnetic resonance imaging (MRI), magnetic resonance angiography (MRA), and conventional angiography are useful adjuncts for specific problems. CT and MRI scans typically provide 2-D planar images that can be reconstructed into any plane. Through computer manipulation, specific structures can be examined in detail and, in some instances, function evaluated.

SPECIFIC PROCEDURES

X-Rays

A X-rays (plain x-rays) are indicated when an immediate radiologic assessment is required, when a patient cannot be moved to a CT or MRI scanner, or when repeated interventions with concomitant assessment are required, for example, during CPR. X-rays are also beneficial when only a limited assessment is required for diagnosis, for a global assessment of fractures, for detecting air or foreign bodies in soft tissues, and for evaluating the patency of large airways and the position of endotracheal or nasogastric tubes. X-ray imaging is less prone to image degradation from metal than CT and MRI. The main disadvantages of x-rays are a limited ability to evaluate soft tissues and the overlapping of 3-D structures when displayed as a 2-D image. Facial fractures are difficult to accurately assess with x-rays, even when multiple images are obtained in different views. However, Panorex and a complete mandible series detail the location and extent of mandible fractures quite clearly.

Computed Tomography

CT is the procedure of choice for evaluating acute, complex trauma of the head and neck. A complete study can be performed in seconds, and images can be reconstructed into multiple planes with resolution as high as 1 mm. Suboptimal exams can be repeated quickly if patient motion degrades image quality.

CT images bony structures in detail but is not as useful as MRI for imaging soft tissues. Contrast CT can significantly improve the soft tissue examination but cannot evaluate the spinal cord unless there is gross trauma or significant bleeding in the spinal canal. Acute hemorrhage, especially in the brain, is readily detected with noncontrast CT, but it often misses acute infarction or brain injury with subtle edema. Metal (bullets, dental amalgam, and surgical hardware) causes image degradation usually confined to the imaging planes in which the metal resides. CT exams can cause significant radiation exposure accelerating the loss of marrow and causing cataracts. Examples of CT scans and their application are described later.

Magnetic Resonance Imaging

B MRI provides superior soft tissue detail compared to CT. MRI is the procedure of choice for evaluating the spinal cord. MRI can assess blood flow without contrast agents (MRA), and exams can be tailored to examine specific aspects of blood flow, for example, magnetic resonance venography (MRV). The main disadvantage of MRI is the time required to image (minutes) compared to CT (seconds) for complete exams. MRI is much more susceptible to artifact from motion than CT. MRI is much less useful for imaging bone (e.g., assessment of fractures), especially bones that contain little marrow like the facial bones. Metal in tissues outside of the scanned structures can produce severe artifacts, which does not occur with CT. MRI can also induce pacemaker malfunction. Because magnetic fields can cause metals to move, MRI is contraindicated when metallic objects are close to arteries, such as aneurysm clips in the brain. While MRI provides excellent contrast between soft tissues (superior contrast resolution), it has poorer spatial resolution (typically 3 to 4 mm) compared to CT (<1 mm).

SPECIFIC INDICATIONS

Soft Tissues of the Head and Neck

For acute trauma, CT is usually adequate to assess important structures, even without contrast. CTA is quickly and easily performed with resolution approaching standard contrast angiography. The entire head and neck can be evaluated in <15 seconds. The venous system can be assessed in the same study although arterial anatomy is better assessed than venous anatomy.

C Soft tissue injuries are assessed with tissue windows looking for asymmetries of the face, head, and neck. The air column should be centrally positioned from the nasopharynx to the laryngopharynx. Most injuries can be assessed without intravenous contrast. Acute hematomas are seen as heterogeneous soft tissue densities while abscesses and cerebrospinal fluid (CSF) leaks have fluid (water) density. Soft tissue air is best assessed with lung windows that provide sharp contrast between air and adjacent fluid and soft tissues.

Cervical Spine Fractures

Plain x-rays are used for the initial evaluation of the cervical spine. Plain x-ray imaging is mandatory if there is any possibility of a displaced fracture, since an adequate exam can be performed without moving the patient. A single crossable lateral view of the cervical spine should nearly always be obtained to evaluate for displaced or unstable fractures before the patient is moved.

D Fractures are seen as discontinuities in cortical bone as well as abnormalities in the shape of the vertebrae. Hyperflexion of the neck can result in the loss of anterior vertebral body height (anterior wedge compression fracture) or displaced fractures of the anterior vertebral body. A characteristic flexion fracture is the teardrop fracture in which a triangular fragment is fractured off the anterior vertebral body. Extension fractures are due to tearing of the anterior longitudinal ligament, which often avulses the superior corner of a vertebral body producing widening of the intervertebral space due to hemorrhage in a disrupted disc. On lateral plain x-rays or sagittal CT images, imaginary lines are used to assess intervertebral relationships. The spinolaminar line is a smooth anteriorly convex curve connecting the anterior portions of the spinous processes in the spinal canal. Loss of this continuity implies disruption of the posterior elements such as spinous process fractures or displacement of one vertebral body on another, which can result in locked facets. Smooth lines also connect the anterior and posterior cortices of the vertebral bodies, and discontinuities in these lines imply fractures or subluxations. Any significant injury to the anterior portion of the cervical spine will cause hemorrhage and edema that displaces the thin ribbon of prevertebral soft tissue anteriorly causing a bulge in the adjacent airway.

Teeth

E CT is adequate for evaluating fractures of teeth. Dental amalgam, however, produces severe artifact, and plain x-rays are much more useful in this situation. CT, however, can simultaneously assess soft tissues and is more useful for detecting dental abscesses and hematomas. Displaced tooth fractures are easily detected on maxillofacial CT scans, especially with simultaneous axial, sagittal, and coronal reconstructions. When

IMAGING OF CRANIOFACIAL TRAUMA

X-RAY

A

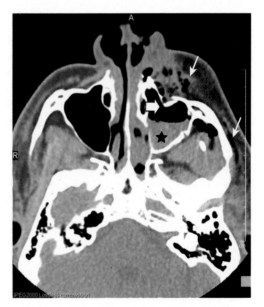

AP x-ray of the facial skeleton. There is a displaced fracture through the right angle of the mandible exiting anteriorly and superiorly at the junction of the mandibular ramus and body posterior to the third molar tooth (white arrows). There is an irregular linear fracture through the left side of the body of the mandible (black arrows).

MRA

B

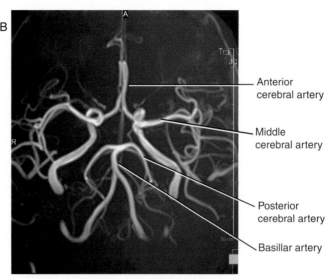

Anterior cerebral artery

Middle cerebral artery

Posterior cerebral artery

Basillar artery

Magnetic Resonance Angiography (MRA) of the intracranial arteries. MRA can readily depict flowing blood in arteries without the use of contrast. The image is a 3-D reconstruction viewed from above centered on the circle of Willis.

SOFT TISSUES

C

Axial CT image through the maxillary sinuses. The anterior wall of the left maxillary sinus shows a depressed fracture (large arrow). There is blood (black star) layering in the posterior portion of the sinus. Thin white arrows point to air in the soft tissues from the maxillary sinus.

CERVICAL SPINE

D

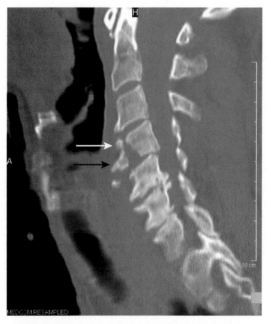

Sagittal CT image of the cervical spine showing a teardrop fracture of anterior body of the fourth cervical vertebra caused by hyperflexion of the neck. An osteophyte has been fractured off the superior endplate (white arrow) along with the anterior inferior portion of the vertebral body (black arrow).

dental amalgam is present, streak artifact is intense in axial sections degrading imaging of adjacent teeth. In sagittal and coronal sections, only a few teeth are seen in each section, restricting artifact to only the sections containing amalgam. When a tooth with amalgam is fractured, plain films are much better for assessing displaced or minimally displaced fractures. Where tooth overlap prevents proper assessment, an orthopantogram (Panorex) allows visualization of individual teeth with minimal overlap. Dental x-rays are useful for the evaluation of the anatomy and injury of teeth.

Mandible Fractures

F–J Mandible fractures are usually assessed with CT although fractures can usually be seen with plain x-rays. Features to assess are disrupted contours of the inferior margin of the body and the smooth anterior and posterior margins of the mandibular ramus and neck. The mandible forms a functionally closed bony ring with the skull base, and significant trauma typically fractures the mandible on opposite sides, for example, right angle and left anterior body. The exception is midline trauma to the chin resulting in a single vertical symphyseal fracture. Parasymphyseal fractures are bony defects between the lateral incisor and canine teeth. Lateral body fractures are seen as bony disruptions between the ramus and the canine tooth. Fractures of the mandibular angle are located at the junction of the ramus and body. Angle fractures commonly involve the bony socket and roots of the third molar. Due to the thickness of the ramus, pure ramus fractures (linear fractures from the posterior to the anterior border of the ramus) are unusual. In the condylar region,* the neck of the mandible directly below the head is most likely to fracture. These fractures are usually horizontal and frequently show lateral displacement of the ramus unless the trauma is directed at the ramus, in which case the ramus is displaced medially. Subcondylar fractures are commonly associated with parasymphyseal fractures. Condylar head fractures occur when an inferior force applied to the body impacts the head on the skull base. These fractures are often nondisplaced, making diagnosis by plain film difficult. Most condylar head fractures are vertical sagittal fractures, best assessed with axial CT images. The glenoid fossa in which the mandibular head resides has medial, anterior, and posterior walls and is open laterally. Thus, lateral displacement is more common and is easily seen on anteroposterior x-ray views. Fractures of the glenoid are usually not present.

Midfacial and Orbital Fractures

CT is by far the best method for accurate assessment of these fractures, especially in cases of multiple fractures. CT is usually quite adequate for assessing soft tissues, especially in the orbits since orbital fat contrasts sharply with muscle, bone, fluid, and hemorrhage. Midface and orbital bones tend to be thin, and because callus formation in old fractures can be minimal, distinguishing acute trauma from old can be difficult. Signs associated with acute trauma include soft tissue swelling adjacent to the fracture, air in the soft tissues adjacent to sinus wall fractures, and blood or fluid in sinuses with fractured walls.

Sinus fractures are readily diagnosed by discontinuities in their walls. Frontal and maxillary sinus fractures are usually obvious because of their large sizes and simple shapes. The sphenoid sinuses have irregular shapes and angles with internal projections complicating assessment. Because of their thin walls and small sizes, isolated fractures of the ethmoid air cells, especially the walls forming portions of the medial walls of the orbits, may be difficult to diagnose. Prominent medial bowing of the medial orbital wall is not uncommon on CT scan. In most of these individuals, no significant history of trauma can be elicited, and it is unclear if these deformities are related to prior trauma. In the setting of trauma, acute fractures should be accompanied by the soft tissue signs listed above.

K Fractures of the nasal bones, orbits, or midface are identified by displacement of bone from its normal anatomic position. Aside from a distorted smooth bony contour, identification of a fracture requires knowledge of the normal shape, position, and relationship of the bony structures to each other. Difficulty occurs in distinguishing acute trauma from old trauma and anatomic variants. In many nontrauma situations, the nasal septum is frequently deviated, angulated, and discontinuous. The nasal bones usually contain prominent symmetric vertical grooves anteriorly, the ethmoidal grooves that contain the external nasal branch of the anterior ethmoidal nerve. They are frequently misinterpreted as fractures, but since the groove thins the nasal bone, it is a frequent site of fracture. Again, soft tissue swelling should be looked for on CT images, and on physical exam, swelling and tenderness should be assessed.

L Trauma to the malar region can fracture the zygoma, maxilla, and orbit. Fractures of one or more of these bones are generically called zygomaticomaxillary complex (ZMC) fractures or orbital maxillary zygomatic (OMZ) fractures. One classic ZMC fracture

---

*The mandibular condyle (condylar process of the mandible) includes the head and neck of the mandible. The subcondylar region refers to that portion of the mandibular ramus immediately inferior to the neck of the mandible.

IMAGING OF CRANIOFACIAL TRAUMA

PANOREX / DENTAL XRAY

E

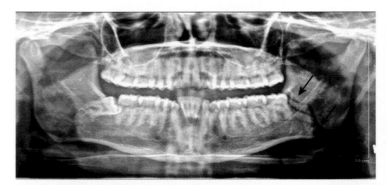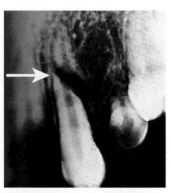

An orthopantogram (Panorex) [left] permits imaging of all the teeth without overlap. Mandibular fractures, such as the fracture of the left mandibular angle indicated by the black arrows, are also well visualized. The dental x-ray on the right shows a fracture of a tooth root (white arrow).

MANDIBLE FRACTURES

F

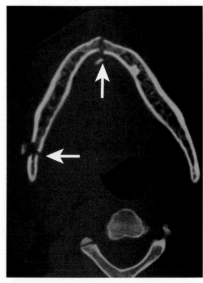

Axial CT image through the mandibular body. The vertical arrow shows a symphyseal fracture. The horizontal arrow shows an associated fracture through the right mandibular angle.

G

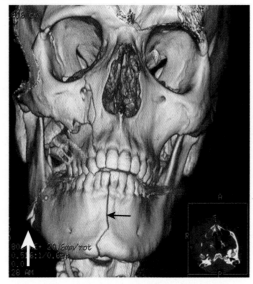

3-D reconstruction of the same study showing the symphyseal fracture (black arrow) and the right mandibular angle fracture (white arrow).

H

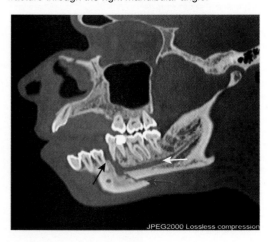

Left mandibular body fracture, oblique sagittal CT image. The black arrow shows the fracture extending into the anterior portion of the socket of first molar tooth. The red arrow points to a fracture through the inferior margin of the mandible. The fracture is displaced with the posterior portion of the mandible superior to the anterior portion. The long linear defect parallel to the inferior margin of the mandible is the mandibular canal (white arrow).

IMAGING OF CRANIOFACIAL TRAUMA

MANDIBLE FRACTURES *(Continued)*

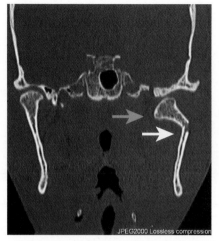

Sagittal CT image of a right mandibular angle fracture. The fracture extends from the angle of the mandible (white arrow) to the base of the coronoid process (black arrow).

Coronal CT image. The white arrow points to an angulated fracture of the left mandibular condyle with the head of the left mandibular condyle (gray arrow) displaced medially.

MIDFACIAL / NASAL FRACTURES

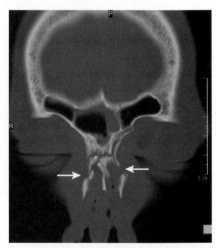

Axial [left] and coronal [right] CT images showing comminuted fractures of the nasal bones (white arrows).

ZYGOMATICOMAXILLARY COMPLEX FRACTURE

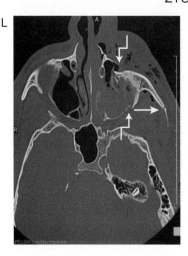

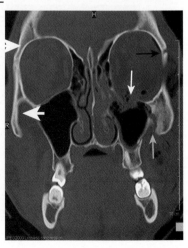

Axial [left] and coronal [right] CT images of a left zygomaticomaxillary complex (ZMC) fracture. The ZMC fracture shown in these images separates the zygomatic bone from the facial skeleton. The three strongest attachments of the zygomatic bone to the facial skeleton are fractured including: the zygomatic arch (straight white arrow, left image), the zygomaticofrontal suture in the lateral orbital margin (horizontal black arrow, right image), and the zygomatico-maxillary suture (vertical gray arrow) which extends anteriorly to the inferior orbital margin. Secondary fractures through thinner bony plates include the orbital floor (white arrow, right image), the anterior and posterlateral walls of the maxillary sinus (jagged white arrows, left image) and the lateral wall of the orbit (not shown).

occurs when the zygoma is fractured off its attachments to the rest of the facial skeleton. The three main components of this fracture include a fracture through the attachment to the maxilla at the zygomaticomaxillary suture extending through the inferior orbital rim, a lateral orbital wall fracture that exits through the lateral orbital margin at the zygomaticofrontal suture, and, lastly, a fracture of the zygomatic arch.

M,N Direct trauma to the anterior portion of the eye may transmit a force to the orbital walls with the thinnest walls fracturing with outward displacement of bone (orbital blow-out fractures). Two common sites of fracture are the medial wall (formed by the thin orbital plates of the ethmoid air cells) and the orbital floor. The weakest point in the orbital floor is the infraorbital groove/canal which transmits the infraorbital vessels and nerve. Floor fractures are often difficult to evaluate in axial sections, and coronal sections should always be examined. A classic fracture is the orbital floor trapdoor fracture in which there are two linear parallel fractures. One fracture is nondisplaced and acts as a hinge about which the fractured bone rotates into the maxillary sinus. With sufficient trauma, the inferior rectus muscle can herniate through the defect in the floor into the maxillary sinus.

Le Fort fractures are fractures of the facial bones that separate portions of the facial bones from the rest of the skull numbered I to III in increasing amounts of facial separation from the skull. All the Le Fort fractures involve the pterygoid plates, the nasal septum, the lateral walls of the nasal cavities, and a variety of buttresses (see Chapter 35 for a description of beams and buttresses of the facial skeleton). The classic Le Fort fractures are bilaterally symmetric fractures that rarely occur as isolated injuries. More commonly, injuries producing craniofacial separation are asymmetric involving various combinations of the Le Fort fractures. In these instances, it is somewhat problematic designating an injury as a specific Le Fort fracture, and a detailed description of the fractures is more informative.

O The Le Fort I fracture is a horizontal fracture through the maxillae just above the hard palate producing a "floating palate." There are circumferential fractures just above the floors of the maxillary sinuses, fracture of the inferior nasal septum, and fractures through the pterygomaxillary junctions.

P The Le Fort II fracture separates most of the maxilla from the rest of the face, producing a "floating maxilla." There are two main fracture lines: one through the anterior orbit and lateral maxilla and the other through the medial orbital wall. Posteriorly, the two lines meet in the posterior wall of the maxillary sinus above the pterygomaxillary junction. Anteriorly,

the fracture lines meet at the frontal process of the maxilla with a fracture extending into the nasal bone. A horizontal fracture through the inferior portion of the pterygoid plates completes the facial separation. Medially, a fracture begins at the frontal process of the maxilla and continues through the medial wall of the orbit. The other fracture line extends from the frontal process of the maxilla through the most anterior portions of the medial wall and floor of the orbit exiting through the lateral portion of the inferior orbital rim. The fracture then extends laterally and posteriorly below the body of the zygomatic bone through the zygomaticomaxillary suture and continues through the posterolateral wall of the maxillary sinus joining the medial fracture above the pterygomaxillary junction.

Q The Le Fort III fracture separates the facial bones from the rest of the skull. Horizontal fractures extend through the medial and lateral walls of the orbits separating the frontal bone from the rest of the facial bones. These two fractures meet centrally in the orbit at the inferior orbital fissure. The lateral wall fracture exits anteriorly through the lateral orbital rim at the zygomaticofrontal suture. The medial wall fracture is continuous with a fracture through or adjacent to the nasofrontal and frontomaxillary sutures. In addition, there is a horizontal fracture through the superior portion of the nasal septum and the lateral wall of the nasal cavity at the same level. There is also a vertical fracture through the zygomatic arch.

The hard palate forms the floor of the nasal cavities and roof of the mouth. It attaches peripherally to the body of the maxilla at the junction of the alveolar ridges with the body of the maxilla. Because of its position deep in the face and its attachment to the maxilla, it fractures in conjunction with other fractures of the maxilla and the alveolar ridge. The hard palate should be examined in coronal and sagittal sections when fractures of the lower maxilla are seen since the hard palate lies in nearly an axial plane, and nondisplaced fracture may be missed when only axial sections are viewed.

Frontal Bone and Nasoorbitoethmoid Fractures

R,S Frontal bone fractures are best evaluated by CT scans, but since the injury may involve the structures in the anterior cranial fossa, MRI scans are a useful adjunct for diagnosis. It is important to note the integrity of the anterior and posterior walls of the frontal sinus and to determine the degree of fracture displacement. Fluid within the sinus may indicate a CSF leak, but further studies are necessary to determine this condition (see Chapter 84). Intracranial air should be an indication of a fracture. Fractures that extend to the frontal sinus floor are important to define

IMAGING OF CRANIOFACIAL TRAUMA

MIDFACIAL AND ORBITAL FRACTURES

BLOWOUT FRACTURE

M

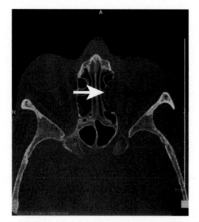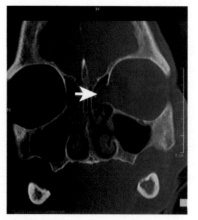

Medial orbital wall blowout fracture. Axial [left] and coronal [right] images. The arrows point to the medially deviated left medial orbital wall. This is an old injury in which soft tissue swelling has resolved.

N

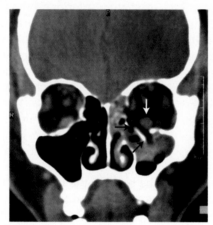

Coronal CT image of a trapdoor fracture of the left orbital floor. The orbital floor is fractured in two places (black arrows). The lower arrow shows that the lateral portion of the fractured floor has rotated inferiorly. The white arrow points to the inferior rectus muscle which lies in the fracture gap but has not herniated into the maxillary sinus.

LE FORT I FRACTURE

O

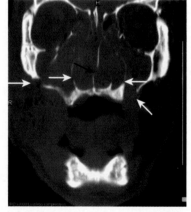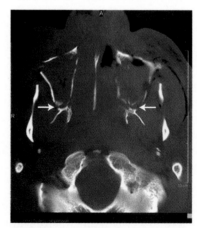

Coronal CT image through the anterior maxillary sinuses [left] showing fractures of the medial and lateral walls of the maxillary sinuses (white arrows) and the bony nasal septum (black arrow). Axial CT image [right] through the lower portions of the maxillary sinuses below the attachments of the zygomas. There are fractures of the posterior attachments of the maxillae to the pterygoid processes at the pterygomaxillary junctions (white arrows). The fractures detach the hard palate from the rest of the facial skeleton.

IMAGING OF CRANIOFACIAL TRAUMA

MIDFACIAL AND ORBITAL FRACTURES *(Continued)*

LE FORT II FRACTURE

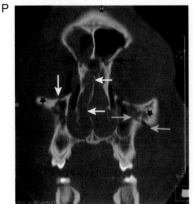

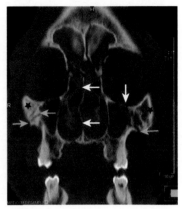

In a Le Fort II fracture, the maxillae and the hard palate are separated from the rest of the facial bones. The primary attachments of the maxilla are to the zygoma, the frontal bone, the nasal septum by the hard palate, and the pterygoid process through the pterygomaxillary junction at the inferior posterior wall of the maxillary sinus. These two contiguous coronal CT images show fractures through the frontal processes of the maxillae (black arrows, left image) that continue through the medial walls of the orbits (black arrows, right image). The attachments to the zygomas are fractured at the inferior orbital margins (left and right images, vertical white arrows) continuing through the zygomaticomaxillary sutures (gray horizontal arrows, right and left images). These fractures converge on the posterior walls of the maxillary sinuses and continue through the pterygoid plates completing the separation. The nasal septum is also fractured (horizontal white arrows). Note that the zygomas (stars) remain attached to the upper portion of the facial skeleton. Fractures through the pterygoid plates are not visualized in these images.

LE FORT III FRACTURE

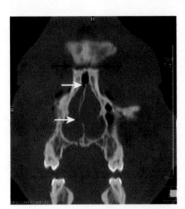

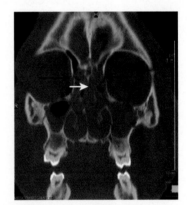

Coronal CT images showing a Le Fort III fracture with fractures through the frontal processes of the maxillae (left image, black arrows), left zygomaticofrontal suture (right image, short black arrow), the medial walls of the orbits and the adjacent lateral walls of the nasal cavities (right image, long black arrows) and the bony nasal septum (white arrows). Fractures through the pterygoid plates are not visualized in these images.

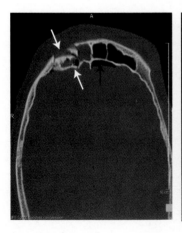

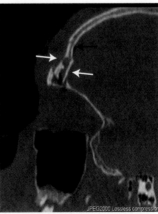

FRONTAL BONE FRACTURE

Axial [left] and sagittal [right] CT images showing a depressed fracture of the anterior wall and a posteriorly displaced posterior wall fracture of the right frontal sinus (white arrows). The posterior wall fractures have lacerated the arachnoid and dura mater, and air from the frontal sinus has entered the subarachnoid space (black arrows).

IMAGING OF CRANIOFACIAL TRAUMA

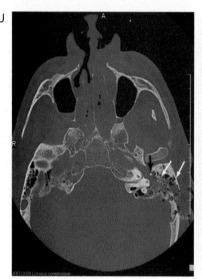

◀S

NASOORBITOETHMOID FRACTURE

Nasoorbitoethmoid (NOE) fracture. Axial CT image. The black arrow point to the fossa for the right lacrimal sac formed by the frontal process of the maxilla anteriorly and the lacrimal bone posteriorly. There are fractures of the right nasal bone and the medial wall of the right orbit which is part of the right orbital plate of the ethmoid bone (short white arrows). On the left, there are fractures through the fossa and the medial wall of the orbit (long white arrows). There are also several fractures of the bony nasal septum (unlabeled).

T

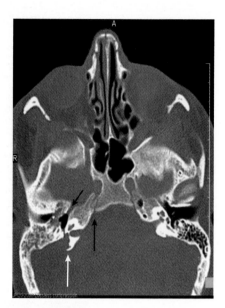

SKULL BASE FRACTURE ▲

Skull base fracture, axial CT image. There are fractures through the mid portion of the petrous pyramid of the right temporal bone through the inner and middle ears (white arrow) and though the right lateral portion of the sphenoid bone (long black arrow) with displacement and rotation of the fractured fragment. There is widening of the bony part of the right eustachian (auditory) tube (short black arrow).

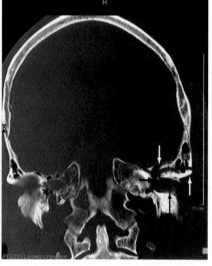

TEMPORAL BONE FRACTURE ▲

Axial [left] and coronal [right] CT images of a fracture along the longitudinal axis of the mastoid and petrous portions of the left temporal bone (white arrows) extending into the middle ear. The short black arrows point to the head of the malleus in the blood filled middle ear. The petrous and the mastoid air cells are also filled with blood. The long black arrow points to the blood filled external auditory meatus.

V ➤

3-D IMAGING

Three Dimensional [3-D] reconstructed CT scan showing a left zygomaticomaxillary complex (ZMC) fracture. This image is a 3-D reconstruction of the ZMC fracture in Figure L. The zygoma has been separated from the rest of the facial skeleton. Fractures include 1) a fracture through the attachment of the zygoma to the maxilla (at the zygomaticomaxillary suture) that continues superiorly through the inferior orbital rim (black arrows), 2) a fracture through the zygomaticofrontal suture in the lateral orbital rim, and 3) a fracture through the zygomatic arch which attaches the zygoma to the temporal bone (white arrow).

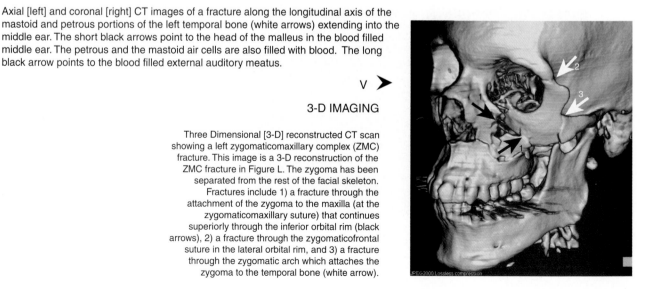

as these fractures can cause problems with nasofrontal duct aeration and drainage of the sinus. Coronal and axial CT images are helpful in evaluating the nasoorbitoethmoid complex and are important in determining medial canthal injury which if unrecognized can cause late epiphora and telecanthus.

Skull Base and Temporal Bone Fractures

CT is the only adequate means for assessing the skull base. Current scanners can produce 0.5-mm sections, with the main limitation being patient motion. At a resolution of 0.5 mm, even undetectable motion, such as motion from the beating heart, can negate resolution at these levels. For trauma, the ability to evaluate brain, bone, and other soft tissues in a single exam makes CT the procedure of choice, and often the only acceptable procedure.

T,U The temporal bones, the sphenoid bone, and the occipital bone comprise the skull base posterior to the orbits. Because the occipital bone is mostly flat, fractures are seen as linear defects in its otherwise smooth surface. The temporal bones, however, are very irregular with numerous internal cavities: inner ears, middle ears, and air cells in the mastoid, petrous, and squamous portions of the temporal bone. The thin walls of these cavities can make detection of nondisplaced fractures difficult. Any fluid in these cavities or intracranial air adjacent to the inner table of the skull in these regions should prompt a diligent search for fractures in the walls of the adjacent air cells. The principal sutures of the posterior skull convexity and posterior skull base are the lambdoid and occipitomastoid sutures, respectively. Any fracture extending to these sutures can propagate through the suture causing a sutural fracture. A fracture though the occipitomastoid suture can extend anteriorly through the inferior surface of the temporal bone to the anterior skull base. A sutural fracture may be difficult to distinguish from a normal suture. Comparison with the contralateral suture helps to distinguish a normal suture from a sutural fracture.

3-D Imaging

V 3-D imaging is a useful adjunct to planar (2-D) imaging. 3-D images provide a more intuitive and more easily interpretable exam obviating the difficult problem of mentally creating a 3-D image from multiple planar images. CT and MRI both allow for reconstruction of 3-D images. CT reconstructions are the gold standard for 3-D imaging of the skull.

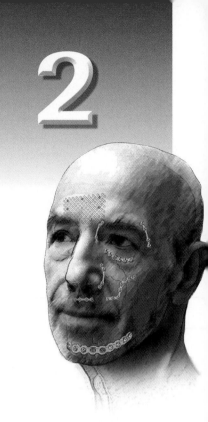

Materials, Plating, and Instruments

In Consultation With Michael A. Carron, MD

INDICATIONS

The goal of the craniofacial trauma surgeon is to restore the anatomic form and physiologic function of the face after injury. Recovery should be as quickly as possible and the repair should be maintained for the life of the patient. In order for this to occur, the surgeon must be familiar with reconstruction of the craniofacial skeleton using both conservative treatment and operative intervention. Familiarity with open reduction and fixation methods and available plating materials and instruments is essential.

Healing of bony fractures requires complex biologic processes. The fracture can be deemed "healed" when the bone resumes its full function and is able to bear the physiologic load placed upon it without the assistance of plates and screws. Until healing is complete, the applied hardware keeps the ends of the fracture(s) in as close approximation as possible. This minimizes the gap between the segments, so remodeling may take place. Remodeling becomes more difficult when the gap between the two fracture segments is increased. For optimal healing, the fracture site should be clean, well perfused, free of infection, and motionless. If these conditions are not met, healing may be delayed (delayed union) or not occur at all (nonunion).

Selecting the appropriate material(s) to stabilize a fracture is important to optimize the healing of the fracture. Different plates and screws are available for various fracture situations. Screws, plates, and mesh used in facial fractures are usually made of titanium, a metal which is biocompatible, minimally corrosive,

nontoxic, and bendable. Recently, absorbable plates, screws, and mesh composed of poly-L-lactic acid have become available and are widely used in pediatric craniofacial procedures, cranial and midface fixation, some mandible fractures, and orthognathic surgery. These materials dissolve by hydrolysis after 12 to 18 months. Essentially, one needs to select a plate that adequately bridges the defect and stabilizes the fixation in conjunction with appropriately sized screws.

PROCEDURE

Materials and Their Application

A Trays. Typical instrumentation trays have most of the materials necessary to reduce and stabilize craniofacial fractures. There are many manufacturers and a variety of devices, but most instruments and supplies are designed to use similar methodology.

B Plates. Fixation plates are classified by profile height; a 2.0 plate is 2 mm in height. Plates are also characterized by their function.

C Reconstruction plates are "Heavy Duty" load-bearing plates. They assume the physiologic stress at the fracture. Reconstruction plates are the highest profile, strongest plates and are commonly used for bridging gaps in resected bone, in severely comminuted, contaminated, or infected fractures. They are used for periods of extended fixation in repair of a fracture of the edentulous mandible and in the treatment of poorly compliant patients (see Chapters 27 and 34).

INSTRUMENT AND PLATE TRAY

A

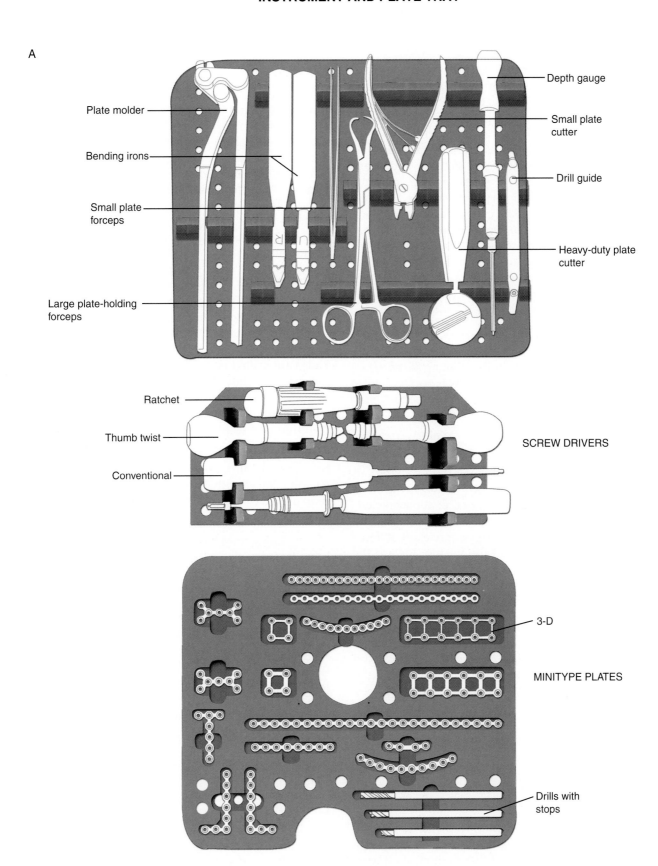

Plate molder

Bending irons

Small plate forceps

Large plate-holding forceps

Depth gauge

Small plate cutter

Drill guide

Heavy-duty plate cutter

Ratchet

Thumb twist

Conventional

SCREW DRIVERS

3-D

MINITYPE PLATES

Drills with stops

Reconstruction plates must be bent exactly to the contour of the bone and may be placed above or below the periostium. Superiorly placed tension bands are not necessary with reconstruction plates.

D Compression plates exert a preloading force that pushes the fractured segments together. Eccentric screw holes and drilling permit this action when screws are placed. Compression increases the friction between fracture ends to minimize movement and the gap that needs to be bridged. Compression plates are used in situations that require increased stability and rapid healing (see Chapter 24). Theoretically, the compression plate provides for primary bone healing, which is more rapid than the secondary type that requires intermediate callus formation. Oblique fractures are not good candidates for compression plating as the fracture segments may slide over one another and come out of reduction when compressed. Compression plates may at times distract the upper part of the mandible and require the application of a tension band or plate.

E Noncompression plates are the "work horse" plate used for most mandible fractures. These plates minimize movement at the site by splinting the two fracture ends once they are reduced. Screw holes are circular and there is no preloading force to push the two ends together. Absorbable plates are a noncompression type.

F Locking plates are also available in which the screw head locks into the plate. This plate has the advantages of preventing the screw from backing out of the plate or having the screw strip a hole in the bone; it also facilities an internal/external fixation precluding the exact contouring of the plate to bone. It should be noted that nonlocking screws can exert a force on the bone, which may pull the fracture toward the plate and out of reduction. The design of the locking plate permits the screw to lock into the plate and not the bone avoiding this potential distraction.

G Miniplates (or microplates) are small nonlocking plates useful for fractures of beams and buttresses of the forehead and midface (see Chapters 45, 69, and 75). Miniplates are low-profile, easy to contour, light, and are available in a variety of geometric shapes. Miniplates are preferred for fixation of the bones of the cranium and midface, which are subject to little or no force when compared to the forces exerted upon the mandible. Thinner microplates are also useful when there is no external force and where the skin is quite thin such as the glabella, frontal bone, cranium, and nasal bones.

H Titanium mesh is employed like a plate to bridge fractures but in a situation where there is a need to cover broad defects of the cranium, skull base, and orbit (see Chapters 62 and 75). Mesh is light, low-profile, and easy to trim and to contour to bony topography. Mesh is designed like a screen with multiple screw whole options.

Screws

I Screws are essential to hold the plate and fracture in fixation. Most screws are placed after drilling a pilot hole through a plate or mesh into the underlying bone. Pilot holes are recipient holes for the screw. Some screws are self-drilling with cutting flutes at the screw tip, which avoids the need for a pilot hole in the bone. Usually, firm pressure is necessary when using self-drilling screws and may not be suitable for thin, unstable bone.

All screws are named according to their "thread" diameter, the absolute width of the screw from thread to thread. The "core" diameter refers to the width of the central core of the screw and corresponds to the size of the drill bit necessary for the pilot hole. The size of the drill bit corresponds to core diameter not the thread diameter. The thread diameter of the screw is always wider than the drill bit (the core diameter). Holes are drilled using drill guides to ensure 90° pilot holes to the plate. Irrigation cools the bone and prevents necrosis around the screw. If drill holes are inappropriately placed or overheated, the fixation may be compromised resulting in a delayed or failed union.

J Special intermaxillary fixation screws are used to establish intraoperative occlusion rapidly (see Chapter 24). Usually two or three screws are placed on both the maxillary and mandibular arches and secured to each other with wire loops.

K Lag screws have the special purpose of pulling bone fragments together (see Chapter 24). The technique is particularly useful for the treatment of oblique fractures of the mandibular body and sagittal fractures of the symphysis. The lag screw is also important for securing bone grafts. Because the entire length of the screw is threaded, a gliding hole must be placed at least as wide as the thread diameter of the screw in the outer layer (first cortex) of bone. The hole in the underlying bone (second cortex) is drilled in the conventional manner with the appropriate bit for that screw size (equal to the core diameter). When the lag screw is seated, the two bones are pulled together. To prevent shearing of the fragments, the lag screw is placed at 90° to the fracture line and equidistant from the two fracture edges.

Drill Bits

L Drill bits bore a hole in the bone and should correspond to the core diameter of the screw. They should be used with drill guides of appropriate size

PLATES

B

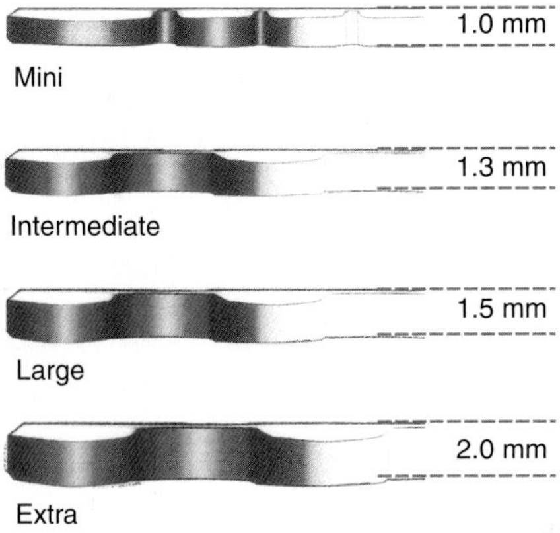
1.0 mm
Mini
1.3 mm
Intermediate
1.5 mm
Large
2.0 mm
Extra

Plate thickness

C

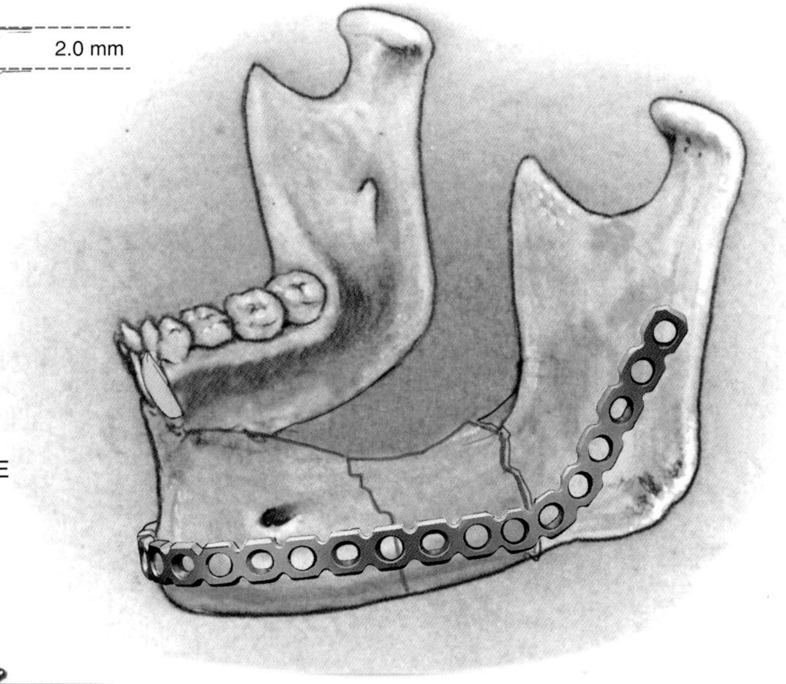

RECONSTRUCTION PLATE

D

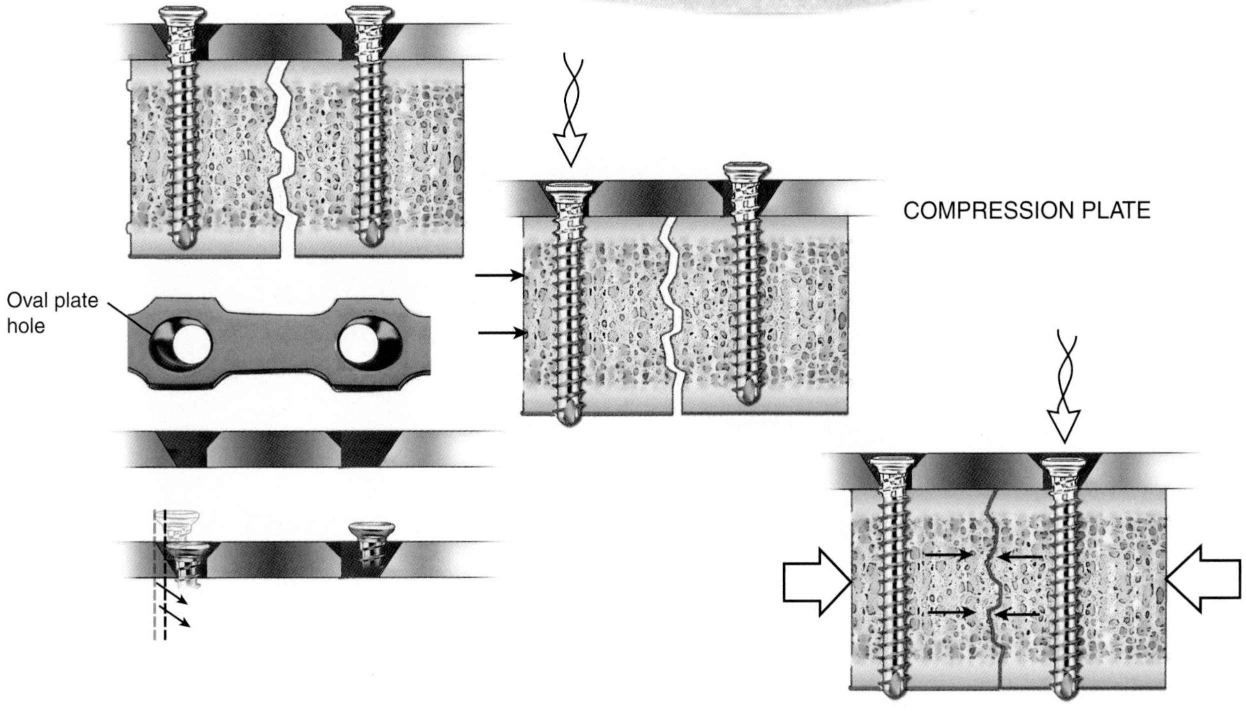
Oval plate hole

COMPRESSION PLATE

PLATES *(Continued)*

NONCOMPRESSION

E

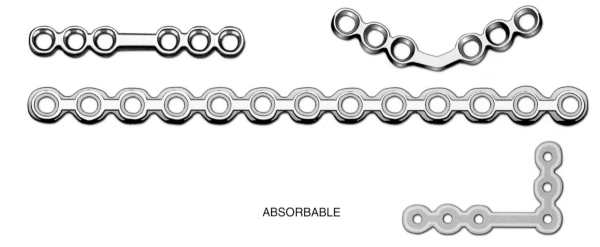

ABSORBABLE

F

Threaded screw ———

Threaded plate ———

LOCKING

G

MINIPLATES

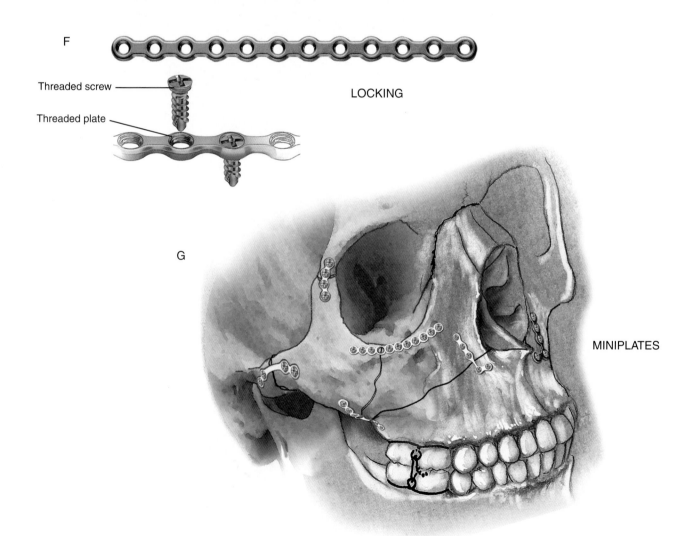

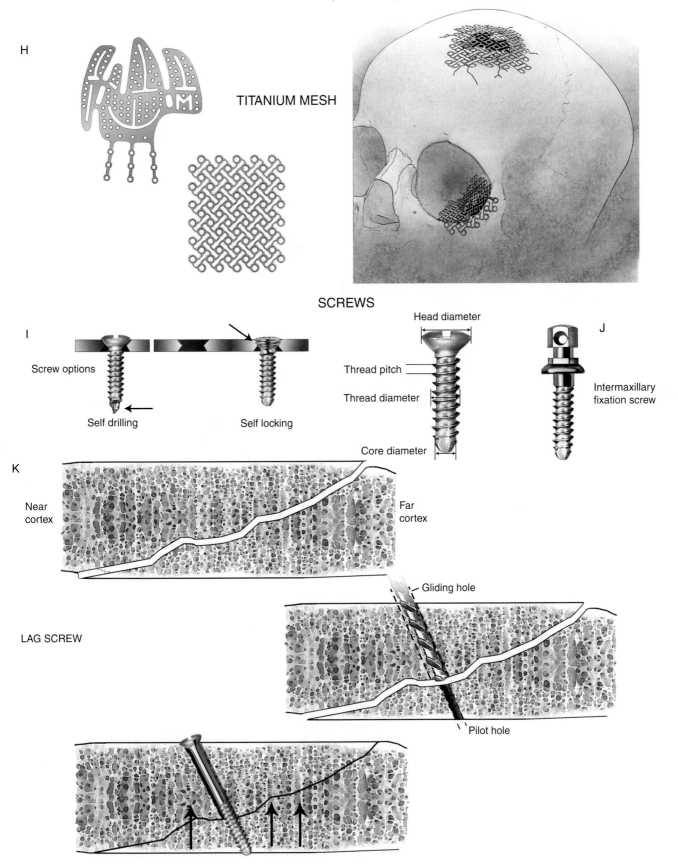

H

TITANIUM MESH

SCREWS

I

Screw options

Self drilling

Self locking

Head diameter

Thread pitch

Thread diameter

Core diameter

J

Intermaxillary fixation screw

K

Near cortex

Far cortex

Gliding hole

Pilot hole

LAG SCREW

(these are color coded to prevent confusion). Irrigation prevents overheating of the bone. The length of the bit is important since too long a bit may wobble and too short a bit may not provide sufficient attachment. A "stop" on the drill bit for thin bones avoids drilling beyond a preset depth. It is important to be aware of important neurovascular structures deep to the area of drilling that may be injured if the drill is advanced beyond the inner cortex.

Depth Gauge

M A depth gauge assures measurement of a hole for proper screw length and insurance that the screw will secure both cortices. The tip of the screw should slightly exit the inner cortex. A slide mechanism allows precise measurement of the depth of the drill hole.

Drill Guides

N Drill guides are used to ensure 90° placement and uniform holes while protecting the surrounding soft tissue. The guide is usually secured to the plate before drilling. A drill guide with an arrow is used when drilling compression plates. The arrow points to the fracture line and allows for offset drilling, one side of the fracture line at a time. For noncompression plates neutral holes are achieved using a nonarrow drill guide.

Screwdrivers

O Screwdrivers have a quick coupling that allows the attachment of various screwdriver blades. The driver may be a traditional, ratchet type or twist type with thumb and forefinger. Blades are of various lengths and widths for different screw sizes and hard to reach areas.

Plate Benders

P Plate benders are used to bend the plate to the 3-D topography of the bony surface. Micro- and mini-plates are contoured by hand or with small plate benders. More rigid plates have heavy-duty benders and rollers to contour the plates.

Plate Cutters

Q Micro- and miniplates are cut to size with small plate cutters. The larger plates are cut with two cutters placed opposite the desired area to cut. A twisting motion will cut the plate, but this varies somewhat with the manufacturer of the set.

Plate Holders

R Once the fracture is reduced and the plate applied, the plate needs to remain stationary with plate holders while drilling occurs. Plate holding forceps have a sharp tip and a ball tip. The sharp tip grasps the bone on its inner cortex while the ball tip fits into the hole in the plate. The holders stabilize the entire complex of the two fracture ends and the plate.

Trochars

S Occasionally, it is necessary to use a percutaneous approach for drilling holes in hard to reach areas. The percutaneous system uses a drill guide over a trochar to pierce the soft tissues and create a tunnel to the plate. The trochar is removed, the guide is inserted, and the screw placed through the guide. A cheek retractor is normally used to maneuver the drill guide over the plate holes.

Arch Bars, External Fixation Devices, Splints, and Mesh

These materials and application are discussed in Chapters 19, 20, 21, 62, and 75.

PITFALLS

1. Failure to adequately reduce the fracture commonly results in movement leading to delayed healing or failure to heal. The gap between segments should be minimized so that healing may occur. Interfragmentary motion should be avoided and is often caused by poor reduction, poor application of the plate, too few screws, or insufficiently large screws for the situation.

2. A fracture may be taken out of reduction if the plate is not bent properly or contoured to the bone that is to be repaired. Because the plate is rigid, the bone will adapt to the configuration of the plate and be drawn away from the opposite fracture segment. Therefore, it is prudent to adapt the plate to the reduced bony topography as precisely as possible before placing screws.

3. Skin thickness varies depending on the facial subunit. Thin skinned areas will have a propensity for plate palpability and show. Only thin plates (microplates) should be used in these thin skinned areas.

COMPLICATIONS

1. Plate extrusion occurs when an overly thick plate is used in thin skinned individuals or when there is osteomyelitis or necrosis of the soft tissues. Patients should be informed of the possibility of these complications, and when the complication occurs, they should be treated aggressively. This may require complete removal of the plate, debridement of the bone, or refixation with or without bone grafts as described in Chapters 34, 35, and 36.

2. Screws may loosen if they are not tightened completely and are overtightened or too short to provide

TOOLS FOR RIGID FIXATION

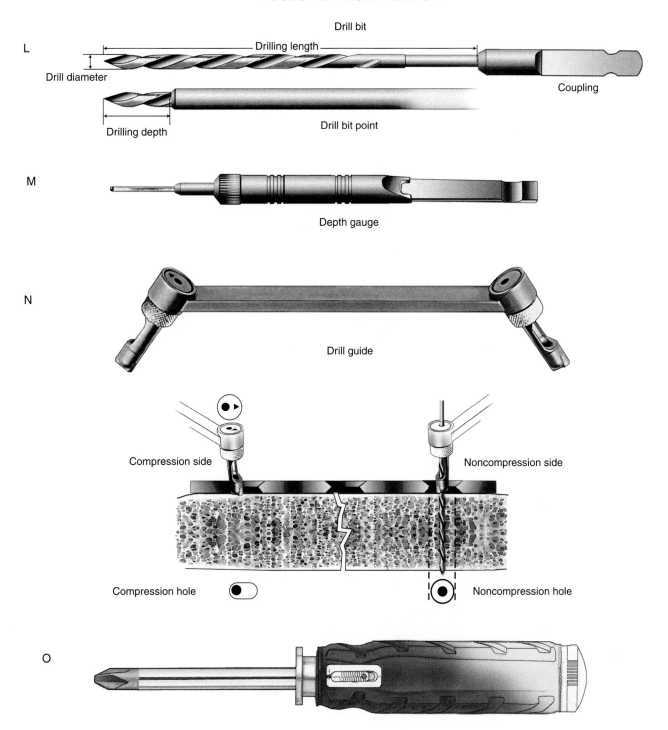

Drill bit

L

Drilling length

Drill diameter

Coupling

Drilling depth

Drill bit point

M

Depth gauge

N

Drill guide

Compression side

Noncompression side

Compression hole

Noncompression hole

O

Ratchet screw driver

Plate benders

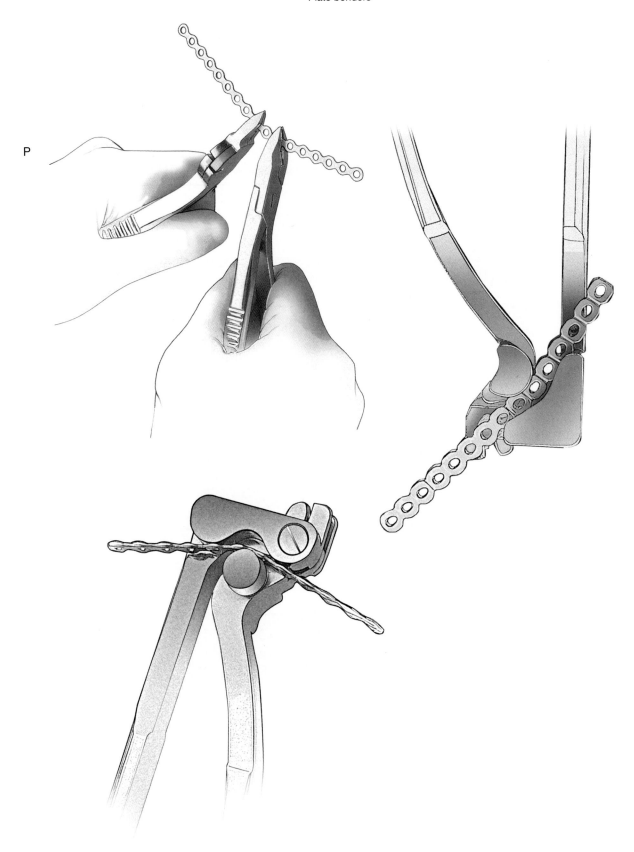

P

Plate cutters

Q

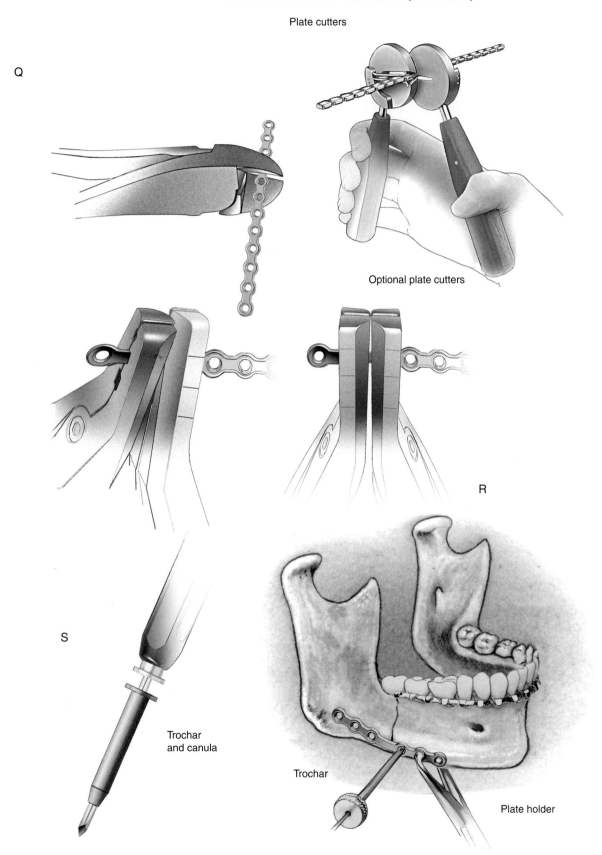

Optional plate cutters

S

Trochar
and canula

R

Trochar

Plate holder

stability. Moreover, failing to irrigate predisposes to bone necrosis and loosening of screws. Screw failure, in turn, may lead to loosening of the plate and loss of fixation.

3. Poorly adapted plates to the bony contour may cause deformity and pull the bone segments out of reduction. Plates are unforgiving, and if this condition occurs, it will require removal of the plate and another attempt at fixation and reduction.

4. As noted earlier, large plates present a risk of palpability in thinned skinned individuals. This can be avoided by using micro- or miniplates in such areas as the nasal bones and orbital rims. Palpable plates may have to be removed.

5. On occasion, plates may cause sensitivity to cold and heat, and in these situations, plates also may require removal.

6. Titanium plates should be avoided in children as they have been shown to migrate from the outer to inner cortex. If such plates are utilized, they should be removed at an early stage. Resorbable plates can avoid this complication.

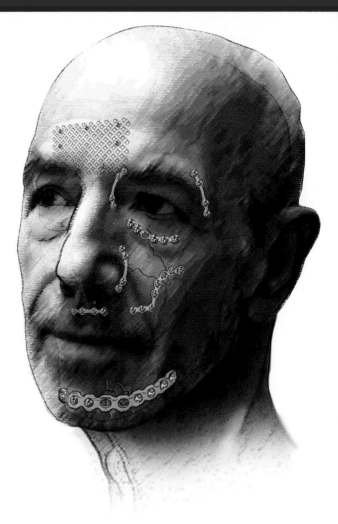

PART TWO

Emergency Measures

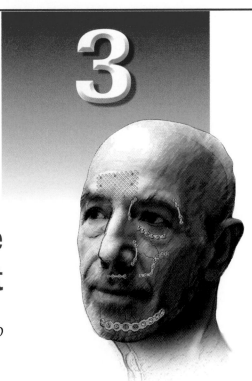

CHAPTER **3**

Evaluation of the Trauma Patient

In Consultation With John Fath, MD

INDICATION

Organizing the initial evaluation of the trauma patient is very important. The reader is directed to the American College of Surgeons' course and publication on advanced trauma life support to learn the appropriate algorithm for the care of injured patient. This protocol focuses on support of the airway, breathing, and circulation, with a diagnostic evaluation of additional injuries taking place in sequential fashion. It is thus important to appreciate potential life threatening injuries and not be distracted by the associated often dramatic facial injuries. Specialists who understand how to manage a polytrauma situation protect both the patient and himself or herself from missed injuries. This chapter focuses on specific problem areas in the care of patients with facial trauma.

PROCEDURES

Airway

Oral tracheal intubation is the primary means to provide a secure airway to the trauma victim (see Chapter 5).

Unfortunately, there are times when control of the airway by intubation becomes problematic due to debris in the oropharynx, bleeding, and altered anatomy. In this instance, one resorts to secondary airway devices such as nasal trumpet, oral airway, and laryngeal mask. Secretions should be suctioned from the oropharynx, and the tongue and mandible should be brought forward. If the airway cannot be controlled by these methods, a rapid cricothyroidotomy is the procedure of choice. It is also possible that after the cricothyroidotomy, the endotracheal tube can be passed and the cricothyroidotomy tube removed.

A–G There are well-documented techniques for cricothyroidotomy using a small size endotracheal or tracheostomy tube (see Chapter 6). Several of the commercial cricothyroidotomy kits are very user-friendly and work well under emergency conditions. Our preference is the Melker Emergency Cricothyrotomy Kit that uses a guide wire technique, which can be taught easily to a variety of different emergency providers. According to this technique, the anatomy of the neck is evaluated and a small vertical incision is made over

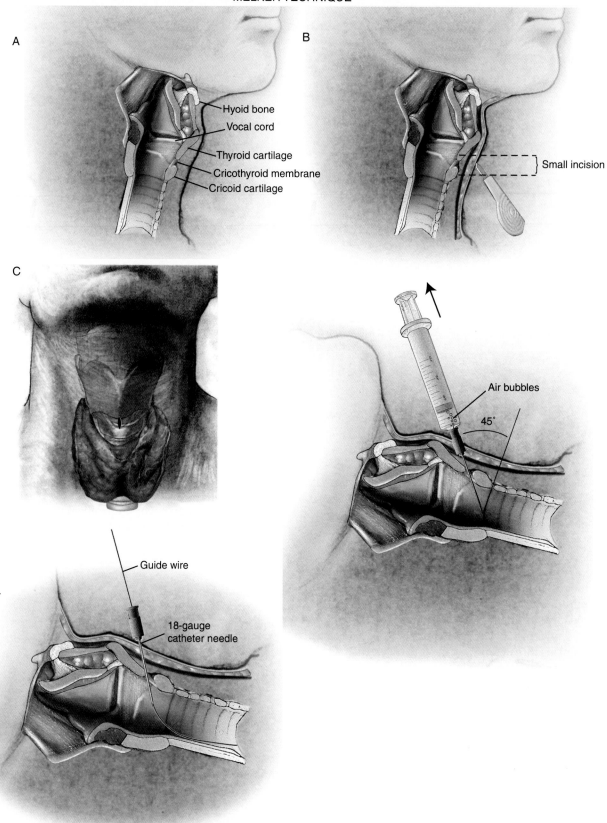

A

Hyoid bone
Vocal cord
Thyroid cartilage
Cricothyroid membrane
Cricoid cartilage

B

Small incision

C

Air bubbles

45°

D

Guide wire

18-gauge
catheter needle

MELKER TECHNIQUE

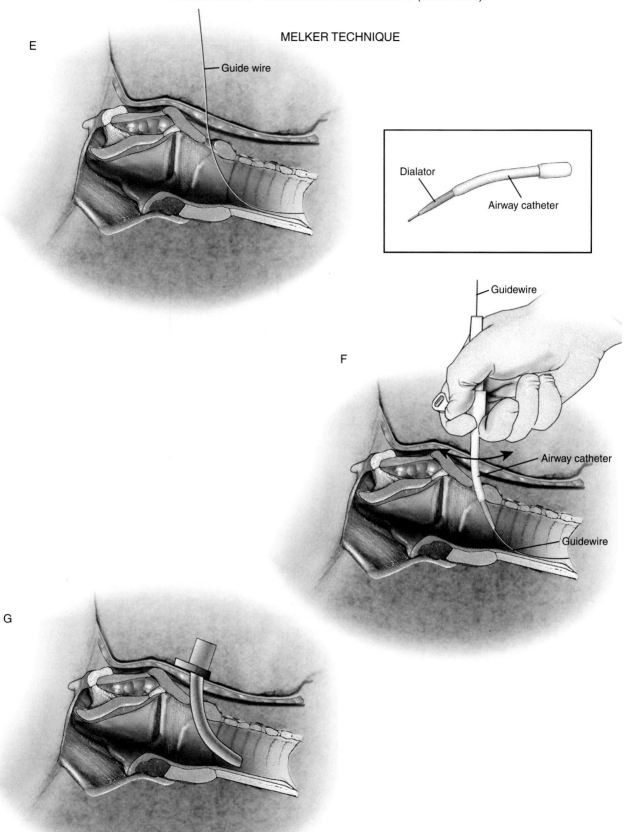

E

Guide wire

Dialator

Airway catheter

F

Guidewire

Airway catheter

Guidewire

G

the cricothyroid membrane. A 10- to 20-mL syringe with an 18-gauge catheter/needle is inserted through the membrane and aspirated to assure that the airway is directly below the chosen area. A guide wire is inserted through the needle, the needle removed, and a dilator attached to an airway catheter inserted over the guidewire. The dilator and guide wire are removed as the airway catheter is inserted into the airway.

Cricothyroidotomy achieves a rapid airway but is not considered adequate for long-term control of the airway. When maintained for the long-term, this procedure is known for tendency to induce subglottic stenosis. A conversion to tracheotomy is standard, especially when many patients have a compromised upper airway from jaw, laryngeal, or cervical fracture and will need long-term airway management. The surgeon may also require appropriate exposure for intermaxillary fixation and establishment of occlusion in the face of multiple facial injuries making tracheotomy a practical consideration.

Breathing

H,I Once the airway is established, it is important to determine the adequacy of respiration. Tension pneumothorax and hemothorax should be addressed in the primary survey by the physician managing the trauma situation. When thoracic computed tomography (CT) scans are performed, they sometimes identify small pneumothoraces that do not require immediate treatment. Usually, these small injuries heal without incident, but when subjected to positive pressure ventilation, they can progress to a large pneumothorax requiring treatment. Erring on the side of caution, some trauma surgeons place tube thoracostomies in asymptomatic patients undergoing positive pressure ventilation for early operative repair of facial trauma. This will help prevent the development of tension pneumothorax during the facial repair. The risks for developing pneumothorax with positive pressure ventilation are not clearly defined. The surgeon, anesthesiologist, and operating team need to discuss how to prevent this complication.

Control of Bleeding and Circulation

Facial hemorrhage can be particularly distressing if the injured vessels are difficult to identify and control. Severe hemorrhage can cause drowning making it mandatory to obtain control of the airway at a very early stage. In some cases, aggressive packing in the oral pharynx may be needed. If a larger vessel is suspected to have been injured, a CT angiogram is very important in identifying the bleeding source and helps to guide management. Often times the bleeding will stop with or without packing and elective repairs can be accomplished (see Chapter 11). If conservative

attempts to control the bleeding fail, then the patient should be considered for angiographic embolization or operative intervention. Ideally, the concept and availability of an endovascular operating room can provide for anesthesia, an evaluation of the area of bleeding, embolization of bleeding vessels, and ultimately ligation if necessary. It is important to avoid blind stabbing in the traumatic field, and every attempt should be made to clearly identify the involved vessel. If this is not possible or there is an involved region of bleeding, one can consider ligation of the external carotid artery.

Facial trauma usually does not require extensive resuscitation, but with large vessel bleeding, prior antiplatelet or anticoagulant therapy, or coexisting injuries, resuscitation can be critical. Resuscitation in trauma patients varies with the extent of blood loss, shock, and age. The endpoint of resuscitation is adequate tissue perfusion. Large volume resuscitation is best performed through large gauge peripheral IV guided by a transfusion protocol that provides a one-to-one ratio of fresh frozen plasma and packed red blood cells. Initial crystalloid boluses of 20 mL/kg can be infused while blood products are being arranged. In previously healthy young people, response to resuscitation is displayed by improved blood pressure, decreased heart rate, and improved urine output. In the older adult, prior use of beta-blockade and anticoagulants and preexisting congestive heart failure complicate the resuscitation and make identification of appropriate response more difficult. Normalization of serum lactate, pH, and HCO_3 are surrogate endpoints for adequate tissue perfusion.

Early evaluation of the injury should consider the possibility of an expanding hematoma or intravascular thrombus. Expanding cervical hematomas can lead to airway compromise. Additional data can be obtained through an angiographic CT. Such a condition will require immediate intervention as described in Chapter 11 with repair or ligation of the involved vessel. The patient should also be monitored for changes in neurologic status as a result of an intravascular thrombus or intimal dissection with occlusion. Angiographic evaluation can allow stenting or guide operative repair.

Operative intervention is through standard access incisions noted in Chapter 11. On the other hand, if the carotid vessels are involved near the base of the skull, there may be need for subluxation or dislocation of the mandible and/or endovascular interventional therapy.

Head Injury

Head injury includes a spectrum of injury from mild concussion to hemorrhage that requires surgery. A standard head injury evaluation should follow ATLS protocol with frequent reexamination. Hourly Glasgow coma scores can help detect deterioration in mental status over time. Elderly patients on various forms of anticoagulation are particularly at risk for deterioration. CT scans and/or MRI scans are essential in detecting intracranial bleeding as well as facial fractures. Physical exam with identification of otorrhea or rhinorrhea can be more sensitive indicators of basilar skull fracture than imaging studies.

While treatment of intracranial bleeding and elevated intracranial pressure is out of the scope of this chapter, facial trauma in these settings has the potential to exacerbate injury due to airway compromise at several stages of postinjury care. The surgeons providing treatment of the facial injuries need to be in frequent communication with critical care and neurosurgical experts to coordinate the operative interventions for facial trauma in the patient with head injury.

Cervical Spine Injury

J,K One of the common complications of head and neck injury that often goes unrecognized is injury to the cervical spine. This type of injury is prevalent especially in the elderly who have arthritis and osteoporosis with fragile bones. The injury is particularly noted following forces to the larynx and occasionally with mandibular fractures. Patients who suffer craniofacial trauma from blunt injuries need to undergo cervical spine clearance, and although routine radiographic evaluation may be helpful, CT scan and MRI are often required. CT scan will determine the degree of fracture and dislocation, while MRI is necessary to evaluate ligament stability. Patients with cervical injury need to be treated with a cervical collar and evaluated further for cord contusion and neurologic stability. Stabilization of the neck is mandatory when moving these patients, and the airway is to be secured when necessary.

Neck Injury

The neck is also prone to injury during craniofacial trauma and must be evaluated for life-threatening sequelae. Neck injury is classified according to three zones of injury, which carry important prognostic and treatment implications. Zone 1 is the area from the thoracic inlet to the cricoid. Zone 2 is the area from the cricoid to the angle of the mandible and Zone 3 from the mandibular angle to the skull base. Penetrating injuries to Zone 1 are probably the most life threatening since they can affect the trachea, lungs, and great vessels. CT Angiography has become the diagnostic modality of choice in that it is rapid and allows evaluation of the path of the penetration as well as diagnosis of specific organ or vessel injury. Operative and endovascular procedures are often necessary. In Zone 3, the injury may involve the carotid arterial system, and evaluation should include an angiogram with the possibility of endovascular intervention. In Zone 2, there is potential injury to the pharynx, larynx, and carotids, and if the platysma is violated, surgical intervention will probably be required. In evaluating all of these neck injuries, the history will be important for changes in swallowing, voice, breathing, and neurologic status. The physical examination should focus on penetrating wounds, swelling of the neck, hematoma, bruits, stridor and breathing difficulty, and subcutaneous emphysema. The patient should undergo direct laryngoscopy, esophagoscopy, and bronchoscopy to evaluate the upper aerodigestive tract. Imaging studies to consider are CT scan, ultrasound, CT angiogram, angiogram, and barium swallow with esophagram.

PITFALLS

1. The airway must be secured early to avoid hypoxia and cardiovascular insufficiency. As noted, there are many different ways to secure the airway, and much will depend upon the available instrumentation and the expertise of the provider. The preferred order would be orotracheal intubation, cricothyroidotomy, and then tracheostomy.

2. Cervical spine precautions should be continued until cleared by the trauma service or spine surgeon. Even after clearance, manipulation of the neck during operative treatment of facial injuries can still lead to cord or spine injury, especially in the elderly population.

3. Monitoring of the circulation is important to maintain perfusion to the body tissues and organs. Any insufficiency should bring attention to the possibility of occult hemorrhage. Appropriate consultation should be obtained to determine the location, degree, and treatment for such a condition.

4. As noted earlier, a small simple pneumothorax may go unnoticed and become a serious problem later. A tension pneumothorax may have to be treated with needle aspiration followed by tube thoracostomy should ventilation become difficult.

5. While the focus of the surgeon caring for facial trauma is clearly on the facial injuries, the care plan should take into account the overall status of the patient and the efforts of the other care providers for a polytrauma patient. This may require operating earlier than convenient block time in the operating room allows, or delaying the procedures due to pulmonary or hemodynamic instability. It may mean allowing endoscopy and gastrostomy placement prior to fixation of a mandible fracture or placing a tracheostomy in a patient with the need for multiple operative procedures rather than risk recurrent intubations. Coordination of multiple operative services providing care becomes a demanding task. A hospital that has a dedicated trauma surgical service is at a great advantage.

ADEQUACY OF RESPIRATION

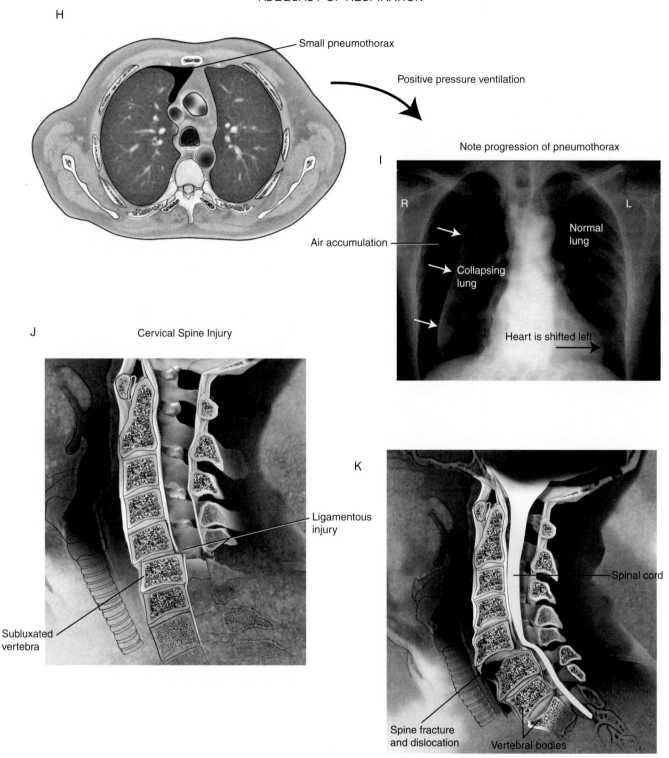

H

Small pneumothorax

Positive pressure ventilation

Note progression of pneumothorax

I

R   L

Air accumulation

Collapsing lung

Normal lung

Heart is shifted left

J   Cervical Spine Injury

Ligamentous injury

Subluxated vertebra

K

Spinal cord

Spine fracture and dislocation

Vertebral bodies

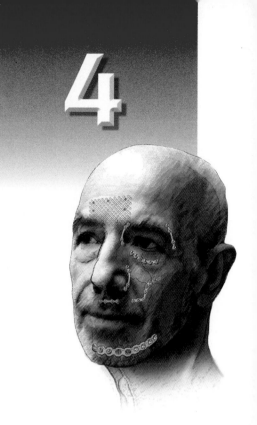

Control of the Airway by Reduction of Facial Fractures or Pharyngeal Intubation

A patent airway with adequate respiration is critical for life processes. Once it is established, attention can be devoted to the cardiovascular, gastrointestinal, neurologic, and other important systems.

In the patient with craniofacial injury, the available options include clearing of secretions, oro- or nasopharyngeal intubation, tracheostomy, or cricothyrotomy. Determining which method is best applied requires an understanding of the respiratory difficulty, site and severity of the injury, level of consciousness, cervical spine stability, and the immediate and long-term objectives. The methods of establishing an airway are highly specialized, and because of the urgency of the situation, they must be performed expediently.

All patients must be treated as if they have a cervical spine injury, and until they are cleared by physical and radiographic examination, the neck must be stabilized (see Chapter 3). For the obtunded patient in whom blood and secretions are collecting in the pharyngeal portion of the airway, the pharynx can be cleared with a Yankauer suction tube. If the patient still shows evidence of obstruction at a high level within the airway, a naso- and/or oropharyngeal intubation can be performed. Sometimes reduction of retrodisplaced facial fractures is indicated. If these methods do not secure the airway and assist with respiration, then oro- or nasotracheal intubation, cricothyrotomy, and/or tracheostomy must be considered (see Chapters 5 through 7).

PROCEDURE

A–C The head and neck of the patient should be stabilized by an assistant, but if no one is available, sandbags can be strategically placed to restrict movement. The pharynx is inspected with a headlight and tongue blade and cleared of secretions with a Yankauer suction tube. If the patient is obtunded and still having respiratory difficulty, the mandible and/or maxilla should be reduced with digital manipulation. The body or parasymphysis of the mandible should be grasped and lifted forward. Alternatively, the lower jaw can be thrust upward with pressure exerted from behind the angles. The maxilla, if retrodisplaced, should be reduced by placing an index finger behind the palate and pulling anteriorly. Impacted fractures may require special hooks or disimpaction forceps (see Chapter 41).

D,E The patient is then immediately reevaluated. If the airway still is not adequate, pharyngeal intubation should be considered. For the nasal route, the nose is sprayed with 1/4% oxymetazoline hydrochloride (Neo-Synephrine); a nasopharyngeal tube is then coated with an antibiotic ointment, and the tube is inserted through the nares into the nasopharynx. For oral intubation, a plastic airway, generally used for anesthesia, can be inserted through the mouth and behind the base of the tongue.

Success is ensured by improvements in the clinical and laboratory evaluations of respiration. Failure to observe normal chest movement and airflow, corroborated

CONTROL OF THE AIRWAY

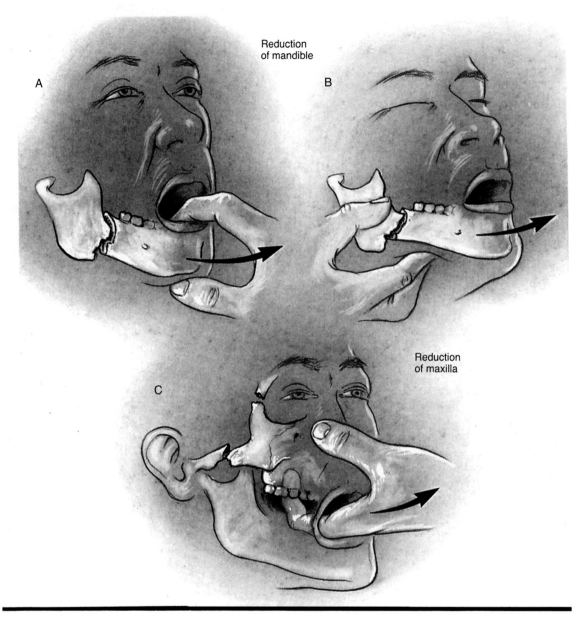

Reduction
of mandible

A

B

Reduction
of maxilla

C

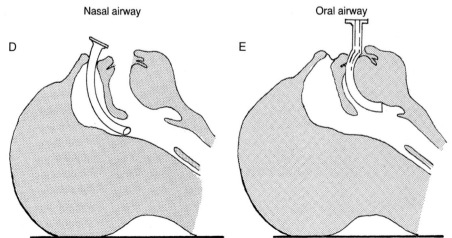

Nasal airway

Oral airway

D

E

by abnormal blood gases, should prompt consideration of other procedures (see Chapters 3 through 7). Also, the oro- or nasopharyngeal airways should be considered temporary, and if the patient is unable to be extubated in a short period of time, alternative methods must be implemented.

PITFALLS

1. Problems with the upper airway should be approached systematically. One should first appreciate that there may be an injury to the cervical spine and that all maneuvers should be carried out with stabilization of the neck. Initially, secretions should be cleared and the facial fractures reduced. Only after these measures have failed is it necessary to insert the naso- or oropharyngeal airway.

2. Remember that the pharyngeal airway is a temporary device. Nasopharyngeal tubes or oropharyngeal airways are often extruded and are easily blocked with blood and pharyngeal secretions. Long-term usage should be avoided.

3. Usually the patient can be temporarily ventilated with positive pressure while the surgeon checks for spinal injuries. Any patient who does not resume unassisted respiration should be considered a candidate for ventilation through oro- or nasotracheal intubation, cricothyrotomy, or tracheostomy.

COMPLICATIONS

1. The main complication of oro- or nasopharyngeal intubation is failure to achieve adequate respiration. This will become evident if there is still labored and noisy breathing, retraction of the chest, poor aeration of the lungs on auscultation, and less than optimal blood gas levels. In such situations, the surgeon can try to replace the tube and again clear secretions, but if this fails, alternative methods of airway control should be considered.

2. Aspiration is a common problem in the obtunded patient with a naso- or oropharyngeal airway. This complication can be prevented by keeping the airway clean or, alternatively, converting to cuffed endotracheal intubation. If aspiration has already occurred, tracheobronchial cleansing and administration of antibiotics are important methods of treatment.

3. Occasionally the cervical spine has been destabilized by the injury, and if the neck is flexed or turned too abruptly, there can be damage to the spinal cord. The surgeon should always be aware of this possibility and keep the patient's neck in a neutral position. If the patient is to be intubated, endoscopic methods are preferred while an assistant should stabilize the neck (see Chapter 5). Cervical spine radiographs should be obtained as soon as possible to help in the evaluation.

4. Insertion of the oro- or nasopharyngeal airway can cause bleeding. Often this bleeding stops in a few minutes, but if it continues, the surgeon should consider placing packing around the nasal tube and/or cauterizing the bleeding sites. If pharyngeal bleeding persists, tracheostomy and direct control of bleeding with cauterization and/or packing are procedures of choice.

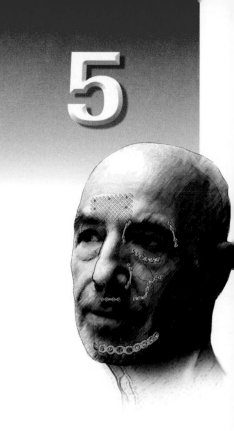

Establishing an Airway With Nasotracheal or Orotracheal Intubation
Alternative Techniques Using Endoscopic Methods

INDICATIONS

Tracheal intubation is an excellent emergency technique with which to establish a controlled airway. It is easily performed and is an efficient method of ventilation. It also provides an opportunity to stabilize the patient and examine for sites and degree of injury.

The main indications for tracheal intubation are breathing difficulty after oro- and/or nasopharyngeal intubation or when there is a known functional obstruction involving the pharynx and/or larynx. Intubation should also be considered in patients with obvious closed head injury (or other associated injuries) necessitating assisted ventilation. Caution must be exercised when there is a suspected cervical spine injury.

Nasotracheal intubation is more difficult to perform than orotracheal intubation but is better tolerated by the patient and provides for a longer period of airway control. Evaluation of occlusion is also possible. Furthermore, after orotracheal intubation, the patient tends to struggle and may bite the tube. However, both oro- and nasotracheal intubation techniques are excellent methods in stabilizing the patient for a tracheostomy.

PROCEDURE

The positioning of the patient is very important for the tracheal intubation procedure. Unless there is evidence to the contrary, the possibility of cervical spine instability should be assumed and precautions taken to stabilize the head and neck. In most patients, the neck should be slightly flexed and the head slightly extended. A stethoscope should be attached to the patient's chest to listen for adequacy of breath sounds.

A–D For the orotracheal intubation, the mouth and pharynx should be sprayed with a topical anesthetic and the pharynx suctioned and cleared of blood and secretions. The individual who is performing the procedure should be standing at the patient's head. A straight-blade laryngoscope is then introduced into the right side of the oral cavity, and the tongue is pushed to the left. The blade is inserted further, and when the epiglottis is visualized, the blade is pushed under it into the vestibule of the larynx. If a curved blade is used, the end of the scope will project into the vallecula. Elevation of the epiglottis with the blade will demonstrate the vocal cords, and the tube can be introduced into the trachea. A No. 7 or 8 orotracheal cuffed tube (with or without a stylet) or ventilating bronchoscope can be inserted. The tube is hooked up to a ventilator bag, and breath sounds are checked. The cuff is then injected with air to an optimal pressure, and the tube is secured to the face with adhesive solutions and plastic tape. Alternatively, a gauze strap can be tied around the tube and then around the head.

E For the nasal intubation, the nose should be sprayed with a vasoconstrictive agent. If the patient is alert, the nose and pharynx should also be prepared with a topical anesthetic. A No. 7 or 8 nasotracheal tube

INTUBATION TECHNIQUES

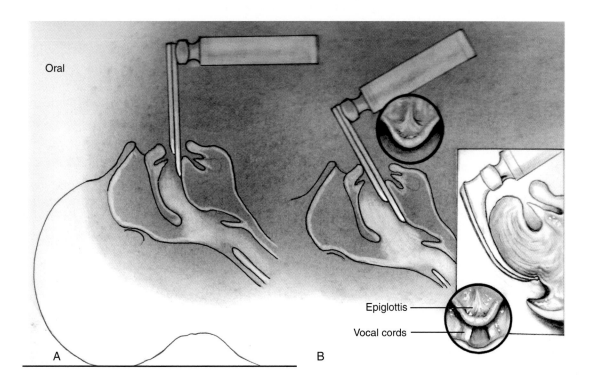

Oral

A

B

Epiglottis

Vocal cords

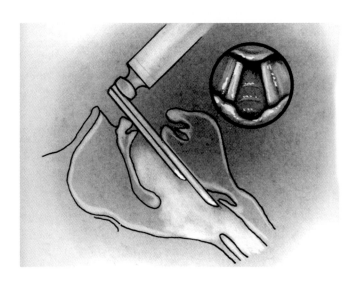

C

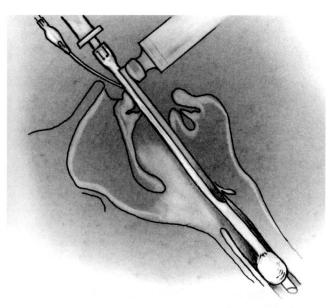

D

is then passed through the nose and into the pharynx. The mouth is opened, and after suctioning the pharynx, the laryngoscope is introduced into the airway. Using a special forceps (Magill), the tube is grasped and placed into the glottic chink. As in oral intubation, the adequacy of the airway should be checked, the cuff inflated, and the tube secured with tape to the face.

Postintubation, cuff pressures must be checked and occasionally relieved to avoid necrosis at the site of contact of the cuff with the wall of the trachea. Secretions should be removed as necessary and the oral cavity kept clean with mouthwashes and suctioning. Prophylactic antibiotics are recommended. Tension on the tube by respirator tubing should be minimized. The tube should not be retained for more than 5 to 10 days, as longer periods of intubation can produce inflammation and cicatrization of the trachea. For prolonged intubation, a tracheostomy should be considered (see Chapter 7).

PITFALLS

1. If the patient's cervical spine status is not known, the head should be slightly extended and the neck slightly flexed. Abrupt and excessive movements of the neck should be avoided. With these precautions, the risk of damage is minimal. Endoscopic intubation provides additional measures of safety.

2. If possible, avoid tracheal intubation in patients with laryngeal injury. Placement of the tube can cause additional damage to the soft tissues and can confound the diagnosis and treatment of the condition. If time permits, the patient should undergo a routine tracheostomy.

3. Do not use the upper dentition as a fulcrum for the laryngoscope. Undue pressure can cause tooth fractures, and portions of the tooth can potentially enter the airway. Placing a moist 4 × 4 gauze pad on the upper alveolus can help prevent this complication.

4. Be prepared for regurgitation of stomach contents during the intubation and for the possibility of aspiration. If time permits, the stomach should be preliminarily emptied with a nasogastric tube. If any material is aspirated into the lungs, the upper respiratory tract should be suctioned and irrigated with normal saline solution.

5. Long-term tracheal intubation should be avoided, as it is associated with potential subglottic stenosis and granuloma formation of the vocal cords. If the patient requires intubation for more than 5 to 10 days, a tracheostomy should be considered.

6. Postintubation care is extremely important. The patient should be watched carefully for displacement of the tube and accumulation of secretions. Suctioning must be performed using aseptic techniques. Cuff pressure must be checked and maintained below levels that would cause necrosis of the adjacent tracheal wall. Ideally the cuff should be deflated for a few minutes every 1 to 2 hours.

7. If the patient receives assisted ventilation, the ventilation tubes must not put undue tension on the intubation tubes. Such pressures can lead to necrosis of the nasal ala and/or septum and cause damage along other portions of the respiratory tract.

COMPLICATIONS

1. Spinal cord injury is possible, especially if the vertebrae are unstable and displaced during the intubation. To avoid this problem, it is advisable to evaluate the neck with computed tomography (CT) scans or radiographs and physical examination. If satisfactory imaging studies cannot be obtained, the neck should be stabilized by an assistant while the intubation is being performed. Maintaining a neutral position will often prevent additional injury. Flexible endoscopic intubation should be considered (see later).

2. Tooth fractures can occur by the scope striking the tooth and/or alveolus. To avoid this complication, the laryngoscope should be introduced into the mouth and pressure exerted by lifting the laryngoscope up against the tongue and mandible. Fulcrum-like effects should be avoided. If a tooth should become fractured, the fragments should be collected and the fracture treated as described in Chapters 31 and 32.

3. Occasionally the laryngoscope and/or intubation tube injure the arytenoid and displace it from its joint. Following such an occurrence, the arytenoid will appear rotated, the patient's voice will be changed, and there can be a risk of aspiration. Early recognition of the complication provides an opportunity to replace the arytenoid to its normal position; later repairs are generally unsuccessful.

4. Crusting, displacement, or kinking of the tube can cause further problems with obstruction. Thus the patient should receive humidified oxygen, and aseptic suctioning should be performed to collect accumulated secretions. The patient must be watched closely for displacement and kinking of the tube.

5. Subglottic stenosis, although uncommon, is most often observed following long-term intubation. It is believed to develop secondarily to pressure necrosis caused by twisting and tension on the tube and by excessive cuff or tube tip pressures aggravated by acid reflux. Such a situation often develops in patients who are obtunded or who do not, or cannot, respond to pain; infection and reintubation are also contributory factors. Many of these conditions can be minimized or avoided. Cuff pressures and tube position should be checked repeatedly, and the patient should be maintained on

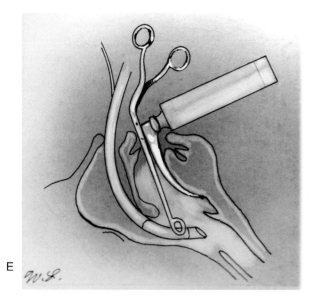

E

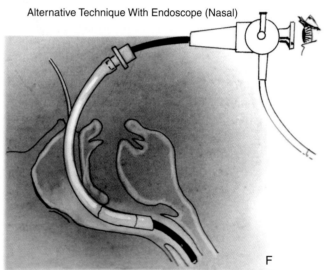

Alternative Technique With Endoscope (Nasal)

F

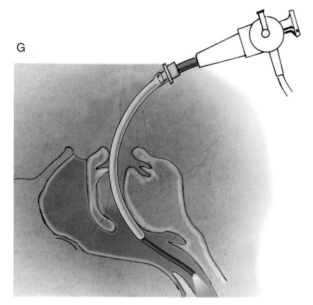

G

antibiotics and antireflux medications. The tube should be replaced by a tracheostomy after 5 to 10 days.

6. Vocal cord granulomas can also develop as a result of intubation. Although it is suggested that repeated motion and trauma by the tube on the vocal cords is significant, the factors that cause this problem are generally unknown. Granulomas are best treated with excision using laser or microsurgical techniques. Voice rest should be implemented. Repeated trauma should be avoided.

7. Sinusitis involving the maxilla and/or other paranasal sinuses is common following nasal intubation. The complication is difficult to avoid, but if it should occur, secretions should be cultured and appropriate antibiotics started. Usually the sinuses clear when the intubation tube is removed. If the tube needs to be in place for long periods of time, it may be more prudent to perform a tracheostomy.

ALTERNATIVE TECHNIQUE USING ENDOSCOPIC METHODS

F,G If there is a possibility that neck extension may cause damage to the cervical spine or it is difficult to open the patient's mouth, then laryngoscopic-guided intubation should be considered. For this technique, the nose is prepared with a vasoconstrictive agent and the nose, pharynx, and larynx with a topical anesthetic. The end of the fiberoptic laryngoscope is first placed through the endotracheal tube. Both laryngoscope and tube should be generously lubricated. The laryngoscope is then inserted through one side of the nose and advanced to identify laryngeal structures. When the glottis is visualized, the scope should be advanced into the upper trachea. The endotracheal tube is then passed over the scope through the nose, pharynx, and larynx into the trachea. The scope is removed and the patient checked for end-tidal volume and carbon dioxide. Postintubation management is the same for patients intubated with other techniques. Intubations may also be accomplished transorally, but in these patients the posterior displacement of the tongue will make the procedure difficult to accomplish, and even when it is successful, patients do not very well tolerate the oral tube.

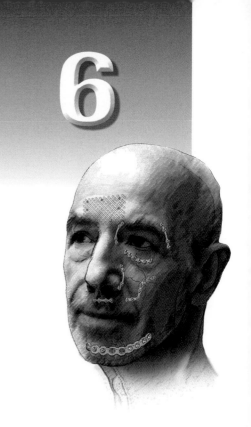

Treatment of Respiratory Difficulty With Cricothyrotomy

INDICATIONS

Cricothyrotomy is indicated for life-threatening situations in which the equipment or expertise to perform intubation is not available or the laryngopharynx is so distorted that intubation would be difficult, if not impossible, to perform. The procedure should be considered when there is insufficient time for tracheostomy. The trauma surgeon has the option of a percutaneous technique described in Chapter 3 or an open procedure described below. However, cricothyrotomy has limitations, and because it can cause progressive damage to the cricoid and subglottic area, it should be converted as soon as possible to tracheostomy.

PROCEDURE

A–E The cricothyrotomy is truly an emergency procedure. The position of the cricoid cartilage and cricothyroid membrane should be determined by palpation, and the larynx should be stabilized between the thumb and index finger. If time permits, the cricothyroid membrane can be marked and the area infiltrated with 2% lidocaine. A horizontal incision (about 2 to 3 cm) is then made with a No. 15 knife blade, cutting through the skin, subcutaneous tissues, the cricothyroid membrane, and respiratory mucosa. Once into the airway, the opening can be enlarged with a small Kelly clamp. A No. 4 tracheostomy tube can then be inserted and tied to the neck with sutures and/or straps.

Postoperatively the cricothyrotomy wound should be cleaned with 3% hydrogen peroxide. The airway should be kept free of secretions, and prophylactic antibiotics should be administered. Ideally, the patient is soon stabilized, and in 24 to 48 hours, a tracheostomy should be performed. The cricothyrotomy tube can then be removed.

PITFALLS

1. Because cricothyrotomy is associated with a high degree of laryngeal and subglottic injury, it should only be performed when other methods are not applicable (see Chapters 4, 5, and 7). To avoid complications, the cricothyrotomy should be converted to a tracheostomy within 24 to 48 hours after the initial procedure.

2. Cricothyrotomy requires accurate placement of the knife, and thus obliteration of the anatomic landmarks with overinjection of a local anesthetic should be avoided. If there is some concern about the position of the cricothyroid membrane, a 16- or 18-gauge needle can be inserted. Once air is aspirated, an incision can be made around the needle and the opening enlarged into the airway.

3. The cricothyroid membrane is small, and a tube should not be forced into it, as this will injure the cricoid cartilage. Usually a No. 4 (rarely, a No. 6) tracheostomy tube fits and will maintain the airway until a more permanent method can be applied.

CRICOTHYROTOMY

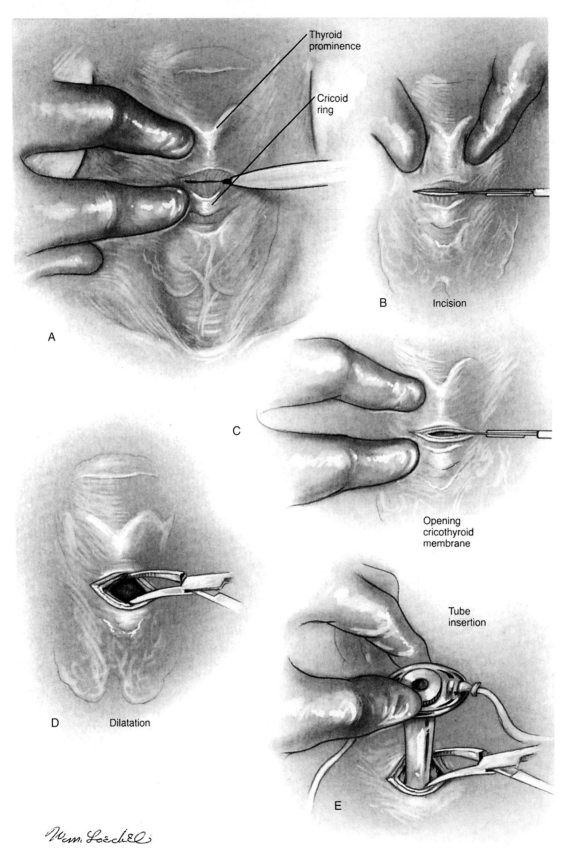

Thyroid prominence

Cricoid ring

A

B   Incision

C

Opening cricothyroid membrane

D   Dilatation

Tube insertion

E

COMPLICATIONS

1. Cricoid injury and subglottic stenosis are common complications following cricothyrotomy. The damage can be minimized by accurate placement of the incision, a small indwelling tube, and a limited time of intubation. Because the procedure is usually performed in life-threatening situations, the surgeon should wait until the patient has been stabilized and then convert the cricothyrotomy to a tracheostomy. The sooner the tracheostomy is performed, the less chance there is of subglottic damage. Conversion of the airway ideally should take place within 24 to 48 hours of the initial procedure.

2. Cricothyrotomy places the patient at risk for the same problems that can occur with any type of intubation. The airway must be maintained with suction, and infection should be kept to a minimum with local wound care and prophylactic antibiotics. Bleeding is rare and usually can be stopped with cauterization and/or judicious use of packing.

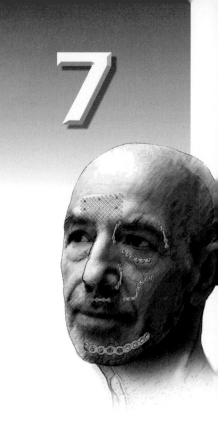

Tracheostomy
Alternative Technique of Björk Flap
Alternative Technique in Children

INDICATIONS

Tracheostomy should be considered in any patient who has sustained craniofacial injury and is not exchanging a sufficient amount of air. However, if the condition of the patient is critical and speed is important, then an emergency cricothyrotomy (see Chapters 3 and 6) is performed.

In most patients, the possibility of cervical spine injury should be assumed and the stability of the neck maintained while establishing an airway. First, there should be an attempt to clear secretions and blood from the pharynx and manually reduce the facial fractures that may be obstructing the airway. In the obtunded patient, an oral or nasal airway should be inserted. If these measures fail to improve breathing, then oral intubation must be considered. Nasotracheal intubation may be indicated when the patient's mouth cannot be adequately opened or in preparation for a procedure that requires occlusal evaluation and adjustments.

Tracheostomy is indicated when intubation is required for more than 5 days or when complex facial fractures require multiple procedures and repeated intubations. The procedure is helpful to relate occlusal surfaces to each other and should be considered when there is a subsequent risk of aspiration. Tracheostomy is a reasonable treatment option when packing of the nose is combined with intermaxillary fixation. The procedure is elective, and for emergency situations in which time is critical, cricothyrotomy or intubation should be used.

PROCEDURE

Ideally, tracheostomy should be performed in the operating room. An initial tracheal intubation is preferred, with the patient either sedated or controlled with a general anesthetic. If the patient is alert and oriented but the situation is such that intubation of the airway may pose a risk, the tracheostomy should be performed under local anesthesia.

A–C The patient should be positioned so that there is a "safe" slight extension of the neck and prominence of the laryngeal cartilages. Useful landmarks are the thyroid lamina projections, the cricoid ring, and the suprasternal notch. Usually, an incision is designed horizontally in a crease halfway between the cricoid and suprasternal notch. The width of the incision is determined by the degree of anticipated difficulty. Usually, a 3- to 4-cm incision is sufficient, but a larger 4- to 6-cm incision should be used in patients with short, thick necks, and in situations in which speed is important. The area of incision should be infiltrated with 1% or 2% lidocaine; the anesthesiologist should approve the use of 1:100,000 epinephrine, which can be helpful for the control of bleeding.

D,E The incision is carried through the subcutaneous tissues. The anterior jugular veins are ligated with 3-0 silk sutures. The investing layer of fascia is cleaned to expose the fine fibrous septum between the strap muscles (sternohyoid and sternothyroid). This septum

TRACHEOSTOMY

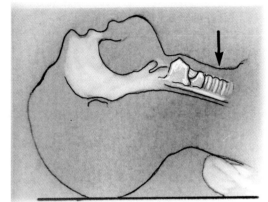

A   Position

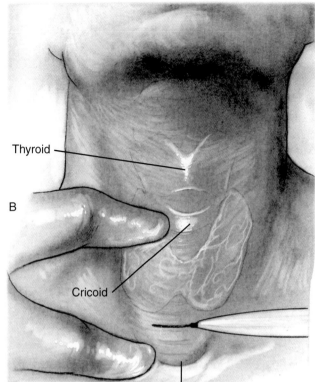

B

Thyroid

Cricoid

Suprasternal notch

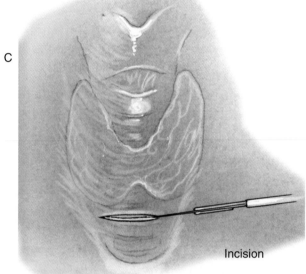

C

Incision

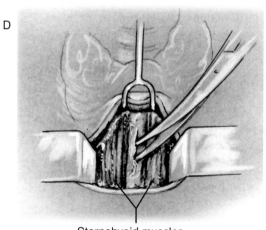

D

Sternohyoid muscles

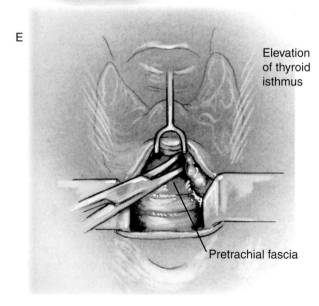

E

Elevation
of thyroid
isthmus

Pretrachial fascia

is incised, and the strap muscles are displaced laterally with Army-Navy retractors. The lower portion of the thyroid gland should be exposed and, beneath it, the pretracheal fat and fascia. The inferior thyroid veins are divided and ligated with fine silk sutures.

F Using a clamp or peanut dissector, the soft tissues overlying the trachea are teased apart. The thyroid isthmus is elevated superiorly with blunt dissection. The surgeon should then be able to visualize the upper tracheal rings and at least palpate the cricoid arch. A cricoid hook is subsequently inserted between the first and second or the second and third rings to stabilize the airway. An incision through the trachea, preferably between the second and third tracheal rings, is made with a small curved knife blade.

G,H The opening is enlarged by resection of a ring (or alternatively by the creation of a Björk flap described later). Usually the lower ring is grasped with an Allis clamp, and the anterior portion of the ring is excised with heavy scissors. The endotracheal tube is advanced to the upper part of the tracheal incision. A tracheostomy tube is then inserted by rotating the tube 90° to the midline and rotating it back into the trachea. There is also the option of widening the airway with a Trousseau dilator before inserting the tube.

I Once assured that the tube is in the airway by suctioning secretions and observing for exchange of air, the surgeon should secure the tube to the neck with umbilical tape. Additional fixation is obtained by attaching the tube directly to the skin with 2-0 silk sutures. The neck should then be gently flexed and the tapes tied with a square knot. A gauze dressing is placed under the flanges of the tube.

Tracheostomy care requires close observation and periodic suctioning for secretions that accumulate within the airway. A postoperative chest radiograph should be performed to ensure that the lungs are well aerated and that there are no intrathoracic complications such as pneumothorax or atelectasis. The cuff of the tracheostomy tube should be inflated according to the directions that accompany the tube. Cuff deflation with suctioning should be performed every hour. The tube should be changed between 4 and 7 days after the tracheostomy and then every other week as needed. The tracheostomy wound should be kept clean with frequent dressing changes.

Decannulation can be carried out when the tracheostomy tube has fulfilled its purpose and the patient is able to breath without assisted respiration. The patient should also be free of aspiration and able to cough out tracheal secretions. There should be no evidence of upper airway obstruction.

The procedure for decannulation should be initiated by changing the cuffed tube to a noncuffed tube and then by changing the noncuffed tube to a tube of smaller size. When a No. 4 or 6 tube size is reached, the tube can then be plugged with a finger and the patient checked for airflow through the nasal or oral airway. If satisfactory airflow is observed, the tube can be plugged for 24 hours and removed thereafter. If there is evidence of respiratory problems, the patient should be evaluated for anatomic or functional obstruction with a laryngoscope. Following removal of the tracheostomy tube, the wound is then covered with a petrolatum gauze dressing and allowed to close by secondary intention.

PITFALLS

1. Recognition of landmarks and anatomic layers is an important part of the surgery. The incision should be long enough to provide adequate exposure. Bright lighting should be available from a source located on the forehead or nasoglabella region.

2. The procedure is best performed with patient cooperation and a local anesthetic block, but if the patient cannot lie still, a general anesthetic is preferred. An agitated, struggling patient makes the procedure extremely difficult and dangerous.

3. Check for pulsations in the suprasternal notch. An abnormally high innominate artery can be injured at the time of dissection, or it can later bleed from pressure necrosis exerted by the bend, cuff, or tip of the tracheostomy tube. Excessive extension of the neck should be avoided, as this can elevate the innominate artery from the chest into the lower portion of the neck.

4. Use vasoconstrictive agents whenever possible to reduce bleeding. Small vessels should be treated with cauterization and/or ligation.

5. Cutting through the thyroid can often cause a bloody field and postoperative bleeding. Thus, elevation of the thyroid isthmus by blunt dissection is preferred over division and ligation of the gland.

6. The trachea should be stabilized while incising the tracheal wall. The trachea can be isolated and held in position with a vein retractor pulling upward beneath the thyroid isthmus or with a tracheal hook secured between the first and second rings. The hook can be used to keep the trachea from moving; it also improves exposure by elevating the trachea toward the surface of the wound.

7. Although there is much controversy as to the best tracheal opening, we prefer, in adult patients, to create a Björk flap (see later) and/or to remove an anterior portion of the third ring. If more exposure is needed, a Trousseau dilator is inserted, and the walls of the trachea are displaced laterally. Extension of the horizontal incisions may also be helpful. In children, a vertical cut through the second, third, and fourth rings provides an adequate opening (see later).

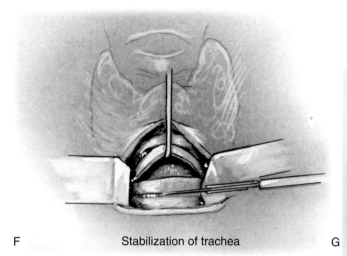

F   Stabilization of trachea

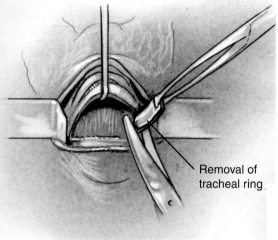

G   Removal of tracheal ring

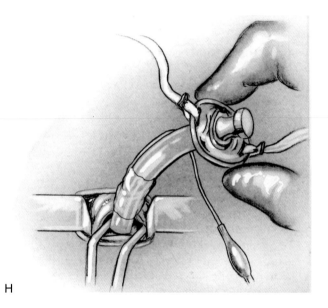

H

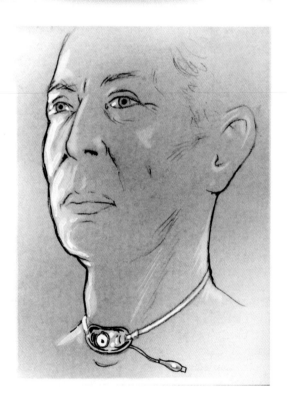

I

8. If there is concern that the tracheostomy tube may become dislodged, the Björk flap becomes important. In children, silk sutures can be applied through the lateral portion of the tracheal rings (see later). These sutures are then tied in loops and secured with tape to the skin of the neck. If the tube should become dislodged, pulling up on the sutures will elevate and secure the trachea for reinsertion of the tube.

9. In attaching the tracheostomy tape, make sure that the head is flexed. If tape is placed around the neck when the neck is extended, the tape will loosen when the head returns to the flexed position. The tracheostomy tube can then slip out of the trachea. The tracheostomy tube can also be secured to the skin of the neck with 2-0 black silk sutures.

10. Avoid a tight closure of the tracheostomy incision. On coughing, air can enter into the tissues and cause a subcutaneous and mediastinal dissection.

11. A chest radiograph should be performed postoperatively to check the position of the tube and aeration of the lungs. A tracheostomy can cause pneumothorax and/or atelectasis, and an early diagnosis is helpful in the treatment of these complications.

12. Check the tracheostomy tube for pulsations and/or obstruction of the mainstem bronchi. A tube that is too short may enter into the pretracheal tissues and be partially obstructed. A tube that is too long will project from the soft tissues of the neck. Pulsations may indicate that the tube is resting near the innominate artery. Should any of these conditions develop, the tube should be changed to one of appropriate size and position.

COMPLICATIONS

1. Postoperative obstructive phenomena should alert the surgeon to the possibility that the tube and/or cuff are not properly positioned. If obstruction is associated with inflation of the cuff, the cuff may be covering the end of the tube, and the tube and cuff should be replaced. Occasionally the tube is too short and is partially inserted into the mediastinal space anterior to the trachea. In such a situation, the tube size and contour should be corrected. Finally, the airway should be checked for obstructive crusts and secretions. This problem can be prevented by cleaning the inner cannula and maintaining high humidity in the airway. Suctioning is also important to prevent secretions from collecting and drying out. Airway patency can be checked by observing the exchange of air or by examining the airway with a fiberoptic endoscope.

2. Early bleeding following tracheostomy usually indicates failure of cauterization and/or ligation to control bleeding from a vessel of the neck or thyroid gland. Oozing of blood around the tube can often be controlled by placing 1/2 to 1-inch gauze packing into the wound. If this does not stop the bleeding, the patient should be returned to the operating room to have the wound explored and bleeding controlled.

3. Postoperative pneumothorax can occur from overzealous retraction and direct injury to the pleura. If this complication develops, immediate insertion of a chest tube must be considered.

4. Atelectasis can also be a problem in the postoperative period. This can usually be treated by suctioning, irrigation, and positive pressure respiration. Occasionally there is obstruction from a tube that is too long and enters one of the mainstem bronchi. If such a situation develops, the tube should be changed and the position of the tube monitored by chest radiograph.

5. Subcutaneous emphysema can occur, especially if the patient is coughing and soft tissue closure around the tube is too tight. Although air can be diverted into the pleura and mediastinum, rarely is there any compression of the airway or spread of infection. Once the air is observed in the tissues, precipitating factors should be corrected.

6. Infection of the wound site, bronchitis, and pneumonia are all possibilities following the tracheostomy. To avoid these sequelae, the tube should be kept clean with proper tracheobronchial care. Cultures should be obtained and appropriate antibiotic treatment instituted.

7. Injury to the esophagus, carotid artery, and innominate artery at the time of surgery can be prevented by accurate, relatively atraumatic techniques. If any of these anatomic structures are damaged, appropriate consultation and therapy should be immediately instituted.

8. One of the most feared delayed complications is erosion of the innominate artery. This problem can be avoided by keeping the dissection superior to the innominate vessels and by avoiding cuff pressures and/or suctioning that will destroy the anterior tracheal wall adjacent to the vessel. Many times the patient will have a sudden, small amount of bleeding. This "sentinel" bleed should alert the surgeon to the possibility of tracheal erosion, and emergency measures should be instituted. The trachea should be examined with fiberoptic endoscopy, and if it is apparent that bleeding is coming from the region of the innominate artery, the region of bleeding should be tamponed with finger or cuff pressure. Ultimately, ligation of the innominate artery or bypass surgery must be considered.

9. Laryngeal and/or tracheal stenosis can develop as a result of tracheal wall injury occurring directly from the tracheostomy tube, cuff, and/or tip pressure (see Chapters 107 through 109). Infection also plays a major contributory role. In the case of early stenosis, removal of granulation tissues and dilatation with

BJÖRK FLAP TECHNIQUE

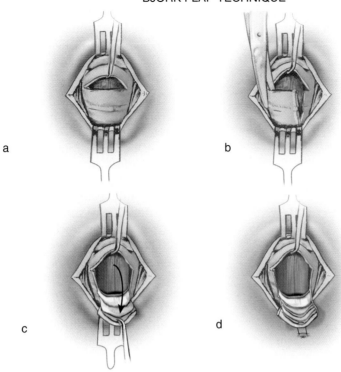

a

b

c

d

ALTERNATIVE TECHNIQUE IN CHILDREN

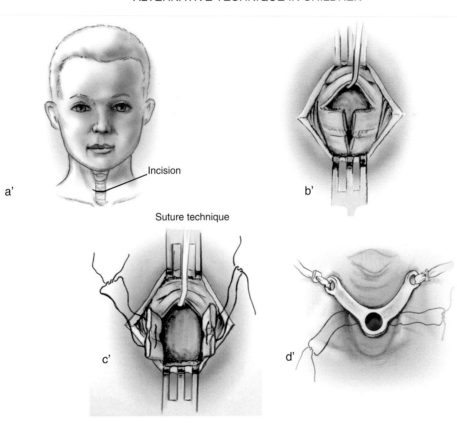

a'

Incision

b'

Suture technique

c'

d'

a bronchoscope or an indwelling T tube can be considered. If the stenosis becomes mature and does not respond to dilatation, then tracheal resection should be considered.

ALTERNATIVE TECHNIQUE OF BJÖRK FLAP

a–d In elective situations the Björk flap should be considered. For this procedure the trachea is stabilized by a hook. The trachea is incised between second and third ring and the lower ring is cut laterally on both sides with a Mayo scissors to develop a 1.5 cm flap of cartilage. This flap is then advanced to the skin and secured subcutaneously with a 3-0 vicryl suture. The tracheostomy tube is then inserted into the trachea and secured to the neck with sutures and straps.

ALTERNATIVE TECHNIQUE IN CHILDREN

a' Modifications in the tracheostomy technique are required in children. Generally children's tissues are very pliable, and coughing can raise the pleura into the neck region. For these reasons, the surgeon must be careful with the retractors; the tracheostomy also should be kept as high as possible, away from the thorax. However, a tracheostomy that is too high should be avoided, as postoperative subglottic narrowing and stenosis can result.

b'–d' The tracheal rings in children are soft, and the tracheostomy tube can usually be inserted through a vertical incision of two or three rings of the trachea (second, third, and fourth rings). The opening is secured with 3-0 black silk sutures, which are placed through rings lateral to the tracheal incision, tied in loops, and subsequently secured with adhesive solutions and tape to the neck. These sutures are also helpful in stabilizing and exposing the trachea and are immediately available should the tube become dislodged.

Postoperative care and decannulation are performed in a fashion similar to that used in adults. Pediatric tracheostomy tubes are usually pliable and do not require cuffs. Nevertheless, many of the complications that occur following adult tracheostomy can also occur in children.

Bleeding

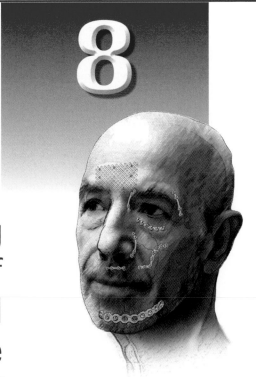

CHAPTER

8

Control of Bleeding
Alternative Techniques of Posterior Packs and Balloon Tamponade Alternative Technique of Endoscopic Control of Bleeding

In Consultation With Adam Folbe, MD

INDICATIONS

Management priorities in the critically injured patient, as discussed in Chapter 3, are to establish an airway and control bleeding. The preferred order of emergency care is to ensure ventilation and, soon after, to stop the bleeding and restore blood volume. The patient should be evaluated for other associated injuries and disorders that can contribute to the bleeding. Once the injured patient is stabilized, the surgeon can diagnose and arrange for repair of facial injuries. In a patient in whom there is evidence of blood loss (i.e., hypotension, oliguria, tachycardia, and gross bleeding), an intravenous large-bore (No. 16 or larger) catheter is inserted into the antecubital veins. Blood should be drawn for type and crossmatch. Normal saline or lactated ringers are infused for expanding the blood volume; however, blood is preferred, and the appropriate matched type should be administered as soon as possible.

Most bleeding sites in the head and neck region can be controlled with digital pressure, packing, or controlled clamping and ligation. Nosebleeds are common with naso-orbital, maxillary, and nasal fractures, and if bleeding does not stop, the nose should be packed with dissolvable or nondissolvable pledgets or with 1/2-inch gauze soaked in antibiotic solution. Most anterior bleeding will respond, but if bleeding continues or is coming from a more posterior location, posterior packs or balloon tamponade is indicated. Bleeding from the ear, which often accompanies temporal bone injuries, can be treated with cotton or gauze packs. Bleeding from the nose and pharynx requires simultaneous control of the airway and respiration with intubation or cricothyroidotomy, and once this is achieved, the pharynx can be tamponed with vaginal packing. Damage to the larger vessels (i.e., carotid artery and jugular vein) can be initially controlled with digital pressure, but definitive treatment can be difficult, and it is important to consult immediately with a vascular surgeon (see Chapter 11).

PROCEDURE

A Packing of the nose is a time-tested procedure that will control most nose bleeds. This also provides an opportunity during preparation to examine the damage to the lateral walls and septum.

The nose should first be sprayed with 1/4% oxymetazoline hydrochloride. Eight small cotton pledgets, soaked in 8 mL of 4% cocaine solution containing five drops of 1:10,000 epinephrine, are strategically placed throughout the nasal cavity. For maximal hemostasis and decongestion, pledgets should be positioned in the nasal vault, behind the middle turbinate, on the floor, and along the septum. The pledgets should be retained for at least 5 minutes.

B Bacitracin gauze, which can be used for packing, is prepared from 1/2-inch gauze treated with Bacitracin ointment. After the pledgets are removed from the nose, the packing is inserted in layers with a bayonet or Hartmann forceps. The first loop is placed directly on the floor, and additional loops are layered horizontally against one another. Blood is suctioned as necessary to observe the orientation of the loops. Once the vault is packed, the loops can be directly inserted into the vestibule of the nose.

Ideally, both sides of the nose should be packed, or the septum will be pushed to one side, and compression will be lost. Adhesive tape can be applied across the middle and lower third of the nose to hold the dressings in place. The patient should be placed on antibiotics. The airway should be evaluated for obstruction, and if necessary, oxygen should be administered or an alternative airway considered. Packing should be removed at 3 to 5 days, and at that time, the nose should be sprayed with 1/4% oxymetazoline hydrochloride. Saline douches should be used to provide a physiologic wash and to prevent crusts from forming.

With lesser bleeds, control can often be obtained by placing soft pledgets to exert pressure directly over the area that is bleeding. Surgifoam or surgicel with hemostatic properties is useful for this procedure and have the advantage of dissolving in approximately 5 days. One also has the option of nonabsorbable sponge-like materials, which primarily work through direct pressure on the bleeding site. These tampons can be trimmed to the desired length, lubricated with ointment, and placed directly along the septum and nasal floor. Once in place, the tampon is injected with Lidocaine containing epinephrine or Afrin to allow it to expand. To prevent toxic shock syndrome, the tampons are removed in 3 days and the patient is kept on antibiotics for the duration of the packing.

Alternatively, the bleeding may be controlled with inflatable balloon tampons. These are carefully inserted along the nasal septum and saline is injected into the port as directed (described later). Balloon tampons expand to exert pressure along the entire course of the septum and not to a particular spot.

PITFALLS

1. If the nasal bones are fractured, it may be more prudent to reduce the nasal fracture before packing the nares (see Chapter 52). Such action may avoid subsequent surgery to the nose and still control bleeding.

2. Beware of making the initial loops of packing too long or too loose. Loops of packing can fall into the pharynx; when this occurs, the patient will start gagging. If such a situation develops, the surgeon can cut off the excess loops in the pharynx and/or remove the gauze and repack the nose.

3. Avoid overpacking the nose which can cause displacement of nasal or facial fractures. If this should occur, the bones should be reduced digitally into an anatomic position and the excess packing removed.

4. If bleeding is not controlled by anteriorly placed nasal packs, then the surgeon should consider either adding more packing, balloon tamponade or administering posterior packs (see later). Maxillary ligation is difficult to perform in acutely traumatized patients and should be avoided. Severe bleeding can compromise breathing and an emergent airway should be considered.

5. Most patients with nasal packing can usually breathe quite well through the oral cavity. However, if the oropharynx is compromised, there may be an obstruction, and an airway may need to be established. In these cases, oral intubation or tracheostomy should be performed.

6. In most cases, epistaxis can be controlled with light packs. As discussed, hemostatic pledgets and/or prefabricated tampons coated with Bacitracin ointment can be used.

COMPLICATIONS

1. Usually persistent bleeding is the result of inadequate anterior and/or posterior packing. This can be corrected by repacking and/or additional packing. Only rarely is arterial ligation necessary. If bleeding continues, it is possible that the patient has a blood dyscrasia that should be evaluated and treated as soon as possible.

2. Excessive bleeding can lead to hypotension and inadequate perfusion of vital organs. Thus bleeding must be brought under immediate control, intravenous lines established, and preparations made for blood replacement. Electrocardiograms and catheterization for monitoring central venous pressure and urinary output are important adjunctive procedures. Ventilation should be evaluated, and because ventilatory insufficiency can compound the problems created by blood loss, respiration should be normalized as soon as possible.

3. Packing of the nose can cause displacement of facial fractures and confound the definitive treatment. To avoid this, nasomaxillary fractures should be reduced and manipulated into anatomic position (see Chapter 52). If there is too much packing, several loops of packing should be removed and the fragments of bone once again reset into proper alignment.

4. Overpacking of the nose can cause displacement of fractured nasal bones and infrequently cause necrosis, loss of tissue, and scar formation. These complications can be avoided by packing just enough to control bleeding and by removing the packs in 3 to 5 days. Prophylactic antibiotics are helpful in reducing the degree of damage.

ALTERNATIVE TECHNIQUE OF POSTERIOR PACKS

Posterior packs are indicated in those patients who have bleeding from the posterior nares or nasopharynx and/or who do not have control of bleeding with the anterior pack method described previously. The posterior pack technique requires patient cooperation; sedation or general anesthesia may be necessary.

a–c The nose should be prepared with 1/4% oxymetazoline hydrochloride and 4% cocaine containing epinephrine, as with the anterior packs. Two or three 2-inch × 2-inch gauze sponges are rolled into a tampon. An assistant then holds the sponges as the physician ties a length of 2-0 silk around the center of the roll. The

ends of the silk should be left long. The ends of the tampon are then tied with additional lengths of 2-0 silk. These strands are placed 5 mm from the edge, and the knots are positioned so that the strands are in a direction opposite to that of the central silks. The tampon is coated with Bacitracin. A second tampon is similarly prepared.

d–f Two 8-french red rubber catheters are then passed through the nose (one on the right, the other on the left) and into the pharynx. With use of a headlight and tongue blade, the catheters are pulled out through the mouth and secured to the center strings. The catheters are pulled and the tampons guided into the posterior nares with the surgeon's finger. The tampons will fold as they become lodged in the posterior nares. The central silk strands are pulled tightly along the floor of the nose; the ends of the other strands are left dangling from the side of the mouth, to be later secured to the cheeks with tape. The nose is subsequently packed anteriorly with gauze, and the silk strands are tied over the gauze or a small dental roll that is placed over the gauze packing.

Postoperatively the patient should be treated with antibiotics. If ties have been used to hold any of the gauze packing, the columella and ala of the nose should be inspected for pressure necrosis, and if this occurs, the tightness of the silk strands should be adjusted. A Telfa bolster placed between the collumella and the sutures before any knots are tied will aid in protecting the skin. Excessive packing can affect the airway by pressing down on the soft palate and thus, the patient should be evaluated for signs of respiratory difficulty. Evaluation of blood gases will help in assessing adequate oxygenation and CO_2 exchange.

ALTERNATIVE TECHNIQUE OF BALLOON TAMPONADE

a'–c' The commercial balloon tamponade technique is time proven and easy to perform for the inexperienced physician. There are many balloon devices and they should be inserted according to the directions. The nose is usually prepared with a decongestant and topical anesthetic. The balloon/catheter is placed into the nose and inserted so that one balloon is beyond the posterior choana and the other in the nasal cavity. The posterior balloon is then filled with saline and brought forward to make sure that it is caught in the posterior choana. The anterior balloon is then inflated to hold both balloons in position. Additional packing may be placed around the catheter anteriorly if necessary. Dye colored water can also be used to inflate the balloons providing a measure of observation for leakage.

In an emergency situation, Foley catheters can be substituted for the commercial balloon devices. The

CONTROL OF BLEEDING

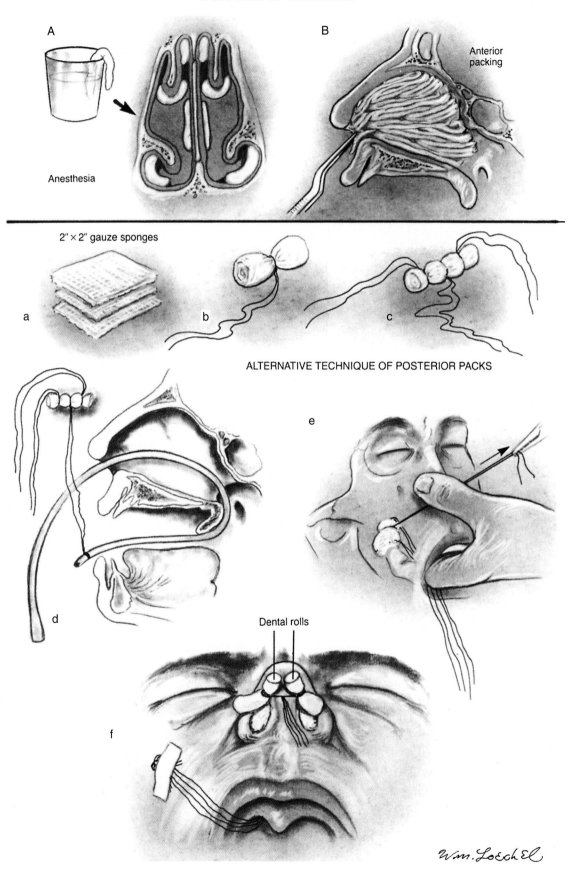

A

Anesthesia

B

Anterior
packing

2" × 2" gauze sponges

a

b

c

ALTERNATIVE TECHNIQUE OF POSTERIOR PACKS

d

e

Dental rolls

f

Wm. Loechel

54

CONTROL OF BLEEDING *(Continued)*

ALTERNATIVE TECHNIQUE OF BALLOON TAMPONADE

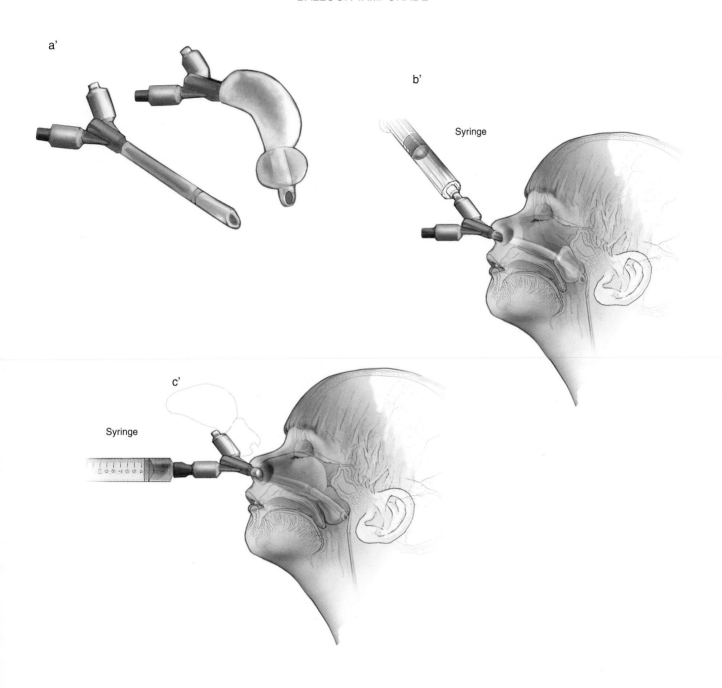

a'

b'

Syringe

c'

Syringe

Foley is lubricated, inserted into the nasal cavity, and directed toward the nasopharynx. The Foley is then filled with saline and pulled tightly against the posterior choana, while the rest of the nasal cavity is packed with antibiotic-impregnated gauze. The catheter is then secured anteriorly with a large knot.

ALTERNATIVE TECHNIQUE OF ENDOSCOPIC CONTROL OF BLEEDING

If vasoconstrictive agents, balloon tamponade, endovascular techniques, or packing fail to control bleeding, then an operation may be indicated. Currently, we prefer an endoscopic approach as opposed to an open or Caldwell-Luc procedure. Knowledge of the nasal blood supply is crucial. Control of posterior epistaxis focuses on the terminal branches of the internal maxillary artery: the sphenopalatine and posterior nasal artery. The sphenopalatine foramen lies just posterior and lateral to the horizontal attachment of the middle turbinate. Also, it is approximately 7 cm from the collumella.

As described in Chapter 86, the nose is prepared with oxymetazoline followed by 4% Xylocaine spray. The lateral wall of the nose posterior and inferior to the middle turbinate is injected with 2% Xylocaine containing 1:100,000 epinephrine.

Before proceeding with the surgical procedure the surgeon should evaluate the bleeding site with a 0° endoscope and evaluate for the use of cautery. If the bleeding site is visualized and can be controlled with a unipolar suction cautery or bipolar cautery, then this method should be applied. If bleeding cannot be completely controlled, then a surgical procedure is employed.

a"–d" There are several options to locate and control bleeding from the sphenopalatine artery. A conservative approach is to push the medial turbinate medially and make an incision below the attachment of the middle turbinate from the posterior part of the bulla ethmoidalis to the undersurface of the horizontal part of the middle turbinate. A mucoperiosteal flap is raised exposing the bone of the middle turbinate, the lateral nasal wall and the dorsal part of the inferior turbinate. The dissection continues subperiosteally and posteriorly to expose the sphenopalatine foramen. The artery is then identified, put on a stretch as it leaves the foramen, and either cauterized or ligated with surgiclips.

e",f" The other method, which we prefer, uses the endoscopic approach described in Chapter 86. The procedure is initiated by pushing the middle turbinate medially followed by a maxillary antrostomy. The inferior, lateral tail of the middle turbinate is removed, and the lateral wall of the nose, posterior to the antrostomy, is taken down to expose the sphenopalatine foramen. Either electrocautery or vascular clips are used to cauterize or ligate the artery/arteries as they exit the foreman. If needed, the bone of medial, posterior wall of the maxillary sinus can be removed, providing exposure and ligation of the internal maxillary artery.

CONTROL OF BLEEDING *(Continued)*

ALTERNATIVE TECHNIQUE OF ENDOSCOPIC CONTROL

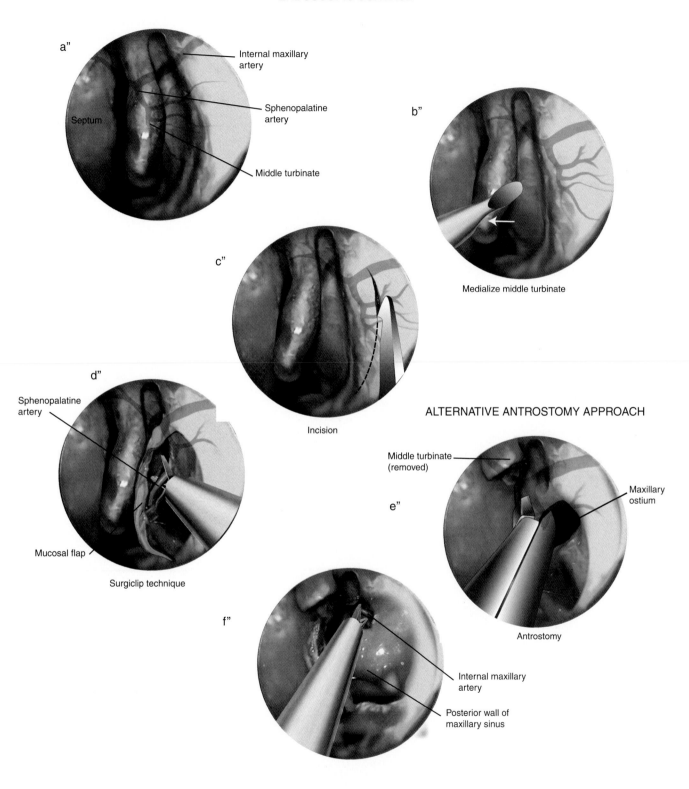

a"

Internal maxillary artery

Sphenopalatine artery

Septum

Middle turbinate

b"

Medialize middle turbinate

c"

Incision

d"

Sphenopalatine artery

Mucosal flap

Surgiclip technique

ALTERNATIVE ANTROSTOMY APPROACH

Middle turbinate (removed)

Maxillary ostium

e"

Antrostomy

f"

Internal maxillary artery

Posterior wall of maxillary sinus

Soft Tissue Trauma

CHAPTER

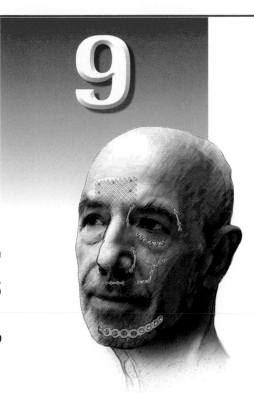

Abrasions, Lacerations, and Avulsions

In Consultation With Michael Carron, MD

INDICATIONS

Knife stabs, automobile and motorcycle accidents, gunshots, assaults, and sports are common causes of skin injury. The size and shape of the striking object and its direction and force will determine the type of injury, that is, abrasion, laceration, or avulsion. The severity and consequence of the injury largely depends upon the area and depth of tissue damage and involved anatomic structures.

The layers of the skin are epidermis, papillary dermis, and the deeper reticular dermis. Beyond this is a fatty subcutaneous tissue which cushions the skin, is mobile and contains blood vessels and nerves. Deep to this is the facial superficial muscular aponeurotic system (SMAS), mimetic muscles, salivary glands, and the facial skeleton. The blood supply of the skin with its subdermal plexus is considerably robust in the face and neck, and the skin often heals without complication.

A Abrasion injuries are the result of shearing forces tangential to the skin. The epidermis and papillary dermis are removed. The reticular dermis and the deeper

structures usually remain intact. The hair follicles will provide the cells necessary to re-epithelialize and resurface the injury. Injury to the reticular dermis or beyond will result in scarring. It is common for debris to be present in these wounds and if not removed, it will cause tattooing or act as a nidus of infection. Properly managed abrasions tend to heal without the formation of scar.

B Traumatic lacerations are unintentional incisions through the skin. The depth of injury will vary and important structures such as nerves, blood vessels, and salivary glands may be injured. In extreme situations, such as saw injuries, bone may be involved. Whether surgically repaired to heal in primary intention or left open to heal secondarily, there will always be some degree of scar formation.

C Like abrasions, avulsions result from shearing forces; however, the depth of injury is beyond the papillary dermis into deeper structures. A significant amount of tissue may be torn from the face leaving tissue voids. If the avulsion lifts up tissues without

ABRASIONS LACERATIONS AND AVULSIONS

A

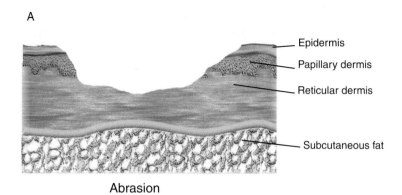

Epidermis

Papillary dermis

Reticular dermis

Subcutaneous fat

Abrasion

B

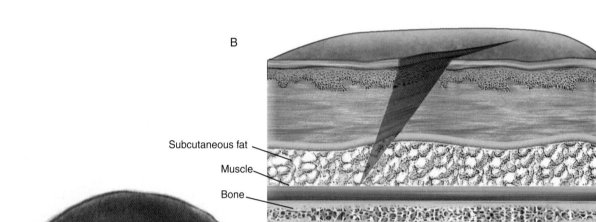

Subcutaneous fat

Muscle

Bone

Laceration

C

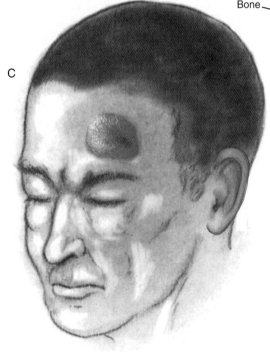

Avulsion

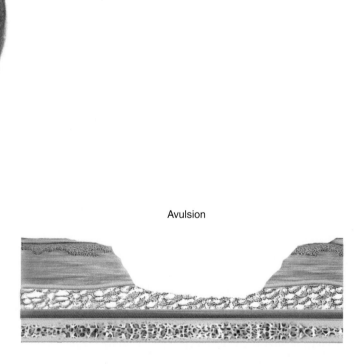

removal of them, it is referred to as a laceration/avulsion. Invariably, these avulsions will heal with scar formation and commonly end up with deformity in the area of injury.

Avulsions have a variable depth of damage and the consequences may be severe in thin structures such as the eyelids. The eyelid skin is flimsy and easily distorted by scar contracture; injury to all layers may affect the globe beneath which is usually protected by these tissues.

The commisures of the mouth and eyelids may be distorted by an avulsion or laceration either directly or secondarily from wound healing and contracture. The scarring can lead to functional impairment of these structures. Finally, the vermillion border and nasal ala are also vulnerable to distortion as a result of contraction of tissues following a laceration or avulsion.

PROCEDURES

Preparation

The objective of treating a wound in the acute phase is to create a wound bed for optimal healing. The wound must be cleaned with removal of debris and necrotic tissues. The reconstruction should achieve anatomic integrity with an adequate blood supply. The wound should be closed in a way to avoid any dead space with appropriate drains to avoid accumulation of blood. The surface of the wound should be managed with a layered closure under minimal tension.

Patients should initially be evaluated for tetanus prophylaxis and cause of injury. Patients with contaminated wounds should be treated with antibiotics.

Photographic documentation is also important. Photographic images should capture the site and extent of injury.

The wound is generally prepared with a slow injection of 2% Lidocaine containing 1:50,000 epinephrine (buffered with 1 mL of bicarbonate for every 10 mL of the solution) to achieve anesthesia and hemostasis. The wound is next copiously irrigated with normal saline and the adjacent area prepared with antiseptic solution. If there is foreign material or necrotic tissue, the wound is scrubbed with a 4 × 4 gauze and/or a sterile scrub brush with irrigation. Also these maneuvers will reduce the bacterial load within the area.

Abrasions

Usually abrasions do not violate the papillary dermis and should heal well in a clean, undisturbed field. The wound is anesthetized, irrigated, and cleansed. Any grossly necrotic tissue should be sharply removed with scissors or scalpel. Necrotic or crushed tissue should be debrided to a point where the tissues are bleeding and appear viable. Antibiotic ointment is applied immediately. Depending on the degree of contamination, the presence of overt infection and the viability of the wound, oral antibiotics may be given. The patient is instructed to wash away any crusts with a mild soap and washcloth and reapply ointment three times a day. Alternatively an antibiotic can be applied covered by a non sticking (Telfa) dressing and changed three times daily. These dressings however must be kept moist to avoid removal of migrating epithelium. Reepithelization occurs more readily if the wound is kept moist with ointment. Patients with type 1 and 2 skin are counseled that redness may persist for up to 3 months. Those with type 3 to 6 skin are counseled about the possibility of hypopigmentation due to melanocyte destruction.

Lacerations

D For lacerations, the wound is anesthetized, irrigated, and cleansed as described earlier. The depth of the wound is probed and a determination is made of whether muscle, nerve, blood vessels and/or salivary gland are involved with the injury. Repair of these deeper structures is covered in great detail in Chapter 10. Debridement of crushed or necrotic wound edges is accomplished with sharp scissors or scalpel. The wound edges should be cleaned and trimmed (squared off) or slightly beveled outward for eversion upon closure. The skin should be undermined to relieve tension from the underlying tissues. The subcutaneous tissue is closed with 4-0 vicryl or chromic (sutures) and the dermis with 5-0 vicryl or chromic sutures. These sutures are important as they obliterate dead space, prevent fluid accumulation, and relieve tension from the skin edges allowing early suture removal. The skin is closed with 5-0 or 6-0 prolene or nylon. Care is taken to evert the wound edges which should lie flat after wound contraction. Ointment is applied to the wound. If swelling or fluid accumulation is a concern a small drain should be applied and/or pressure dressing for at least 72 hours. Antibiotics are used in contaminated wounds or in wounds with questionably viable tissue or a tenuous blood supply. If a laceration enters the oral cavity antibiotic treatment should be directed to the anerobes in this area.

Avulsions

E In avulsions, the wound is anesthetized, cleansed, and debrided. The depth of the wound is probed for any neurovascular injury. The underlying muscles and salivary glands should also be assessed and their status documented. If the skin can be undermined and the wound closed without excessive tension,

D

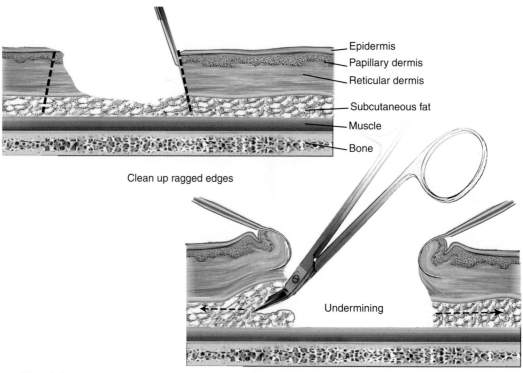

Epidermis
Papillary dermis
Reticular dermis
Subcutaneous fat
Muscle
Bone

Clean up ragged edges

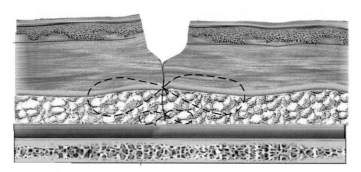

Undermining

Wound closure

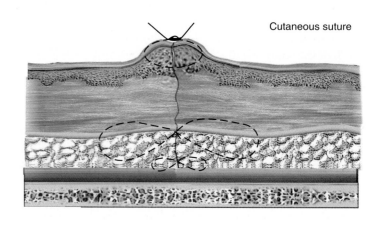

Intradermal suture

Subcutaneous suture

Cutaneous suture

E

FLAPS

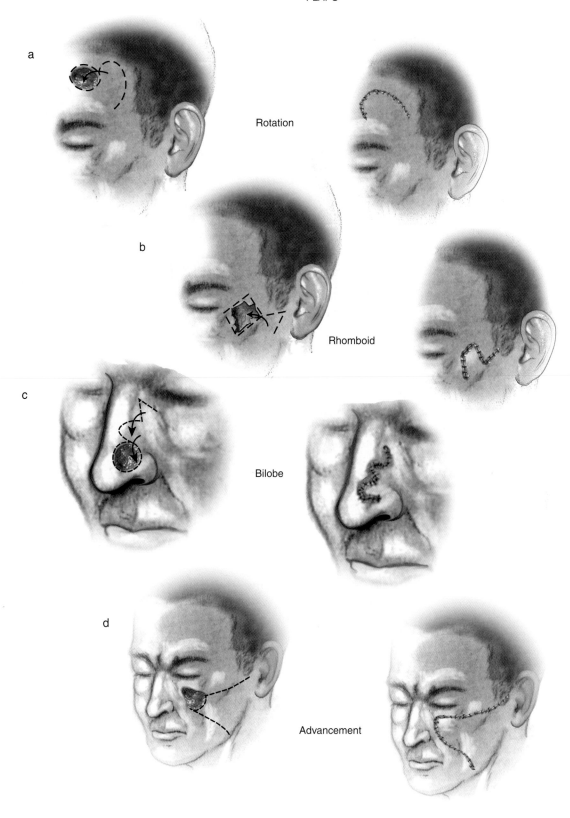

a

Rotation

b

Rhomboid

c

Bilobe

d

Advancement

primary closure is the simplest method of repair. If the size of the injury prohibits primary closure, a split thickness skin graft can be employed for temporary coverage with a thought of later reconstruction using a regional or free flap. If the defect is such that a flap is needed immediately, advancement and rotation flaps are desirable. Rotation, rhomboid, bilobed, forehead, and cervicofacial advancement flaps work well (see *a–d*). For more severe types of injuries such as those seen in gunshot wounds and high-speed power tools, larger flaps such as the pectoralis major, temporalis muscle, trapezius, and nape of neck may be required. Some large avulsive injuries will require microvascular reconstruction with free tissue and bone (see Chapter 36).

PITFALLS

1. Debris and necrotic tissue within the wound predispose to inflammation, wound breakdown, and scarring. It is thus important to prepare the wound bed with adequate cleansing, debridement, and antibiotic coverage.

2. Meticulous wound preparation is critical. Removal of vital tissues during debridement should be avoided as it is more difficult to replace missing tissue than it is to revise or debulk a wound closed previously.

3. The management of a wound requires an understanding of the anatomy of the craniofacial region especially the layers of the face. Bear in mind that you should be ready to evaluate injuries to deeper structures and determine the type of injury and the need for reconstruction involving the nerves, ducts, bone, and mucosa.

4. Injury involving the eyelids, lips, and ala require special consideration. The lips are a complex structure and require repair of mucosa, muscle, and surface skin. The eyelids are extremely thin and it is necessary to restore this thin tissue retaining the mobility and function of the eye covering. The nasal ala constitutes an important unit of the face and this must be restored to proper position and appearance. Failing to properly repair these wounds can result in serious cosmetic and functional impairment such as ectropion and epiphora, difficulty with speech and smell, and nasal obstruction and deformity.

COMPLICATIONS

1. The most common complication from abrasions, lacerations, and avulsions are usually wide, depressed, or contracted scars. The assessment, management, and repair of these squeal are covered in Chapter 13.

2. It is important to prevent infection since infection will cause further destruction of tissues and provide for excessive scaring. Cleaning, debridement, and preparation of the wound will help avoid the infection from occurring. It is also important to obliterate any dead space and drain any area that will accumulate fluid or blood.

3. Sometimes the patient will not remember or understand the degree of injury. Photographs should be taken before embarking upon the reconstruction and become a part of the patient's record. Photographic documentation can also be useful in medical legal decisions.

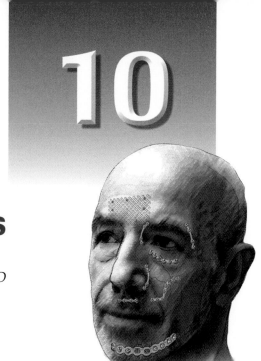

Penetrating Injuries

In Consultation With Giancarlo F. Zuliani, MD

INDICATIONS

General Considerations

The initial treatment of a victim with penetrating trauma is often performed by the emergency room physician and/or trauma surgeon. Once the patient is stabilized, the craniofacial surgeon may be called to address any relevant injury. To treat victims responsibly, the craniofacial surgeon should have mastered head and neck anatomy, the ATLS trauma protocol, and an understanding of high- and low-velocity ballistics.

Mechanism of Injury

In urban areas, the incidence and severity of penetrating injuries to the craniofacial region are high. These injuries are typically a result of stab or bullet wounds, but impaling injuries also occur with automobile, motorcycle, snowmobile, or farm injury. Stab wounds often occur in the neck, while slash wounds to the face are more common. Facial prominences such as the nose, eyelid, ear, or lip may be avulsed from the body (see Chapter 9).

The location and severity of a knife wound depend on the length, shape, and contour of the blade (serrated or smooth), and handedness and gender of the assailant. Because of the much higher velocity, bullet wounds cause more tissue damage than knife wounds. In general, stab wounds or slash wounds are almost never self-inflicted. Bullet wounds to the face are usually from suicide attempts, and neck wounds are more often due to attempted homicide or shooting in

self-defense. Suicides result in massive tissue loss and collateral damage due to close proximity of the weapon to the face. These injuries are often fatal. Survivors have massive bone and soft tissue avulsion with maxillary, palatal, and mandibular composite defects.

A The kinetic energy of the missile is the main determinant of injury. Kinetic energy is defined as $1/2\ mv^2$. As the velocity of the projectile increases, so does energy squared. High-velocity missiles (above 2,000 ft/s) from rifles create more damage and tissue loss than low-velocity handguns (below 1,000 ft/s). Shotgun injuries are variable in terms of tissue damage. As the shot exits the barrel, it begins to scatter and lose velocity and energy. Therefore, close range shotgun wounds are especially devastating as the shot has not scattered, the mass of the load is high and the velocity is maximal. At further distances, the wounds are less severe because the shot has scattered and the velocity has diminished considerably.

B A missile damages tissue directly as it cores through the tissue causing temporary and permanent cavitation and transmission of shock waves. High-velocity missile injuries, as those incurred with game rifles, AR-15's or AK-47's generate high-velocity wounds with cavitation (intense and rapid expansion of surrounding tissues) and shockwave propagation leading to intense tissue damage.

C,D Most bullets are made of lead because lead is a heavy metal and imparts more (mass) kinetic energy to the target. The lead core of most bullets is protected

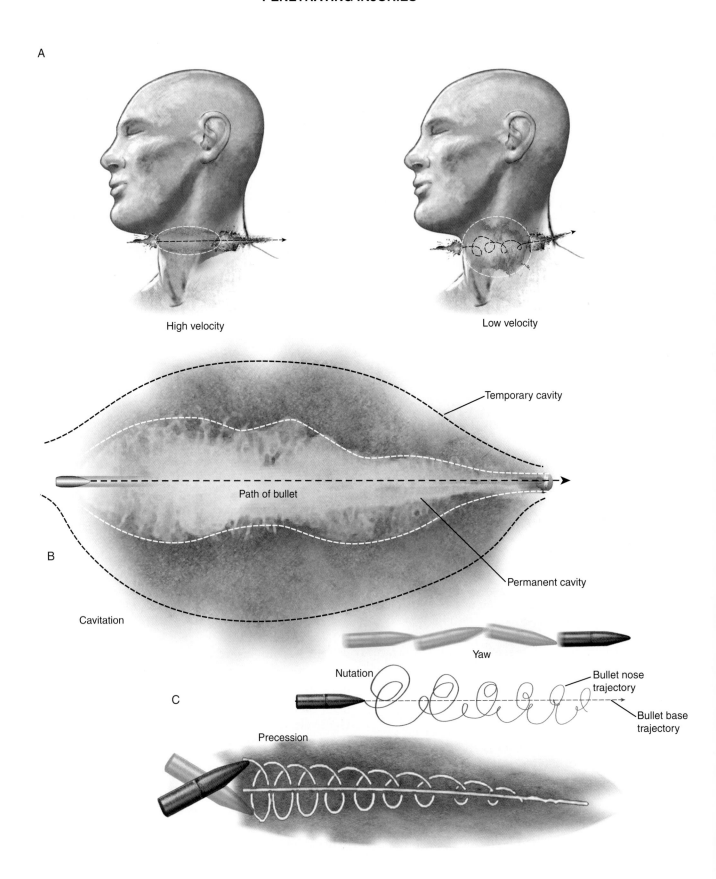

A

High velocity

Low velocity

B

Temporary cavity

Path of bullet

Permanent cavity

Cavitation

Yaw

Nutation

Bullet nose trajectory

Precession

C

Bullet base trajectory

by a jacket of copper to prevent disintegration of the soft lead as it spirals through the barrel's rifling. Full metal jacket bullets minimally expand when they hit tissue creating small entrance and exit wounds. If these bullets tumble through the tissue as in yaw, precession, and nutation, destruction can be quite sizeable and the exit wound enormous. Bullets such as hollow-point, flat-head, or semijacketed are designed to expand rapidly (mushroom) and fragment with the goal of maximal tissue damage and cavitation. Buckshot or birdshot injuries may retain the wadding from the shotgun and if left in the wound may serve as a source of infection.

PROCEDURE

Resuscitation and Initial Evaluation

Emergency care is discussed in Chapter 3. Of primary importance is maintenance and stabilization of the airway, diagnosis and control of vascular injury, and determining whether the larynx, pharynx, or esophagus is involved. Endotracheal intubation, cricothyroidotomy, or emergency tracheostomy must be considered (see Chapters 4 through 7). One must always assume and evaluate for cervical spine injury. As noted previously it is important to control bleeding, detect expanding hematomas, bruits and/or neurologic damage. Blood and fluid replacement is employed when necessary. ATLS protocol is followed, and once the patient is stabilized, an examination including imaging studies is required.

Knives buried in the face or neck should not be removed in the emergency department, nor should any wound be probed as severe hemorrhage or air embolism may occur. These injuries should be evaluated with vascular studies, and knives should only be removed in the operating room where emergency intervention can be safely performed.

Management

Protocols for managing penetrating craniofacial trauma are often in place at major trauma centers. The goal is to identify patients who need emergent surgery and those requiring further workup or transfer to a different facility. Vascular and thoracic surgeons should be available for consultation in addition to ophthalmologic and neurosurgical expertise.

Injuries that do not penetrate the platysma can be managed with removal of foreign material, vigorous cleaning, and debridement. Wounds contaminated with clothing, vegetable matter, or debris are cleaned, debrided, and allowed to granulate. Wounds that appear clean can be closed but on occasion may require grafting or flap closure (see Chapter 9). Scarring can be managed electively once the acute process has subsided (see Chapter 13). Tetanus prophylaxis must be considered when appropriate.

Patients with subcutaneous emphysema, hoarseness, stridor, and crepitance should undergo laryngoscopy and esophagoscopy. If no tear is found, the patient is kept NPO, closely observed and serially examined. Laryngotracheal injury usually requires local tracheotomy and repair via thyrotomy for mucosal lacerations followed by reduction of fractures (see Chapters 96 through 102). Small pharyngeal injuries can be repaired primarily.

E A useful classification system for predicting the degree and site of injury divides the craniofacial area and neck into three Zones (see Chapter 3). Injuries in Zone I, which extends from the thoracic inlet to the inferior border of the cricoid, often presents with morbid and potentially fatal consequences. Patients with Zone I injuries should undergo vascular imaging and a contrast swallow to rule out major vessel damage and tears or perforations of the pharynx or esophagus. CT Scans are also important for evaluation of occult pneumothorax. Injuries in Zone II, which extend from the cricoid to the angle of the mandible, carry the best prognosis as critical structures are readily accessible through the neck. Injuries in Zone III, which extends from the angle of the mandible to the skull base, are more precarious because vessels are in proximity to the skull base and more difficult to access emergently. Zone I and Zone III injuries also have the highest incidence of occult injury, and injuries in these zones warrant aggressive workup, inpatient observation, repeat physical exam, and imaging with angiography.

F–H A long neck incision, parallel to the medial border of the sternocleidomastoid muscle, can be used for most zone II injuries. The same incision can be extended superiorly or inferiorly for zone III or I injury. Exploration should ensure preservation of important structures such as the jugular vein and carotid artery and the hypoglossal, phrenic, vagus, and spinal nerves. Laryngeal and/or pharyngoesophageal structures should be repaired. The incision may be duplicated on the opposite side of the neck for bilateral injury.

In a deep penetrating wound, a cautious debridement should spare neural, vascular, muscular, and glandular structures. If mucosa is involved, it is closed first with chromic or vicryl interrupted sutures. If primary closure is not feasible, relaxation flaps, rotation flaps, and even regional flaps may be necessary to replace missing tissue. After closure of the mucosa, muscles are reapproximated in an anatomic position. Large vessels are checked for adequacy of ligation and for overall hemostasis. If severed nerves are identified, they should be repaired with or without grafting as soon as possible (see Chapter 14). The parotid duct injury is identified,

D

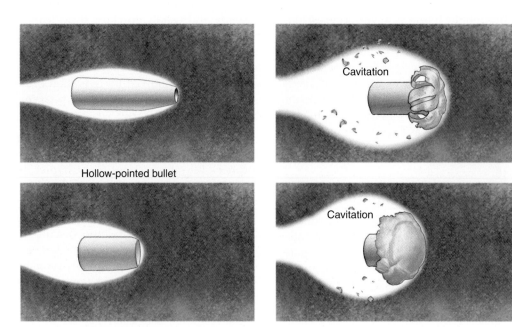

Hollow-pointed bullet

Cavitation

Flat-nosed bullet

Cavitation

E

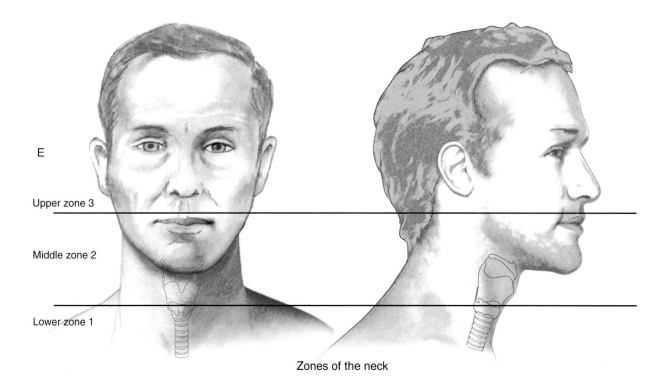

Upper zone 3

Middle zone 2

Lower zone 1

Zones of the neck

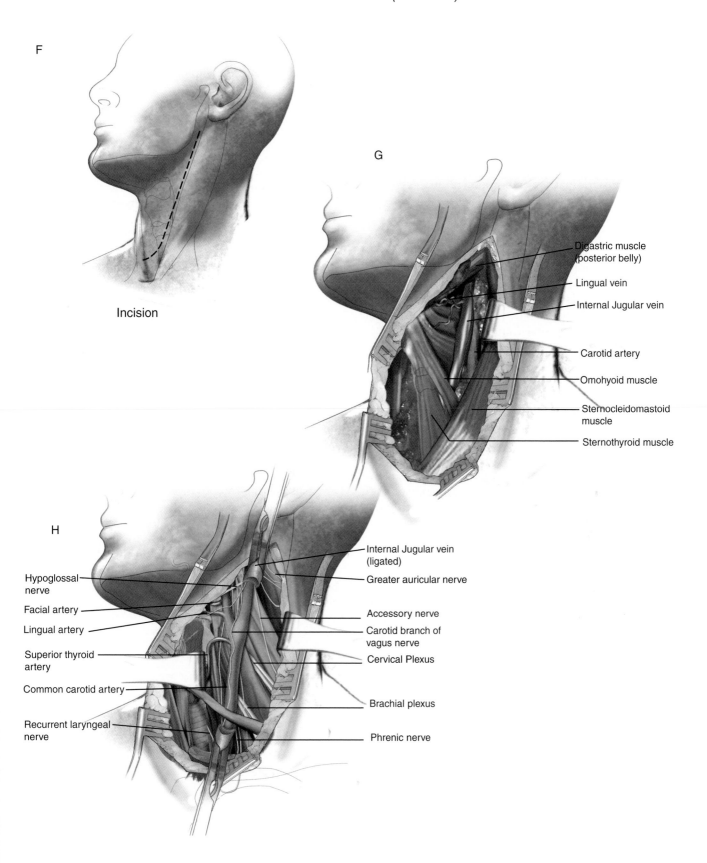

F

Incision

G

Digastric muscle (posterior belly)

Lingual vein

Internal Jugular vein

Carotid artery

Omohyoid muscle

Sternocleidomastoid muscle

Sternothyroid muscle

H

Hypoglossal nerve

Facial artery

Lingual artery

Superior thyroid artery

Common carotid artery

Recurrent laryngeal nerve

Internal Jugular vein (ligated)

Greater auricular nerve

Accessory nerve

Carotid branch of vagus nerve

Cervical Plexus

Brachial plexus

Phrenic nerve

repaired, and stented as outlined in Chapter 16. Finally, soft tissues are closed as described above with appropriate drains, and dressings and compresses.

Facial fractures are diagnosed and repaired as described in later chapters. Avulsion of bone requires free tissue transfer or can be managed with closure of the wound and bone grafting at a future date (Chapters 35 and 36). Adequate reduction and fixation of fractures is important to obtain functional and cosmetic results.

The patient must be observed during the postoperative period for infection and necrosis of tissues with debridement and reconstruction as necessary. Continuous evaluation and interventions even at a later time must be considered.

PITFALLS

1. Identification of pharyngeal or esophageal injury is important. If repair of these injuries is neglected or delayed, infection, abscess, and sepsis may ensue. Laryngeal injury. If not treated early, can lead to airway compromise and voice problems.

2. Identify and repair the facial nerve within 72 hours. Beyond this period finding distal branches by electrical stimulation may not be possible.

3. In the appropriate injury setting, periodically remove the cervical collar and inspect the neck while maintaining in-line stabilization. The collar, if not removed for serial examination, may conceal impending airway compromise or signs suggestive of injury.

4. Do not send a patient with a compromised airway to a darkened, poorly equipped radiology or angiographic suite. The airway should be secured before the patient leaves the trauma bay.

5. If the condition of a patient with a penetrating neck wound continues to deteriorate despite resuscitation, consider an intrathoracic injury, such as a massive hemothorax or tension pneumothorax.

6. Injuries to the face require immediate repair. Use conservative techniques to close and repair defects while planning for continuous evaluation and additional measures if necessary.

7. Serial examination is important to monitor infection or tissue necrosis. Be prepared for debridement and/or change in antibiotics. Wound repair and scar revision can be completed once infection or necrosis has ceased.

COMPLICATIONS

1. Scars are inevitable. The goal of wound management is to close tissue deficits with minimal tension while obliterating dead space and using drains appropriately. Coaptation of skin edges with a slight eversion will avoid depressed scar lines. Residual scarring can be optimized with revisional techniques.

2. Soft tissue deficiency may be noted following repair. In such cases, the patient should be evaluated for flap reconstruction, injection of autogenous materials, or application of grafts.

3. Pharyngeal and esophageal injury can result in stenosis. It is important to monitor for narrowing, progressive dysphagia, and possible dilatation. Swallowing rehabilitation may be necessary.

4. Laryngeal injury may lead to voice problems. Anatomic abnormality and dysfunction may require surgical correction by vocal cord injection, thyrotomy, or thyroplasty depending on the pathology (see Chapters 103 and 104).

5. Airway obstruction may develop insidiously. Nasal obstruction from valve collapse, septal deviation, or nasal fracture can be corrected by septorhinoplasty. More serious and potentially life-threatening laryngeal, subglottic, or tracheal stenosis may require interventions as described in Chapters 103 through 108.

6. Ophthalmic and neurologic complications will require specialty consultation. Such consultants should be part of the evaluation and treatment team and be ready to manage these complications should they arise.

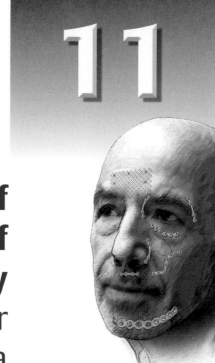

Treatment of Penetrating Injuries of the Carotid Artery
Alternative Technique for Blunt Trauma

In Consultation With Jeffrey R. Rubin, MD

INDICATIONS

Trauma to the carotid artery may result from either penetrating or blunt injuries. Penetrating injuries usually result from a knife or firearm or, rarely, from a bony fragment from facial bone or skull fractures. Injuries to the carotid artery maybe manifest as tense and expanding hematomas of the neck or brisk external bleeding, or there may be no apparent evidence of arterial and/or venous injury. The most commonly associated injury is a tear of the internal jugular vein. Other frequently noted injuries are located in the pharynx, larynx, esophagus, brachial plexus, and spinal cord. Traumatic brain injuries may also be encountered. The patient may be neurologically intact or may present with unilateral symptoms or coma.

Blunt carotid artery trauma is less common than penetrating and it frequently occurs with multiple other injuries. The most common blunt vascular injuries include carotid artery dissection, pseudoaneurysm, and intimal injuries resulting in arterial thrombosis.

Penetrating injuries to the carotid artery are often divided, according to the site of penetration, into three zones: zone 1, below the cricoid; zone 2, from the cricoid to the angle of the jaw; and zone 3, above the angle of the jaw (see *A*).

In the past, open surgical repair was the only option available for the treatment of carotid artery injury. Absolute indications for surgery included active hemorrhage from the neck, wound, a history of hemorrhage with hypotension, active bleeding from the mouth, and expanding cervical hematoma. With the advancement of endovascular technology, especially in the last decade, indications for the use of minimally invasive surgery including stenting for carotid artery traumatic injury have been expanded and in selected patients may actually be the preferred treatment modality. Therefore, there are two treatment regimens that depend upon not only the type, location, and severity of the arterial injury but also physician experience and availability of endovascular resources as well as patient stability.

PROCEDURES

B The first priority in patients with suspected injuries to the carotid artery is to obtain hemodynamic stability and control of the airway. In patients with active bleeding from a neck wound, the bleeding may be controlled by manual pressure while endotracheal intubation is performed. Two large-bore intravenous lines are established. A jugular or subclavian line is indicated but should be avoided on the side or in the path of injury. A large-bore intravenous line may be placed in the femoral vein that avoids the area of trauma entirely. Following intubation, the patient may be taken either to the operating room or to another appropriate department for additional diagnostic studies and/or intervention. Once the patient is placed on the operating room table, the neck and chest are prepared as a sterile field. While this is being done, an arterial line is started in the radial artery contralateral to the site of injury. A nasogastric tube is placed so that the surgeon can decompress the stomach and identify the esophagus during exploration. We also recommend that both thighs be sterilely prepared as well as the left arm, for angiographic access as well as to harvest saphenous vein or femoral artery grafts, which may be needed for open repair of the carotid artery. Intravenous antibiotic therapy is started.

Once the patient is stable, angiography via a femoral or brachial artery approach is used to study the supraaortic trunk and all branches in the zones of injury, in order to identify arterial injuries that may or may not be apparent on examination. Intimal tears, arterial dissections, pseudoaneurysms, transsections, and fistulas may be treated using endovascular stent technology. This minimally invasive modality often eliminates the need for emergent open operations for active hemorrhage and/or acute neurologic deficits. At times, additional advanced endovascular therapy may be needed, especially in zone 1 and zone 3 injuries. These techniques fall beyond the scope of this chapter.

Once the arterial component of surgery is completed, bronchoscopy, laryngoscopy, and esophagoscopy may be carried out as indicated, in a more relaxed setting in order to identify other areas of injury.

If endovascular support is not available, open intervention is indicated. After hemodynamic stability is achieved and endotracheal intubation is carried out, a neck incision is made along the anterior border of the sternocleidomastoid muscle. The muscle is retracted posteriorly, and branches of the anterior jugular vein are divided and ligated. This permits entry into the carotid sheath and dissection of the common carotid artery, its bifurcation, and external and internal carotid arteries. Control of bleeding can be achieved using digital pressure and/or application of double Silastic loops below and above the injury. Haphazard clamping with nonvascular clamps should be avoided. Commonly associated internal jugular vein tears can be handled by a lateral repair (in the case of a knife wound) or by ligation above and below the destroyed wall (in the case of a firearm injury).

C,D In the midneck, the dissection of the common carotid artery is kept close to its wall. In the lower portion of the neck, the surgeon should avoid injury to the vagus nerve that lies in close proximity to the common carotid artery. If the common carotid artery injury is low in the neck, and proximal control is difficult, the neck incision may be lengthened with a median sternotomy, to expose the supraaortic trunks.

Once proximal and distal control is achieved, repair of common carotid injuries employs standard vascular techniques. Prudent use of systemic or local anticoagulation during arterial clamping should be based upon the presence of concomitant injuries and complexity of the vascular repairs, and the benefits and risks should be considered. Small injuries, such as those caused by sharp penetration, may be repaired by arterial wall debridement, lateral arteriorrhaphy autologous tissue patch angioplasty, or resection and anastomosis. For repair of a lateral defect, the artery is cross-clamped, and the clean tear is sutured with 6-0 or 7-0 monofilament vascular sutures (after ensuring by direct inspection that there is no intimal damage, such as a tear in the opposite wall creating an intimal flap). For injuries other than a partial and clean cut that do not involve more than an inch of common carotid artery, the artery may be amply freed, cross-clamped, and repaired by an end-to-end anastomosis. In such cases, the edges of the artery should be freshened sharply and the vessel repaired. A continuous suture (made with a double-armed suture) is placed at the midpoint of the posterior wall. Both ends of the suture usually meet at the midpoint of the front wall. Eversion of the sutured ends of the artery needs to be insured.

E If tension is anticipated with an end-to-end anastomosis management should consist of an interposition saphenous vein graft. A saphenous vein graft, which is <3.5 mm in diameter, is inadequate to bridge a common carotid artery defect. If there is a serious disparity in size between the common carotid artery and the saphenous vein, the repair can still be made by closing both ends of the common carotid artery and bridging the defect with a vein graft anastomosed end-to-side to both ends of the common carotid artery. If the common carotid artery injury is extensive and there is no associated visceral injury or significant contamination, the repair of the common carotid artery may be made with an 8-mm-diameter polytetrafluoroethylene (PTFE) prosthesis.

Another option, if contamination is present and the saphenous is of inadequate size, is to fashion a "panel graft," or "spiral vein graft" from the saphenous vein. This is carried out by vertically opening the vein graft and then resewing it using an anvil of appropriate diameter as the support structure for the newly created graft. Lastly, a superficial femoral artery may be harvested for use as an autologous conduit for

TREATMENT OF CAROTID ARTERY INJURIES

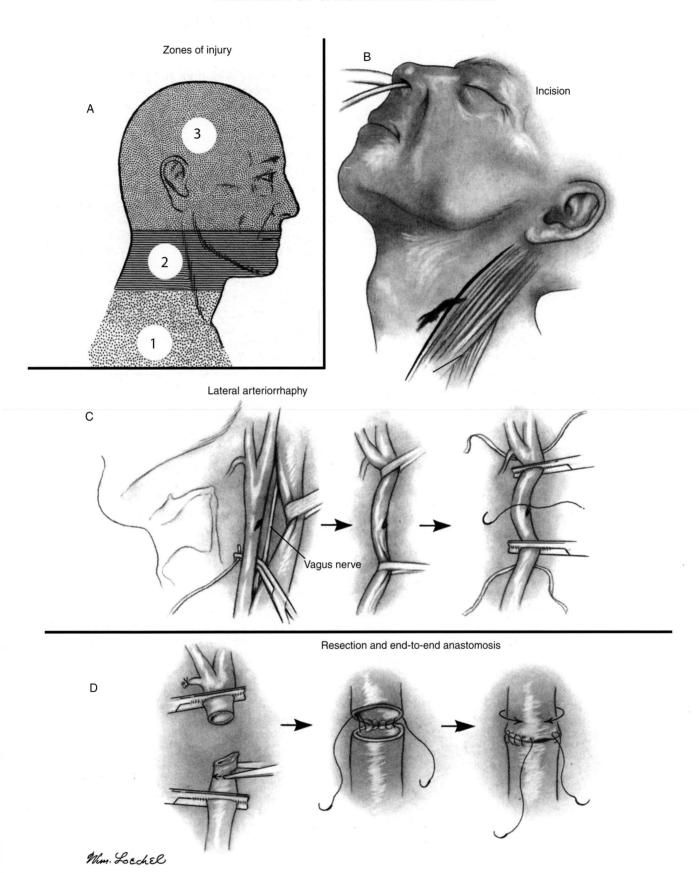

Zones of injury

A

B
Incision

Lateral arteriorrhaphy

C
Vagus nerve

Resection and end-to-end anastomosis

D

Wm. Locchel

carotid reconstruction. This requires femoral artery reconstruction and is therefore more time consuming and thus a less attractive alternative.

F A low common carotid artery injury near its origin can also be repaired by ligating its proximal stump and anastomosing the distal common carotid artery to the second portion of the subclavian artery creating a transposition. This procedure is easier on the right side of the neck than the left. To obtain exposure, the phrenic nerve is identified and dissected free of its bed, followed by division of the underlying scalenus anticus muscle. An end-to-side anastomosis is subsequently carried out. The subclavian artery has an extremely thin wall and tears easily, and this should be borne in mind when dissecting the artery and applying clamps to it. Bleeding from a damaged subclavian artery will often have to be controlled by proximal and distal ligation of the artery, a procedure in itself fraught with the risk of further tear and life-threatening hemorrhage.

Repair of External and Internal Carotid Arteries

G,H Injuries to the bifurcation of the carotid artery are repaired by lateral arteriorrhaphy or bypass grafting from the common carotid artery to the internal carotid artery with a saphenous vein inter position graft. Depending upon the complexity of the injury, the internal carotid artery may also be mobilized and resected, and an end-to-end anastomosis may be performed.

If the injury involves the external carotid artery, this may be repaired with lateral arteriorrhaphy. If the injury is complex and would require extensive repair, ligation above and below the point of injury is acceptable.

Injuries to the internal carotid artery, which require open operations, are managed according to the level of injury. The digastric muscle serves as a recognizable anatomic landmark to separate the two surgical approaches. Injuries below the digastric muscle are treated with standard vascular techniques. Digital pressure over the transverse process of C1 and over the origin of the internal carotid artery will generally slow the bleeding enough to permit dissection of the injured internal carotid artery. The origin of the external carotid artery is clamped, and care is taken to avoid damage to the hypoglossal nerve and the superior laryngeal nerve. Injury to the hypoglossal nerve is avoided by a positive identification of this structure, which may be covered by an anterior branch of the internal jugular vein. The superior laryngeal nerve does not need to be identified. It is usually injured either by blunt dissection behind the carotid bulb or by clamping the superior thyroid artery away from its origin. The internal carotid artery is then clamped. If there are no other associated injuries, 5,000 units of heparin are given intravenously at that time. Repair of the internal carotid artery is usually carried out by means of a vein graft. If a vein graft is not available and the internal carotid artery injury involves the bulb, the skeletonized external carotid artery may be transposed to the internal carotid artery to bridge the defect.

If the carotid artery is thrombosed at the site of injury but has brisk antegrade and retrograde bleeding after removing the thrombus plug at the site of the injury, the artery is reconstructed with a vein graft. An intimal injury present at the site of distal anastomosis is a contraindication and requires further resection of the artery until uninjured intima is identified. If retrograde bleeding is not observed, after reasonable surgical efforts are employed, the thrombosed carotid artery is ligated. The use of balloon thrombectomy catheters high in the neck or in the intracranial segment, should be avoided.

I Injuries to the internal carotid artery above the digastric muscle are more difficult to control. If the level of injury to the internal carotid artery has been determined by arteriography to be high, it is advantageous to convert to a nasotracheal intubation; this will permit bite closure and anterior advancement of the angle of the jaw, the main obstruction met by the surgeon when trying to reach the high cervical carotid (at or above C1). Proximal common carotid or internal carotid artery control is obtained by clamping the corresponding vessel. Digital pressure over C1 may provide distal control. For exposure, the digastric muscle is divided. The occipital artery, which crosses the internal carotid artery below the posterior edge of the digastric artery, is also divided. Our preference is then to reconstruct the distal internal carotid artery from behind, rather than from in front of the jugular vein, and for this approach (which we use routinely in distal vertebral bypass operations), the dissection proceeds between the jugular vein and the sternocleidomastoid muscle. The spinal accessory nerve is identified and gently retracted with a Silastic loop. The jugular vein and vagus are reflected anteriorly to the internal carotid artery, and the latter is exposed between C3 and C1. Again, care must be taken not to injure the hypoglossal or vagus nerve during this maneuver. The superior laryngeal nerve that exits the vagus above and behind the carotid bulb must be preserved. Care must be taken with retraction since stretch injuries of the nerves is also not uncommon.

In those cases in which it is impossible to obtain proper distal control of high internal carotid injuries, ligation is the advisable form of therapy. If the associated injuries and general condition of the patient permit, the internal carotid artery ligation should be treated with heparin for approximately 5 days postoperatively. This is done to curtail the extension of the thrombus into the segment of the intracranial internal

TREATMENT OF CAROTID ARTERY INJURIES *(Continued)*

SAPHENOUS VEIN GRAFT REPAIR

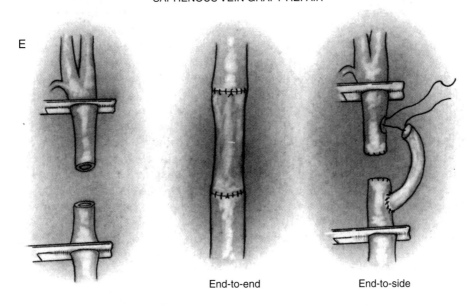

E

End-to-end   End-to-side

ANASTOMOSIS OF COMMON CAROTID TO SUBCLAVIAN

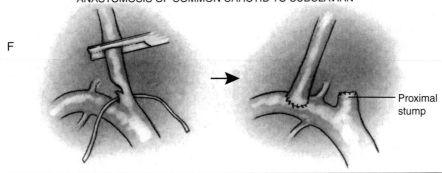

F

Proximal
stump

BYPASS GRAFT FROM COMMON TO INTERNAL CAROTID

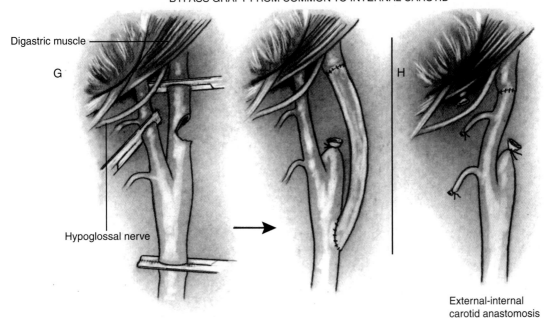

Digastric muscle

G

H

Hypoglossal nerve

External-internal
carotid anastomosis

carotid artery and into its main branches, the anterior and middle cerebral arteries. Due to the complexity of high carotid artery reconstruction, endovascular techniques, if available, would be preferred in this region.

In general, postreconstruction intraoperative completion imaging is carried out based upon the surgeon's general practice. This includes intraoperative angiography or duplex imaging. Follow-up imaging is recommended 8 weeks following primary intervention, for all reconstructed patients, and is carried out in a noninvasive vascular laboratory.

Postoperative antibiotic therapy is indicated when there is gross contamination of the wound or associated injury of the aeroesophageal tract and whenever a prosthetic graft is used. In arterial reconstruction, where a prosthetic graft is employed, intravenous antibiotic therapy is maintained for 3 to 5 days. When there is an esophageal fistula, evidence of inflammation, or sepsis, antibiotic therapy should be prolonged. In most vascular reconstructions, drains are left for <24 hours. Dressings are light and may be removed within 24 hours as well.

PITFALLS

1. An endovascular approach to carotid artery injury, if available, is the preferred method of treatment for blunt and penetrating carotid artery injury. This is especially the case with zone 2 and zone 3 injuries.

2. The saphenous vein graft diameter should be consistent with the diameter of the artery to be repaired and that the valves do not interfere with blood flow.

3. If the carotid artery injury is associated with atheroma of the carotid wall, care should be taken to include the full thickness of the wall with the suture. All arterial repairs should be done with interrupting sutures from the inside out. Eversion of the walls of the artery is preferred, as this prevents intraluminal dissection beneath the plaque or fragmentation of the plaque into the lumen.

4. Care should be taken to avoid missing intimal injuries especially with blunt injury trauma.

5. Injuries to the external carotid artery can be managed with ligation. The technique for repair of injuries to the internal carotid artery, if not amenable to endovascular therapy, is determined by the level of internal carotid artery injury.

6. If a common carotid artery injury is low or associated with a subclavian or innominate artery or a brachiocephalic vein injury, the sternocleidomastoid incision is lengthened to include a median sternotomy; partial sternotomy should be avoided. The sternotomy, however, should not be used in patients who have had previous aortocoronary bypass grafting. Under these circumstances, resection of the clavicle and control of the common carotid artery from the neck is a safer approach.

7. Subclavian artery injuries may be associated with common carotid artery injuries. Injuries in the first portion of the right subclavian artery are controlled by midsternotomy; injuries on the left require a fourth-space anterior thoracotomy. Injuries to the second portion of the subclavian artery require division of the scalenus anticus muscle for exposure. The phrenic nerve, which rides over the scalenus anticus, must be carefully preserved. Because the subclavian artery has a particularly thin wall, direct repair of injuries to the artery may be impossible or hazardous. If this is the case, we advise ligation proximally and distally to the site of injury and restoration of the blood supply to the arm by means of a common carotid artery to axillary or brachial artery bypass.

8. Concomitant vertebral injuries are common in penetrating neck trauma. These are also frequently noted in acceleration/deceleration injuries. Injuries to the first segment of the vertebral artery, from the origin of the subclavian to the transverse process of C6, present with active bleeding and are treated by ligation. Associated injuries of the vertebral artery in its intraspinal portion (C1–C6) have a tendency for spontaneous hemostasis and for the formation of a false aneurysm or an arteriovenous fistula. This is the result of the vertebral artery running through a tight osteomuscular compartment surrounded by a plexus of veins that are intimately associated with the artery and are therefore injured with it. In such cases, the vertebral artery should be explored and ligated or clipped above and below the point of injury. Once again, endovascular vertebral artery repair, in competent hands, would be the primary procedure of choice. The establishment of uninterrupted flow via the use of stents would preclude tedious dissection and complicated arterial reconstruction.

COMPLICATIONS

1. One of the most dreaded complications with injuries to the carotid artery is hemorrhage. Often, the patient has lost large amounts of blood, which must be replaced utilizing blood products and non–blood volume expanders. Large-bore access lines inserted into the femoral or opposite jugular and/or subclavian arteries are used. A radial artery line is placed in the arm opposite to the site of injury for monitoring of central venous pressure. Active bleeding may be frequently controlled with digital pressure, vascular clamping, or vessel loops that are doubly looped around arteries for control. One must avoid vigorous and aggressive dissection and clamping, which may result in more severe arterial, peri arterial venous, and nerve injuries.

2. Postoperative hematomas present as an expanding firm mass of the deep neck tissues. The most significant complication from a hematoma include compromised airway leading to respiratory arrest. Bradycardia, hypotension, and hypoxemia are the direct result of large hematomas that have been allowed to compromise the airway. In such situations, reintubation may be extremely difficult and/or impossible due to a tracheal deviation. Fiberoptic reintubation, drainage of the hematoma, and control of the bleeding site are indicated. These are best accomplished in a controlled environment and if time allows the patient can be transported back to an operative suite. In an extreme condition, in the ICU or in a floor bed, reopening of a neck wound followed by a careful expert reintubation may be indicated.

3. Embolism and arterial thrombosis are potential complications of arterial injury. Signs of endoluminal defects include transient central nervous system deficits such as aphasia, hemiparesis, and impaired vision. These patients should have a prompt return to the operating room for immediate reexploration. In the operating room duplex ultrasonography, intraoperative angiography or open exposure of the carotid artery may be indicated. Intimal injuries, the presence of a thrombus and/or embolus, a technical repair complication, and other etiologies may be identified. These should be removed by reconstruction. Anticoagulation therapy may or may not be indicated depending upon the complication and comorbidities.

ALTERNATIVE TECHNIQUE FOR REPAIR OF BLUNT TRAUMA

a–c Blunt trauma to the carotid artery may be the result of a direct blow from the outside or of an impact on and stretching of the vessel by the transverse process of C1 or a fragment from a fracture. On rare occasions, the internal carotid artery may be contused as a result of intraoral trauma, as seen in children who fall with a pencil or lollipop in their mouth.

Blunt trauma often produces a characteristic clinical picture. An intimal tear and an intramural hematoma or dissection are common consequences. These lesions may eventually lead to distal embolization of the brain or *in situ* thrombosis of the carotid artery. This process and the subsequent appearance of neurologic symptoms may take minutes, hours, or days. The delayed appearance of symptoms is the most common presentation of blunt trauma to the carotid artery. In addition, mural contusion with hematoma or dissection of the carotid may result in a stenosis, which may produce neurologic symptoms years later from compromised flow dynamics.

The possibility of blunt trauma to the carotid artery should be suspected in patients who have undergone direct blows to the neck or have trauma of the head and neck associated with the appearance of neurologic symptoms. These patients are candidates for immediate noninvasive vascular testing and arteriography, depending on the results of the noninvasive testing. At the time of arteriography and once the arteriogram has defined the arterial lesion suspected to be secondary to trauma, endovascular therapy is indicated. This generally involves the placement of a stent across the lesion via a femoral or brachial artery approach. If endovascular therapy is not possible because of an inability to cross the lesion with a guide wire or because the damage is too massive to be repaired using endovascular techniques, surgical exploration will be required. If the injured vessel has resulted in subsequent thrombosis and/or spasm and the distal portion of the internal carotid artery is accessible through the neck, an immediate exploration with resection and grafting of the carotid artery using a saphenous vein graft can be employed. If a saphenous vein is not available, a thin, 6-mm PTFE graft will provide an acceptable substitute.

In patients in whom the internal carotid artery is thrombosed and the arteriogram shows the petrous and cavernous portion of the carotid to be patent by a collateral flow, from the opposite internal carotid or from the ipsilateral external carotid, an exploration is advised. The exploration is done through the standard incision anterior to the sternocleidomastoid muscle, exposing the common carotid bifurcation and internal carotid artery. The retrojugular approach, described earlier, provides improved access to the distal cervical internal carotid artery. The internal carotid artery is then opened at the level of C1 through a longitudinal arteriotomy. Thrombus is cleared by insertion of a short length of a balloon (Fogarty) embolectomy catheter, which must not reach the intracavernous carotid. The intima of the distal cervical internal carotid is inspected. If it is intact at this level, plans are made for a common-to-distal cervical internal carotid artery saphenous vein bypass. At the conclusion of this grafting procedure, a clip is placed immediately below the anastomosis to exclude the proximal internal carotid artery and transform these into functional end-to-end anastomoses. In children with extensive damage requiring grafting, the surgeon may consider an end-to-end transposition of the external to the internal carotid artery or the use of a free arterial graft from a segment of superficial femoral artery that can itself be replaced with a 6-mm PTFE tube.

If the limited insertion of a Fogarty catheter does not clear the carotid satisfactorily and brisk backflow is not obtained, no distal manipulation of the intracranial carotid with a Fogarty catheter is advised. In such a case, it is better to ligate the internal carotid artery and maintain the patient on intravenous heparin for at least 5 days. This should help avoid progression of the internal carotid artery thrombus into the anterior and medial cerebral artery branches.

TREATMENT OF CAROTID ARTERY INJURIES *(Continued)*

EXPOSURE OF INJURIES ABOVE THE DIGASTRIC MUSCLE

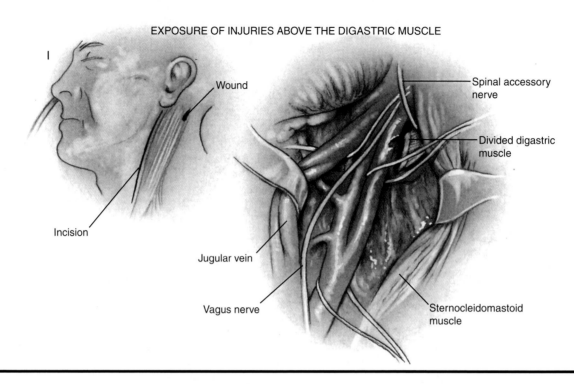

l

Wound

Incision

Spinal accessory nerve

Divided digastric muscle

Jugular vein

Vagus nerve

Sternocleidomastoid muscle

ALTERNATIVE TECHNIQUE FOR REPAIR OF BLUNT TRAUMA

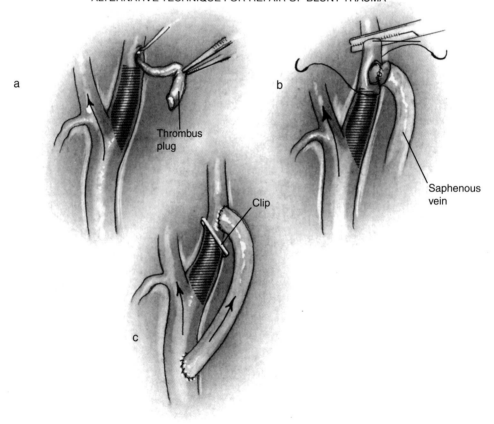

a

Thrombus plug

b

Saphenous vein

Clip

c

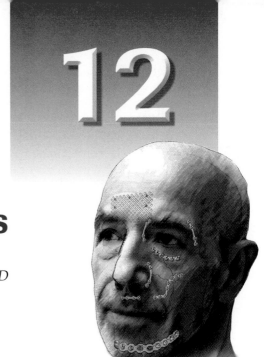

CHAPTER

12

Animal Bites

In Consultation With Chenicheri Balakrishnan, MD

INDICATIONS

Threatened animals often respond by biting. The attack may occur unprovoked without warning or by an animal that was provoked by teasing or taunting. Most bites occur in the summer months with dogs and cats accounting for the majority. Rodents, horses, and humans constitute the rest. Treatment goals are to eliminate infection, prevent rabies transmission, and repair wounds to prevent functional impairment and disfigurement.

The risk of infection is high in the bite injury, and infection may spread quickly through the face. Aside from direct inoculation of bacteria, the type and location of the wound, immunocompromised states such as diabetes, vascular disease, cancer and HIV, delay treatment and the presence of foreign bodies or necrotic tissue predisposes to wound infection.

Bacteria present in the saliva of the animal are usually responsible for contaminating the wound leading to infection. The most common organisms are *Staphylococcus*, *Streptococcus*, *Pasteurella*, and anaerobes. Sequelae range from mild discomfort, cellulitis, abscess formation, and necrotizing fasciitis. Self-limited lymphadenopathy occurs with cat scratch disease, an infection caused by Bartonella henselae present in the cat's saliva.

Dogs, cats, foxes, raccoons, skunks, and bats have been linked to rabies exposure. Rabies is a rhabdovirus transmitted through breaks in the skin. After inoculation, the rabies virus is contained at the entrance site

and is virtually undetectable. The incubation period may be from weeks to months. During this period, the virus can be thwarted with postexposure prophylaxis. Prophylaxis is recommended when the animal is not available for observation and/or the attack was unprovoked.

Bite injuries result in abrasions, lacerations, avulsions, laceration-avulsions, or puncture wounds. Dogs are prone to crush injury because the strength of their jaws and rounded teeth deliver very high pressure per square inch. Cat bites tend to result in deep puncture wounds into which bacteria are inoculated on their long-sharp teeth. Cat bites generally develop infection earlier than those of dogs. Rodents produce small puncture wounds or laceration-avulsions with their long curved incisors. Bat bites may be overlooked because their small puncture wounds tend to be inconspicuous.

PROCEDURES

Wound management involves vigorous cleaning and debridement to remove foreign debris, devascularized and necrotic tissue, and the burden of bacteria. This is accomplished with copious saline irrigation under pressure. Betadine paint may be used as an antiseptic agent, but Phisohex and chlorhexidine (which some believe can kill rabies) must be kept away from the eyes. Tetanus and rabies prophylaxis are administered when appropriate. The most common complication of an animal bite is infection. Antibiotics are recommended in dirty wounds, those involving bones or joints and when the host defenses are compromised.

Laceration

A It is often appropriate to delay the immediate closure of grossly contaminated wounds. Once the infection is cleared with wound care and antibiotics, the reconstruction may take place. Local anesthesia with epinephrine buffered with bicarbonate allows for excellent anesthesia and hemostasis. After the wound is anesthetized, it is washed with copious amounts of normal saline. Necrotic edges and tissue are debrided and hemostasis is obtained. Closure is carried out in layers where the muscle and dermis are closed with 4-0 vicryl. Skin is closed with 5-0 or 6-0 prolene depending on the thickness of the skin and relative motion of the area. Puncture wounds are cleansed and ointment is applied. They are permitted to heal secondarily.

Avulsion

Avulsion occurs when there is full-thickness loss of the skin. The repair can be accomplished with secondary healing, skin grafts, or local flap closure.

B Full-thickness grafts have a better appearing texture, thickness, and color match than split-thickness grafts. Postauricular skin provides excellent donor tissue with good color match in addition to hiding the scar well. The postauricular area is injected with 1% lidocaine and 1:100,000 epinepherine. A template of the defect is obtained with foil from a suture pack or a strip of telfa and used to mark the area for harvest. Once the graft is harvested, the defect is undermined and closed with 4-0 vicryl for the deep layers and 5-0 prolene for the skin. The graft is sutured into the defect and a Xeroform bolster dressing is applied and left in place for one week to prevent fluid accumulation and shearing.

Most defects of the face can be repaired with local tissue transfer. Deciding on which flap to use depends on the location of the wound, direction of the skin creases, size of the defect, and potential distortion of structures such as the eyelid, mouth, or brow. Because of the robust blood supply of the subdermal plexus in the skin, a length to width ratio of 3:1 is acceptable.

C ROTATION FLAP. These flaps are useful to close most defects of the face. Skin laxity, tissue availability, and direction of skin creases are taken into consideration when designing the flap. With the classic rotation flap, the defect is incorporated into the arc of the flap. The arc is four or five times the length of the defect. Marking solution is used to design the arc coming off the defect. Once anesthetized, the flap is incised, elevated with scissors and skin hooks, and

finally rotated into the defect. Dermis is closed with 4-0 vicryl and skin is closed with 5-0 or 6-0 prolene. Lines of rotation should follow the contours of the face and the creases of the skin.

D TRANSPOSITION FLAP. Like rotation flaps, transposition flaps are versatile as they may be designed in various shapes, sizes, and direction of closure. The rhomboid flap consists of two triangles each with angles of 60° and 120°. The bases of each triangle are overlapped to create the shape of a diamond. A straight limb is drawn off the 120° angle with a second limb off the end of the first at 60°.

The point of maximal tension should be in the natural skin creases to optimize the scarring. Double and triple rhomboids may be used to close rectangular and large circular defects.

E BILOBED FLAP. This is two transposition flaps with a common base. The primary flap, which fills the initial defect, is the same size as the defect. The secondary flap, which fills the primary flap defect, is slightly smaller than the void created by the primary flap. The secondary flap defect is closed primarily. Each flap rotates though approximately 45°. Bilobed flaps are excellent for small defects of the dorsum and nasal sidewall. Some potential pitfalls include length of scar, pin cushioning, and skin deformity.

Auricular Injury

The goals of auricular wound management are coverage of exposed cartilage and prevention of hematoma. When repaired appropriately, ear lacerations heal well due to a rich blood supply. Hematomas are secured by bolstering the anterior and posterior leaves of the auricular skin together with Telfa and through-and-through nylon mattress sutures.

F For small auricular defects (<0.5 cm) of the helix or anti-helix in which the skin does not approximate, a wedge excision and closure can be done. Although the ear is slightly smaller, this method maintains the helical contour, which is critical for a normal appearance.

G For defects up to 2.5 cm, a chondrocutaneous composite advancement flap can be used. For helical defects, an advancement flap can be used. The helical rim skin is elevated superiorly, inferiorly, and posteriorly over the conchal cartilage. Elevation proceeds to the elastic skin of the lobule. The cartilage is closed if possible. The envelope is then advanced and rotated to cover the cartilage defect. Elevation into the lobular skin is often necessary because of its ability to reach long distances. Vicryl sutures are used for the deep closure, while 5-0 or 6-0 prolene sutures are used for the auricular skin of the helix, antihelix, and postauricular skin.

ANIMAL BITES

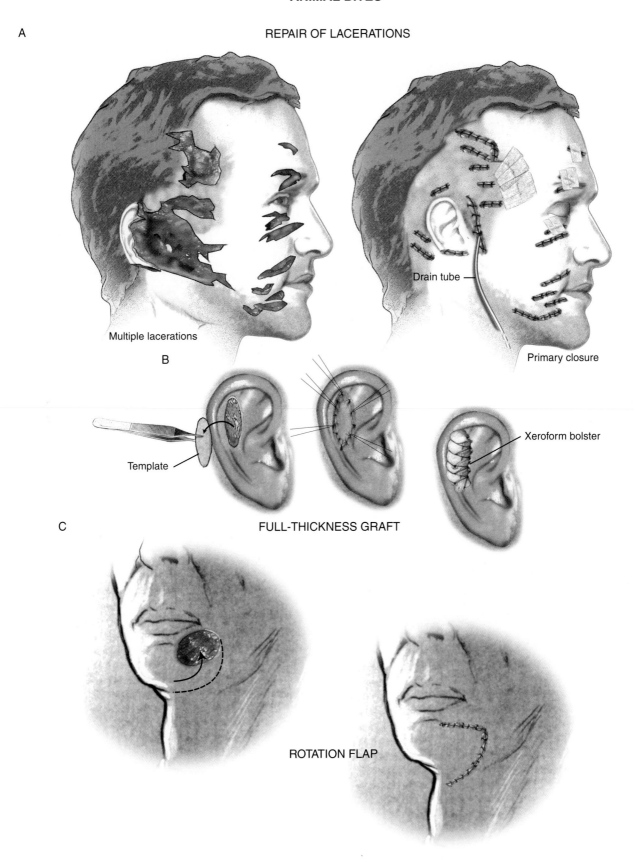

A

REPAIR OF LACERATIONS

Multiple lacerations

Drain tube

Primary closure

B

Template

Xeroform bolster

FULL-THICKNESS GRAFT

C

ROTATION FLAP

TRANSPOSITION FLAPS

D

Rhomboid flap

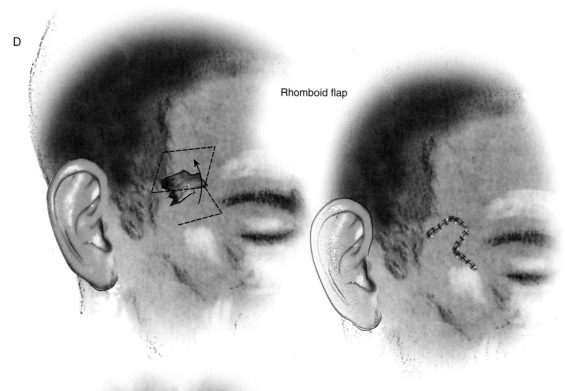

Bilobed flap

E

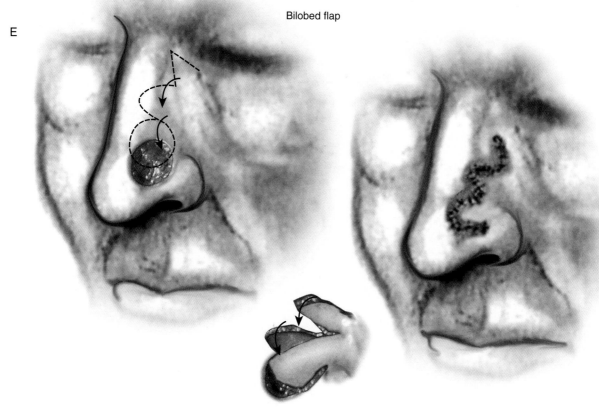

AURICULAR INJURY

Wedge excision and closure

F

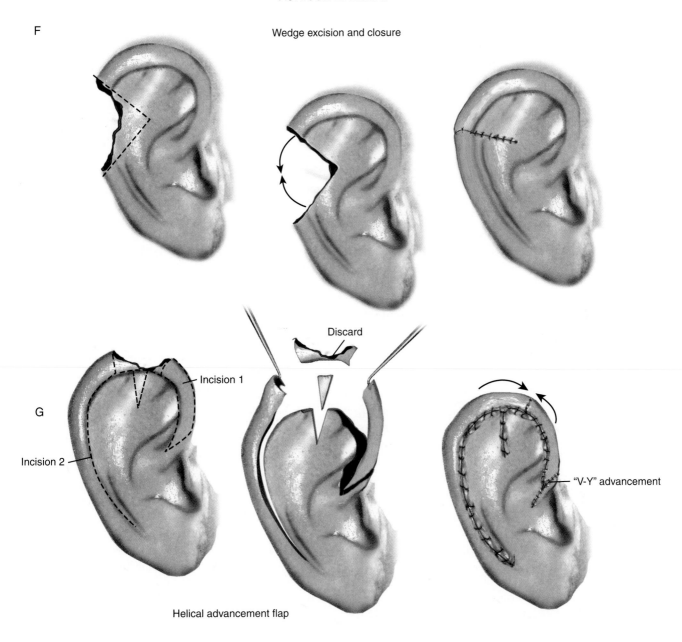

Discard

Incision 1

G

Incision 2

"V-Y" advancement

Helical advancement flap

H For anterior defects of the conchal bowl skin a post-auricular or pre-auricular flap can be used. Based on the postauricular vessels, a template of the defect is marked out, the flap is elevated and either advanced or rotated to cover the defect. The flap traverses through a defect in the cartilage or over the helical rim to reach the defect site. The bare area of the pedicle is either wrapped with Xeroform or cadaver dermis is sewn to it for protection. The pedicle is divided at 4 weeks.

Complete and near-total auriculalar avuslsions are best repaired with microvascular anastamosis and replantation. Recipient vessels are usually located on the posterior surface of the ear. Techniques for revascularization are primary anastamosis, vein grafting, and transposed superficial temporal vessels. Microvascular techniques are discussed further in Chapter 32.

I When microsurgical replantation is not feasible, the denuded cartilage framework is sutured to the remaining stump of the auricular cartilage. The free portion is then buried in a posterior-superior pocket with small round drains in place for 72 hours. The cartilage is kept in the pocket for 3 months while the overlying skin attaches to the framework. The pocket is ultimately released, and a full-thickness skin graft is secured to the defect.

Nasal Injury

Full-thickness nasal defect reconstruction should involve restoration of the inner lining, intermediate cartilaginous framework, and external skin covering. Although large full-thickness skin grafts are easily employed, these can be disfiguring and result in nasal obstruction from severe graft contraction.

J Composite grafts from the ear may be used for defects of the alar rim when <1.5 cm. The composite graft is harvested as a wedge from the root of the helix or the helix per se'. The donor site cartilage is closed with 4-0 vicryl to the cartilage and skin is closed with 5-0 or 6-0 prolene. The composite graft is sutured to the defect using 5-0 interrupted prolene sutures. The maximum alar rim defect that can be reliably reconstructed with a composite graft from the ear is 1.5 cm.

K The dorsal nasal or Reiger flap provides nasal skin from the dorsum and glabella to repair defects of the dorsum, supratip, and tip. The blood supply is based on the angular artery and the descending branches of the supratrochlear artery. The artery's location is the medial canthal area and nasal sidewall and provides the majority of the blood supply. The flap is designed in the loose skin of the nasal root area which permits the skin to cover most defects up to the tip. Marking solution is used to design the flap, incisions are along the nasal subunits as the incisions for this flap tend to be long. Every effort is made to camouflage the incisions along the nasal subunits and any natural skin creases. Flap contraction may cause retraction of the tip or nasal ala if the defect approaches the edge of the structures.

L For defects of the nasal ala, tip, supratip, soft triangle, or columella, a nasolabial flap provides a reasonable color match and coverage for any cartilage grafts. Although there is no direct pedicle, the blood supply is from the proximal and middle portion of the angular artery. A foil or Telfa template of the defect is made. The template is then positioned over the skin superior and lateral to the nasolabial groove. Silk suture is used to measure the necessary length of the pedicle. The flap is incised, elevated, and transposed into the defect. Vicryl and prolene sutures are used to secure the flap into the defect. The pedicle is replaced at 4 to 6 weeks in the nasalabial fold.

M,N Some defects are very large and occupy an entire subunit or multiple subunits. In this situation the paramedian or median forehead flap provides a large quantity of tissue. The flap is designed with its pedicle on the supratrochlear artery. A pedicle whose width is 1.7 cm and 2.7 cm from the midline is marked. Alternatively, the course of the artery can be marked with the aid of a Doppler. A template of the defect is made with foil from a suture pack or from Telfa. The template is situated on the forehead and silk suture is used to measure the required length of the pedicle. The flap is elevated in the subgaleal plane. Distally, it can be thinned to the level of the subcutaneous tissue because at this point, the artery runs in the subcutaneous portion of the flap. Cartilage defects may be replaced with grafts from septum, conchal bowl, or rib. Parietal or rib bone may be necessary to reconstruct resected nasal bones. Internal lining may be replaced with septal mucosal flaps or a split skin graft to the back of the paramedian flap. The flap is inset and closed in layers with 4-0 vicryl and 5-0 prolene. After wide undermining, the donor site is closed with 3-0 vicryl for the frontalis muscle and 4-0 prolene for the skin. Vertical mattress sutures of 2-0 prolene may be used to assist with the closure. Any small areas that fail to close primarily usually granulate in quite well. Transection of the pedicle, defatting, and contouring can be done at 4 weeks.

Lip Injury

Most defects up to one-third of the lip may be closed primarily after the edges are freshened. On occasion, the defect is converted to a "V" or "W" and then closed

ANIMAL BITES

AURICULAR INJURY

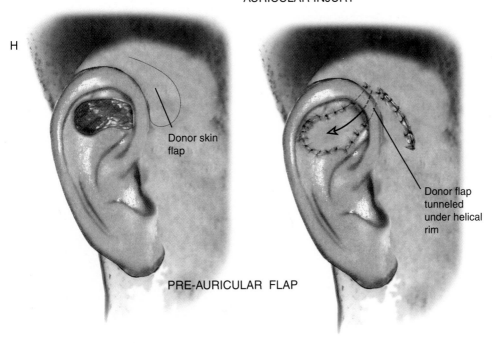

H

Donor skin flap

Donor flap tunneled under helical rim

PRE-AURICULAR FLAP

BURIED FLAP TECHNIQUE

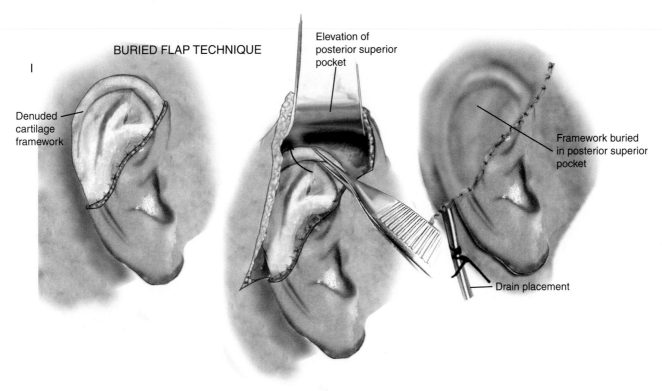

I

Denuded cartilage framework

Elevation of posterior superior pocket

Framework buried in posterior superior pocket

Drain placement

ANIMAL BITES

NASAL INJURY

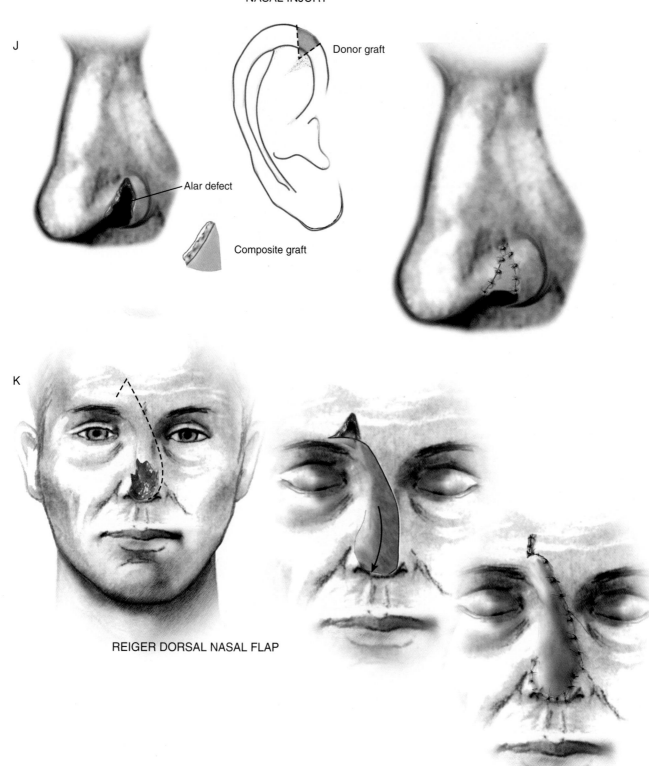

J

Alar defect

Donor graft

Composite graft

K

REIGER DORSAL NASAL FLAP

ANIMAL BITES

NASAL INJURY

NASOLABIAL FLAP

L

PARAMEDIAN FOREHEAD FLAP

M

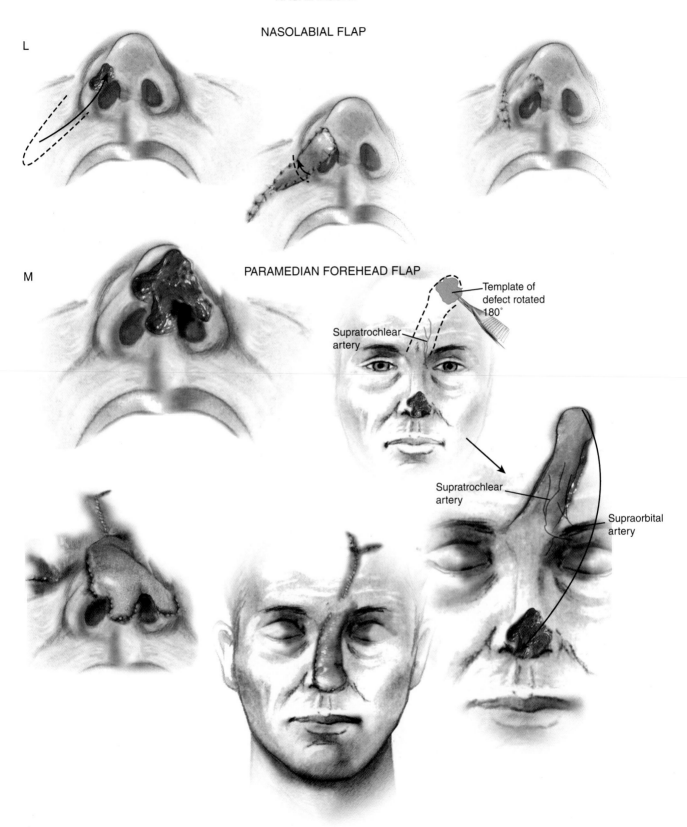

Template of defect rotated 180°

Supratrochlear artery

Supratrochlear artery

Supraorbital artery

THREE LAYER REPAIR

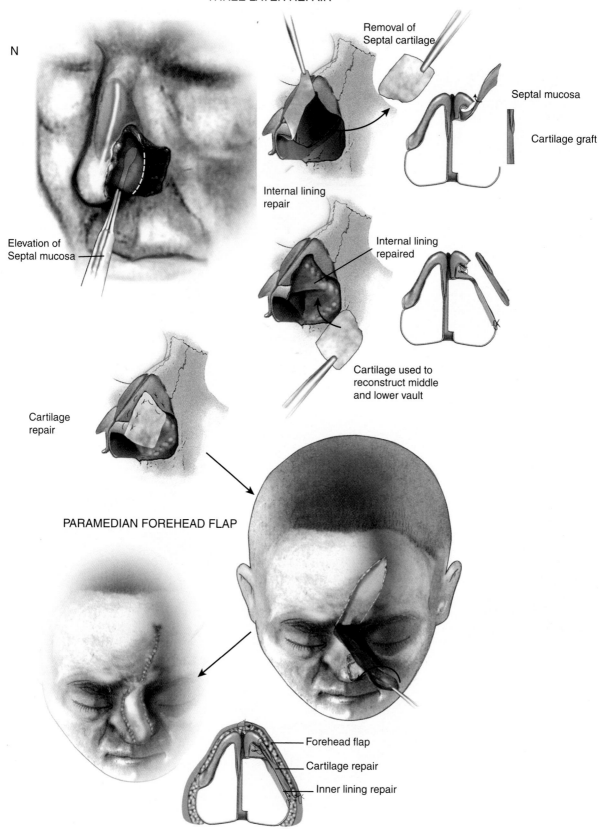

N

Removal of
Septal cartilage

Septal mucosa

Cartilage graft

Internal lining
repair

Elevation of
Septal mucosa

Internal lining
repaired

Cartilage used to
reconstruct middle
and lower vault

Cartilage
repair

PARAMEDIAN FOREHEAD FLAP

Forehead flap

Cartilage repair

Inner lining repair

primarily. These repairs are cosmetically appropriate when the vermilion is properly aligned.

O,P Defects between one-third and two-thirds of the lip are frequently closed with a cross-lip flap. The Abbe' flap is for defects of the middle of the lip while the Abbe-Estlander modification is used for the lateral lip and commissural area. These flaps are designed to rotate into the defect on a narrow but robust pedicle based on either the superior or inferior labial artery. The donor lip is from the lip opposite the defect. The flap is designed, incised, and elevated with the orbicularis muscle and the overlying mucosa. The flap is rotated and inset into the opposite lip defect and closed in layers. Mucosa is repaired with 5-0 Vicryl sutures, muscle with 4-0 vicryl sutures, dermis with 5-0 vicryl sutures, and skin with 6-0 prolene sutures. Disadvantages include having a portion of the lips sewn together for 2 to 3 weeks and a second stage for flap takedown. In the Abbe-Estlander flap, the pedicle of the flap becomes the region of the commissure of the mouth which may require further revision for functional and cosmetic purposes.

Cheek Injury

Designing a flap to reconstruct a missing portion of the cheek depends on the location of the wound, skin crease, and proximity to the free-edge of a fixed structure such as the lip or eyelid. A rhomboid flap with its relatively short, angular lines is a major workhorse for repairing small and medium sized cheek defects (see Figure *D*).

Q For larger defects, the cervicofacial flap is used. Incisions placed adjacent to the nasolabial fold, nasojugal fold, and infraorbial rim. If the defect is extremely large, an incision may extend all the way to the pre-auricular crease. The flap is elevated just deep to the superficial muscular aponeurotic system (SMAS), and it is rotated and advanced to fill the defect. Multiple, deep sutures are necessary to counteract gravity. The deep portion of the wound is closed with 4-0 vicryl for the SMAS and subcutaneous tissue. The dermis is closed with 5-0 vicryl and the skin with 5-0 or 6-0 prolene.

Scalp Injury

R Scalp rotational flaps can be used to close both small and medium defects of scalp. It is often necessary to use a rotation flap on the scalp because the tissues have little stretch and a large flap is required to close even a relatively small defect. An arc or curvilinear design is made off the defect. The diameter of the arc is approximately five times the size of the defect and may need to be extended when the flap is inset.

A small back-cut may be necessary to assist with the rotation and insetting. The wound is closed in layers with 3-0 vicryl for the galea, and 3-0 prolene for the skin and subcutaneous tissue.

S A massive rotation flap or even multiple flaps may fail to close a scalp defect. In this situation, the defect can be covered with a temporary split skin thickness graft or xeroform gauze and tissue expanders employed. The strategy is to stretch the scalp sufficiently so it can eventually be closed with a flap. Tunnels are created away from the defect in the subgaleal plane and a pocket is created adjacent to the defect. To prevent exposure of the expander, it is prudent to leave 2 cm of undisturbed tissue adjacent to the defect. Expanders three or five times the size of the defect are usually employed with the injection ports far from the defect. The pockets are made just large enough to accommodate the expander. The port can be external or hidden beneath the surface of the skin. Normal saline is injected to just eliminate the deadspace after insertion. The wound is allowed to settle for 2 weeks and expansion is begun. Every week the expander is inflated with normal saline. The expander is filled until the scalp slightly blanches. The steps are repeated until the expander is completely filled, followed by removal of the expander and flap closure using the newly expanded tissue.

For massive scalp avulsions, an attempt should be made to replant it. The blood vessels are isolated and if necessary, vein grafts harvested to ensure adequate length. Microvascular anastomosis is carried out under the microscope with 10-0 micro sutures.

COMPLICATIONS

1. The most common complication of a bite wound is infection. Most infections are a localized cellulitis but may progress to an abscess or lymphadenitis. Although uncommon, it is certainly possible to be infected with the tetanus or rabies virus. Human bites carry a risk of infection from blood-borne viruses, such as hepatitis B, hepatitis C, or HIV.

2. Auricular hematomas occur when a shearing injury separates the auricular cartilage from the perichondrium. If neglected, blood accumulates in the potential space ultimately causing fibrosis of the cartilage and cauliflower ear deformity. Auricular hematomas should be drained and treated with a compression dressing.

3. Scar contractures can restrict function around the eyes and lips by distorting the free edge of these structures. Correction may entail excision or release with z-plasty or local flaps (see Chapter 13). Full-thickness skin grafts may be necessary in some

ANIMAL BITES

Lip Injury

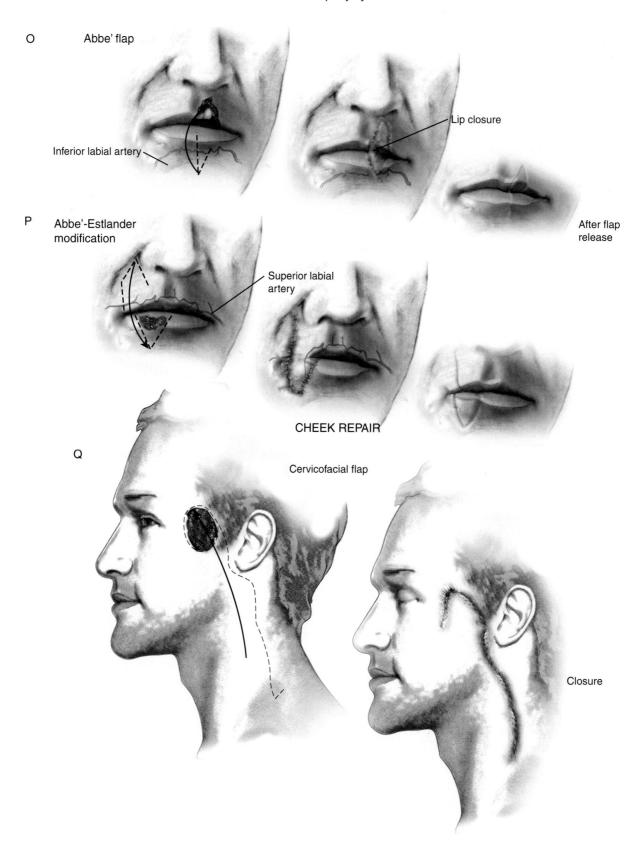

O   Abbe' flap

Inferior labial artery

Lip closure

After flap release

P   Abbe'-Estlander modification

Superior labial artery

CHEEK REPAIR

Q

Cervicofacial flap

Closure

SCALP INJURY

R   Scalp flap

Rotational flap

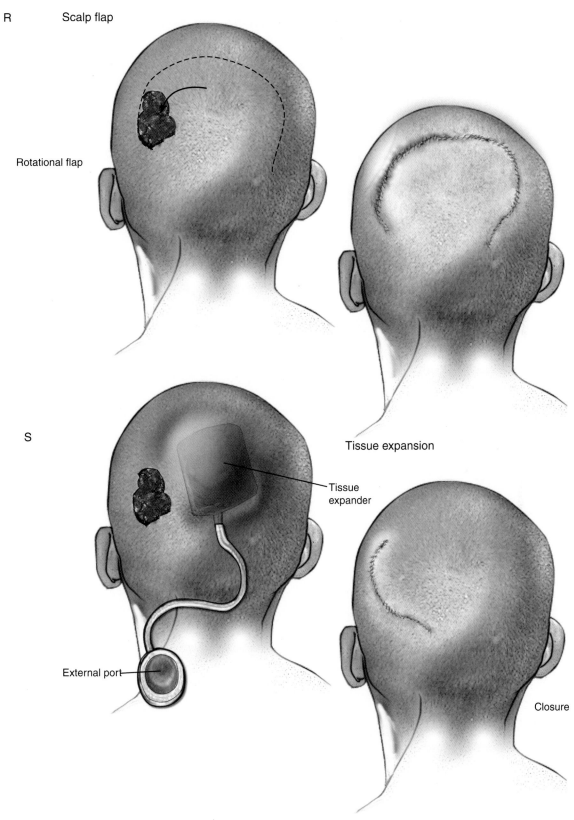

S

Tissue expansion

Tissue
expander

External port

Closure

instances. Keloids and hypertrophic scars can be source of great distress for the patient and should be recognized early. Triamcinilone injection and silicone gel can be used early. If this is ineffective, excision, meticulous closure, and steroid injection can be done.

4. Flap necrosis may occur secondary to hematoma formation. A large or persistent fluid collection may require a return to the operating room for wound exploration and control of bleeding. Poor flap design, excessive wound tension, and insufficient blood supply are common mistakes leading to flap loss.

5. Complications of microsurgical replantation may also occur. Venous insufficiency is the leading cause of free tissue loss. Inadequate venous drainage leads to flap congestion, poor perfusion, and necrosis. Warning signs are flap congestion and blue discoloration. Necrosis does not occur immediately and there may be development of natural collateral drainage in the ensuing days. Leech therapy has been advocated as an adjunct in salvage of flaps suffering from venous congestion.

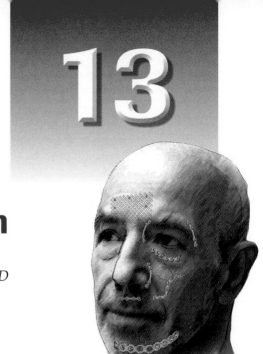

Scar Revision

In Consultation With Michael Carron, MD

INDICATIONS

Wounds that violate the papillary dermis heal with scar. The degree of scar formation will depend upon the efficacy of healing and the condition of the wound with regard to devitalized or crushed tissue, bacterial infection, or foreign debris. Wounds closed under tension are notorious for obtrusive scars. Conversely, favorable scars form under conditions associated with minimal inflammation and optimal conditions of healing.

A favorable scar is one that is barely noticeable and does not affect dynamic structures such as the eyelid or lip. Such a scar is flat and narrow and level with the skin. Favorable scars also fall into natural crease lines; they are short or broken lines that do not involve adjacent facial aesthetic units. Although scars are permanent, they may be optimized with regard to width, direction, elevation, and shape. Unless a scar is healing with an obvious deformity or causing a functional impairment, it is desirable to wait for the scar to mature, which will be approximately 6 months in adults and later in children. Occasionally, the maturation of the scar will lead to thinning and a color change, which will preclude a revision. Scars that are too wide, too long, or running across flat surfaces are good candidates for revision. Moreover, scars that are depressed, elevated, or against natural skin creases should equally be considered for revision. Distortion of the commissures at the eyelids and lips may also require correction. Scars may cause psychological and social reactions demanding close follow-up in the office, psychological support and education about healing.

PROCEDURE

A Delicate handling of soft tissues improves the chance for a favorable outcome. Quality instruments make the operation much easier. A meticulous closure with minimal tissue damage is possible and necessary for a good result. Often trauma to the skin edges can be avoided by using single- or double-pronged skin hooks or gently grasping the tissues with Brown-Adson forceps. An 11 blade is useful for making accurate incisions and creating geometric designs. Wound closure should be without tension and is accomplished by undermining the subdermal and subcutaneous tissues with a layered closure. The subcutaneous tissues should be advanced with buried interrupted absorbable suture. Closure of the dermis with 5-0 vicryl, chromic or mersilene sutures placed away from the skin edge strengthens the repair and relieves tension. Closure of all layers should be accurate so that the skin edges can be coapted with 5-0 or 6-0 prolene (or nylon) depending on skin thickness and regional animation.

Eversion of the skin edges will reduce tension and favor a level scar once the contractile forces of healing have subsided. Postoperative care is important to prevent infection and inflammation. Antibiotic ointment should be applied for 14 days. Hydrogen peroxide may be used to keep the surface of the wound free of crusts. If there is a possibility of fluid accumulation, drains and/or pressure dressings should be applied.

Fusiform Excision

B An unsightly scar may fall in a natural skin crease, but it will remain obvious if it is too wide, too depressed, elevated, or has uneven edges. A simple elliptical excision of the scar with angles of approximately 30° should provide improvement, especially if the scar remains concealed in a natural skin crease. This is the simplest method of scar revision. Leaving the deep margin of the scar intact minimizes depression of the wound. Even though a scar may lie in a natural crease, lengths >2cm may be noticeable. In this instance, a zigzag plasty (geometric broken line) will break the pattern and aid in the camouflage of the revision (see later).

Scar Repositioning

C As noted scars that fall into natural skin creases or along borders of facial subunits like the alar-facial crease or preauricular crease are less obvious. To achieve this result, scars near these areas are excised elliptically, but with the revision, removal of tissue is designed so that the new line is located into the desired area. Closure and postoperative care are as noted earlier.

Serial Excision

D Large wide scars present a different problem. These types of scars, when excised, will often generate excessive wound tension and again heal with a wide scar. Such scars are best treated by serial excision. For this procedure, an ellipse is designed with marking solution to remove scar adjacent to normal tissue. A portion of the scar is excised, and the remaining scar and adjacent skin are undermined and approximated in layers. Once the excision and repair are complete, and the wound has matured, the process is repeated in a similar fashion. Scars should be sequentially replaced with normal elastic skin. Alternatively, the process can be hastened by the use of tissue expanders in the adjacent tissues. Balloon expanders will increase the amount of skin over the expander and when the scar is excised this lose skin can be advanced to cover the defect.

Zigzag plasty

E Scars running against natural skin creases, curvilinear scars, or long and straight scars across flat surfaces are easily noticeable. Dispersing the contractile forces into multiple vectors and breaking up a long straight line into multiple small lines makes the scar more difficult to perceive. This is the principle of the zigzag plasty, which creates a series of irregularly arranged geometric forms that are interposed advancement flaps fitting lock and key. These small geometric flaps are designed to interdigiate into the tissues to the side of the scar. Common shapes are rectangles, squares, and triangles, and they are best designed with widths of 3 to 5 mm and side lines placed along relaxed skin tension lines. The scar is then excised with the incorporated geometric elements, the wound edges are undermined and the wound closed as noted earlier.

Z-plasty

F–H The Z-plasty is a powerful tool that uses two adjacent triangular transposition flaps to increase the length of a tightly contracted scar, change the direction of the scar line, change the location of tissues and efface webs. The Z-plasty has three limbs and two angles. The degree of tissue lengthening depends on the designed angles. The most common z-plasty has angles of 60° and when designed as such, the central member will rotate 90°; angles <60° are useful when you need thin flaps such as in eyelids, noting that the rotation of the central member will be <90°. Angles >60° are used in expanding the space around the vertical limb, but the rotation of the transposition flaps will often cause significant dog ears. The Z-plasty is also indicated in transposing tissues that are in poor anatomical alignment such as a drooping lid or disrupted mucosal border or hairline. Multiple Z-plasty is useful in increasing the length of a long contracted scar.

To create a z-plasty, the limbs and angles are marked and the skin is prepared as usual with an antiseptic wash and a local anesthetic. The wound edges are slightly beveled outward to aid in the final wound eversion. Using fine sharp scissors, the two transposition flaps are undermined in a subcutaneous plane. The flaps are transposed and closed in layers and managed as described earlier.

PITFALLS

1. Mark out areas of incisions before applying the local anesthetic. The anesthetic can blanch the scar and distort the anatomy making it difficult to define the area of excision.

2. Grasping skin edges forcefully with forceps may cause a crush injury with skin necrosis, inflammation, and scarring. Skin hooks or Brown-Adson forceps are desirable. If crush injury occurs, the resulting scar may need dermabrasion or secondary revision.

3. Poor hemostasis can result in the formation of hematoma causing pressure necrosis and/or infection of the skin. Similarly, failure to obliterate dead space may result in fluid accumulation, inflammation, and

SCAR REVISION

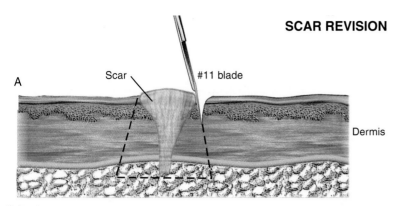

A

Scar

#11 blade

Dermis

Subcutaneous
tissue

Beveled incision

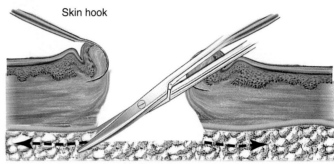

Skin hook

Undermining

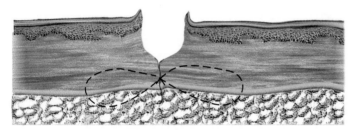

Intradermal suture

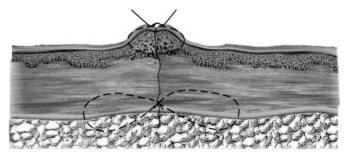

Wound closure

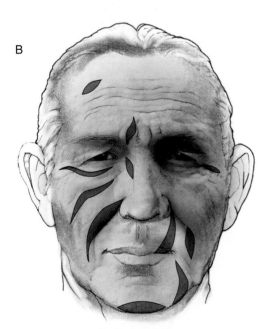

B

Fusiform excisions

SCAR REVISION

SCAR REPOSITIONING

C

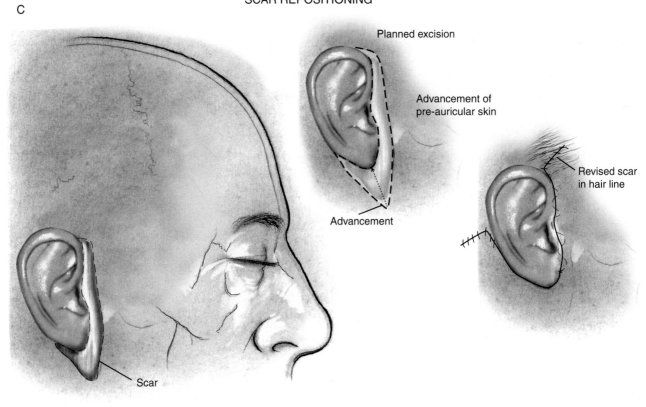

Planned excision

Advancement of pre-auricular skin

Advancement

Scar

Revised scar in hair line

SERIAL EXCISION

D

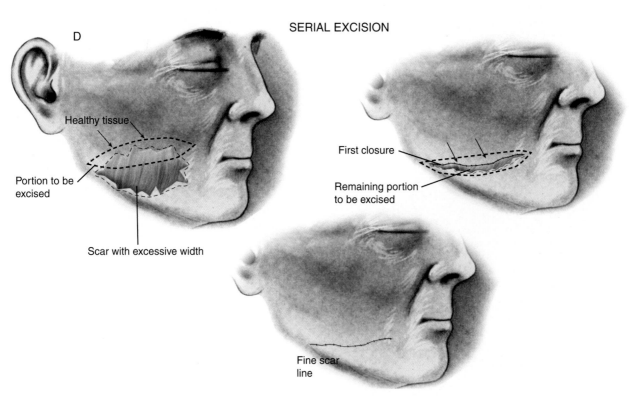

Healthy tissue

Portion to be excised

Scar with excessive width

First closure

Remaining portion to be excised

Fine scar line

Final scar after two excisions

SCAR REVISION

ZIG ZAG PLASTY

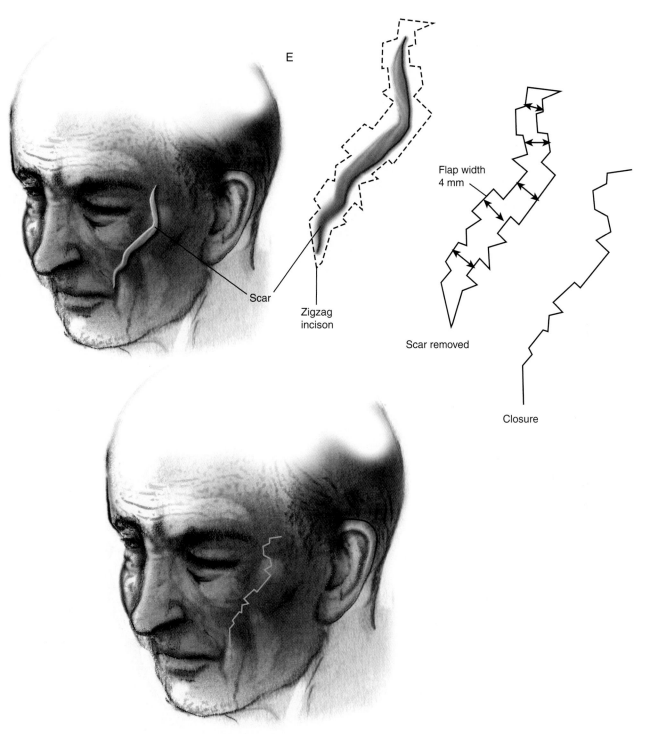

E

Scar

Zigzag incison

Flap width 4 mm

Scar removed

Closure

Scar irregularity breaks up line

SCAR REVISION

Z - PLASTY

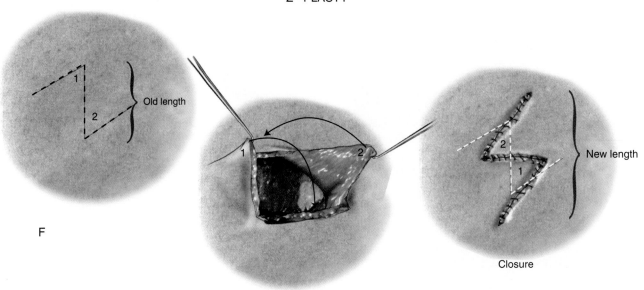

F

Old length

New length

Closure

Z - Plasty used to reposition
malpositioned oral commisure

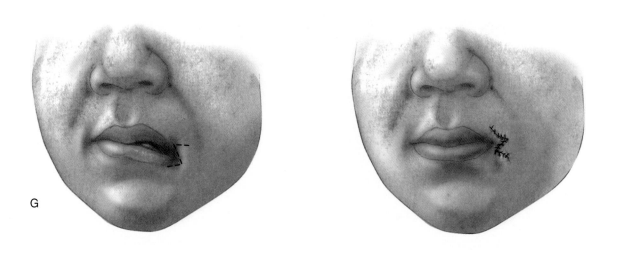

G

SCAR REVISION

MULTIPLE Z - PLASTY

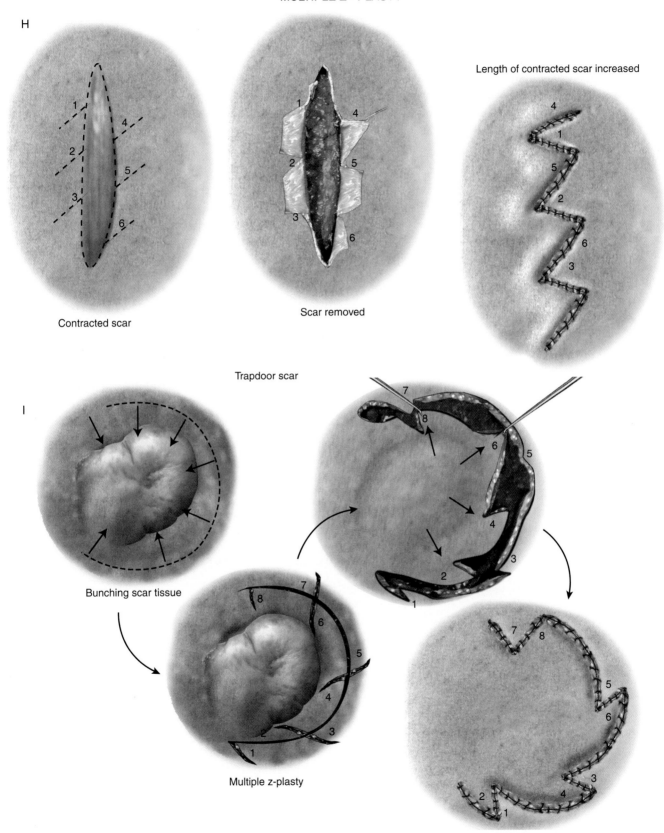

H

Contracted scar

Scar removed

Length of contracted scar increased

I

Trapdoor scar

Bunching scar tissue

Multiple z-plasty

scarring. Rubber band drains and/or compression dressings as noted earlier will help avoid these problems.

4. Designing ellipses and flaps with angles of <30° will likely lead to tip necrosis, inflammation, and scarring. Therefore, flaps should be at least 3 to 4 mm in width and of sufficient thickness to maintain blood supply to the margin.

5. Excessive angulation should be avoided. Too much angulation or rotation can twist the pedicle affecting blood supply and healing potential.

6. If the patient requires multiple procedures in a defined region, it is prudent to stage the revisions. Revising one scar may affect the revision of adjacent scars and should be avoided.

7. It is important to reduce wound tension as this is one of the major causes of a wide scar. Tension also incites inflammation and healing by secondary intention with an increase in scarring. Adequate undermining, layered closure of wounds, and eversion of skin edges will reduce tension and affect a more desirable scar.

8. Depressed or puckered scars may occur if wound edges are secured at different levels. To avoid this problem, skin must be closed in layers and the edges everted so that as the wound settles there is a secure underlying foundation of tissue and the edges are even.

COMPLICATIONS

1. Depressed scars are unsightly and need to be revised. Some of these scars can be raised by injection of filling materials but, usually the scar needs to be reexcised leaving the deep portion of the scar as the skin is advanced over the defect or by advancing the subcutaneous tissues before skin closure. Advancing subcutaneous tissues, one layer over the other—that is, (pants over vest) will increase the thickness of the deficient area. If after the scar revision, there is still some unevenness in the area, dermabrasion can be used to level the surface.

2. Widened scars are the result of tension, poor blood supply, inadequate eversion, insufficient undermining, lack of deep closure, and other factors such as diabetes, smoking, and poor nutritional status. Gentle handling of tissues and appreciation of protocols described to reduce tension with patient optimization should help.

3. Trapdoor scars occur in wounds that are oblique or semicircular because of centripetal force distribution with resultant bunching of the tissues. The trapdoor scar is corrected with excision of the scar, layered closure, generous undermining of adjacent tissues and geometric design or multiple Z-plasties. Occasionally debulking the elevated portion and lifting the depressed portion by sliding subcutaneous tissue under it are useful techniques (see Figure *1*).

4. Excessive scarring is sometimes observed in areas around the ear, neck upper chest, and shoulders. If these scars extend out of their boundaries they are then referred to as keloids. In these patients the scar can be managed often by injection of 20 to 40 milligrams of triamcinolone. Pressure treatment may be effective. If the scars do not respond to conservative management, it is best to reexcise the scar, close the wound without tension, and serially inject steroids into the healing area.

5. Scars that penetrate deep into the muscle or mucosa require special consideration. Such injuries are seen in children who bite on an electrical cord and sustain an electrical burn. These types of scars must be treated with excision of the skin, mucosa, and underlying muscle. Reconstruction will require advancement or rotation of skin and/or mucosa into the defect.

6. Suture marks occur if the suture material used in the skin closure causes inflammation such as silk or vicryl. Also if the suture is left in place too long or is too thick, marks will be made. Sutures used in the skin should be no more than a size 5-0 or 6-0 and as inert as possible. Suture marks may be gently dermabraded for concealment.

CHAPTER 14

Early Facial Nerve Injury
Neurorrhaphy for Facial Nerve Injury
Alternative Technique of Interposition Nerve Graft
Alternative Technique of Gold Weight and Lateral Canthoplasty
Protection of the Eye

INDICATIONS

Immediate facial paralysis after trauma suggests a partial or complete transection of the facial nerve. Paralysis associated with a wound lateral to the nasolabial fold carries a poor patient prognosis; more medially oriented wounds, on the other hand, are associated with transient weakness and usually good return of function.

The history, physical findings, and laboratory tests are important. An immediate loss of function usually means an interruption of the nerve, whereas a delayed onset often indicates a neurapraxia and a reversible phenomenon. For those patients in whom the onset and duration of paralysis are not clear, facial nerve stimulation and electromyographic studies should be performed. If the threshold for stimulation of the affected side exceeds that of the normal side by 3.5 mA or, on electromyography, action potentials are replaced by fibrillation potentials, then there

is degeneration and the possibility of a transection. A continuation of action potentials usually denotes a good patient prognosis and probable return of function. Electroneurography may also provide information on the degree of injury.

When findings indicate a disruption of the nerve, exploration and repair should be considered. In general, the earlier the exploration, the better the chance to find the ends of the nerves and effect an anastomosis. Loss of neural tissue requires nerve grafts, and for most patients, the great auricular nerve is the ideal donor. For injuries occurring within the temporal bone, the reader is referred to Chapter 93.

PROCEDURE

Surgery is usually performed under general anesthesia, with the head of the patient facing toward the anesthesist. Paralyzing agents are avoided, especially if intraoperative testing is anticipated. A preliminary injection of 1% lidocaine containing 1:100,000 epinephrine to the incision and operative site will assist in hemostasis.

A Our preference is to explore the facial nerve by way of a superficial parotidectomy. An incision is first marked in a preauricular crease. It is then extended below the earlobe in the form of a lazy S to join a line in the neck crease, about 3 cm below the angle of the mandible. The skin is incised, and the superficial layer of fascia (superficial musculoaponeurotic layer) is exposed. The flaps are developed in a subcutaneous plane anteriorly to the nasolabial fold, superiorly to the posterior half of the zygoma, and inferiorly to the level of the hyoid bone.

B The preauricular incision is then deepened to separate the parotid from the tragus. The triangular portion of the tragal cartilage will "point" toward the facial nerve. A plane is developed between the mastoid tip and the parotid gland and deepened to the level of the digastric muscle. Superiorly the superficial temporal artery and vein are identified, and if they are in the way, they are either ligated or retracted from the field.

Several important landmarks should be noted. The nerve lies directly beneath the tympanomastoid suture at a level about 1.5 to 2 cm below the mastoid prominence. The digastric muscle, which inserts on the deep aspect of the mastoid, is directly inferior and deep to the nerve. Several fibrous attachments are noted just lateral to the facial nerve as it exits the stylomastoid foramen.

C Once the facial nerve is identified, the nerve trunk is followed anteriorly into the parotid gland. Using a blunt and sharp dissection, the superficial lobe is separated from the deep lobe of the gland (i.e., a parotidectomy is performed). The major divisions of the nerve (superior and inferior) are traced into the area of injury. A useful technique is to spread the soft tissues along the nerve with a fine clamp and incise those fibers that lie posterior to the main nerve pedicle.

As the surgeon approaches the periphery of the gland, several landmarks should be appreciated. The mandibular branch of the facial nerve lies just above or below the posterior facial vein. The buccal branch of the facial nerve parallels the parotid duct. The frontal branch crosses the zygoma at a point one-half the distance from the root to the orbital rim.

D–F Once the superficial lobe of the parotid gland is removed and the area of damage is isolated, both proximal and distal branches of the nerve should be identified and freshened by cutting the ends with a No. 11 knife blade over a wooden tongue blade. Using microscopic control, the nerve is then anastomosed with 7-0 nylon sutures. We prefer the "halving" technique, so that once the suture is placed through the perineurium, it is tagged with a microvascular clamp, and the nerve is rotated 180°.

Another suture is then placed, followed by additional sutures between the attachments. The sutures will then be located clockwise at 12, 3, 6, and 9 o'clock, respectively. The larger nerve trunks require three to four sutures, whereas the smaller branches can be repaired with two sutures. The repairs should be without any tension.

The wound is closed with three Penrose drains: one anterior to the tragus, a second beneath the earlobe, and a third along the cervical incision. The subcutaneous tissues are closed with 3-0 chromic sutures and the skin with interrupted 5-0 nylon sutures. A light pressure dressing of stretch gauze and fluffs is then placed over the ear in a figure-of-eight design that includes both the eye and forehead and the neck and jaw region. The eye is protected with eye ointment and an eye patch. Prophylactic antibiotics are used for 5 to 7 days. The drains are removed when drainage has ceased, and the sutures are usually removed at 7 days.

PITFALLS

1. Early exploration and repair of a neural discontinuity is desirable. Late repairs are made more difficult by the appearance of inflammatory tissues, which tend to bleed and obscure details of the reconstruction.

2. The surgeon should be aware of the facial nerve anatomy and the landmarks available to find the nerve roots and branches. Paralytic agents should be avoided, as there will be opportunity during the operative procedure to also stimulate the peripheral branches and identify their locations.

3. Nerve repair should be accomplished without tension. We prefer an epineural anastomosis using 7-0 nylon sutures. The edge of the epineurium should be held with jeweler forceps, and the needle should just penetrate the epineurium (about 2 mm from the edge). Injury to the fascicles should be avoided. The "halving" technique should be used, placing enough sutures to approximate the ends without tension.

4. Return of function should not be expected for at least 4 to 6 months, as the neural tissues grow about 1 mm per day in length. Some weakness and synkinesis should be expected.

COMPLICATIONS

1. Hematomas, seromas, and salivary gland fistulae are possible complications of the surgery. For these reasons, the entire superficial lobe of the parotid should be removed, the wound should be adequately drained, and the drains should not be removed until all drainage has ceased. A light compression dressing will help prevent accumulation of blood or serum beneath the flaps.

2. Gustatory sweating (Frey's syndrome) is a common sequela. It is believed that this condition

NEURORRHAPHY FOR FACIAL NERVE INJURY

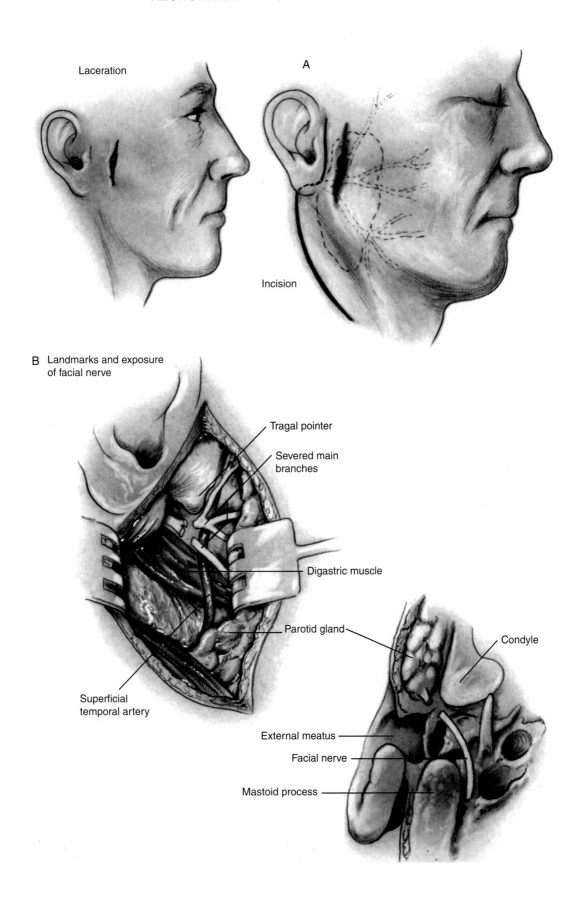

Laceration

A

Incision

B Landmarks and exposure
of facial nerve

Tragal pointer

Severed main
branches

Digastric muscle

Parotid gland

Condyle

Superficial
temporal artery

External meatus

Facial nerve

Mastoid process

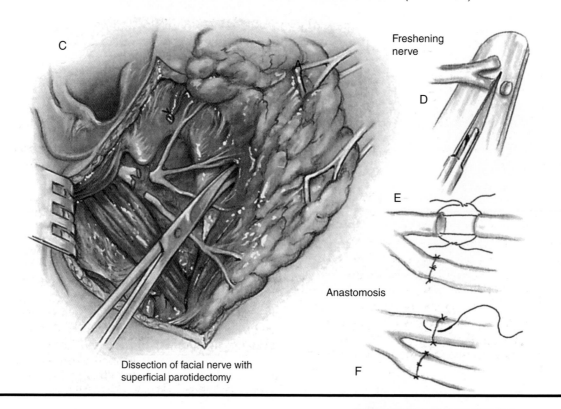

Freshening nerve

Anastomosis

Dissection of facial nerve with
superficial parotidectomy

ATERNATIVE TECHNIQUE OF INTERPOSITIONAL NERVE GRAFT

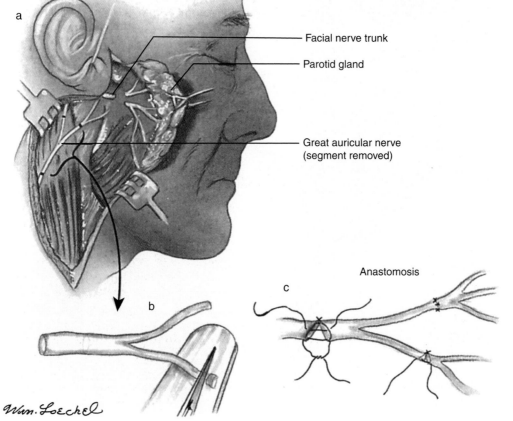

Facial nerve trunk

Parotid gland

Great auricular nerve
(segment removed)

Anastomosis

Wm. Loechel

develops as the parasympathetic fibers reinnervate the overlying skin. If the sweating becomes incapacitating (which is rare), the surgeon can place a piece fascia between the skin and overlying tissues. Alternatively, the parasympathetic supply delivered by the chorda tympani and Jacobson's nerve can be lysed or temporarily denervated with botulinum injections.

3. A depression of skin over the parotid gland should be expected. This can be avoided by rotating a sternocleidomastoid/platysma flap into the defect prior to closure. A later correction is also possible, but because the nerve is very close to the skin, there is a risk of injury to the nerve.

4. Continued paresis and/or paralysis are also a possibility. The surgeon should consider a temporary tarsorrhaphy or gold weight implant (see later) to protect the eye. If nerve function does not return, reexploration and repair or, alternatively, interposition and/or hypoglossal grafts should be considered. Once atrophy has occurred, muscle flaps and transposition procedures should be used (see Chapter 15).

ALTERNATIVE TECHNIQUE OF INTERPOSITIONAL NERVE GRAFT

If the nerve injury is characterized as penetrating and avulsive and the destruction between the neural segments exceeds 5 mm, the surgeon should consider a great auricular nerve graft interposition. The great auricular nerve is close by and in the same surgical field, and its thickness resembles that of the facial nerve. The disadvantages of using the great auricular nerve are that (1) it is a sensory nerve and (2) the fascicles will not match.

a For the procedure, the surgeon should isolate the facial nerve and then develop subcutaneous flaps inferiorly to expose the great auricular nerve. Usually the great auricular nerve penetrates the platysma and fascia just lateral to the upper portion of the sternocleidomastoid muscle. More inferiorly, it passes from the deeper tissues behind the sternocleidomastoid muscle about 6 cm caudal to the mastoid tip. The main branch spreads out into smaller branches in the preauricular and infraauricular space. A secondary branch usually transverses the sternocleidomastoid muscle and continues across the neck. At least 8 to 10 cm of nerve should be harvested. This means that the nerve must be carefully dissected from the superficial layers of tissue and from those tissues that are deep to the sternocleidomastoid muscle. After the nerve is removed, the edges should be sharpened with a No. 11 knife blade; the nerve should be kept in physiologic solution or left to lie in the tissues until it is used for grafting.

b,c The neurorrhaphy technique resembles that used for the primary anastomosis. Tension should be avoided. The use of microscopic control, 7-0 nonreactive sutures, and "halving" techniques is desirable. Drains and soft compression dressings are applied, and the wounds are closed in layers. Postoperative care is essentially the same as that used for the direct anastomosis technique.

ALTERNATIVE TECHNIQUE OF GOLD WEIGHT AND LATERAL CANTHOPLASTY PROTECTION OF THE EYE

When the facial nerve is injured, closure of the eye may be compromised, and in older patients, this can cause desiccation and erosion of the cornea. To protect the eye and assure closure, a gold weight implant to the upper eyelid is very effective.

a' For this procedure, the face is prepared and draped as a sterile field. The supratarsal fold is identified, and if not easily seen, a mark is made for a 2 cm incision, central to the position of the pupil and 7 mm from the lower edge of the eyelid. The area is infiltrated with 1% lidocaine containing 1:100,000 epinephrine.

b' After adequate time for vasoconstriction to occur, an incision is made through the skin and the orbicularis oculi muscle to the levator fascia. Following a plane above the levator, a flap is elevated inferiorly to expose the tarsal plate. The dissection should continue to the inferior border of the plate taking care not to perforate the overlying tissues.

c',d' A gold weight of approximately one gram is held with a forceps while a 5-0 clear vicryl suture is passed through one of the lower holes. The implant is then positioned under the flap and over the tarsal plate; the suture is subsequently passed through perichondrium and cartilage of the lower part of the tarsal plate. Another suture is passed through the tarsal plate and other lower hole, and both sutures are tied to secure the lower part of the implant to the lower border of the tarsal plate. The upper border of the implant is subsequently secured to the upper border of the tarsal plate. The skin and orbicularis are closed with fine nylon sutures. Ophthalmic ointment is applied.

e' For the lateral canthoplasty, a simple wedge resection and upward lateral displacement of the canthal ligament is preferred. After injection with a local anesthetic, the lateral canthus is severed and a wedge is inferiorly directed to remove a portion of skin overlying the lateral canthal ligament. The periosteum over the lateral orbital rim is elevated superiorly. The lateral canthal ligament is then mobilized and pulled up laterally and superiorly to be secured to the periosteum with a 4-0 merseline suture. The orbicularis is closed with a 4-0 chromic suture and the skin with 6-0 nylon sutures, carefully approximating the free edge of the eyelid.

ALTERNATIVE TECHNIQUE OF GOLD WEIGHT IMPLANT

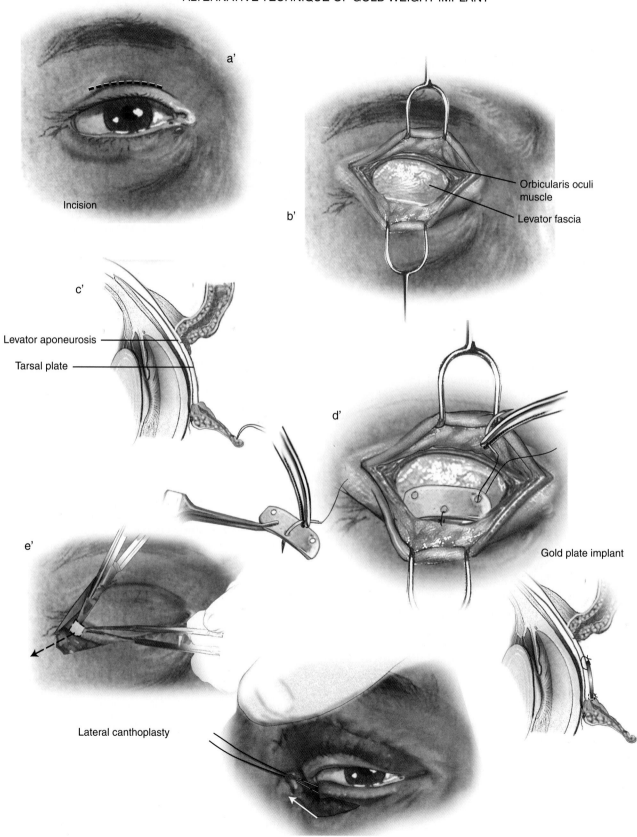

a'

Incision

b'

Orbicularis oculi muscle

Levator fascia

c'

Levator aponeurosis

Tarsal plate

d'

Gold plate implant

e'

Lateral canthoplasty

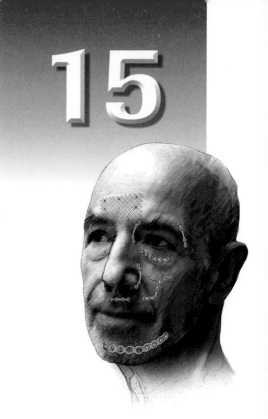

Late Facial Nerve Injury
Reanimation of the Paralyzed Face With a Temporalis Muscle Galea Flap

INDICATIONS

Interruption of the facial nerve often leads to paralysis of the face and, depending on the degree and location of muscle weakness, a dysfunction of the eye, mouth, and nares. When the nerve is completely severed, the best method of repair is an early exploration, freshening of the ends of the nerve, and a direct anastomosis. If there is a neural deficit of several centimeters, great auricular nerve grafts are indicated (see Chapter 14). Occasionally, crossover nerve techniques using the hypoglossal or branches of the opposite facial nerve are indicated, but these methods are rarely used in injuries following trauma.

Long-standing facial paralysis, however, is different. With time, there is an atrophy of muscle and neural tissues. In such situations, the surgeon must test for residual nerve function, and if it is insufficient for reanimation, a muscle transposition technique must be considered. The temporalis muscle galea flap provides an opportunity to transfer functional muscular units to different areas of the face. The method is particularly useful when there are accompanying craniofacial defects and/or destruction of the peripheral branches of the nerve.

PROCEDURE

In preparation for surgery, the patient's scalp is shaved, and the skin is treated with a standard antiseptic solution. The face and one-half of the scalp are then draped as a sterile field.

A Skin incisions are first outlined with a marking solution and then infiltrated with 1% lidocaine containing 1:100,000 epinephrine to help in hemostasis. A line is then drawn along the preauricular crease and extended upward several millimeters behind the temporal hairline. A horizontal limb is fashioned about 2.5 cm above the pinna and, starting from the anterior line, drawn toward the occiput. Additionally, the surgeon can draw another horizontal line beneath the earlobe, just beyond the cervical hairline, and connect it to the upper horizontal limb with a vertical line, but for many cases, the superior and anterior lines will be sufficient.

B,C The preauricular incision is used to elevate the skin in a subcutaneous plane as in a classic rhytidoplasty procedure. The skin of the face is retracted to expose the fibers of the orbicularis oris, depressor groups, zygomaticus, levator labii superiorus, and orbicularis oculi. The plane of dissection around the eye is facilitated by additional upper and lower eyelid incisions through crease lines. This exposure will help at a later time with the attachment of the muscle flaps to the orbicularis oculi musculature.

The temporalis muscle galea flap is exposed by elevation of superficial scalp flaps at a level just beneath the hair follicles and external to the superficial temporal artery. This artery should be identified and maintained within the deeper tissues, as it will nourish primarily the galea flap. The extent of the superior and posterior part of the flap is determined by the length of the temporalis muscle and galea needed for reconstruction.

Once the design of the muscle galea flap is complete, a curvilinear incision is made along the galea from the frontal to the occipital region. Working in a plane between the galea and pericranium, the galea is elevated to the level of the temporalis fossa, at which point the pericranium is incised, and the pericranium and temporalis muscle are elevated from the fossa. Nerve and vascular injuries are avoided by a dissection close to the skull.

D,E Rotation of the flaps should provide complete coverage of the hemiface. Additional length can be achieved by incisions strategically placed along the zygomaticofrontal process and along the pretragal root of the zygoma. The galea can then be split into three to five compartments, the lower two of which can be placed below and above the lips, the middle one at the midface, and the upper two below and above the eyelids. Excess galea should not be excised, but rather folded onto itself and sutured to the base of each compartment with 3-0 chromic or vicryl sutures.

With the flap in appropriate position, each extension is sutured with 3-0 vicryl to the appropriate facial muscles. Ideally the lower compartments are secured to the lateral and middle thirds of the orbicularis oris, the middle to the levator labii superioris muscle, and the upper to the inner aspect of the orbicularis oculi of the upper and lower eyelids. The tension of each flap segment should be adjusted to obtain a slight smile and almost complete closure of the palpebral fissure.

All wounds are treated with multiple small Penrose drains. Skin flaps are sutured into position with a layered closure. Prophylactic antibiotics are desirable. A light decompression bandage is applied for 24 to 48 hours.

PITFALLS

1. The temporalis muscle galea flap is best used when there is no longer any opportunity for neural repair (i.e., the muscle and/or nerve have undergone atrophy or there are large defects of the face in which it is not possible to repair nerve segments). Neurorrhaphy, if indicated, is described in Chapter 14.

2. The muscle galea technique is time consuming and requires a meticulous dissection to avoid injury to the muscle, arterial supply, and overlying hair-bearing tissues. The surgeon should study the anatomy of the superficial temporal artery and be prepared to follow the artery to the periphery. Preoperative Doppler studies are helpful in determining the location of the vessels as well as their integrity regarding vascular flow.

3. Flaps should be designed to provide appropriate length and compartmentalization. Each segment can potentially operate as an independent neuromuscular unit, and if independent eye and lip movements are to be achieved, these segments must be separated from each other. To preserve viability, each segment should be 2 to 3 cm in width and no longer than 5 to 6 cm in length.

4. The tension provided by the muscle galea slings will temporarily establish facial "tone." Ideally the surgeon should strive for a half closure of the palpebral fissure and a slight smile. As the muscle begins to function, tension and relaxation should increase, and additional reanimation should become apparent.

5. The patient should be instructed to practice movements of the face. Biting down on the jaws should cause contraction of the muscles. Changes in the bite will cause certain muscle groups to become more activated than others.

COMPLICATIONS

1. Alopecia will occur if the hair-bearing follicles are injured during elevation of the flap. The dissection is therefore carried out in a plane just deep enough to avoid the follicles, but not so deep as to injure the superficial temporal artery. The wound should be drained and closed without tension. If alopecia develops, small areas of hair loss may be excised; larger areas require tissue expansion and advancement techniques.

2. Rotation of the temporalis muscle flap will cause a depression over the parietal region and a bulge along the zygomatic arch. The deformity will become less noticeable over time as the tissues atrophy. Removal of the zygoma and/or placing implants above the bulge may help to camouflage the irregularity.

3. Although reanimation is to be expected, it is not as "natural" as that seen with the neurorrhaphy technique. If more tension is needed in the tissues, the method can be augmented with tarsorrhaphy, gold weights, facial slings, and Z-plasty. However, these techniques should be applied only after the patient has had sufficient time for rehabilitation.

TEMPORALIS MUSCLE GALEA FLAP REANIMATION PROCEDURE

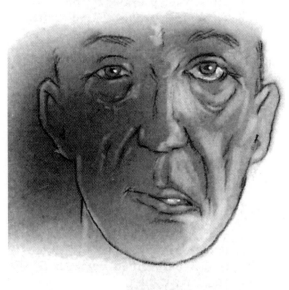

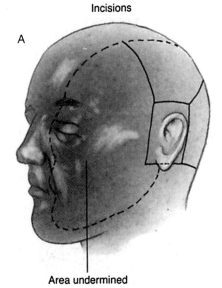

Incisions

A

Area undermined

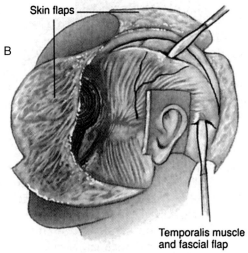

Skin flaps

B

Temporalis muscle
and fascial flap

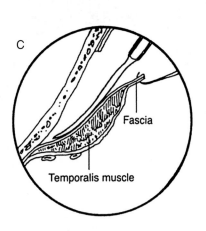

C

Fascia

Temporalis muscle

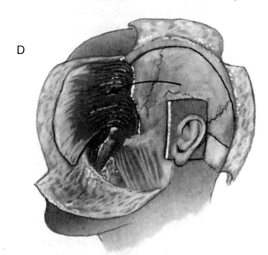

D

Rotation of flap

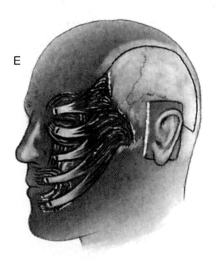

E

Compartmentalization
and attachments

Wm. Loechel

Parotid Duct Injury
Open Repair of Parotid Duct Injury

INDICATIONS

Penetrating wounds of the cheek can injure the parotid (Stensen) duct and cause a leakage of saliva into the soft tissues. Although parotid gland drainage will stop with pressure, leakage from the parotid duct will persist, often causing accumulation of fluids and/or a fistula. Early recognition and repair is desirable.

Several options for treatment of a parotid duct injury are available. For a laceration or avulsion injury that occurs proximal to the anterior portion of the masseter muscle, an end-to-end anastomosis should be considered. For those injuries closer to the duct orifice, a new opening should be created into the oral cavity. Frequently, the duct injury is associated with a facial nerve injury, and duct repair is carried out at the same time as a neurorrhaphy or grafting (see Chapter 14).

PROCEDURE

The location of the duct and the site of injury should be mapped out on the face. The area is then prepared and draped as a sterile field. Paralytic agents should be avoided since this will provide an opportunity to stimulate and find the position of the branches of the facial nerve, which will be an excellent guide to the duct system.

The main parotid duct travels along the buccal branch of the facial nerve. The nerve can be located with a facial nerve stimulator, and once this branch is found, it will be easy to define the proximal and distal ends of Stensen duct and carry out the repair.

Another method of finding the duct is with intubation. For this technique, the duct orifice is cannulated with a lacrimal probe. Pulling the cheek laterally will help straighten the duct and assist with the cannulation.

A–D After the duct is isolated, a small polyethylene tube should be placed through the proximal and distal segments. The long end of the catheter should be brought out through the oral cavity and fixed to the oral-buccal mucosa with sutures and to the corner of the mouth and cheek with adhesive tape. The duct is then closed around the tubing, using 6-0 or 7-0 nylon sutures and atraumatic needles. The wound is closed in layers. The catheter should be retained for approximately 10 days. Prophylactic antibiotics are administered for the duration of intubation.

PITFALLS

1. The duct can be tortuous and difficult to cannulate. Pulling the duct and gland laterally will straighten the duct and provide for an easier passage of the intubation tube.

2. Dislodgement of the intubation tube is common and can be avoided by securing the tube to the cheek tissues with tape and directly to the oral mucosa with sutures.

3. Avoid any additional injury to the facial nerve. The buccal branch should be identified. If the nerve has been injured, it can be treated at the same time as duct repair (see Chapter 106).

REPAIR OF PAROTID DUCT

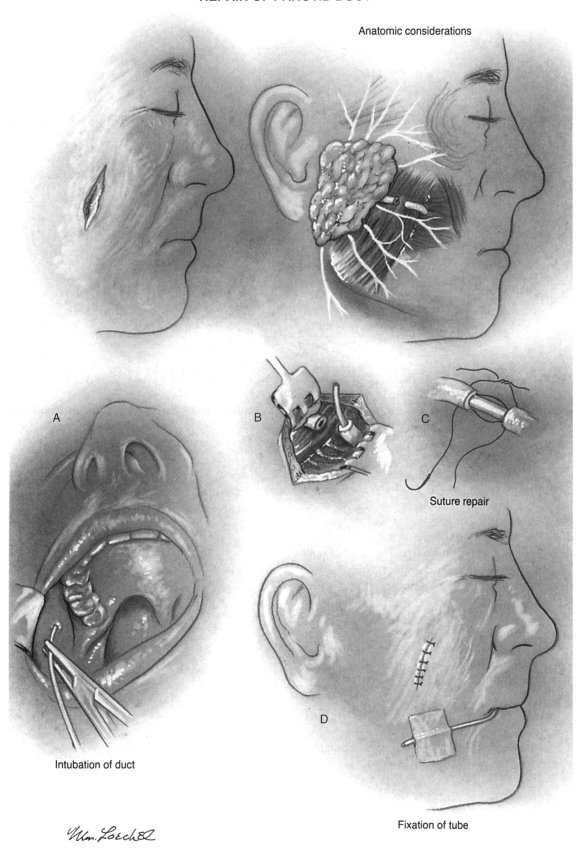

Anatomic considerations

A

B

C

Suture repair

Intubation of duct

D

Fixation of tube

COMPLICATIONS

1. Accumulation of fluid and fistulization can occur in spite of carefully applied reconstructive techniques. If such complications develop, the surgeon can attempt packing and/or pressure dressings. Salivary flow can be diminished by lysing the chorda tympani and/or Jacobsen nerve. If these procedures are unsuccessful, ligation of the duct and/or radiation must be considered.

2. Parotitis is always possible, especially when the flow is obstructed and associated with stasis of secretion. Antibiotic treatment and generous use of sialagogues are indicated. However, if the condition persists, the surgeon can consider denervation by way of resection of the chorda tympani. Failure of this technique should prompt removal of the gland (superficial parotidectomy).

PART THREE

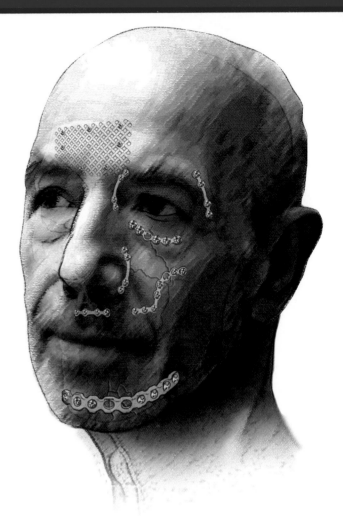

Mandibular Fractures

Classification and Pathophysiology of Mandibular Fractures

CHAPTER **17**

General Considerations

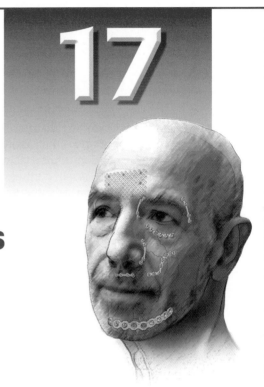

Patients with mandibular fractures can present with a myriad of signs and symptoms related to the type of fracture, pull of muscles of mastication, and the preexisting dentition. Swelling, tenderness, and ecchymoses are often accompanied intraorally by fractured teeth, lacerations, and exposure of bone fragments. Speech and swallowing are impaired, and saliva collects in dependent areas. In severe cases, the tongue is displaced posteriorly and can be associated with respiratory obstruction. The patient complains of pain, and with displacement of the fracture, there is an inability to occlude and approximate the upper jaw to the lower one. Premature contact of the molars often causes an open bite deformity. Unilateral injuries may cause deviation of the jaw and a crossbite appearance. To recognize these conditions, the surgeon must have a complete understanding of the types of fracture and of those pathophysiologic processes that produce each clinical picture. This information is also essential in designing the best treatment program.

CLASSIFICATION

A Fractures of the mandible are classified according to both anatomic location and the specific characteristics of the fracture. Most adult fractures are classified according to the area of involvement (i.e., condyle, coronoid, ramus, angle, body, and parasymphysis). The most common areas of injury are in the condyle and angle, followed by the body, and parasymphysis; rarely is the coronoid process involved. The alveolar ridge fracture is a subtype that can occur in one or several regions. Mandibular fractures may be isolated or multiple and unilateral or bilateral.

B Other descriptions of mandibular fractures consider the extent of injury. In the *simple* fracture, the mucosa and skin are intact. When the fracture is *compound* (or *open*), there is an exposure of bone, either into the oral cavity or extraorally, by way of a laceration or avulsion. The *greenstick* fracture, which often occurs in children, is an incomplete fracture in which only one cortical surface is involved. The *comminuted* type is characterized by several small fragments of bone. The fractures can also be *complex*, in which the fracture is associated with fractures of other areas of the mandible, or *complicated*, in which the fracture involves both the mandible and maxilla.

The presence or absence of teeth can also provide an important classification. A Class I fracture has teeth on both sides of the fracture line (dentulous), a Class II fracture has teeth on one side (partially edentulous), and a Class III fracture (edentulous) has no teeth adjacent to the sides of the fracture. Often Class III fracture patients are completely edentulous.

STABILITY CONCEPTS

The various directions and planes of fracture, coupled with the forces exerted by the muscles of mastication, affect displacement and either assist or interfere with the stability of fixation. Other factors that can affect stability are the presence of contralateral or ipsilateral fractures, comminution, and the presence or absence of teeth. In general, fractures that are deemed unstable (or unfavorable) are best treated with open methods of reduction and fixation, whereas those that are stable (or favorable) are usually managed with conservative techniques.

C,D Fracture lines can be extremely important, especially if they allow the muscle groups to pull the fragments from each other. Fractures of the body and the anterior portion of the angle are often unstable because the direction of the fracture line allows depression by the digastric, geniohyoid, genioglossus, and mylohyoid muscles. At the same time the ascending ramus and the upper portion of the angle are elevated by the temporalis and masseter muscles and, to some extent, by the medial and lateral pterygoid muscles. A vertically directed angle fracture that traverses from the posterior portion of the body superiorly to the third molar tends to be held in a normal position. In the horizontal plane, the pterygoid muscles are unopposed, and if a fracture extends from the lateral part of the angle anteriorly to the inner cortex, the posterior segment will be unstable and displaced inward. Fractures from the lateral portion of the angle directed posteriorly to the inner cortex will be pulled together.

E At the parasymphysis, a relatively vertical line of fracture predisposes to instability. The digastric and mylohyoid muscles tend to pull the hemimandible downward, causing one half of the jaw to be distracted from the other. Obliquity of the fracture may or may not lead to instability; this will depend on the direction of the fracture and on whether the mylohyoid muscle brings the fragments together or apart.

F At the condyle, the line of fracture also determines the degree of instability. Because the lateral pterygoid muscle inserts high into the neck of the condyle and into the capsule of the temporomandibular joint, high fractures are associated with minimal displacement. On the other hand, fractures in the subcondylar area are often associated with medial dislocation of the head and neck of the condyle.

G Multiplicity of fractures is also a factor in determining stability and treatment options. Parasymphyseal fractures commonly occur with angle or condylar fractures of the opposite side. Angle fractures are often seen with opposite condyle, parasymphysis, or body fractures. These multiple fractures can also be associated with a depression and rotation of the intervening segment. If the fractures happen to be ipsilateral, as in a parasymphyseal and subcondylar fracture, then the mylohyoid and pterygoid muscles tend to rotate and pull the fragments medially. The same effect can be seen in ipsilateral, parasymphyseal, and angle fractures. For these reasons, multiple fractures commonly lead to unfavorable forces at the fracture site.

Comminuted fractures of the angle also tend to cause instability. Several fractures in the area of the angle will tend to prevent "locking" of the fragments. Internal and/or external fixation thus becomes important in developing a solid union.

H Loss of teeth also creates additional stability problems. Second or third molar contacts on the posterior segment prevent upward rotation of the posterior fragment. When these teeth are missing (on either the upper or lower jaw) there is no "stop," and the posterior fragment tends to be more mobile. Occasionally a molar is involved with the fracture, and when the tooth is loose and carious or devitalized from injury to the pulp and/or root, the surgeon must extract the tooth and then select an appropriate method to treat the destabilized segment.

Completely edentulous patients present even more of a problem. For this condition, there is no dentition with which to guide the "fit" of the upper and lower jaws. Also, the option of using the upper dentition to stabilize the lower (through intermaxillary fixation) is not available, and other methods of fixation must be used.

PEDIATRIC CONSIDERATIONS

Fractures of the mandible are treated more conservatively in children than in adults because of the growth characteristics of the jaw and the risk of injury to developing teeth (see Chapters 110 and 111). Healing of bones is very efficient in children, and even if the fragments are not lined up perfectly, there can be

MANDIBULAR FRACTURES

A

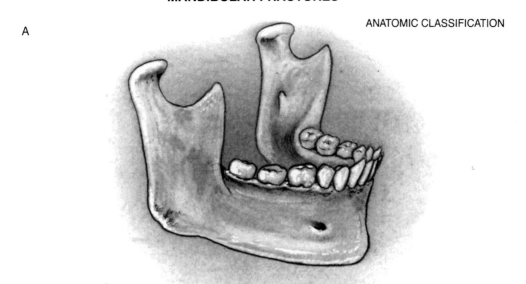

B   CLASSIFICATION BY TYPE OF FRACTURE

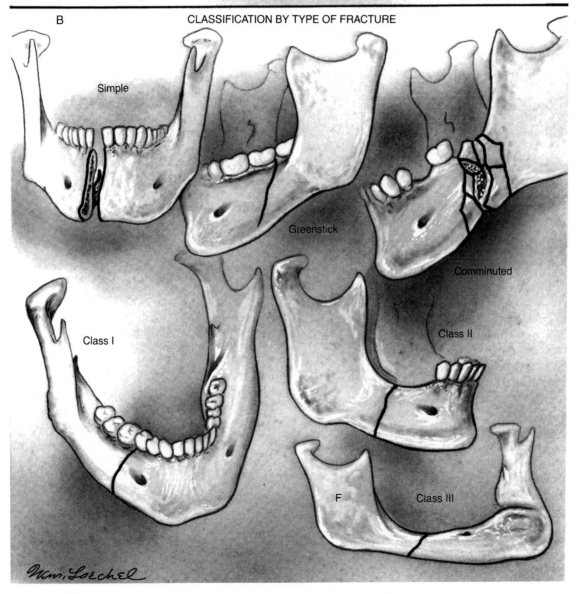

Simple

Greenstick

Comminuted

Class I

Class II

F   Class III

Wm. Loechel

STABILITY CONCEPTS

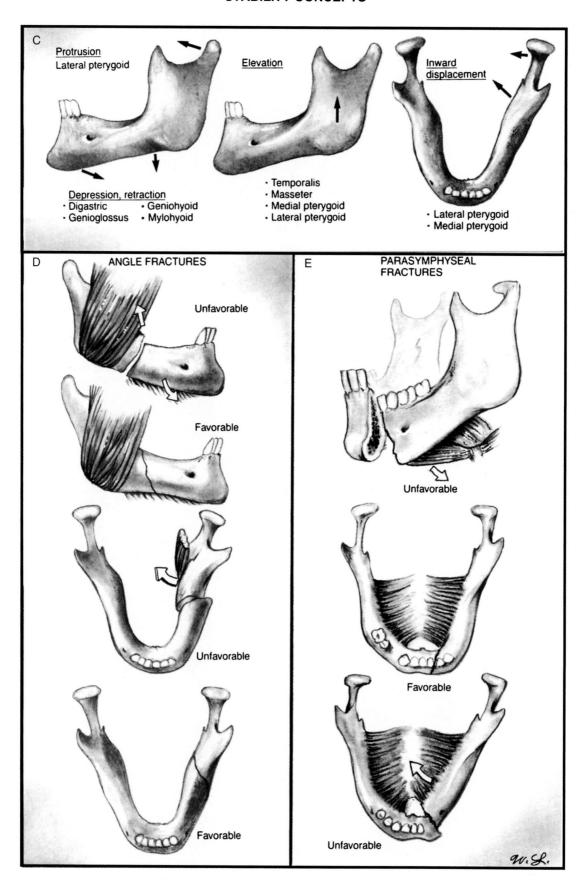

C

Protrusion
Lateral pterygoid

Elevation

Inward displacement

Depression, retraction
· Digastric   · Geniohyoid
· Genioglossus   · Mylohyoid

· Temporalis
· Masseter
· Medial pterygoid
· Lateral pterygoid

· Lateral pterygoid
· Medial pterygoid

D   ANGLE FRACTURES

Unfavorable

Favorable

Unfavorable

Favorable

E   PARASYMPHYSEAL FRACTURES

Unfavorable

Favorable

Unfavorable

F   **CONDYLAR FRACTURES**

Unfavorable   Favorable

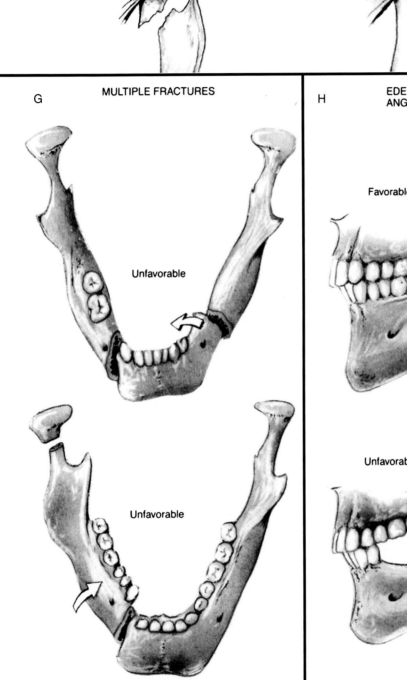

G   **MULTIPLE FRACTURES**

Unfavorable

Unfavorable

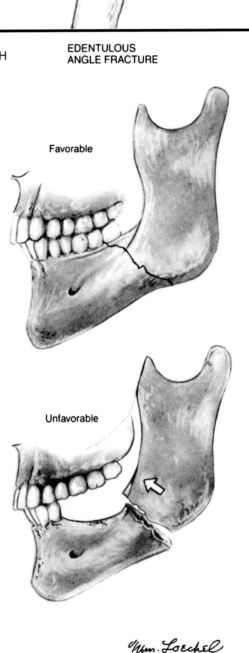

H   **EDENTULOUS ANGLE FRACTURE**

Favorable

Unfavorable

Wm. Loechel

rapid healing across the gaps, with new bone formation and a remodeling that restores normal anatomic configuration.

I In children, the surgeon must also be aware of the growth of the mandible. Essentially, the ramus and body are remodeled by resorption and deposition processes, whereas the rest of the jaw elongates in response to growth at the condylar region. Injury to the growth area (center) can occur with condylar trauma and/or surgery and, for this reason, open reduction and fixation of the condyle is controversial, although not contraindicated under conditions requiring an open procedure. (see Chapter 21) If there is damage, the jaw will have limited growth, especially in the condyle-ramus region. This can cause a dysfunction, and later the jaw, on opening, will deviate to the side of the injury.

The temporomandibular joint can also be indirectly affected. In such patients, there can be a fibrous fixation of the joint and secondary growth deficits. The complication can develop rapidly in children, and early mobilization of the jaw should be attempted to prevent this from occurring. The mandible should be held in intermaxillary fixation for no more than 2 weeks, and if it is necessary to add additional fixation, it should be performed at intermittent periods. Occasionally patients can be treated in a "halfway" manner with loose rubber bands, allowing them a limited use of the joint.

J,K Knowledge of the anatomy and position of teeth is also important. If holes are drilled in the lower portion of the mandible for screws or plates, there can be injury to the primordium of the teeth. For these reasons, the objective in children is to align the fragments in the best manner possible without injury to the growth potential of teeth.

Specific methods that should be applied in young children include the following:

1. Try to avoid open techniques

2. Consider the use of lingual splints.

3. Intermaxillary fixation can be maintained, but the surgeon must be certain to place the ligatures around sound teeth. Strategically placed Ivy loops are excellent alternatives to the arch bar technique.

4. Avoid prolonged fixation, especially if there is a suspicion of injury to the condyle or temporomandibular joint.

5. Internal fixation is best accomplished with miniplates at the inferior border of the mandible, preferably using absorbable types.

PEDIATRIC MANDIBLES

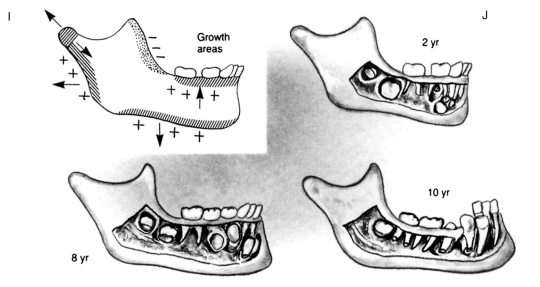

I — Growth areas

J — 2 yr

8 yr

10 yr

ERUPTION

K

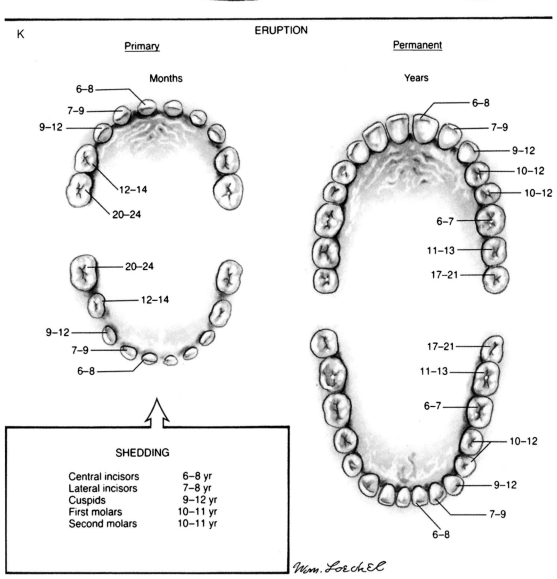

Primary

Months

6–8
7–9
9–12
12–14
20–24

20–24
12–14
9–12
7–9
6–8

Permanent

Years

6–8
7–9
9–12
10–12
10–12
6–7
11–13
17–21

17–21
11–13
6–7
10–12
9–12
7–9
6–8

SHEDDING

Central incisors	6–8 yr
Lateral incisors	7–8 yr
Cuspids	9–12 yr
First molars	10–11 yr
Second molars	10–11 yr

Wm. Loechel

Condylar Fractures

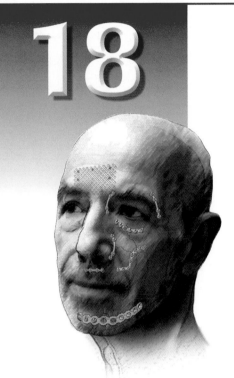

Closed Reduction for Simple Dislocation of the Condyle
Alternative Technique of Condyloplasty for Recurrent Dislocation

INDICATIONS

Acute dislocation of the condylar head from the temporomandibular joint without fracture is not common and can develop from any sudden, forceful opening of the jaw. During the dislocation, the condyle usually rotates forward, breaking the adjacent ligaments. The head of the condyle, under the pull of the pterygoid muscles, then leaves the glenoid fossa, crosses the articular eminence, and becomes locked in front of it. The dislocation is often bilateral. It is associated with pain and difficulty in management of the saliva, speech, and swallowing. The condition can become chronic and recurrent if not treated appropriately.

PROCEDURE

A–C Reduction of the condylar head can be achieved with manual pressure exerted at the angle of the jaw. The muscles of the patient should be relaxed with a tranquilizer, and pain should be controlled with an analgesic prior to the reduction. To achieve the correct force for reduction, the surgeon should stand behind the seated patient. The surgeon's thumbs should then be placed at the junction of the body of the ramus just lateral to the molar dentition. The jaw is pushed down while rotating the chin upward. Constant pressure will eventually break the "spasms," but this process may take 5 to 10 minutes. Alternatively, reduction can be performed from the front, but the surgeon will have to

TREATMENT OF CONDYLAR DISLOCATION

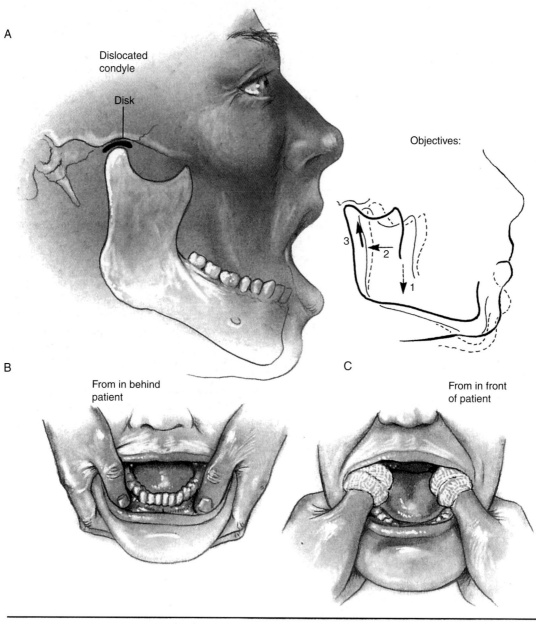

A

Dislocated
condyle

Disk

Objectives:

B

From in behind
patient

C

From in front
of patient

ALTERNATIVE TECHNIQUE OF CONDYLOPLASTY

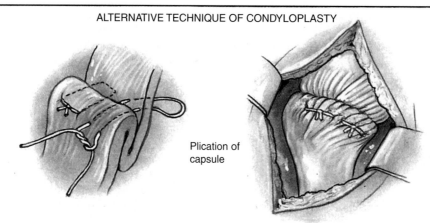

Plication of
capsule

use more thumb and hand pressure. During the postreduction period, excursion of the jaw should be limited. If this is the first time for dislocation to occur, intermaxillary fixation (Chapter 19) for a few weeks should be considered. The patient should be placed on a liquid diet and told to avoid any chewing of foods for at least 10 days. Pain can be controlled with analgesics.

PITFALLS

1. Be sure that the condylar dislocation is not part of a fracture of the condyle and/or glenoid fossa. Such injuries can be associated with damage to the auditory system and intracranial complications. These problems should be recognized and treated accordingly.

2. A search for factors leading to occlusal disharmony is often beneficial. Some patients have a myofascial pain syndrome or may be taking drugs, such as phenothiazides, that induce extrapyramidal effects and spasms of the muscles of mastication. Such a condition should be referred to the neurologist for appropriate control.

3. Proper sedation will expedite the reduction process. The addition of a tranquilizer can promote relaxation of the spastic musculature.

4. Reduction of the dislocation in a noncompliant, noncooperative patient is difficult, and in such situations, general anesthesia is preferred.

COMPLICATIONS

1. Recurrence of the dislocation is easy to diagnose because of the characteristic history. Intermaxillary fixation will limit movement of the condyle and encourage fibrosis of the capsule, but results are quite variable. Frequently, something more definitive must be done. Shortening of the capsule with a "pants-over-vest" technique is helpful (see later). Enlargement of the articular eminence with an allograft or autogenous bone graft may control anterior excursion of the condyle. In the noncompliant patient, removal of the lateral third of the articular eminence may be the more prudent course.

2. Injury to the meniscus can occur as a result of temporomandibular joint dislocation and/or fracture involving the condylar head. Several types of injury can be defined: inflammation, complete or partial severing of the meniscus from its attachments, or tearing of the meniscus itself. Inflammation alone is diagnosed when the pain responds to analgesics and jaw motion improves within 10 days. The more severe injuries associated with tearing will have persistence of trismus, deviation of the jaw on opening of the mouth, and limitation of excursion of the head of the condyle. The inflammatory condition is treated with a soft diet and analgesics. More serious injury to the joint is treated with intraoral splints and jaw exercises. If conservative approaches are unsuccessful, the surgeon must consider surgical reattachment (or reconstruction) of the soft tissues, meniscectomy, or prosthetic substitution. For indications and details of these procedures, the reader is referred to Chapter 38 and appropriate oral surgery texts.

ALTERNATIVE TECHNIQUE OF CONDYLOPLASTY FOR RECURRENT DISLOCATION

Chronic dislocation may be treated simply by strengthening the loosened capsule over the condylar head and neck. This method is conservative, and therefore, if it is not successful, the surgeon can proceed to a more aggressive approach. Exposure is similar to that obtained in Chapter 21. The capsule is identified and tightened by simply plicating the lower portion of the capsule over the upper portion and securing the plication with two 3-0 nonabsorbable mattress sutures. Excursion of the mandible is limited for 2 weeks, and the patient is subsequently treated with active opening and closing exercises.

CHAPTER 19

Closed Reduction and Immobilization of Condylar Fractures With Intermaxillary Fixation

Alternative Techniques of Ivy Loops, Intermaxillary Fixation Screws and Molar Wafers

In Consultation With Mark T. Marunick, DDS

INDICATIONS

Most condylar fractures can be treated with closed methods of intermaxillary fixation. Contact of the teeth in the molar region drives the mandible downward; this, together with the anterior medial pull of the pterygoid muscles, tends to reduce the fracture. There can also be a remodeling of the condylar neck that reestablishes normal anatomic relationships. In adults with an intact dentition, intermaxillary fixation is carried out with arch bars, intermaxillary screws, or Ivy loops; in the edentulous patient, these arch bars can be secured to dentures, which, in turn, are secured to the upper and lower jaws and to each other by intermaxillary fixation (see Chapter 20). In children, fixation need only be temporary and is often achievable with strategic placement of Ivy loops.

PROCEDURE

Intermaxillary fixation with arch bars can be carried out using general or local/topical anesthesia. Good lighting is important. An assistant is necessary to help in retraction of the lips and cheeks and to aid in the suctioning of blood and saliva from the field.

A,B For usual fixation, a pliable Erich arch bar is satisfactory. These bars are designed with small hooks that should be directed toward the gums on each dental arch. The bar can be cut to the correct size by placing the bar on half of the arch and counting the number of hooks. The bar is then cut at twice the number of hooks to cover the entire arch. The posterior portion of the bar should be bent inward to avoid unnecessary injury to the mucosa.

C,D The arch bar can be applied first to either the upper or lower jaw. Regardless of which jaw is selected, the bar should initially be affixed to the first premolar tooth. For this technique, a 6-inch length of 25- or 26-gauge stainless steel wire is passed above the bar and between the teeth in the interdental space to the lingual surface. The wire is then fed back between the teeth so that it exits below the bar on the buccal surface. The wire is then twisted down across the bar and

INTERMAXILLARY FIXATION FOR CONDYLAR FRACTURE

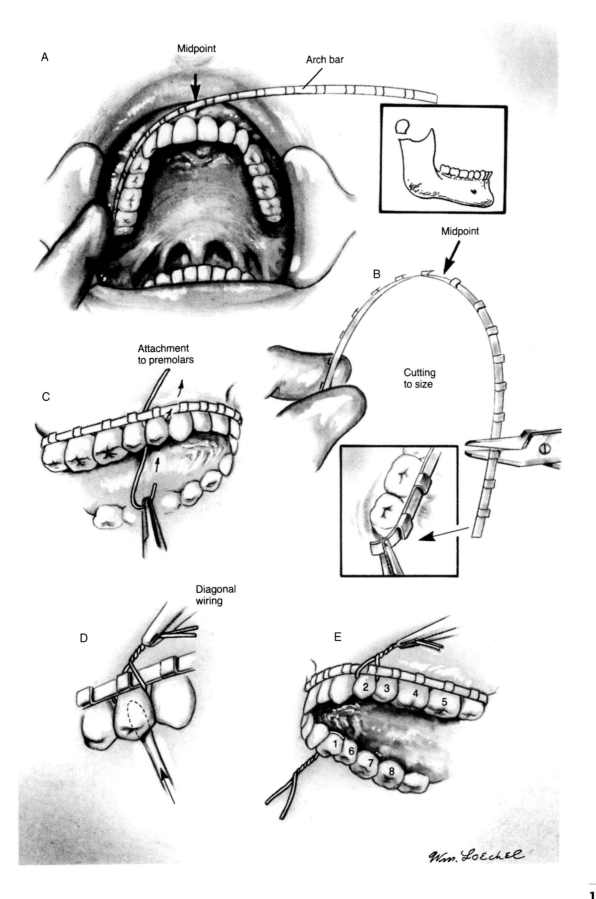

A

Midpoint

Arch bar

Midpoint

B

Cutting
to size

Attachment
to premolars

C

Diagonal
wiring

D

E

Wm. Loechel

tooth in a clockwise diagonal fashion and is secured as high as possible on the crown by pushing the wire with a Freer elevator toward the gum line. The curvature on the crown will keep the wire from being displaced toward the occlusal surface of the tooth. All wires should be pulled while twisting in the same direction (i.e., clockwise). The wires should be temporarily left long and secured with a clamp to help in the retraction of the lip.

E After the bar is attached to the premolar of one side, it is affixed to the first premolar on the opposite side. It is important that the bar be held firmly against the dental arch so that when the second wire is placed, there is no space between the arch bar and the teeth. Subsequently the bar is secured to the other molars and to the canine teeth.

F Because the canine tooth is cone-shaped, special techniques must be applied. As described by Dingman and Natvig (1964), the wire should be passed above the arch bar toward the lingual surface and returned around the tooth (still above the arch bar) to the buccal or lateral surface. One end of the wire is then looped around the arch bar, and the ends are twisted horizontally around the tooth. These techniques can also be used when there is an isolated molar next to an edentulous area or when the surgeon is forced to use the incisors for additional fixation.

G,H During the process of applying the wires, there is a tendency for the wire to stretch. This can cause some loosening, and to avoid this problem, the surgeon should twist the wires tightly once more later in the procedure. Alternatively, the wire can be pre-stretched prior to use. The twisted ends of the wire are cut at 1.0 to 1.5 cm, and with the same clockwise rotation, the wire is turned with a hemostat into a sharp curve directed toward the gingival mucous membrane. The other (upper or lower) arch bar is applied in a similar fashion.

I Arch bars can be secured to each other with elastic bands or wires. Elastic bands can be made easily by cutting a No. 14 elastic catheter into thin sections. The elastic bands have the advantage of providing for dynamic reduction and are easily adjusted by incorporating more or fewer loops on the bars. Wires will occasionally need to be tightened or removed and replaced in new positions. Wire cutters should be available should the patient vomit in the postoperative period.

J,K As the rubber bands or wires are applied, occlusion should be checked in the molar region. Wear facets should be in contact with one another, and centric occlusion should be established. Excessive traction

should be avoided on the incisors, as such forces can cause a partial or complete extraction of the teeth.

Postoperative radiographs are useful in evaluating the reduction and fixation. Hygiene of the teeth and gingiva is maintained with a water irrigation device or gentle brushing. When the arch bars are to be removed (2 to 6 weeks later), the bands are first taken off, and the patient is asked to bite on a tongue blade. If there is discomfort at this time or during the next week, or if jaw movement does not return to normal, then the patient must be reevaluated for malunion, delayed union, or nonunion.

PITFALLS

1. Avoid injury to the interdental papillae. Try to pass wires between the teeth, rather than through the gingiva. This will keep the teeth healthier during the period of fixation and avoid permanent injury to the periodontia.

2. Check the arch bar for slippage postoperatively. On occasion, the wires will loosen; when this occurs, they should be tightened with additional turns. If they are not tightened, the arch bar can become dislodged from the dentition.

3. Avoid wire ligatures around the incisors, as they can pull the incisors from their sockets. However, if there are many missing teeth and the incisors can help with the fixation, they should be used. In such a case, the vertical traction should be kept to a minimum.

4. If a segment of jaw is edentulous, it is possible to bridge this gap with a strong arch bar and a more secure ligature to the remaining teeth. Often this can be accomplished with a heavier Jelenko bar and a Dingman wire ligature applied to the premolar or molar teeth.

5. The surgeon must be sure that the condylar fracture is not associated with another fracture. If this should occur, one or both fractures will usually require open stabilization.

6. Be careful when applying arch bars in children with deciduous teeth, as the bar can prematurely extract the tooth. The teeth should thus be carefully studied for maturity (see Chapters 17 and 110). Alternatively, Ivy loops can be secured to selected groups to maintain adequate intermaxillary fixation (see later).

7. Arch bar fixation for condylar fractures should be limited to just enough time for healing to take place. If the time of fixation is prolonged, ankylosis can result. In children, intermaxillary fixation should be removed in 2 weeks, and in adults, within 4 weeks. When intermaxillary fixation is used for other types of mandibular (e.g., condyle, body) and maxillary fractures, the arch

Attachment to canine
(horizontal wiring)

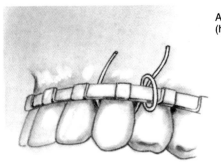
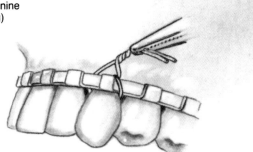

F

Cutting and twisting ends

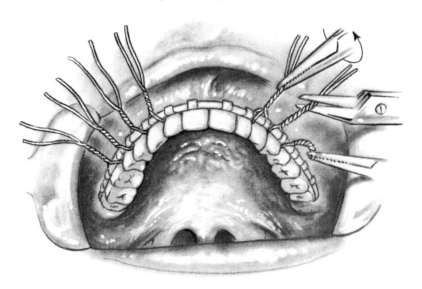

G

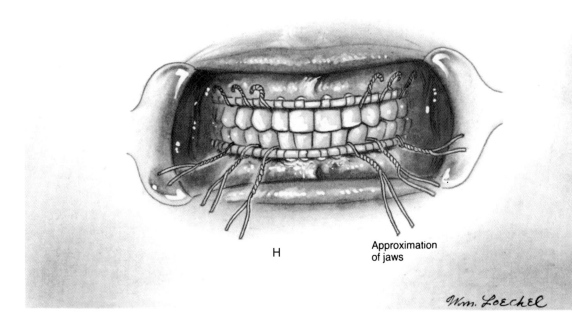

H

Approximation
of jaws

Wm. Loechel

I

Elastic band traction in occlusion

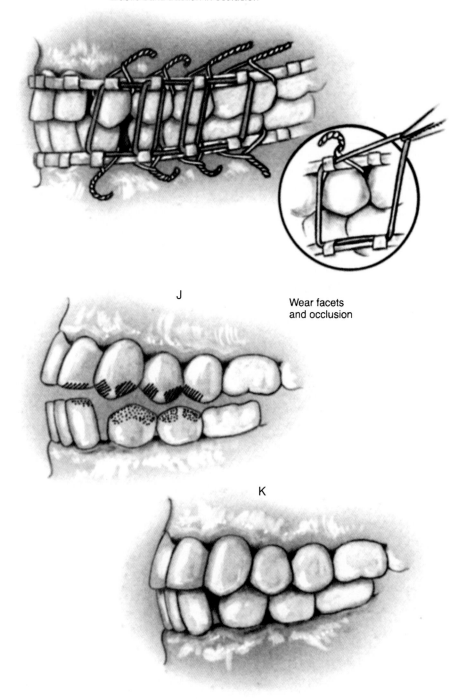

J

Wear facets
and occlusion

K

Wm. Loechel

bars should be retained for 4 to 6 weeks in children and 6– to 8 weeks in adults.

8. If wires are used to attach the bars to each other, the surgeon has to be prepared for possible postoperative vomiting and the need for an emergency cutting of the wires. In anticipation of such an event, wire cutters should be available at the bedside.

COMPLICATIONS

1. Injury to the condyle is often associated with tearing of the ligamentous capsule and/or displacement or tearing of the meniscus of the temporomandibular joint. Often, appropriate fixation and reduction will provide for satisfactory healing. If this does not occur, the surgeon must reevaluate the injury and treat the condition. Management includes nighttime head bandages, soft diet, and analgesics; in other patients, it may be necessary to consider interocclusal splints and even reconstruction of the joint space.

2. Displacement of the condyle can result in bony auditory canal wall fractures and/or penetration of the middle fossa. An accurate diagnosis is essential if appropriate treatment for these complicating injuries is to be provided (see Chapter 18).

3. Failure of the condyle to heal will lead to a nonunion or pseudarthrosis. If the fracture is high, the pseudarthrosis will have negligible effects. It may cause short periods of pain and, on opening, a deviation of the jaw to the affected side. However, if nonunion complicates mastication and causes excessive pain, exploration of the condyle and condylectomy or reconstruction of the joint must be considered (see Chapter 38).

4. Ankylosis of the condyle is a serious complication and may lead to failure of growth of the mandible in children and/or major dysfunction of the jaw. In the adult, mastication is usually impaired, and as a result of inability to open the mouth, problems with oral hygiene and/or oral intake resulting in inadequate nutrition may develop.

Ankylosis can be treated with several techniques. Early, the surgeon should attempt jaw prying by sequential placement of increasing numbers of tongue blades, or alternatively, by application of dynamic expansion devices (Therabite or Dynasplint) between the dental arches. If these are unsatisfactory, then surgical intervention is necessary. If the joint has been irreversibly damaged, it is possible to restore it with a new joint surface made of metal or plastic. If the entire joint has been destroyed, condylectomy or a planned pseudarthrosis may be advisable. In some patients, condylectomy and reconstruction with rib graft or a prosthesis is desirable (see Chapter 38).

ALTERNATIVE TECHNIQUE OF IVY LOOPS

The Ivy loop is an important alternative method for closed reduction and fixation. Although it is not as strong as the arch bar, it is useful in selectively bringing occlusal pairs of teeth together. It is used in children who have a mixed dentition, in partially edentulous patients who will have additional forms of fixation, and in individuals who need temporary occlusion while other methods (i.e., biphase or plates) are being applied.

a,b The Ivy loop is constructed of a 25- or 26-gauge stainless steel wire. The wire is cut to approximately 16 cm. It is then wound around the tip of a small clamp, and a small loop is formed with two to three twists of the end of the wire. The ends are inserted between two suitable teeth. Each wire is wrapped around the neck of the adjoining tooth, and the wire is brought out to the labial/buccal surface.

c–e A mesial wire is then inserted through the loop, and both wires are twisted around the more distal tooth. A Freer elevator should be used to push the wire closer to the neck of the tooth while additional twists are applied to the wire. A final tightening occurs when the loop is grasped with a needle holder, pulled laterally, and twisted one to two turns around the external wire.

f Additional Ivy loops are placed on opposing pairs of occluding teeth. The jaws can be held in fixation by applying fine wire ligatures (No. 28) through the eyelets (loops).

The loops must be checked often for displacement of the wires, and if this occurs, appropriate adjustments should be made. The dentition must be kept clean with a soft toothbrush or water irrigation device.

ALTERNATIVE TECHNIQUE OF INTERMAXILLARY FIXATION SCREWS

Specially designed bone screws are available to obtain intermaxillary fixation. For this technique, a small stab incision is made just lateral and above the canines on the upper jaw and lateral and below the canines on the lower jaw. If the screw is not of the self-drilling variety, drill holes are then placed and the screws secured to

ALTERNATIVE TECHNIQUE OF IVY LOOPS

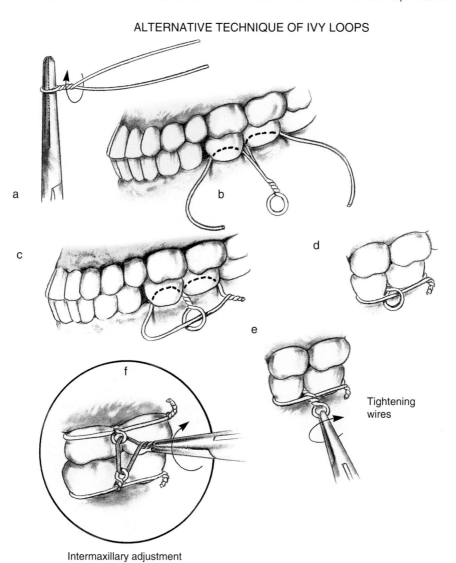

a

b

c

d

e

Tightening wires

f

Intermaxillary adjustment

ALTERNATIVE TECHNIQUE OF INTERMAXILLARY FIXATION SCREWS

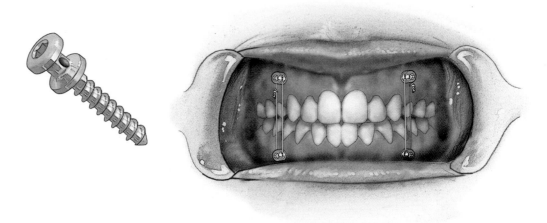

the alveolar bone. Most systems have a hole through which the wire can be placed, or alternatively, the wire can be affixed circumferentially around the head of the screw. The wires are tightened as the jaws are reduced and placed into proper occlusion.

ALTERNATIVE TECHNIQUE OF MOLAR WAFERS

If the condyle does not become reduced with time, adjunctive reduction techniques can be considered. Appropriate imaging studies should be obtained 2 weeks following reduction and fixation. If the condyle is still displaced, the situation must be evaluated for addional reduction and fixation. For closed gradual reduction an interocclusal acrylic wafer can be made and placed between the molars to provide additional downward traction on the mandible. If unsuccessful, one must consider the open technique described in Chapter 21.

a',b' The wafer can be fabricated in two ways. The best (and preferred) method is to make stone dental casts (see Chapter 20) and fabricate the wafer on these casts. The wafer is built up approximately 2 to 5 mm to provide more downward stress on the posterior

fragments. To achieve these relationships, the casts should be mounted on an articulator and the articulator adjusted to increase the vertical distance between the teeth. The wafer can be developed in wax at this position and processed in heat-cured acrylic.

c'–e' The wafer can also be made by coating the cast with petrolatum. Autocure or light-cured acrylic, in a viscous state, is adapted to the lower cast, and the articulation is closed to the predetermined vertical opening. After appropriate polymerization, trimming, and adjustment, the splint is placed into the mouth and held by intermaxillary fixation.

If the surgeon is seeking a reduction only, a splint can be designed so that an incline is exerted on the posterior dentition. However, this splint should be used for only 7 to 10 days.

f' A rapid, but less exact, method is to make a splint directly on the teeth. This can be accomplished by applying petrolatum to the posterior maxillary and mandibular molars, having the patient bite down on the viscous autocure material, removing the material, and allowing it to harden. Excess acrylic can be trimmed from the splint. The splint should be secured tightly with intermaxillary fixation.

ALTERNATIVE TECHNIQUE OF INTEROCCLUSAL WAFER

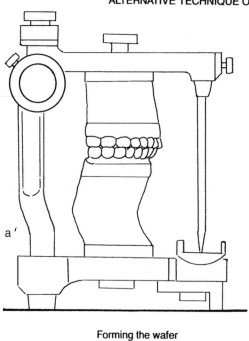

a′

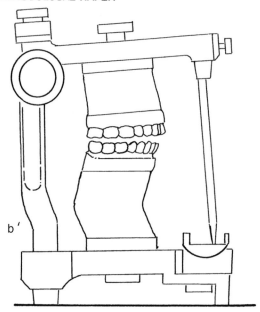

b′

Forming the wafer

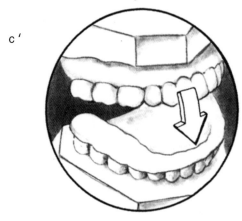

c′

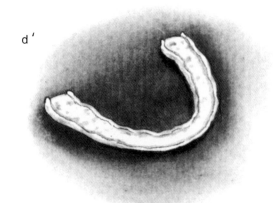

d′

e′

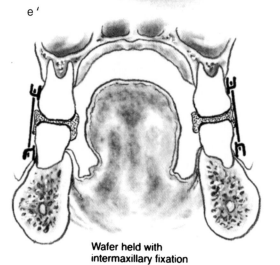

Wafer held with intermaxillary fixation

"Direct" method

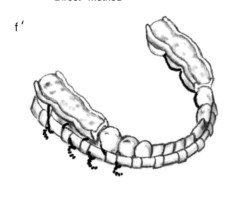

f′

Closed Reduction of Condylar Fractures in the Edentulous Patient With Circummandibular and Circumzygomatic Splint Fixation

In Consultation With Mark T. Marunick, DDS

INDICATIONS

Simple isolated condylar fractures can often be treated with intermaxillary fixation or Ivy loops. However, if the patient is edentulous, it becomes necessary to use other fixation methods. Most commonly, the dentures are secured to the mandible and the zygoma by circumosseous wiring and then to each other with intermaxillary wires. For patients who do not have dentures, there is the option of making splints (Gunning type), which are also secured to the upper and lower jaws. In severely displaced condyles, often associated with other mandible fractures, open techniques must be considered (Chapter 21). With splint fixation, the period of fixation is variable, depending on the age of the individual. In children, fixation is employed for a 2-week period; in adults, it is used for a 2- to 4-week period. Consultation and collaboration with a maxillofacial prosthodontist to fabricate and apply these devices are highly recommended.

PROCEDURES

Preparation of the Splint

The splint is made from either an autopolymerizing or a heat-cured acrylic resin. Most dental laboratories will make the splint, provided they are given satisfactory casts, appropriate instructions, and authorization. The principal aspects of the technique are discussed in the text that follows.

To make the impressions, stock plastic dental or metal edentulous impression trays are used. In selecting trays, the lower tray is identified by its U shape, which provides space for the tongue. The upper tray is ovoid or square to cover the region of the hard palate. The selected trays should fit the alveolus comfortably.

A–D The impression is made using type I, normal-set, alginate material mixed to the manufacturer's specifications. Equal parts by volume of water and powder are mixed in a flexible bowl until the mixture is uniform and smooth. The material is then placed into the upper tray with a spatula to the height of the flanges of the tray. Prior to mixing the alginate, the oral cavity is rinsed with water and dried with 2 inch × 2 inch cotton gauze pads that are placed in the buccal and lingual sulci. The lips are lubricated with petrolatum. The gauze pads are removed, and the loaded tray is centered over the edentulous ridge and carefully seated. Digital pressure is maintained until the mixture "sets" (approximately 3

SPLINT FABRICATION

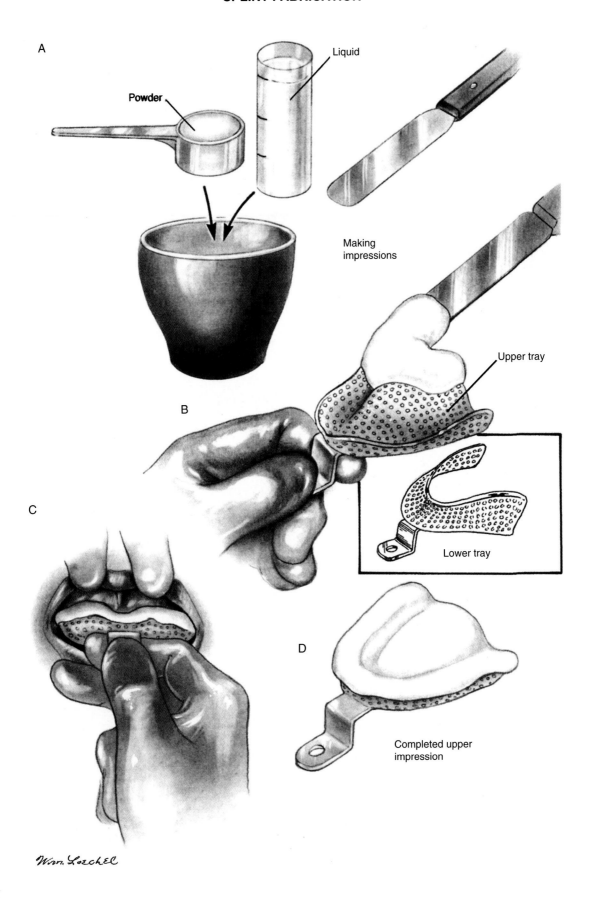

A

Powder

Liquid

Making impressions

B

Upper tray

Lower tray

C

D

Completed upper impression

Wm. Loechel

minutes). The tray is then removed and the impression inspected. If the impression is acceptable, it is washed, wrapped in a moist paper towel, and placed into a plastic bag. The lower impression is made and handled in a similar fashion. When making the impressions, care must be taken to minimize extrusion of impression material from the posterior part of the tray. This can elicit a gag reflex and pose a risk of aspiration.

E–G The material chosen for the cast (made from the impression) can be plaster, stone, or combinations of the two. Ideally, the stone (or plaster) should be mixed with the correct water-to-stone ratio and spatulated under vaccuum before pouring with the aid of a vibrator. If these instruments are not available, the stone and water can be hand-mixed in a flexible bowl with a spatula. To minimize voids, the mixed stone should be carefully placed in the impression in small increments on a vibrator, or alternatively, the handle of the tray can be tapped on the top of the table. When the stone has set, the impression is separated from the cast, and the cast is trimmed appropriately.

H–J The next step is to coat the cast with petrolatum and to fabricate autopolymerizing acrylic resin record bases. The stone cast must be carefully evaluated to limit the extension of the record bases where tissues were displaced by the impression. Wax rims are placed on the record bases, and these same record bases are used for facebow registration. The facebow is then transferred to the articulator. An appropriate clinically determined occlusal vertical dimension and centric position are recorded and used to relate the casts on the articulator.

K–M With the cast and record base on the articulator, the record bases can be waxed to the appropriate design. To expedite intermaxillary fixation, arch bars are imbedded into the labial aspect of the wax rims. Lateral stability is provided by grooves placed on the top of the lower wax rim; extensions are then waxed on the upper rim so that when it is occluded with the lower, the extensions engage the grooves, relate the two splints to one another, and prevent lateral displacement. Separate grooves are also placed on the lower rim to aid in circummandibular wiring of the lower splint. The anterior portions of the wax rims are cut away, providing access for the intake of food and liquids. The separate upper and lower splints are processed in acrylic resin, finished, and polished. Holes are placed in the flanges of the upper splint, several on each side, for circumzygomatic wiring. The splints should be checked and adjusted in the mouth prior to surgical placement.

Denture Preparation

a–f For those patients with adequate dentures, the preparation process is quite easy. If damaged, the dentures should be repaired with an autopolymerizing acrylic resin. A channel can be cut in the labial aspect of the base of the denture just above the teeth in the upper denture and below the teeth in the lower denture. The channel should be large enough to accommodate a segment of arch bar, which is properly positioned and secured with autopolymerizing acrylic resin. Access to the loops must be maintained. If the flange is too thin, shallow recesses can be cut and stainless steel wire loops secured with autopolymerizing acrylic resin. Grooves or holes are placed on the occlusal surfaces of the lower denture to facilitate circummandibular wiring. Anterior teeth should be removed for intake of food and liquids. Holes are drilled, several on each side of the flanges of the upper denture, to allow circumzygomatic wiring. With such modifications to the dentures, most patients will require new dentures after healing.

If the teeth are not made out of porcelain, a more expedient option is available. After the denture is repaired, an arch bar can be directly applied to the denture with loops of 26-gauge wire. Usually two sets of holes placed in the molar regions are sufficient to hold the wires, which are secured diagonally to the arch bar. In making the holes, the surgeon must be certain that the holes are not placed near the gingiva of the alveolus. A wire through this area can cause damage to the mucosa, and such wires should not be in contact with the jaw.

Application of Splint or Denture

a'–d' The methods for applying the splints and dentures are similar. For attachment to the mandible, a small incision through the skin is made beneath the jaw, and a passing awl or large needle is passed to the gingivolingual sulcus. A 24- or 25-gauge stainless steel wire is attached to the end of the awl. The instrument is then pulled down along the inside of the mandible, rotated around the mandible, and pushed out through the gingivobuccal sulcus. The wire is removed from the awl, pulled back and forth to seat on the mandible, and subsequently secured through the preformed hole or groove in the splint. The procedure is performed in an identical fashion on the opposite side of the jaw. One or two wires per side can be applied. The wires are then twisted, cut to size, and bent onto the external surface of the prosthesis.

e' For the upper denture or upper part of the splint, a passing awl is placed through a small stab incision made above the zygomatic arch and passed on the medial surface of the zygoma to the upper

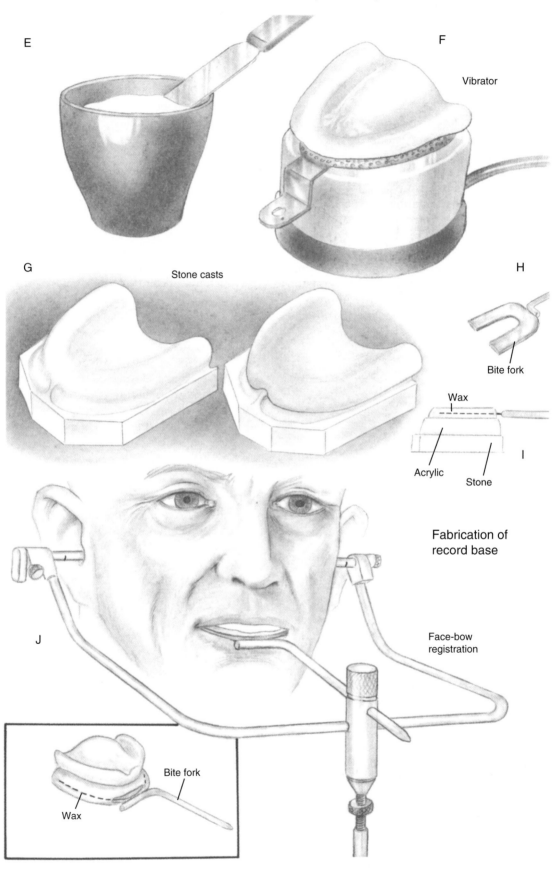

E

F

Vibrator

G

Stone casts

H

Bite fork

Wax

Acrylic

Stone

I

Fabrication of
record base

J

Face-bow
registration

Bite fork

Wax

SPLINT FABRICATION (Continued)

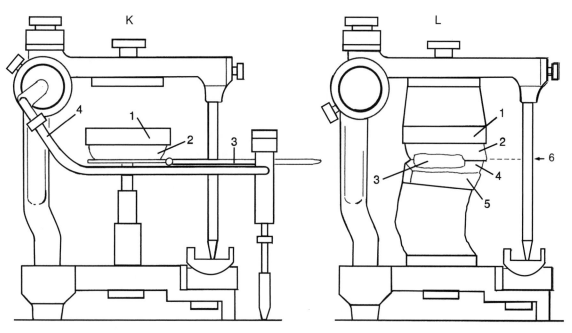

K

1- Maxillary cast
2- Record base with
   wax rim
3- Bite fork
4- Face bow

L

1- Maxillary cast   4- Wax rim
2- Wax rim   5- Record base
3- Wax registration   6- Incisal pin

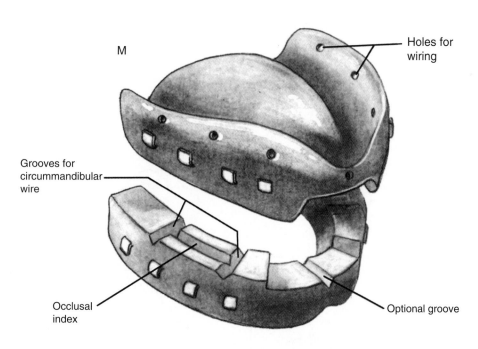

M

Holes for wiring

Grooves for
circummandibular
wire

Occlusal
index

Optional groove

Completed acrylic splint

DENTURE PREPARATION

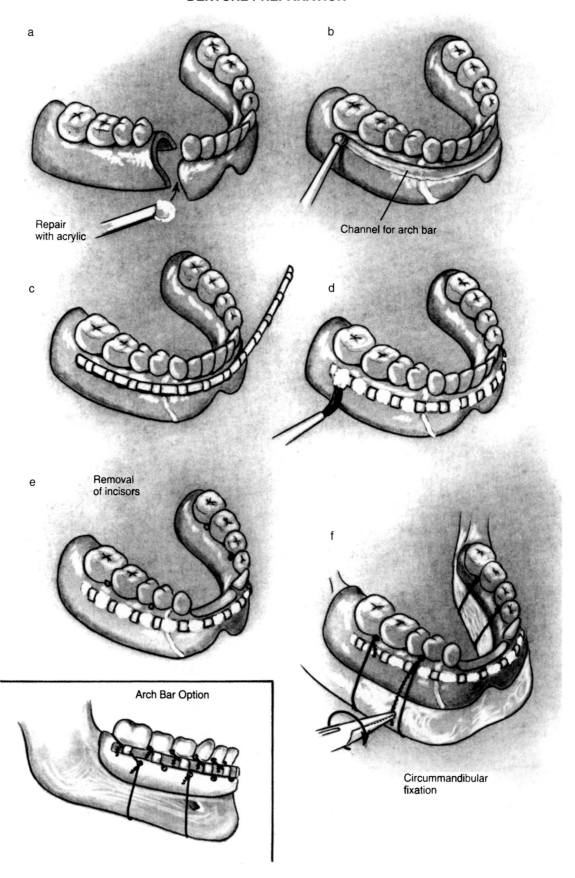

a

Repair
with acrylic

b

Channel for arch bar

c

d

e

Removal
of incisors

f

Arch Bar Option

Circummandibular
fixation

gingivobuccal sulcus near the area of the first molar. A 25- or 26-gauge wire is attached to the awl, and the awl is pulled to the level of the arch. At the superior border of the arch, the awl is rotated downward, lateral to the arch, carrying the wire into the oral/buccal cavity. Clamps are then placed on the wire, and with a sawing motion, the wire is seated as far anteriorly as possible on the zygoma.

f' The ends of the circumzygomatic wire are held with a clamp and twisted on each other to form a loop within the oral/buccal cavity. A second loop of 28-gauge wire is attached to the molar flanges, and the 25-gauge circumzygomatic wire is affixed through this loop.

g' Often circumzygomatic wires are sufficient to secure the prosthesis, but if the prosthesis or denture is loose, it is necessary to place additional drop wires in the region of the anterior nasal spine. For this procedure, a small incision is made in the gingivolabial sulcus through the frenulum, and the periosteum is elevated off the anterior nasal spine. A small hole is then made through the spine, and a 26-gauge wire is dropped through this hole and passed through holes in the anterior flange of the denture or splint. The splint is thus secured at three points to provide maximum fixation.

h' Another method of fixation to consider uses bone screws. For this technique, holes are strategically placed in the prosthesis so that the holes can be drilled through these holes into the palate and/or alveolus. Using a lag screw technique, screws are then applied through the prosthesis and into the bone pulling the prosthesis into a secure position with the palate and alveolus. Screw length should be sufficient to engage both cortices even if the screw should penetrate the nasal cavity or sinuses.

i' For fixation between splints or dentures, elastic bands can be applied to the arch bars (see Chapter 19). Occasionally Gunning splints are made as one unit composed of both upper and lower segments, but this limits options in adjustment and should be avoided.

Postoperative Care

Splints and dentures are kept as clean as possible by daily use of a soft toothbrush and/or a water irrigation device. Additional oral hygiene is effected by chlorhexidine oral rinses. Patients are maintained for 5 to 7 days on prophylactic antibiotics. Patients should be seen weekly to check occlusal relationships, fixation, and reduction. The period of fixation will depend on the age of the patient. Radiographic evaluation should be performed after reduction and prior to the removal of the prosthesis.

PITFALLS

1. The denture or splint can efface the surface of the mandible. This complication often results when there is a laceration or avulsion of the alveolar ridge. Occasionally the prosthesis does not fit properly and may cause an erosion. If this occurs, the prosthesis should be relined with tissue conditioner liner material.

2. For the prosthesis to fit firmly, the circummandibular and circumzygomatic wires must be placed appropriately. The circumzygomatic wires should be dropped as perpendicular as possible; for this to occur, they must be placed anteriorly on the zygomatic arch. The hook or hole for attachment to the upper prosthesis must also be sufficiently posterior to obtain the proper direction of pull of the wire. The anterior nasal spine is useful for providing anterior fixation, but if the anterior nasal spine is small, wires can be dropped from the piriform aperture. For the lower jaw attachment, circummandibular wires can be applied.

3. Check the prosthesis weekly to see if there is any pain or increased mobility of the prosthesis or denture. If increased mobility is noted, the wires should be tightened. Radiographs may be helpful in evaluating for bone healing.

4. The denture is often ruined during the procedure. Moreover, oral relationships will have changed, and for these reasons, patients may have to have a new set of dentures.

COMPLICATIONS

1. Erosion of mucosa with exposure of the mandible and resulting osteomyelitis is one of the most feared complications. If the patient complains of atypical pain, swelling, or redness around the jaw area, the prosthesis must be removed and the area inspected. This complication is prevented by a good fit of the prosthesis and a padding of gutta-percha or tissue conditioner material.

2. Because fixation of a splint or denture is not as tight as that using direct osseous methods, there is a possibility of developing a nonunion or malunion. If this occurs in the subcondylar area, a pseudarthrosis may cause minimal functional sequelae. Failure to heal in other parts of the jaw must be dealt with accordingly.

3. Nonunion (pseudarthrosis), ankylosis, and temporomandibular joint dysfunctions are potential complications. These conditions are addressed in Chapters 34 through 38.

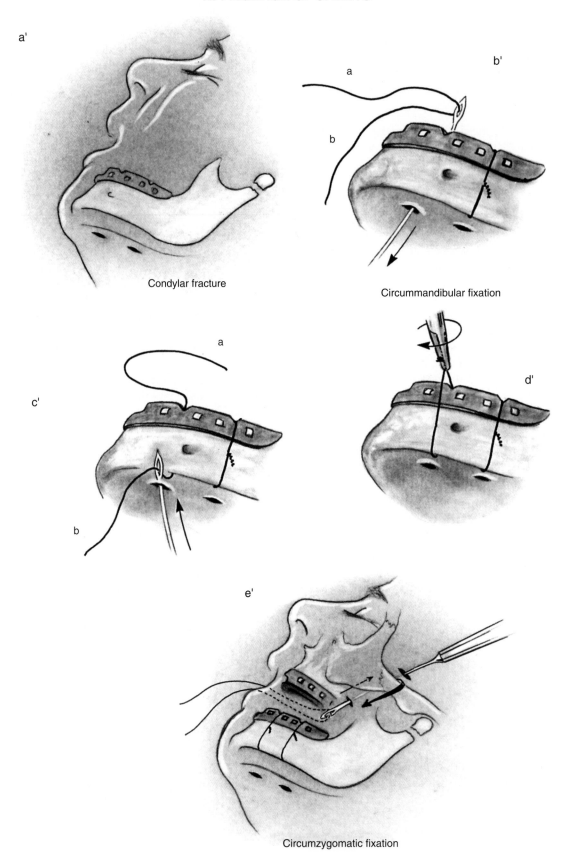

a'

Condylar fracture

b'

Circummandibular fixation

c'

a

b

d'

e'

Circumzygomatic fixation

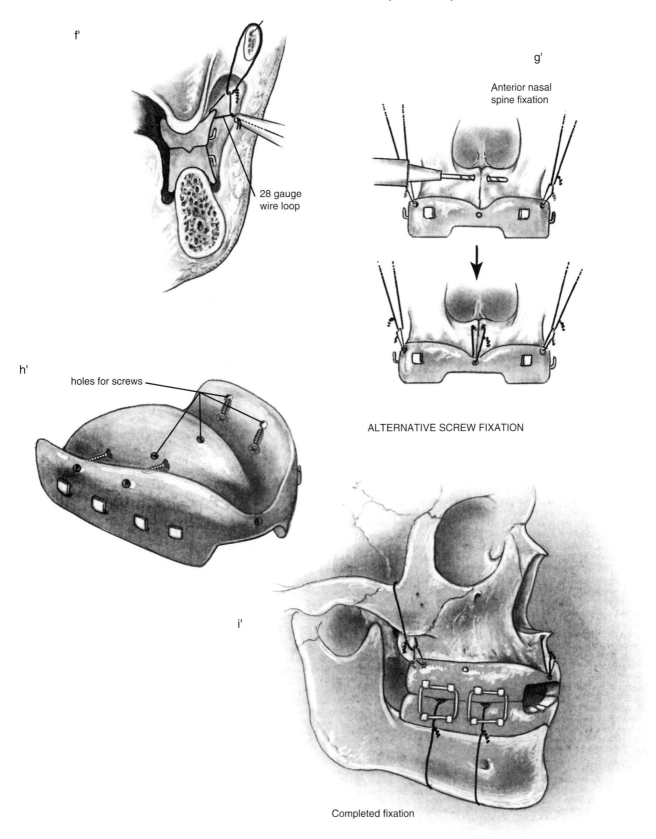

f'

28 gauge
wire loop

g'

Anterior nasal
spine fixation

ALTERNATIVE SCREW FIXATION

h'

holes for screws

i'

Completed fixation

Wm. Loechel

CHAPTER 21

Open Reduction of Condylar Fractures
Alternative Technique Using External Pin Fixation

INDICATIONS

Open reduction may be indicated in patients with severely injured and displaced condylar fractures and in patients with a combination of maxillary and condylar fractures. The technique should be considered when the condyle is displaced into the external auditory canal or middle fossa, also when it is subluxated almost completely in a medial direction at right angles to the neck or when it is displaced in the opposite direction, projecting laterally toward the zygoma. Exploration should be performed when there are foreign bodies, such as bullets or glass fragments, in or near the joint space. Open reduction should be considered when closed methods are unsuccessful in reduction of the fracture. This can occur especially in edentulous patients with bilateral condylar fractures or in patients with multiple ipsilateral fractures. Of the many methods that are available, miniplate or external pin fixation has the advantage of direct approximation of fragments with limited trauma to bone and soft tissue. Both methods provide for a relatively rigid fixation with mobility of the joint during the healing process. Endoscopic techniques have also been reported as a reasonable approach.

PROCEDURE

In preparation for open reduction of the condyle, the upper and lower jaws should be placed into optimal occlusal relationships. Downward digital pressure on the permanent molar region will help in the reduction process. In the dentulous patient, short-term or routine intermaxillary fixation should be obtained with intermaxillary screws, arch bars, or Ivy loops (see Chapter 19). In the edentulous patient, the relationships should be evaluated and the jaws manipulated into the best reduced position. The surgeon should also outline with a marking solution the angle of the jaw, the zygomatic arch, and the expected position of the facial nerve as it exits the stylomastoid foramen.

A The incision is made in a preauricular crease line from the lobule to the zygoma. If additional exposure is needed, the incision can be extended several centimeters upward and curved into the temporal hairline. Just anterior to the incision, the superficial temporal artery and vein will be evident, and to prevent troublesome bleeding, the vessels should be identified and ligated.

B–C The dissection should be performed in such a way as to avoid risk of injury to the main trunk and divisions of the facial nerve. The parotid gland should be separated from the tragus, carefully avoiding extension of the incision inferiorly beyond the "tragal pointer." The dissection should be continued upward to the periosteum of the zygomatic process of the temporal bone and extended no farther forward than a line drawn approximately one-half the distance from the tragus to the outer canthus of the eye. The periosteum of the zygoma can then be followed inferiorly, just anterior to the tympanic plate, to expose the capsule of the temporomandibular joint. The elevation of tissues should be extended to the neck of the condyle to expose the fracture site. Staying lateral to the condyle should avoid damage to the middle meningeal, deep auricular, and anterior tympanic arteries, which are on the deep aspect of the bone.

D–E If the fracture is not already reduced, the condyle should be grasped with a Kocher clamp, reduced and held securely in the proper position. Occasionally a small incision is necessary below the angle of the mandible to expose the angle which is subsequently grasped with a clamp or secured with a wire and pulled downward. When reduction is achieved, a small four hole miniplate is placed over the fracture and the holes drilled with an appropriate instrument. Screws are then used to secure the plate.

PITFALLS

1. The open technique should be avoided in patients with fractures confined to the intracapsular head of the condyle. This type of injury is made worse by opening the capsule and growth centers within the area can be adversely affected.

2. To avoid injury to the facial nerve, the surgeon must understand the location of the nerve and its branches. The nerve exits the stylomastoid foramen, which will be several centimeters deep to the tragal pointer. The branch going to the forehead travels across the zygomatic arch between the lateral canthus of the eye and midportion of the arch. Thus by keeping the dissection posterior to the middle portion of the arch and above the tragal pointer, the nerve can be protected.

3. A dissection deep to the condylar neck can injure branches of the maxillary artery, and fairly brisk bleeding may occur. This problem can be avoided by elevating only those tissues that are lateral to the condyle. If the surgeon must work on the deep aspect of the condyle, the dissection should be performed subperiosteally.

4. At least two screws inserted into the distal and proximal segments of the condyle are necessary for stabilization. If only one screw is used, the fragments will tend to rotate. The screw will also become loose and be separated from the bone.

COMPLICATIONS

1. Nonunion is possible, especially if the screws and plate are displaced from their original position. If this is suspected either clinically or radiographically in the postoperative period, the surgeon can reoperate and reinsert the screws/plate; removal of the fixation and acceptance of the nonunion or pseudarthrosis can also be considered.

2. Infection of the fracture site is a possibility, but the fracture usually heals with conservative measures (i.e., antibiotics, drainage, and continued immobilization).

3. Facial nerve injury is an uncommon sequela. If damage is suspected as a result of blunt injury (e.g., pressure from a retractor), then watchful waiting is encouraged. However, if disruption of the nerve is suspected and confirmed by neurodiagnostic testing, the nerve must be explored and repair accomplished (see Chapter 14).

ALTERNATIVE TECHNIQUE USING EXTERNAL PIN FIXATION

a–d An alternative technique for open reduction and fixation of condylar fractures is external pin fixation (see also Chapter 34). The exposure is the same as that obtained using the reduction and miniplate fixation described earlier. A small incision is then made through the skin just lateral to the area selected for fixation. A threaded Kirschner (Steinmann) pin, 5/64 inch in diameter is placed through the incision and drilled into the neck of the condyle with a K-wire minidriver. In most patients a second pin can be applied through a separate incision. Biphase pins are subsequently applied in a standard fashion to the other fragments of the jaw. All pins are secured with an acrylic bar. At least two pins must be placed in each fragment to prevent rotation. The reduction is then visualized and a piece of acrylic prepared to cover the pins. The acrylic is made by mixing a liquid with a powdered mixture until it becomes the consistency of putty. Acrylic is then molded to resemble a rod or cigar and then placed over the tops of the pins. The acrylic and pins are held into position until the acrylic has hardened. Kirschner pins, being relatively sharp can catch on objects and cause damage to the patient. Thus these pins should be bent over or covered with a piece of cork or vacuum container tube tops. Avoid undue pressure on the pins. Patients should be reminded not to sleep on the pin side and to avoid any physical contact sports. Pins may be associated with leakage of saliva but this usually will stop when the pins are removed. Scars from pins are usually not noticeable, but if they are conspicuous, scar revision should be considered (see Chapter 13).

OPEN REDUCTION OF CONDYLAR FRACTURES

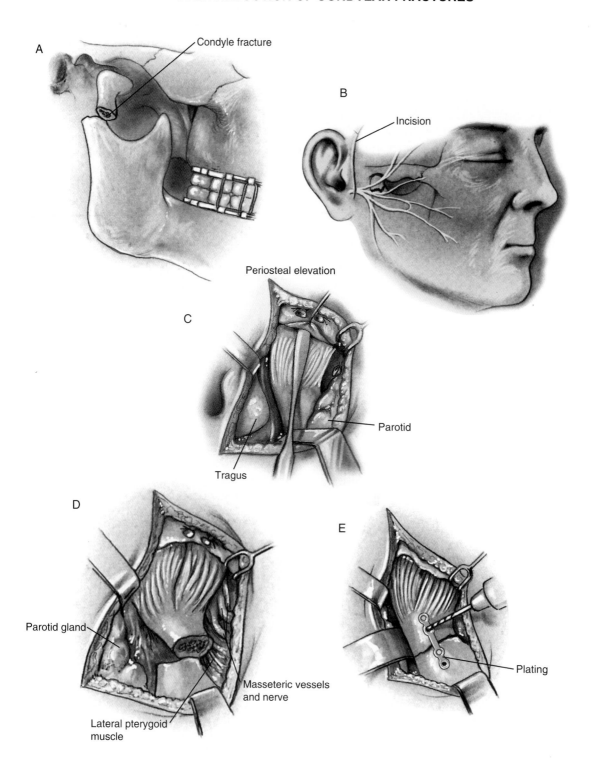

A

Condyle fracture

B

Incision

Periosteal elevation

C

Parotid

Tragus

D

Parotid gland

Masseteric vessels
and nerve

Lateral pterygoid
muscle

E

Plating

ALTERNATIVE TECHNIQUE USING
EXTERNAL PIN FIXATION

a

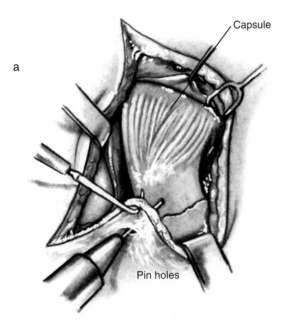

Capsule

Pin holes

b

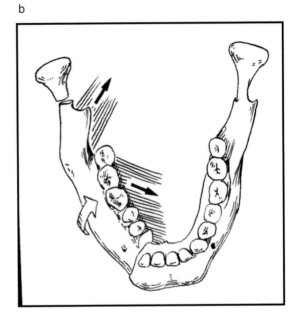

c

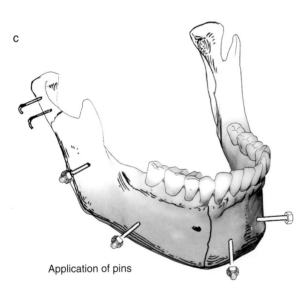

Application of pins

d

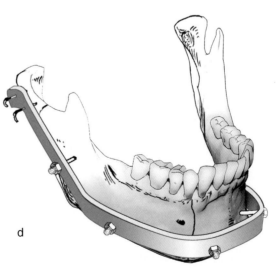

Completed biphase fixation

Coronoid Fractures

CHAPTER

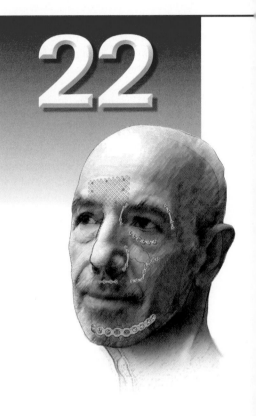

Closed and Open Treatment of Coronoid Fractures
Alternative Technique of Coronoidectomy

INDICATIONS

Coronoid fractures are extremely rare. They often produce minimal symptomatology and can be easily missed on radiographic evaluation. Usually there is transient pain and swelling, but if the coronoid is displaced and comes in contact with the zygoma, limitation of jaw movement can result. Most coronoid fractures can be managed with close observation. Fractures characterized by displacement and/or continuation of pain should be treated with intermaxillary fixation.

PROCEDURE

Intermaxillary screws, Erich arch bars, or Ivy loops can be used for the fixation. The procedure can be performed using general anesthesia and nasotracheal intubation or local anesthesia with sedation. The methods for applying the intermaxillary screws, arch bars, or Ivy loops are described in Chapter 19.

A The jaws can be held together with either elastic bands or loops of 28-gauge stainless steel wire. A postoperative radiograph should be obtained at 10 days, and fixation should be maintained for 6 weeks. Examinations should be carried out weekly for displacement of bars and/or breaks in the fixation devices. Dental hygiene is maintained with gentle brushing and/or with a water irrigation device.

B Intermaxillary fixation is removed at 6 weeks. The patient is then tested, and if there are no problems, the fixation can be removed. Active exercise with application of tongue blades or a dynamic spreader device between the incisors will help expand the interincisor distances.

PITFALLS

1. Following fixation, the position of the coronoid should be improved. If radiographs do not confirm reduction of the fracture, it may be necessary to perform an open reduction. Removal of the coronoid (see later) may be warranted and is more easily performed than a direct wiring procedure.

2. Following removal of intermaxillary fixation, there will be some limitation of jaw movement. Active exercises are encouraged. The tongue blade technique, in which the jaws are pried open with an increasing number of tongue blades between the incisors, is helpful. Dynamic spreader devices are available.

3. Coronoid fractures are rare, but when they do occur, they are often associated with zygomatic and maxillary fractures. This relationship can predispose to a malposition of the fragments and ankylosis. To prevent this from occurring, all facial fractures must be recognized and treated appropriately.

4. The edentulous patient with a coronoid fracture usually can be treated with a soft diet and analgesics. However, if a closed reduction becomes necessary, then application of dentures, splints, and intermaxillary fixation must be considered. These techniques are described in Chapter 20. Postoperative care is similar to that used in the treatment of other types of mandibular fractures.

COMPLICATIONS

1. Malunion with fixation to the zygoma is a debilitating complication. If this develops early, it is possible that the jaw can be opened with tongue blades interposed between the incisors or with dynamic spreader devices and 40 mg/mL of triamcinolone injected into the coronoid/ramus area. If this technique is not successful, a coronoidectomy should be performed.

2. Malunion of the coronoid can also cause problems with denture placement. Projections of the coronoid should be shaved transorally and the denture refitted for proper occlusion.

ALTERNATIVE TECHNIQUE OF CORONOIDECTOMY

a,b A transoral open approach to the coronoid process is a direct, simple method to treat malunion of the coronoid process or a marked displacement of the coronoid fracture. Usually the procedure is performed using general anesthesia. To control bleeding, the coronoid/ascending ramus area should be infiltrated with 1% or 2% lidocaine containing 1:100,000 epinephrine. Exposure is obtained by placing an interocclusal bite block on the opposite side. The coronoid can usually be palpated with the mouth open, and an incision is then made over the prominence of this process and the adjoining ramus. A Joseph elevator is used to elevate the periosteum and the attachment of the temporalis muscle. The coronoid is then removed piecemeal with bone-cutting rongeurs. The bite block is removed, and jaw mobility is tested. The incision is subsequently closed with several 2-0 chromic sutures.

Postoperatively the patient is treated with a 3- to 5-day course of antibiotics. For the first day, the patient is given liquids; then the diet is advanced as tolerated. The patient should be evaluated for contracture in the area of surgery, and if this occurs, intralesional steroids should be injected and jaw-opening exercises instituted.

TREATMENT OF CORONOID FRACTURES

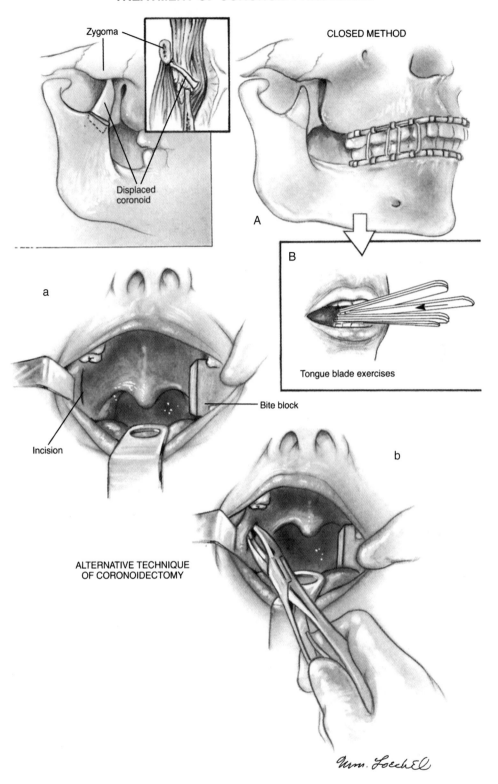

Zygoma

Displaced coronoid

CLOSED METHOD

A

B

Tongue blade exercises

a

Incision

Bite block

b

ALTERNATIVE TECHNIQUE OF CORONOIDECTOMY

Wm. Loechel

Ascending Ramus Fractures

CHAPTER

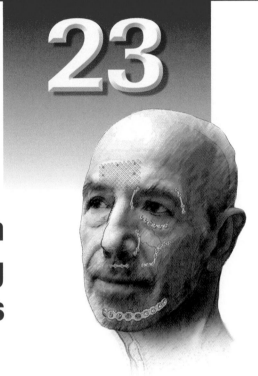

23

Closed and Open Treatment of Ascending Ramus Fractures

INDICATIONS

Fractures isolated to the ramus of the mandible are uncommon. The ramus is protected by the zygoma and by a "sling" of the pterygoid and masseter muscles. Moreover, displacement of the fracture fragments is usually minimal, and the majority of the fractures can be managed by closed techniques. An open method is necessary only if there are multiple fragments or marked displacement of the fragments.

PROCEDURE

The ramus fracture is traditionally treated by intermaxillary fixation with intermaxillary screws, Erich arch bars, or Ivy loops. The technique is identical to that described for the condylar fracture (see Chapter 19).

A If the ramus must be opened for fixation, the same exposure applicable to the angle fracture should be used (see Chapters 24 and 25). The technique is modified by elevating the periosteum of the mandible to a higher level. The fracture can then be easily stabilized

by a single plate (compression or noncompression) across the fracture line.

B For intermaxillary fixation without plating, the jaws are held together with elastic bands or loops of 28-gauge wire. Antibiotics are administered for 5 days. Fixation is checked radiographically, and dental health is maintained by appropriate prophylaxis. Intermaxillary fixation can be removed at 6 weeks.

PITFALLS

1. Intermaxillary fixation often reduces the ramus fracture and provides sufficient fixation for satisfactory healing. If there is displacement of the fragments on a postoperative radiograph, then an open method must be considered.

2. Comminuted ramus fractures in dentulous patients are ideally treated with intermaxillary fixation. However, if the patient is edentulous, other methods must be considered (see Chapter 20). Marked comminution can be managed by open techniques (see Chapters 24 and 25)

TREATMENT OF RAMUS FRACTURE

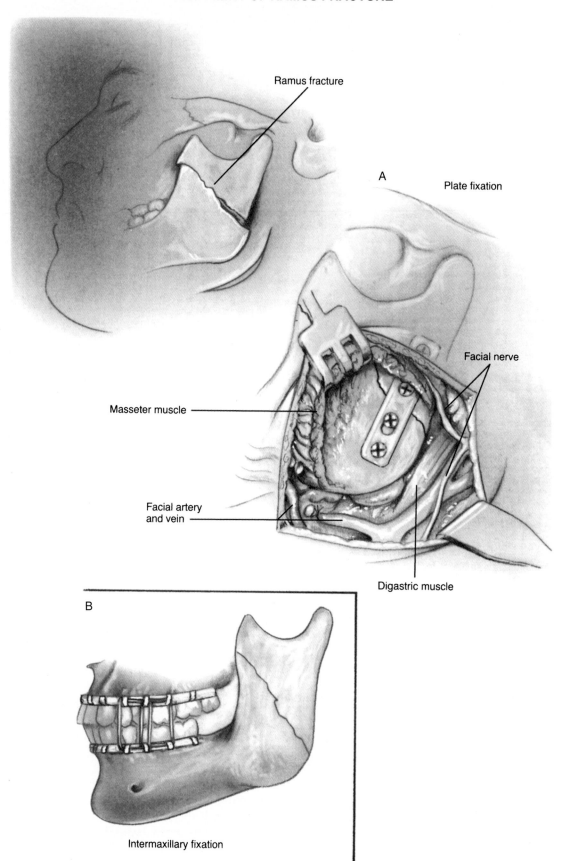

Ramus fracture

A

Plate fixation

Masseter muscle

Facial nerve

Facial artery
and vein

Digastric muscle

B

Intermaxillary fixation

Mandibular Angle Fractures

CHAPTER

24

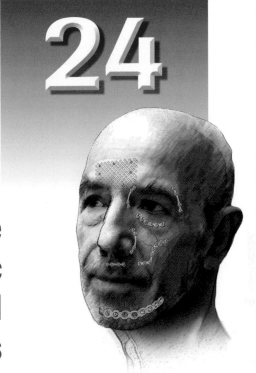

Open Reduction of Angle Fractures Using Dynamic Compression Internal Rigid Plating Systems
Alternative Techniques Using Tension Bands, Noncompression Plates, Miniplates, and Lag Screws

INDICATIONS

The rigid plating technique has become one of the more popular methods for open reduction and fixation of angle fractures. It is particularly useful for edentulous patients with unfavorable lines of fracture and/or multiple fractures. The method is also applicable when there is limited comminution of fragments such that the small pieces of bone can be wedged between solid pieces of ramus and body. A major advantage of the technique is that it provides for early oral intake (especially helpful in elderly and/or debilitated patients), and for early mobilization of the condyle, to avoid ankylosis.

PROCEDURE

A Ideally, dental occlusion and normal jaw relationships should be obtained through intermaxillary screws, temporary arch bars, or Ivy loop fixation (see Chapter 19). A 5-cm curvilinear incision in a crease line is marked at two to three finger breadths below the angle of the mandible. The line is injected with 1% lidocaine containing 1:100,000 epinephrine. The surgeon should wait 10 minutes for maximal vasoconstriction.

B The dissection is carried through the subcutaneous tissues and platysma to the superficial fascia. Just anterior to the sternocleidomastoid muscle, the surgeon should identify the cervical branch of the facial nerve. More superiorly, the marginal mandibular branch of the facial nerve can be noted and preserved. A helpful technique is to identify a branch of the anterior or posterior facial vein system. Because the marginal branch lies superficial to these structures, elevation of the vein during the superior dissection should theoretically protect the structure.

C,D The fascia overlying the submandibular gland is incised inferior to the marginal mandibular nerve, and the dissection is continued beneath the fascia toward the lower margin of the angle of the mandible. The periosteum is stripped on the inferior and outer surfaces of the mandible to demonstrate the fracture line. The masseter muscle is elevated with the periosteum, helping to relieve some of the forces displacing the posterior fragment. The fracture is reduced with small Lane or Dingman bone clamps.

E A 2.4 compression plate with at least four holes is then fitted so that two holes are placed to each side of the fracture. The plate should be oriented perpendicular to the fracture at least 5 to 7 mm above the inferior border of the mandible and held into position either manually or with a special plate holder. Depending on the line of the fracture, curved or straight plates can be used. It is important that the plate have the same contour as the surface of the mandible. This can be achieved with bending clamps or if necessary, the initial bending of a template followed by the bending of the mandibular plate.

The compression plate is secured by drilling a hole at the outer edge of the eccentric compression hole with a 2.1-mm-diameter drill bit. The hole should encompass both cortices. Protection of soft tissues is achieved with an inferiorly placed malleable retractor.

F The depth of the drill hole is measured with a special device, and a screw of appropriate length, held with a screw holder, is then inserted. The screw is tightened just enough to hold the plate in approximate position.

G Attention is then turned to the opposite fragment, and the procedure is repeated, with application of the screw to the outside of the other inner eccentric compression hole. Both screws are tightened completely so that compression is obtained on the fragments. Application of two additional screws, placed through the holes at the outer portion of the plate, stabilizes the system (fixation screws). If one of the screw holes should be stripped during the procedure, the screw can be replaced with a larger diameter screw.

H The periosteum is approximated over the fracture site with several 3-0 chromic sutures. The platysma is closed with an absorbable suture and the skin with a nonabsorbable suture. If the wound is not dry, drains should be placed and utilized for 24 to 48 hours. The patient is placed on prophylactic antibiotics for 5 to 7 days and encouraged to use a soft diet. Postreduction radiographs are obtained, with weekly follow-up maintained for 6 to 8 weeks.

PITFALLS

1. Severe comminution can prevent secure placement of screws. In such cases, a longer plate should be used with a longer incision. If the patient has teeth and the bone comminution is extensive, the surgeon should consider the possibility of intermaxillary fixation. The mandibular reconstruction plate may also be used (see Chapter 27).

2. Infection can have a serious detrimental effect on healing. Open reduction and fixation with plating techniques should be delayed until infection is brought under control.

3. Over- or undercompression can cause displacement of the fragments from each other. If this occurs, the plate should be reapplied in a new position. If the condition cannot be corrected, the physician must consider relocation of the plate with a simple tension band at the alveolar margin (see later discussion).

4. An oblique fracture can cause the compression screw to push away the deeper segment. In such a situation, the physician should change the position of the plate or consider the lag screw technique described later.

COMPLICATIONS

1. The compression plate technique is "unforgiving." If the mandible is placed in an inaccurate position, malunion will result.

2. Screws can penetrate the inferior alveolar nerve and cause pain and hypoesthesia. If such a situation develops, the screws and plate must be removed.

3. Some plates are associated with increased sensitivity, especially when exposed to cold temperatures. When the bone is sufficiently healed, the plates should be removed.

PLATING OF ANGLE FRACTURES

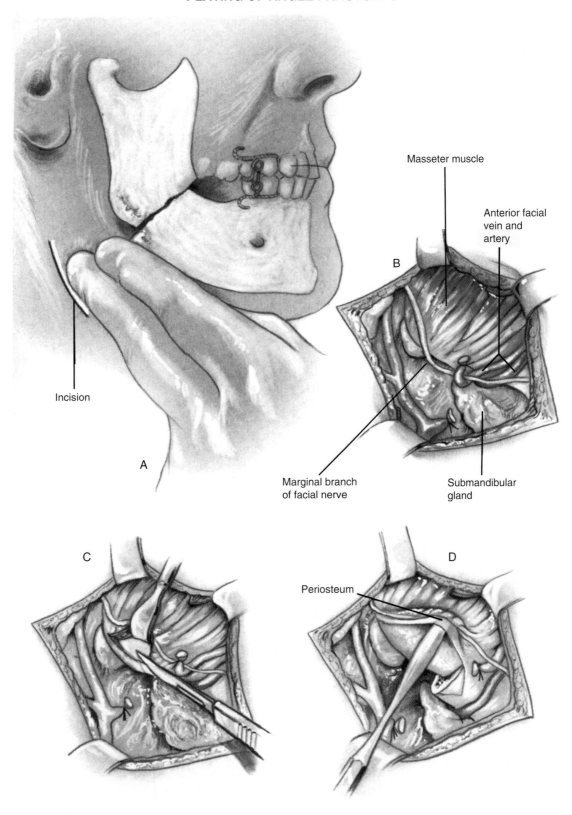

Incision

A

B

Masseter muscle

Anterior facial
vein and
artery

Marginal branch
of facial nerve

Submandibular
gland

C

D

Periosteum

Elevation of masseter muscle

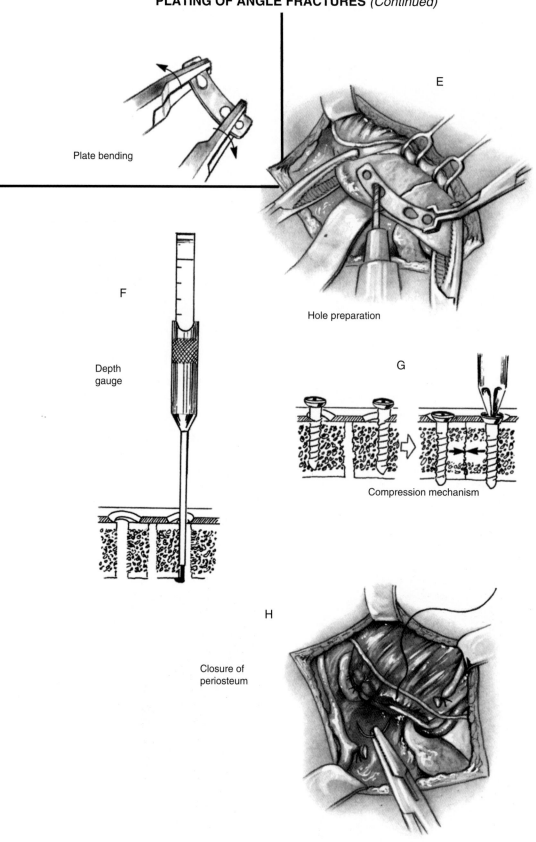

Plate bending

E

Hole preparation

F

Depth
gauge

G

Compression mechanism

H

Closure of
periosteum

Wm. Loechel

4. As with all fractures, infections can occur. Adequate drainage, antibiotics, and removal of devitalized teeth should encourage healing. If the infection does not respond to these maneuvers, debridement, removal of the plate, and external fixation must be considered.

ALTERNATIVE TECHNIQUES USING TENSION BANDS, NONCOMPRESSION PLATES, MINIPLATES, AND LAG SCREWS

Other options are available for stabilizing angle and other mandible fractures.

a Compression plates as described above may on occasion distract the upper portion of the fracture line. If this occurs, the procedure should be stopped, a tension band applied, and the compression reapplied. This tension band can be a four or two hole mini plate, or if teeth are available an arch bar applied across the area of fracture. The compression plate is again applied as described above observing the upper edge of the fracture line for dislocation.

b Noncompression plates, in which all screw holes are neutral, can also be applied to the lower portion of the mandible. In this situation, healing will occur by secondary intention but should still be effective.

c Two miniplates can also be placed across a fracture line on the mandible: one superiorly and one inferiorly carefully avoiding the inferior alveolar nerve and artery.

d The lag screw technique can be useful for the oblique horizontally directed fractures. First, the outer segment of bone is drilled with a 2.7 mm drill. The hole should be accurate, and to avoid wobbling, a drill guide should be used. The drill bit will jerk as it penetrates the inner cortex; at this point drilling should be stopped. Subsequently a 2-mm drill bit is applied, again with a guide, and a hole is made through the inner cortex. The deep hole is then tapped. A gauge is used to measure the depth, and a screw slightly larger than 2 mm is applied. Tightening the screw forces the outer fragment against the head; the deep fragment is then brought up into contact with the outer fragment.

The same technique is useful when applying a rigid plate to oblique fractures. If one is not careful, the bicortical screw will push the deeper segment away from the outer segment, and to prevent this from occurring, the outer segment hole must be made with a drill diameter larger than used in the deeper segment. The applied screw will then pull the segments together as well as the plate against the outer cortex.

TREATMENT OF ANGLE FRACTURES

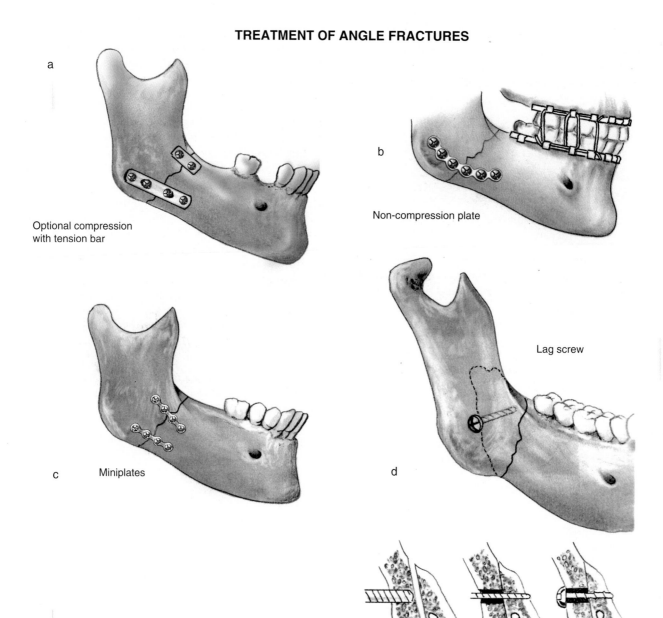

a

Optional compression
with tension bar

b

Non-compression plate

c   Miniplates

d

Lag screw

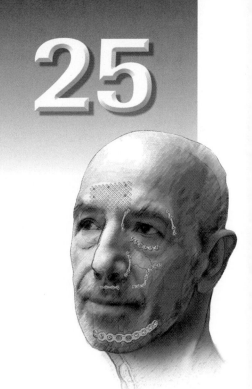

Open Intraoral Approach for Angle Fractures Using Rigid Plate Fixation
Alternative Techniques Using Champy Miniplate Fixation

INDICATIONS

The intraoral approach may be indicated when it is important to avoid external scars and potential injury to the marginal mandibular nerve. The technique is also useful when the surgeon must remove a molar tooth from the fracture site and, in doing so, essentially perform the elevation of the periosteum required for the exposure of the fracture. On the other hand, the method provides limited exposure and requires special instrumentation.

PROCEDURE

A Fractures should be manually reduced to achieve normal occlusal relationships. The angle fracture can be exposed while the jaws are in intermaxillary fixation, but better exposure can be obtained by taking the patient out of intermaxillary fixation and applying a medium-sized bite block to the opposite side.

The alveolus is infiltrated with 1% lidocaine containing 1:100,000 epinephrine. An incision is then carried out along the oblique ridge of the mandible and extended into the buccal sulcus near the second molar. The periosteum is elevated off the side of the mandible to expose the fracture.

B–D A four hole rigid fixation plate is then bent to accommodate the anatomy of the inferior border and held in position while screws are applied. The plate should be placed as close as possible to the inferior border of the mandible to avoid injury to the inferior alveolar nerve. A stab incision is made externally just posterior to the area of fracture. The tissues are spread bluntly in the direction of the facial nerve with a small clamp. Exposure is facilitated by a nasal speculum. A special drill guide is inserted, and a hole is created through both cortices just posterior to the fracture line. The screw hole depth is then measured, and with the screw driver placed externally, the appropriate size screws are placed through the plate holes. Alternatively, the drill hole can be made with a dental offset drill and screws placed directly with downward traction on cheek tissues. Also it is possible with a longer incision and retraction of cheek tissues to obtain exposure for a direct approach.

Following fixation of the fragments and intermaxillary fixation, the periosteum is closed with 3-0 chromic sutures. The patient is treated for 5 days with prophylactic antibiotics and a radiograph is obtained to verify reduction. Dental hygiene can be maintained with frequent brushings or applications of a water irrigation device. The patient is evaluated

INTRAORAL APPROACH FOR ANGLE FRACTURE

Transcutaneous Approach

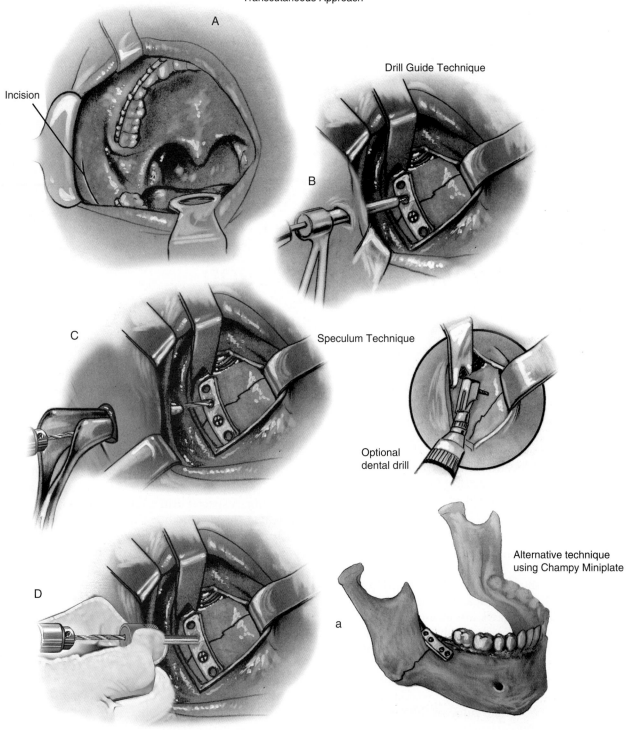

A

Incision

Drill Guide Technique

B

C

Speculum Technique

Optional
dental drill

D

Direct Approach

Alternative technique
using Champy Miniplate

a

weekly, and when there is clinical stability, the arch bars can be removed.

PITFALLS

1. The exposure provided with this technique is not as good as that obtained with an external approach. Moreover, it may be difficult to achieve fixation. If there is still some question of the reduction and fixation, the surgeon should proceed to an external approach (see Chapter 24).

2. The intraoral method should be avoided in patients with comminuted and multiple fractures. Other techniques, such as biphase, mesh, or reconstruction plate, provide much better stability and are more suited for these conditions (see later).

3. Splints or dentures should be avoided. These can wear against the incision and cause subsequent chronic contamination and osteomyelitis. The technique thus becomes limited when it is applied to the edentulous patient.

COMPLICATIONS

1. Malunion can occur with the transoral approach, especially if there are inadequate reduction and fixation of the fracture. Treatment for malunion is described in Chapters 34 and 37.

2. Nonunion can occur following treatment of any mandible fracture. Once recognized, infection must be brought under control and devitalized bone removed from the fracture site. Usually another fixation method, such as a biphase apparatus, is required. Defects of the bone are corrected by the techniques described in Chapters 34 to 36.

3. Hypoesthesia and paresthesia are potential problems, especially if a plate screw is placed too close to the inferior alveolar nerve. By keeping the plate near the alveolus or near the lower border of the mandible, these complications can be avoided.

ALTERNATIVE TECHNIQUE USING CHAMPY MINIPLATE FIXATION

Another alternative is the noncompression miniplate. This plate utilizes a different principle, reinforcing lines of tension and distraction along the mandible. For this technique, a plate is applied subapically and medially to the oblique line of the mandible. This position provides a biomechanical advantage and prevents diastasis of the alveolus. The monocortical screws can be placed over the alveolar canal without injuring the nerve. The plates are usually 0.9 mm thick and 6 mm wide, with screw holes of 2.1 mm diameter. The core of the self-tapping screw is 1.6 mm. Usually one plate is sufficient; however, if stability is not sufficient, another plate can be applied more laterally and inferiorly to provide additional support.

Body Fractures

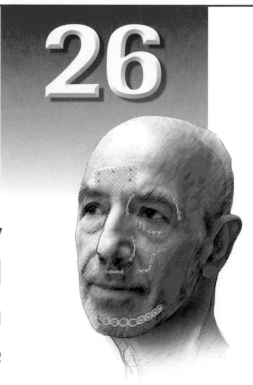

Open Reduction of Body Fractures Using Internal Rigid Plate Fixation
Alternative Technique Using Intraoral Reduction and Fixation

INDICATIONS

Internal rigid fixation is one of the most popular methods to treat unstable fractures of the body of the mandible, particularly when there are edentulous segments and/or multiple fractures. The technique is suitable for the edentulous patient with bilateral mandibular body fractures or body and parasymphyseal fractures of the contralateral or ipsilateral side. The rigid plate can also be used to cross over and stabilize small defects. An important advantage of this method is that it achieves early mobilization of the jaw, which is important for rapid restoration of masticatory, swallowing, and speech functions.

PROCEDURE

A–C Anesthesia is usually obtained with nasotracheal intubation. Ideally a temporary occlusal relationship is achieved by bringing opposing pairs of teeth together with intermaxillary fixation screws, Ivy loops, or intermaxillary arch bar fixation. If the jaws are edentulous, occlusion can be approximated by a manipulation of the fractures into appropriate intermaxillary relationships.

The mandibular body fracture is approached by a curvilinear incision of approximately 8 to 9 cm in a neck crease two to three finger breadths below the middle of the jaw. The incision should be centered

OPEN REDUCTION AND FIXATION OF BODY FRACTURE

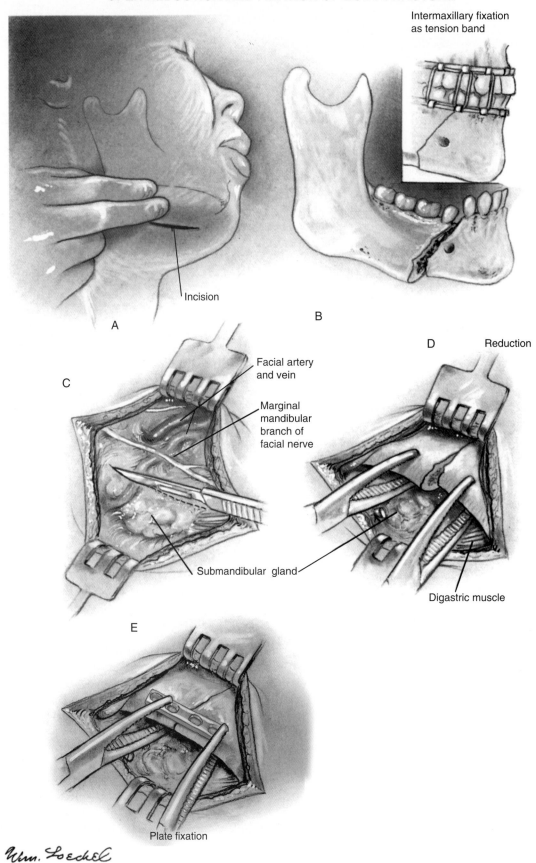

Intermaxillary fixation as tension band

Incision

A

B

C

Facial artery and vein

Marginal mandibular branch of facial nerve

Submandibular gland

D   Reduction

Digastric muscle

E

Plate fixation

approximately at the level of the inferior border of the submaxillary gland. The area is infiltrated with 1% lidocaine containing 1:100,000 epinephrine. The surgeon should wait 10 minutes to achieve maximal vasoconstrictive effects.

The incision is carried through the skin, subcutaneous tissues, and platysma to the superficial layer of fascia. While spreading the fascia with a hemostat, the surgeon should try to define the marginal mandibular branch of the facial nerve. At this level the nerve is near the inferior border of the mandible but can be retracted into the upper neck if the neck is overextended. Because the nerve often lies lateral to the anterior facial artery and vein (at the inferior border of the mandible), it is possible to ligate these vessels external to the submaxillary gland and, by lifting the fascia associated with these vessels, safely retract the nerve upward.

The dissection should be just external to the fascia covering the submaxillary gland. Working cephalad, the surgeon should identify the inferior border of the mandible and its periosteal covering. The periosteum is then incised and elevated to show the fracture site and the area that will be covered by the plate.

D,E The fracture is reduced and fragments are mobilized with bone holding clamps or forceps. A four-hole dynamic compression plate is fitted by bending the plate with a curvature that approximates the outer cortex of the mandible. A holding forceps holds the plate firmly over the area of fracture.

F A malleable retractor is then slipped beneath the mandible for protection of soft tissues. One of the oblique holes next to the fracture site is selected, and an appropriate size drill bit is used, with a drill guide, to create a hole. The drill guide with arrows should be pointing toward the fracture site.

G,H A depth gauge will determine the appropriate length of screw needed so that the screw will engage both lateral and medial cortices. The screw is then loosely applied. A second drill hole is drilled on the opposite side of the fracture closest to the fracture, and again, a screw is loosely placed into position. The plate holder can be removed and the screws tightened down to compress the fracture fragments. The outermost screw holes are then drilled with the holes in neutral position, the arrows should be pointing upward toward the alveolus. The two outer screws are placed and secured.

The wound over the plate is closed in layers. First the periosteum is closed with interrupted 2-0 or 3-0 chromic sutures. The platysma is approximated with 4-0 chromic sutures. Excellent hemostasis should

preclude the use of drains. The skin is coapted with a running 5-0 nylon suture. The patient is placed on a 5- to 7-day course of prophylactic antibiotics and advanced to a soft diet. A radiograph is obtained to check reduction. The patient should be followed weekly for 6 to 8 weeks.

PITFALLS

1. The plate technique should be avoided in young children, in whom there is a potential for injury to the developing dentition. If the patient has an atrophic jaw and the plate occupies the height of the fragment, a smaller compression plate must be considered.

2. Plate bending must be exact. If the plate is not bent enough, the inner cortex will be retracted as the screws engage the bone. Overbending will have the effect of compressing the opposite cortex.

3. Screw holes that are stripped present a problem. One option is to remove the plate and drill new holes at a different level. Another alternative is to employ a larger bore emergency screw. This screw, placed in the same hole, will usually provide sufficient stability to the plate.

4. If a four-hole dynamic compression plate does not provide rigid fixation, the surgeon should consider a dynamic compression plate and tension band or a larger reconstruction plate (see Chapter 27).

5. Do not injure the inferior alveolar nerve or unerupted teeth. This complication can be avoided by placing the plate within 1 to 2 cm of the inferior border of the mandible.

6. Often the screws of the compression plate will not fix small fragments. If there are areas of extensive comminution, it is better to use a reconstruction plate, titanium mesh, or a biphase apparatus (see Chapters 28 and 34).

COMPLICATIONS

1. Malunion can occur if the plate is improperly placed and the jaw heals in an abnormal position. This complication can be avoided by bringing the jaws into the proper occlusal relationships prior to fixation. In the edentulous patient, minor discrepancies can be corrected by modifications in denture fabrication. In the dentulous patient, the surgeon can consider occlusal adjustment at the surface of the teeth. Last, there is always the possibility of osteotomy and reconstruction of the mandible (see Chapter 37).

2. Osteomyelitis can occur at the site of the fracture and must be recognized and managed appropriately. The area of infection must be debrided of foreign

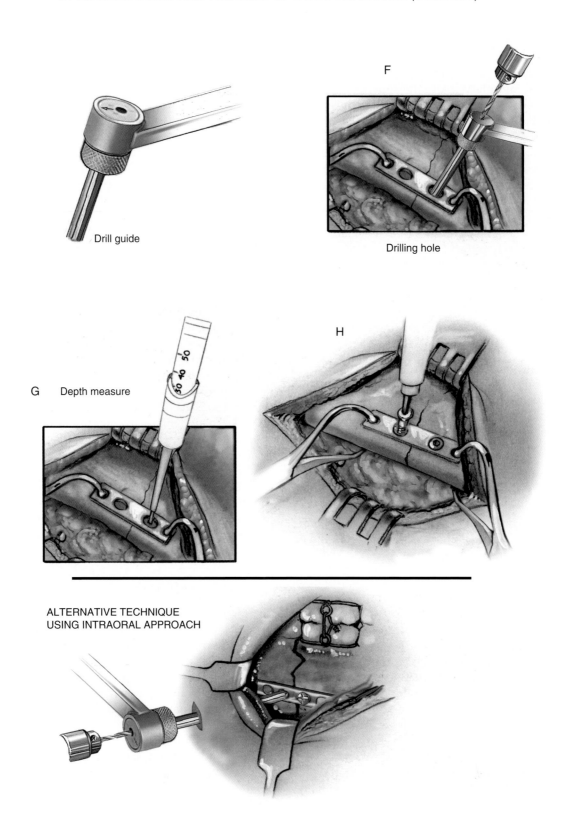

Drill guide

F

Drilling hole

G   Depth measure

H

ALTERNATIVE TECHNIQUE
USING INTRAORAL APPROACH

bodies, and the offending pathogens should be identified and treated with intravenous antibiotics. Plate fixation can continue, but if the infection does not come under control, the plate should be removed and the fracture immobilized with an occlusal splint or external biphase apparatus.

3. Nonunion is uncommon (incidence <2%), but if it occurs, the plate should be removed, the edges of the fragments debrided, and the plate reapplied for rigid fixation. Defects of the mandible must be treated with a bone-grafting technique (see Chapters 34 to 36).

4. The plate may be palpable and noticeable in the thin-skinned individual. It may also project intraorally, affecting the fit of the denture. If this occurs, the plate can be removed through the original exposure several months later. Some patients complain of pain in the area, and if there are no other causes for the pain (e.g., infection, nonunion), the plate should also be removed.

5. Injury to the marginal mandibular nerve is possible and can be avoided by knowledge of the anatomy of the area and an atraumatic dissection technique. Considering that repair of the nerve is difficult and often unsuccessful, conservative management is a more prudent course.

ALTERNATIVE TECHNIQUE USING INTRAORAL REDUCTION AND FIXATION

A rigid fixation plate can also be applied intraorally. This technique requires adjustment of the jaw into occlusal relationships, some type of temporary intermaxillary fixation, and manual reduction of the fragments. The intraoral approach precludes the use of reduction forceps. Similar methods are described in Chapter 25 for the treatment of the mandibular angle fracture.

An incision is made 5 to 7 mm below the gingiva through the gingivobuccal sulcus, and the periosteum is elevated toward the inferior border of the mandible. The plate is then bent into an appropriate position and drill holes are placed. For this portion of the technique, the surgeon can use offset drills or small stab incisions made over the approximate area of the hole. The tissues can then be spread in the direction of the marginal mandibular nerve and a drill inserted through a guide or speculum. The screws can also be placed and twisted by a driver applied through the same hole. The mucosa is closed with chromic sutures and the patient treated as discussed earlier.

27

Open Reduction of Atrophic Body Fractures With Reconstruction Plate Fixation

Alternative Technique Using an Onlay Rib Graft
Alternative Technique of Splint Fixation

INDICATIONS

The edentulous mandible can present as an atrophic body fracture in the elderly patient. Special techniques must be considered. Incisions should be limited and periosteum should be retained as much as possible to provide an adequate blood supply to the underlying bone. Long-rigid plates covering wide areas on each side of the fracture encourage stabilization and healing of the bone. The reconstruction plate, with or without locking screws, seems to be advantageous in these patients.

PROCEDURE

A–F Nasal intubation is desirable and the face and neck should be prepared with an antiseptic solution. Since there are few if any teeth for establishing occlusion, the mandible is manipulated digitally into a position that appears best for occlusion. The face and neck incision is described in Chapter 26 exposing the inferior portion of the body of the mandible. In the area of fracture, the periosteum is elevated judiciously to just identify the fracture of the mandible and allow the positioning of a plate. The mandible is then held in position with bone clamps and a reconstruction plate is bent to the shape of the jaw. A template can be used to assist in developing the correct contour. The plate is then applied and held in position with plate clamps. Holes are first drilled to the sides of the fracture, the depth of the holes evaluated with a gauge and screws applied. A screw is applied first to one side near the fracture and then to the other side securing the fragments. Additional stabilization is obtained by outside holes that are drilled and secured additionally with screws.

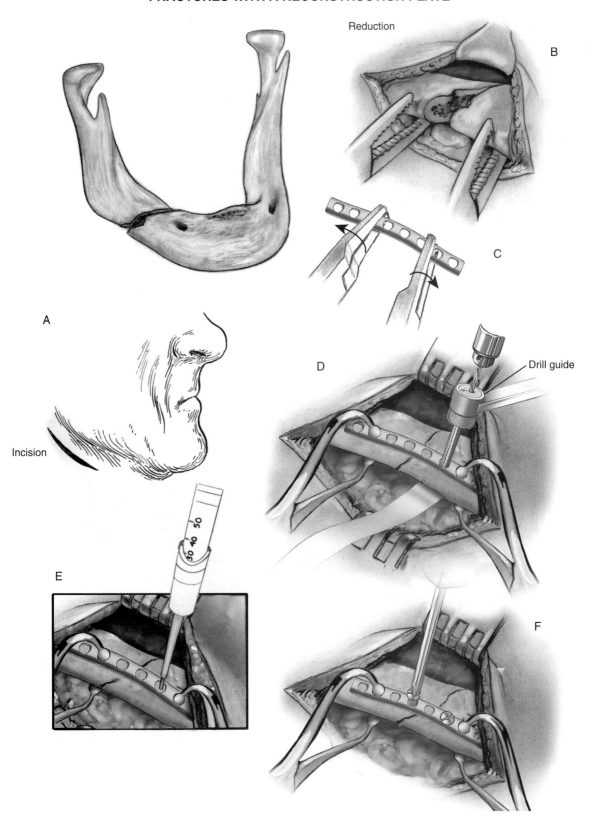

Reduction

B

C

A

Incision

D

Drill guide

E

F

PITFALLS

1. Try to avoid excessive dissection and stripping of the mandible. The blood supply of the atrophic edentulous mandible is limited and the surgeon should handle the tissues gently and try to retain as much periosteum as possible.

2. Avoid elevating intraoral mucosa. When this occurs, carefully close the mucosa with chromic sutures and irrigate the wound.

3. Make sure there are at least three screws securing the plate on each side of the fracture. This is the minimal number of screws necessary to obtain stabilization and rigidly fixate the atrophic bone.

4. Institute oral intake as soon as possible to avoid nutritional deficiencies and dehydration.

COMPLICATIONS

1. Nonunion of the mandible is a rare complication. Postoperatively the patient should be evaluated for pain and inflammation. The fracture should also be evaluated radiographically for accurate reduction and fixation. Healing problems should prompt immediate evaluation and possibly a revision of the technique. The treatment for nonunion is described in Chapters 34 through 37.

2. If the patient develops osteomyelitis at the fracture site the area of infection should be drained and devitalized bone removed. New cultures should be obtained. When such a situation develops, a biphase apparatus is an excellent alternative to hold the fragments in appropriate position and avoid the effects of the plate as foreign body (see Chapter 31).

ALTERNATIVE TECHNIQUE USING AN ONLAY RIB GRAFT

A displaced fracture of an atrophic, pencil-thin mandible in a debilitated and elderly patient presents a formidable problem. In such a situation, the surgeon should avoid denture fixation and apply more stability directly to the mandible. Reconstruction plates can be used, but occasionally the plate is too large for the area to be fixed, and application will cause severe damage to the periosteum and inferior alveolar nerve. If this possibility is a concern, the fracture site should be reinforced with a fresh bone autograft.

a–c Although a variety of donor sites can be considered, rib grafts are ideal because of their length, contour, and ease of harvest. For this procedure, the patient is placed in a lateral thoracoplasty position; the seventh rib is palpated, and a curvilinear incision is made over the angle of the scapula to the anterior axillary line. The latissimus dorsi muscle, the lower edge

of the trapezius muscle, and the serratus anterior muscle are cut, and the periosteum is incised and elevated off the lateral aspect of the rib. Using Freer and Doyen elevators, the periosteum is elevated off the surface of the rib and then off the deep portion, carefully avoiding injury to the pleura.

d A side-cutting forceps is used to resect the appropriate length of rib. The periosteum is closed with 3-0 chromic sutures and the other soft tissues are closed in layers. If the pleura has been punctured, a chest tube must be used.

e The rib is held by an assistant. Using a sharp osteotome and mallet, the rib is split down the center. After the split has started, further splitting can be accomplished with heavy scissors or a knife.

f The mandible is approached as described in Chapter 26. In addition to the usual elevation of the periosteum near the fracture site, additional elevation is used to relax the periosteum that covers the alveolar ridge. The fragments are held together, and the rib is placed into a subperiosteal pocket below the alveolus. The rib is held in position by two lag screws (see Chapter 24). The wound is closed in layers. Usually the graft provides sufficient support so that splints and dentures are not necessary. Moreover, if a splint or denture is applied, it may cause an erosion on the surface of the graft, creating the potential for contamination and breakdown of the wound. The patient should be maintained on a liquid nutrient diet during the 6 to 8 weeks of postoperative care. Prophylactic antibiotics should be administered for 10 to 14 days following the procedure.

ALTERNATIVE TECHNIQUE OF SPLINT FIXATION

Although the rigid plate technique is one of the more popular methods of treating the edentulous patient, occasionally there may be a need to apply splints or dentures to maintain reduction and some degree of stabilization of the fracture. The splint method is a conservative, proven approach to mandibular fractures, but if reduction cannot be maintained, additional fixation is required (i.e., plate or lag screw).

The manufacture of splints and the adjustments necessary for dentures are discussed in detail in the chapter on condylar fractures (Chapter 20).

a'–c' For the body injury, the circummandibular wire must be placed away from the fracture site, and for most patients, one circummandibular wire is placed to each side of the injury. One wire is thus wrapped around the proximal segment and the other wrapped around the distal segment. Circumzygomatic

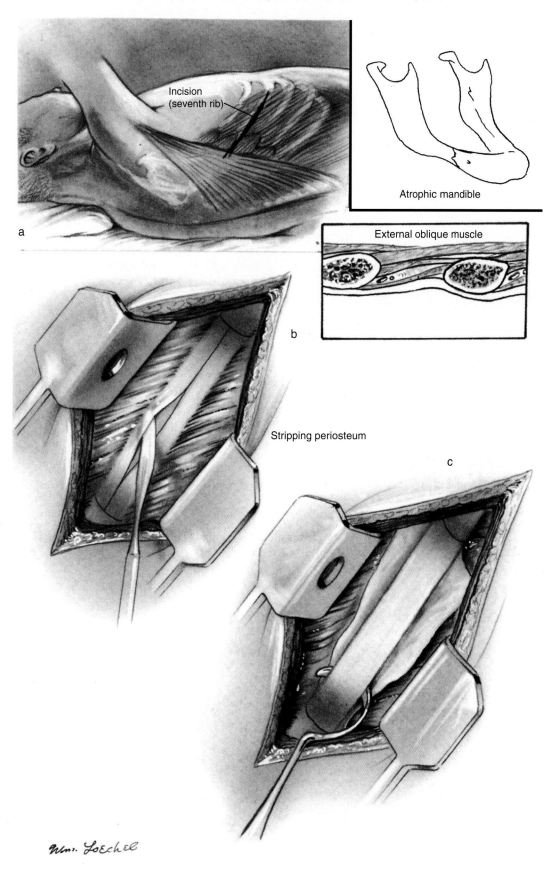

Incision
(seventh rib)

a

Atrophic mandible

b

External oblique muscle

Stripping periosteum

c

Wm. Loechel

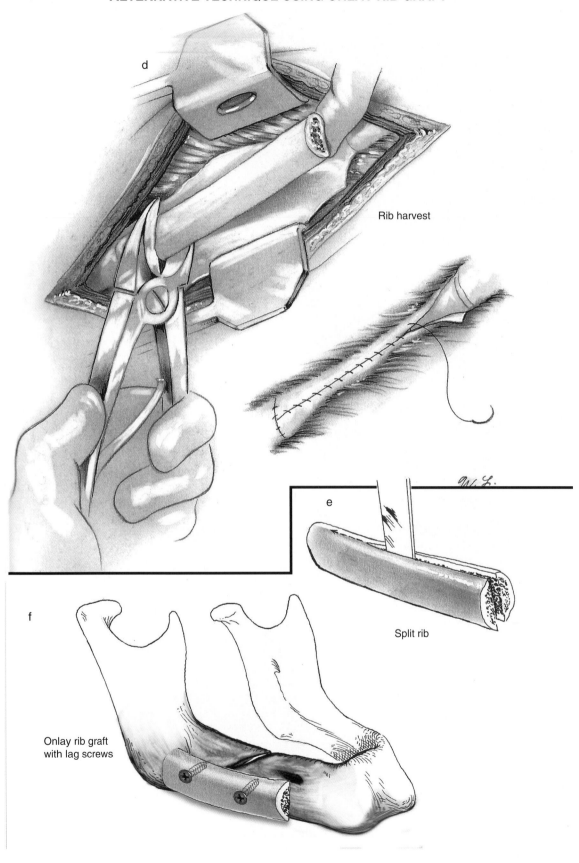

d

Rib harvest

e

Split rib

f

Onlay rib graft
with lag screws

ALTERNATIVE TECHNIQUE OF SPLINT FIXATION

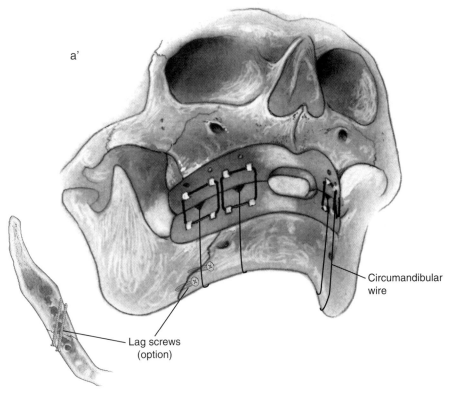

a'

Circumandibular
wire

Lag screws
(option)

MAXILLARY SPLINT FIXATION
WITH LAG SCREWS

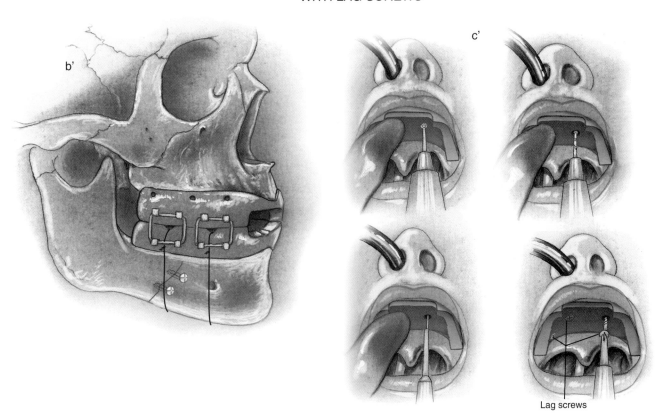

b'

c'

Lag screws

wires or palatal/alveolar screws (see Chapter 20) are applied in a standard fashion.

If there is concern regarding the reduction, the fracture should be inspected as described earlier. Unstable fragments can be further immobilized with plate(s) or in the case of an oblique fracture with lag screws.

The dentures (or splints) are secured and held together with elastic bands. A postoperative radiograph is obtained to evaluate the reduction. The patient is treated with prophylactic antibiotics for 5 to 7 days and evaluated weekly for healing and complications. Healing should be evident in 6 to 8 weeks, at which time the splints can be taken out of intermaxillary fixation and tested for removal.

The use of loose-fitting dentures or splints should be avoided. The fixation should be checked weekly and adjustments made to the circummandibular-circumzygomatic wires and intermaxillary bands.

The manufacturing of splints and adjustments of dentures can be costly and time consuming. The surgeon must consider the resources available and the cost of this method before selecting this technique.

This technique should be avoided in patients with an atrophic, pencil-thin mandible. The anterior segment will not be sufficiently stabilized and will tend to pull downward, away from the posterior segment of the jaw. In such situations, the surgeon should probably use a plate or a rib onlay technique, discussed earlier.

The body fracture can be associated with a laceration of the alveolar ridge. If this is the case, the denture or prosthesis can retard healing, and there can be a continuous contamination of the region by saliva. Should this complication develop, a rigid plate or external fixation technique should be applied.

Parasymphyseal Fractures

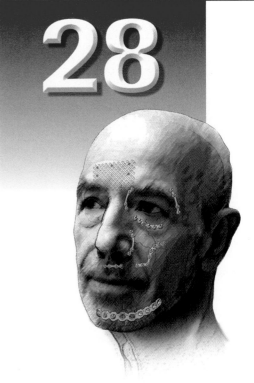

Open Reduction of Parasymphyseal Fractures With Intermaxillary Fixation and Internal Rigid Plate Fixation
Alternative Technique Using External Pin Fixation

INDICATIONS

Because of the distracting forces of the suprahyoid musculature, the parasymphyseal fracture is relatively unstable, and the surgeon should be prepared for open reduction and fixation. The fracture becomes even more unstable when it is combined with other fractures of the mandible, and under these conditions, the mylohyoid, geniohyoid, and genioglossus muscles tend to rotate and pull the intervening fragment medially, posteriorly, and inferiorly. Stability can often be obtained with internal rigid plate fixation or external pin fixation. For the severely comminuted fracture, as seen with gunshot wounds, the reconstruction plate or external pin fixation technique is preferred.

PROCEDURE

A–B General anesthesia with nasotracheal intubation provides for evaluation of intraoperative occlusion and an excellent approach to the submental area. If the dentition is adequate, distraction of the alveolar ridge can be corrected temporarily with the application of a loop of 26-gauge wire around the incisor teeth. The surgeon should then establish intermaxillary fixation with intermaxillary screws, Ivy loops, or arch bars that will bring the fragments into appropriate position (see Chapter 19).

177

OPEN REDUCTION OF PARASYMPHYSEAL FRACTURES WITH INTERMAXILLARY FIXATION AND INTERNAL RIGID PLATE FIXATION

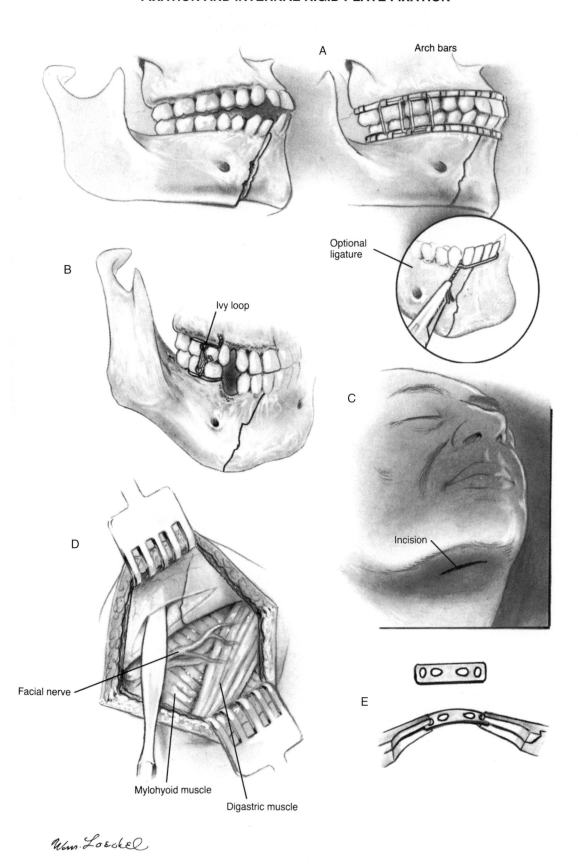

A

Arch bars

Optional ligature

B

Ivy loop

C

Incision

D

Facial nerve

Mylohyoid muscle

Digastric muscle

E

Wm. Loeckel

C The incision (4 to 5 cm) should be hidden beneath the chin. If the fracture lies to one side or the other, the incision can be made from the midline to a point just anterior to the submaxillary gland. The area should be infiltrated with 1% lidocaine containing 1:100,000 epinephrine, and the surgeon should wait 10 minutes to obtain maximal vasoconstriction for hemostasis.

D The subcutaneous tissues and platysma should be incised and the outer surface of the mandible exposed. The periosteum should be elevated, which in turn will release the insertion of the digastric muscle and show the fracture site. Injury to the mental nerve as it exits just inferior to the apices of the first and second premolars should be avoided. If the fragments are distracted, the fracture should be placed into an exact, interlocking position with Dingman or Lane bone-holding forceps.

E–H A dynamic compression plate is then bent to appropriate contour and applied to the surface of the bone. Holes are drilled and screws applied as in Chapter 24 carefully evaluating the lingual portion of the mandible or the alveolar ridge for displacement. Tension bands can be used rather than dental ligatures if the alveolar portion of the fragment becomes distracted. The periosteum is closed with 3-0 chromic sutures. The platysma and subcutaneous tissues are approximated with 3-0 and 4-0 chromic sutures and the skin with a nonabsorbable suture. Drains should be avoided.

For most adults, healing will take place in 6 to 8 weeks. Intermaxillary fixation can be removed at the surgeon's discretion. The patient should be kept on antibiotics for 5 to 7 days and evaluated weekly for displacement of the elastic bands and/or of fragments of the mandible. A postoperative radiograph should be obtained to verify adequate reduction and fixation. Oral hygiene is maintained with a toothbrush and/or water irrigation device.

PITFALLS

1. The fracture site can be misleading on radiographs. Triangular lines can suggest either a fracture extending through both cortices or a triangular free fragment. Failure to recognize the free fragment will cause instability and failure to heal. In such a case, the surgeon must ensure stabilization on both sides of the fragment. Reconstruction plates are helpful when there is a need to stabilize multiple fragments. During these procedures a maximum blood supply should be retained and periosteal elevation limited to the area of fracture.

2. Accurate bending of the plate is very important. If the plate is bent too much, the outer cortex will be distracted. If the plate is not bent enough, the inner cortex will be distracted. Either situation can cause mechanical problems at the tempomandibular joint.

3. Overtightening of the inferior edge of the symphysis can cause distraction of the alveolar ridge. To avoid this problem, make sure that the arch bar is tightened to the lower dentition. A loop of wire (a bridle) temporarily applied to the incisors will often keep the fracture tight at the alveolar ridge while the wire (or plate) is adjusted below. If distraction occurs, a tension band should be applied superiorly.

COMPLICATIONS

1. Malunion of the parasymphyseal fracture can present as an over-, under-, or crossbite. Malposition of the front teeth can affect the biting of food and the general appearance of the lips. If such malocclusion or deformity develops in the early postoperative period, the fracture should be reduced and fixed again. After healing has taken place, the surgeon must consider orthodontic and/or orthognathic surgery.

2. Because the parasymphyseal fracture is relatively unstable and is probably the most distant from the inferior alveolar blood supply, it is prone to the unfortunate sequela of nonunion. This complication is often associated with infection, which must be identified and treated with appropriate antibiotics. Devitalized fragments of bone should be removed and major portions of the mandible stabilized with intermaxillary and/or external rigid fixation. If there is a defect, this should be treated as discussed in Chapters 35 and 36.

3. Hypoesthesia or paresthesia secondary to injury to the mental nerve is usually managed conservatively. Because this is a terminal nerve, sensation often returns. Injury to the nerve is avoided by understanding its location (below the apices of the first and second molars) and by applying atraumatic techniques during the surgery.

ALTERNATIVE TECHNIQUE USING EXTERNAL PIN FIXATION

External pin fixation is a consideration in those patients that have comminuted and contaminated fractures (see Chapters 21 and 34). The technique is useful when the surgeon wants to avoid using splints or dentures.

The biphase pins should be placed on each side of the area of fracture. Stab incisions should be made in the direction of the facial nerve and the pins applied so that they are perpendicular to the plane of the mandible. Several comminuted pieces of bone can be compressed between the more solid pieces of bone. A tight periosteal closure will also help hold the fragments in anatomic position.

OPEN REDUCTION OF PARASYMPHYSEALFRACTURES WITH INTERMAXILLARY FIXATION AND INTERNAL RIGID PLATE FIXATION (Continued)

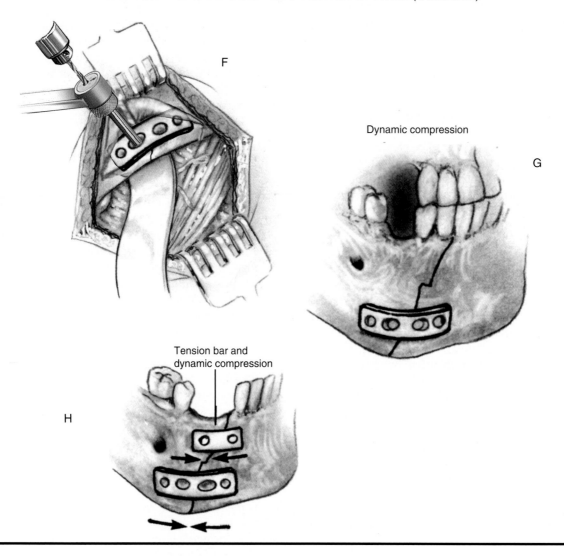

F

Dynamic compression

G

Tension bar and dynamic compression

H

ALTERNATIVE TECHNIQUE USING BIPHASE FIXATION

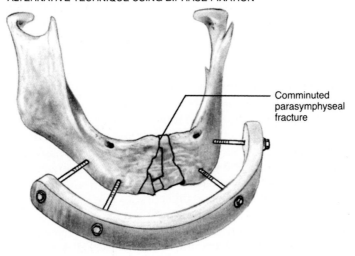

Comminuted parasymphyseal fracture

Wm. Loechel

Closed Reduction of Parasymphyseal Fractures in Children Using Prefabricated Lingual Splints

Alternative Technique of Fabricating the Splint on the Patient's Dental Arch

In Consultation With Mark T. Marunick, DDS

INDICATIONS

The growth and development characteristics of children demand special consideration in the treatment of craniofacial injury (see Chapters 110 and 111). Pediatric fractures tend to heal rapidly, and even if the segments are not perfectly aligned, bone remodeling can bring about normal anatomic relationships. Furthermore, open reduction and fixation put the developing teeth at risk and should only be applied very judiciously. For these reasons, parasymphyseal fractures usually are treated by closed methods and the lingual splint method is an excellent method to use in small children. It is also well tolerated and easy to maintain.

PROCEDURE

A A lingual splint can be made with the techniques noted in Chapter 20. For this method, an impression of the lower jaw is obtained with alginate.

The impression is then poured in plaster or stone to make a cast, and from this cast, a splint is fabricated.

B,C When displaced segments are encountered, cast surgery should be performed. For this procedure, the base of the involved cast should be trimmed with a divergent angle from bottom to top. The cast and entire base are duplicated. A flexible base former is lubricated and filled with a very watery mix of plaster. The base of the cast is lubricated and placed in the plaster. The lubricated tapered base will allow removal of the entire lower cast from the plaster boat.

D,E Cast surgery can then be performed in the area of displacement. The cast is cut along the lines of the fracture and the segments are repositioned in the plaster boat. The segments are subsequently secured with wax.

F–H The stone cast is carefully removed from the plaster boat and a duplicate is made of the cast. The lingual splint is fabricated on the duplicate. To ensure

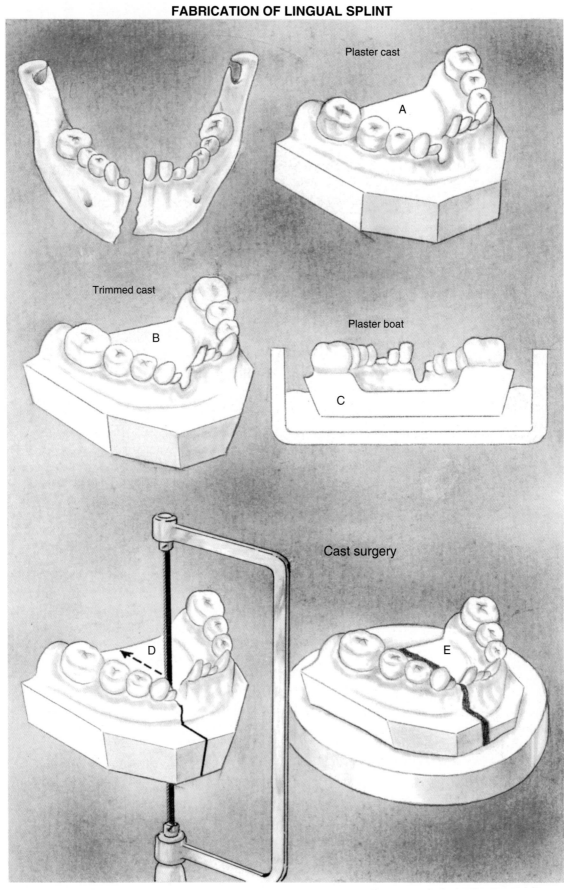

Plaster cast

A

Trimmed cast

B

Plaster boat

C

Cast surgery

D

E

the rigidity of the lingual splint, a heavy-gauge stainless steel wire or a preformed stainless steel lingual bar is adapted to the lingual sulcus of the cast, 3 to 4 mm below the free gingival margin. The wire or bar is luted to the cast with a few beads of wax. A separating medium (petrolatum) is carefully applied to the cast. Care is taken to keep the lubricant off the wire or bar. Autopolymerizing acrylic resin is mixed, and when it thickens, it is adapted to the lingual aspect of the teeth and sulcus and around the wire. The acrylic should not extend over the occlusal surface of the teeth. After the acrylic is set, it is removed, trimmed, and polished. Small holes are directed through it to hold strategically placed circumdental wires. The splint should be 1.5 to 2 mm thick. If it is too thin, it can be reseated on the cast and additional acrylic added. Light activated resin may also be used for the fabrication of the lingual splint.

I The splint should be applied under general anesthesia. If sufficient teeth are available, the lips are retracted, and ligatures of 26-gauge wires are applied through the splint and between the adjacent teeth to be twisted at the buccal or lateral gingival surface. The wires are then tightened, cut, and bent toward the gum area. Usually four wires placed around "solid" molar teeth are sufficient to hold the splint to the teeth. The relationship of the upper and lower jaws is then evaluated for satisfactory occlusion.

Postoperatively the splint is checked daily to make sure that there is no loosening. The jaw is evaluated radiographically and clinically to verify reduction and fixation. Because healing is quite rapid, the splint can often be removed in 2 to 4 weeks. Antibiotics are provided for 5 to 7 days following the procedure.

PITFALLS

1. When treating symphyseal fractures, make sure there is not an associated condylar injury. If such a situation exists, the physician must check the state of the condyle every 2 weeks with appropriate diagnostic imaging to ensure that the condyle can be adequately mobilized. Short periods of intermaxillary fixation may be necessary to achieve adequate rehabilitation of the joint.

2. Because the deciduous teeth can be easily extirpated or loosened by the splint, the splint should be checked daily. If there is a loss of stability, new holes and wires must be applied. If there are no other teeth that can be ligated, the surgeon must consider new holes and circummandibular wires to hold the splint firmly to the alveolus (see Chapter 20).

COMPLICATIONS

1. Although nonunion and malunion are rare in children, the surgeon must be aware that they can

occur and if they do, then treat with appropriate methods (see Chapters 34 through 37).

2. The most unrecognized complication of fracture in children is injury to the condyle with subsequent ankylosis and alterations in growth and development of the jaw. To avoid this problem, the surgeon should obtain radiographic analysis of the temporomandibular joint at the time of injury. If there is any suspicion of injury, the patient should be followed with appropriate diagnostic imaging every 2 weeks. In some condylar injuries, intermaxillary fixation may be necessary for short periods of time. As soon as intermaxillary fixation is completed, the child should be evaluated clinically and radiologically for healing.

3. Tooth injury can also occur in children. If the injury involves the deciduous teeth, it will probably not be a problem. On the other hand, if it involves the permanent dentition, consultation is advisable (see Chapters 31 and 32).

4. If the child has not developed teeth, the splint can be made to conform to the alveolar ridge. Grooves are made in the splint for the circummandibular wires.

5. If parasymphyseal and symphyseal fractures are associated with other fractures, there can be a marked displacement of intervening segments. In such a situation, the surgeon cannot be sure of the reduction or fixation, and an open method must be instituted. If this is necessary, then a miniplate is placed as close as possible to the lower edge of the jaw (Chapter 111). If more stabilization is needed, it may be possible to combine the technique with a lingual splint.

ALTERNATIVE TECHNIQUE OF FABRICATING THE SPLINT ON THE PATIENT'S DENTAL ARCH

If a prosthodontist is not available, there are "shortcuts" to making adequate splints. One way is to apply the autopolymerizing acrylic resin directly to the dentition or alveolar ridge. The technique is performed under general anesthesia. The teeth and/or alveolar ridge are reduced manually and coated with petrolatum. The acrylic is mixed, and when it becomes thick and can be handled, it is applied to the area while the jaw is held in a reduced position. As the acrylic is polymerizing, it must be removed, the tissues irrigated with cold water, and the acrylic readapted. Prior to final set, the splint is removed and placed in a bowl of water. These procedures will minimize heat transfer to the tissue and prevent the acrylic from getting locked into undercuts. The set acrylic is then carefully trimmed to remove overextensions into movable tissues. The peripheries of the splint are smoothed and holes are appropriately drilled for application of wires.

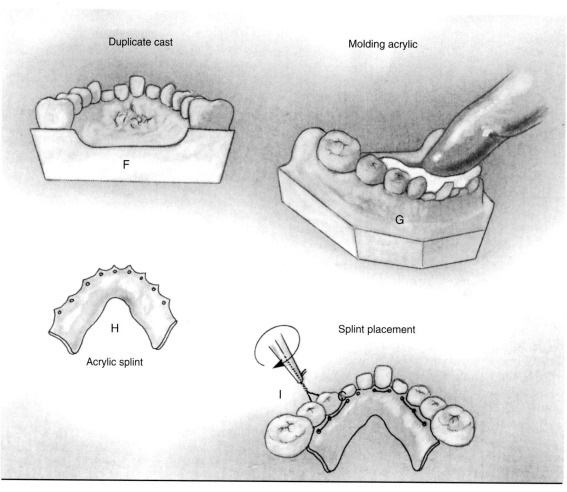

Duplicate cast

F

Molding acrylic

G

H

Acrylic splint

Splint placement

I

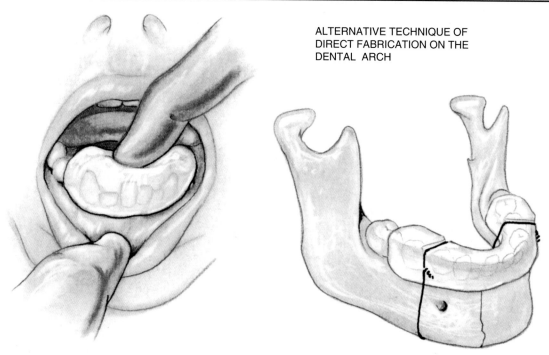

ALTERNATIVE TECHNIQUE OF
DIRECT FABRICATION ON THE
DENTAL ARCH

Open Intraoral Reduction of Parasymphyseal Fractures With Internal Rigid Plate Fixation

INDICATIONS

Because most parasymphyseal fractures are relatively unstable, open reduction and fixation must be considered. Usually an external approach is used (see Chapter 28), but if the surgeon wants to avoid external scars, the fracture can be approached directly through a gingivolabial sulcus incision. This technique provides a direct route to the fracture and an excellent exposure of the external cortex. One can then evaluate the contact of the fragments and the adequacy of the reduction from the lower border of the mandible to the alveolar ridge. Moreover, fractures involving the incisors and the alveolar ridge will not be missed and can be treated appropriately.

PROCEDURE

A Initially the surgeon should achieve normal occlusal relationships by loose application of intermaxillary fixation with intermaxillary screws, Ivy loops, or arch bars to the upper and lower dentition. The arch bar or, alternatively, a transdental loop of wire across the incisors also tends to stabilize the parasymphyseal fracture so that when the inferior portion is reduced, there is no distraction of the fracture at the alveolar surface (Chapter 28).

B–E Following infiltration with 1% lidocaine containing 1:100,000 epinephrine, an incision is made in the gingivobuccal sulcus above the fracture site. This incision should be 5 to 7 mm below the gingival margin, but not so low that it injures the mental nerve. The periosteum is then elevated inferiorly and a periosteal flap held with Senn retractors. Care is again taken to avoid injury to the mental nerve, which exits between the apices of first and second premolars. The fracture is reduced manually and a rigid plate with four holes is bent to appropriate shape and placed on the reduced fracture site. The plate must be bent so that it fits snugly along the surface of the bone. The bending can be assisted by a template that is first fitted to the bone and then contoured to the template. The bending should not distort the cortical surfaces on either side of the mandible. Screw holes are drilled through both cortices. If the option is a compression plate, the screw holes must be placed at the outer most portion of the hole (often assisted be a guide) so that the screw will slide the bone medially (Chapter 24). The holes are measured for depth and the screws placed one at a time to the sides of the fracture. The alveolar portion of the fracture is examined for distraction. The mucosa is closed with chromic sutures, and the arch bar is then tightened.

Postoperatively oral hygiene is maintained with frequent brushings and/or regular use of a water irrigation device. A radiograph should be taken to verify adequate fixation and reduction. Prophylactic antibiotics are taken for 5 days and the jaw evaluated on a weekly basis. Following a test of jaw strength and

OPEN INTRAORAL REDUCTION OF PARASYMPHYSEAL FRACTURES WITH INTERNAL RIGID PLATE FIXATION

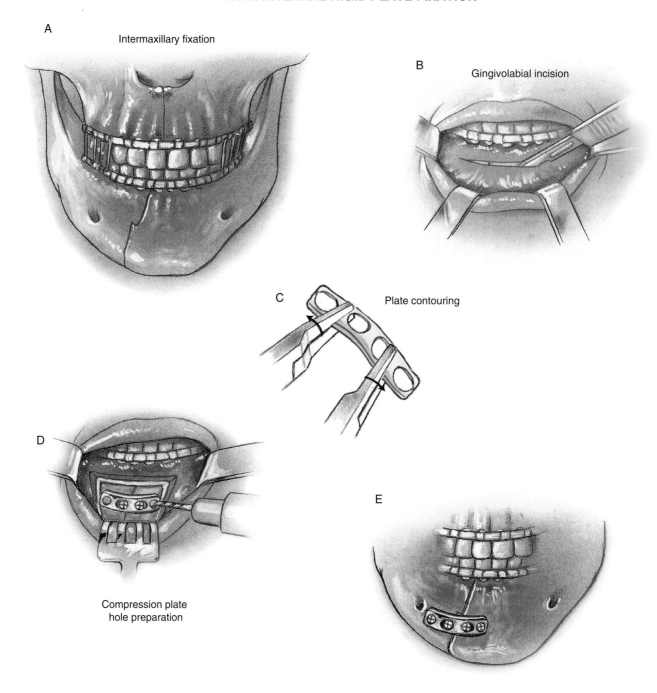

A   Intermaxillary fixation

B   Gingivolabial incision

C   Plate contouring

D   Compression plate hole preparation

E

stability at 6 to 8 weeks, the intermaxillary fixation can be removed.

PITFALLS

1. Avoid overreduction of the alveolar portion from an overtightening of the arch bar. If this occurs, the plate will not bring the fragments together, and the fracture will remain unstable. This problem can be avoided by loosely applying the arch bar and then tightening it after the plate has been applied.

2. The plate must fit accurately the contour of the outer cortex. A plate that is bent too little or too much will distract the inner or outer cortex and displace the mandibular arch.

3. Keep in mind that the mental foramen exits just beneath the apical portions of the first or second premolars. The incisions and/or periosteal elevation must be limited if injury to the nerve is to be avoided.

COMPLICATIONS

1. As with any mandible fracture, there is a potential for malunion. This complication can be avoided by accurate reduction and fixation and verification of preinjury occlusion. Treatment for this complication is described in Chapter 37.

2. Nonunion can occur and must be avoided. The physician must ensure that the fracture is accurately reduced and eventually shows signs of healing. The patient should be examined for evidence of infection, and if present, cultures should be obtained and appropriate antibiotics administered. Fragments that become devitalized must be removed. Further treatment for this complication is discussed in Chapters 34 through 36.

3. Paresthesias involving the lower anterior dentition and chin are possible from injury to the inferior alveolar and/or mental nerve. If this becomes a problem, the plate can be examined for compression of the nerve and can be removed through the same intraoral incision.

4. Hypoesthesia resulting from injury to the mental nerve is usually transient; there is an excellent chance that sensation will return. This complication can be prevented by avoiding any direct trauma to the nerve.

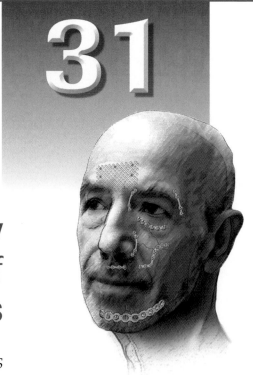

CHAPTER

31

Repair of Tooth Injury
Alternative Technique of Orthodontic Brackets

In Consultation With Lynne Moseley, DDS

INDICATIONS

Injury to the dentition commonly occurs with mandible and/or maxillary fractures. Treatment of this injury depends on whether the tooth involved is deciduous or permanent, the severity of injury (including the number of teeth affected), the health of the injured tooth (or teeth), the overall condition of the noninjured dentition, the cost-effectiveness of the planned repair, and the need to retain affected teeth for a prosthesis or for the stabilization of a mandibular or maxillary fracture. If time permits, consultations with specialists such as dentists, endodontists, orthodontists, and oral surgeons are helpful.

In general, tooth fractures limited to the enamel should be managed electively; those injuries that penetrate the dentin may require dental dressings. When the injury involves the dental pulp and/or root, some form of endodontic therapy will need to be employed. Avulsed teeth require stabilization techniques, often in concert with endodontic procedures.

PROCEDURE

Incisal Edge Injuries Not Involving the Dentin

A For injuries involving the incisal edge but not the dentin, the teeth of the primary and permanent dentition are treated conservatively. The enamel can often be smoothed with an abrading disk or fine diamond bur. In cases of significant loss of tooth substance, a definitive dental restoration is indicated.

Incisal Edge Injuries Involving Enamel and Dentin

B Teeth with incisal edge injuries involving the enamel and dentin can generally be salvaged. First, unsupported enamel is removed by rotary instruments or dental chisels. The tooth is then pumiced, and if the injury is well within the dentin or is thermally sensitive, a dressing of calcium hydroxide or a layer of glass

REPAIR OF TOOTH INJURY

ENAMEL INJURY

A

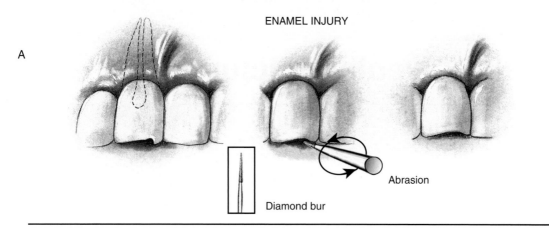

Diamond bur

Abrasion

ENAMEL AND DENTIN INJURY

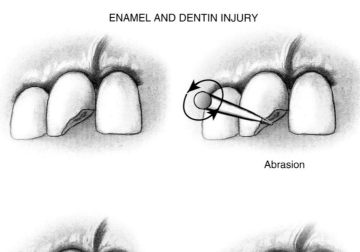

Abrasion

B

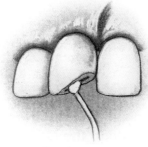

Dressing

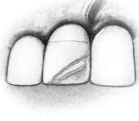

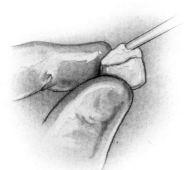

Cement

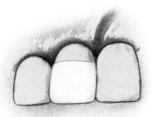

Temporary crown

ionomer liner base is placed over the exposed tooth. An acrylic crown form can be cemented with any temporary dental cement or a build up can be accomplished with composite restorative material.

Enamel, Dentin, and Pulp Injuries

C For complicated crown fractures involving the enamel, dentin, and pulp, much will depend on when the fracture is treated. Generally an uncomplicated fracture of the coronal portion of a tooth involving the pulp can be managed with direct pulp capping with calcium hydroxide and application of a temporary acrylic crown if performed within a few hours. If treatment occurs within 6 to 24 hours, extirpation of the coronal pulp should be completed (pulpotomy), a calcium hydroxide dressing placed on the root stump, and a temporary crown fabricated. After 24 hours, a complete endodontic procedure should be performed. For a deciduous tooth, a nonvital dressing should be placed after pulpotomy (formocresol).

Root Injuries

D For root fractures, the more apical the fracture, the better the patient prognosis. Root fractures in the apical third of the tooth are often stable, and conservative measures, such as fixation with acrylic or composite splints, can retain pulp viability. For these procedures, the tooth is coated with petrolatum; the acrylic is then molded and removed prior to curing. The acrylic should then be smoothed and replaced onto the tooth with a dental cement and/or the tooth can be bonded to the adjacent one. If the tooth later becomes devital, appropriate endodontic therapy should be employed.

E Root fractures in the middle third and the coronal third carry a poorer patient prognosis. In most patients, if the fracture is close to the crown, the outlook is dismal, and extraction is usually the treatment of choice. The crown is removed, and the root is extracted through a small flap in the gingiva. The lateral alveolar bone is cut away as necessary and the root is elevated with a downward (and/or upward) movement.

For fractures in the midportion of the root, rigid fixation with carefully fashioned acrylic or composite splints should be employed. If pulpal death ensues, either endodontic therapy or extraction will have to be performed.

Displacement, Partial Avulsion, or Impaction Injuries

F In displacement, partial avulsion, or impaction injuries, the periodontal space, membrane, and pulp can be affected. A conservative approach is to regain the normal anatomic position of the tooth with careful manipulation and then to fix the tooth by means of a splint or orthodontic ligation.

Total Avulsion Injuries

G A permanent tooth that is completely avulsed is best reset within 30 minutes. Replantation of an avulsed tooth more than 2 hours after injury can result in resorption, infraocclusion, and a variety of inflammatory responses that will require ultimate extraction. Briefly, the technique to be followed for replantation is as follows: the socket and tooth should be freely irrigated with normal saline for removal of foreign material. Using local anesthesia, lightly aspirate any remaining blood clot. If the tooth has been out of its socket <15 minutes, take it by the crown, drop it in a tooth preservation solution of sterile saline and reimplant the tooth. Secure it to adjacent teeth with wire arch bars or acrylic splint. Endodontic therapy will likely need to be initiated within 2 weeks. If the tooth was out 30 minutes to 2 hours, soak for 30 minutes to replenish nutrients. Local anesthesia will probably be needed before reimplanting. If the patient is between 6 and 10 years old, also soak the tooth for 5 minutes in 5% doxycycline to kill bacteria that could enter the immature apex and form an abscess.

PITFALLS

1. The diagnosis of tooth injury is very important in treatment planning. If the deciduous dentition is involved and the tooth is severely injured, it is probably more prudent to extract the tooth than to repair the injury.

2. If a tooth is severely carious or involved with significant periodontal disease, it should be considered for extraction. An exception may be a second or third molar that stabilizes the angle fracture and is not directly involved in the fracture. Extraction techniques are described in Chapter 32.

3. If the tooth is subluxated, displaced, or partially avulsed and is expected to exfoliate within 6 months, any efforts to retain it are not warranted, and the tooth should be extracted.

4. Patient attitudes are an important consideration. Many patients require revisional treatment, pulp testing, and delayed permanent restoration. If the patient is uncooperative and/or noncompliant, extraction may be the treatment of choice.

5. Avoid leaving nonvital teeth in fracture lines, as they are associated with portals of infection. Nonvital teeth can also act like foreign bodies and predispose the patient to osteomyelitis and, ultimately, nonunion of the fracture. The diagnosis can be made by dental radiographs and pulp testing. The tooth should also

ENAMEL, DENTIN, AND PULP INJURY

C

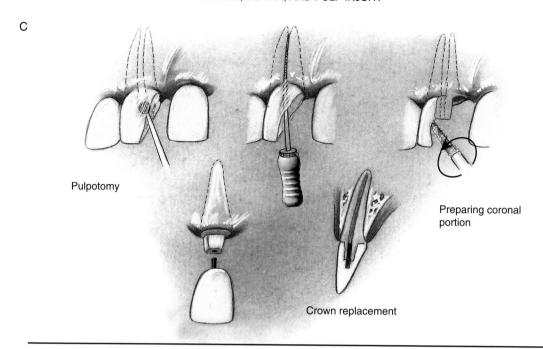

Pulpotomy

Crown replacement

Preparing coronal portion

ROOT INJURY

D

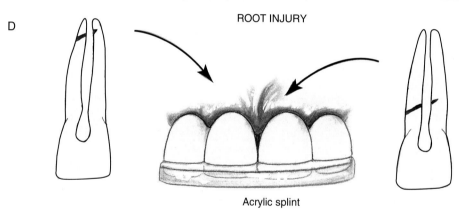

Acrylic splint

E

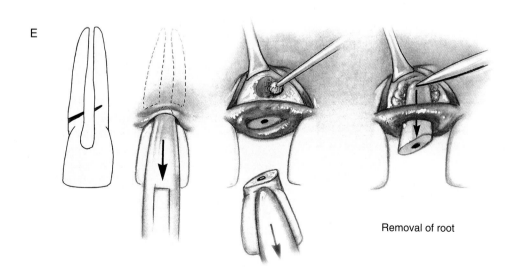

Removal of root

REPAIR OF TOOTH INJURY *(Continued)*

DISPLACEMENT

F

Replacement

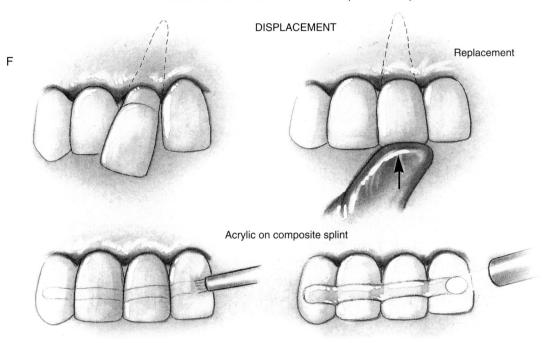

Acrylic on composite splint

AVULSION

G

Replantation

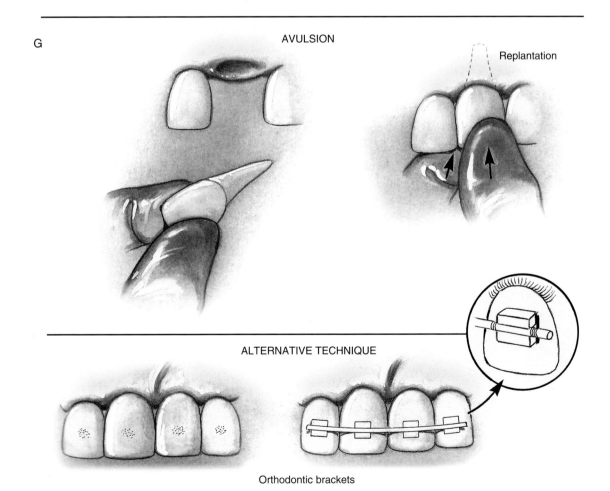

ALTERNATIVE TECHNIQUE

Orthodontic brackets

be evaluated for caries and periodontal disease. If the fracture line involves the tooth or is very close to the adjacent periodontal structures and the tooth is not necessary for stabilization, extraction must be considered.

COMPLICATIONS

1. Tooth injuries that are not successfully treated may cause the tooth to become nonvital and ultimately pose problems with resorption and/or infection. These teeth should be evaluated every few months with inspection and pulp testing. Radiographs should be obtained at least twice a year. Endodontic therapy can not only eliminate infectious processes, but also set the foundation for dental procedures to restore function and cosmesis.

2. Resorption of a tooth can occur following replantation. This process may be slow or accelerated. If there is no inflammation or infection accompanying the resorption, the tooth should be retained until function or appearance is compromised.

ALTERNATIVE TECHNIQUE OF ORTHODONTIC BRACKETS

Avulsed or displaced teeth can alternatively be stabilized by application of arch bars or orthodontic brackets. The arch bar is sufficient in teeth that are displaced laterally or lingually, but it will not give sufficient holding strength to a tooth that is being extracted; the orthodontic band is ideal for this condition.

For use of the band, the surgeon first applies dental etching acid to a 5-mm^2 area in the center of the tooth and to the two teeth on either side. An arch wire-accepting bracket is then attached with orthodontic bonding cement. Care should be taken to ensure that the brackets are aligned for easy placement of the arch wire. The arch wire is subsequently shaped and placed into the cemented brackets and the ends of the arch wire ligated to their appropriate brackets. The splint is retained for a minimum of 2 months. A radiograph should be obtained at the time of splint placement and then every month until the tooth is stable.

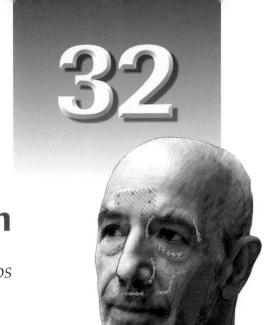

Tooth Extraction

In Consultation With Lynne Moseley, DDS

INDICATIONS

Teeth that will compromise reduction and fixation of fractures should be considered for extraction. Usually these teeth have been assessed as nonsalvageable and are considered potential foreign bodies. If they are in or near a fracture line of the supporting jaw, they should be extracted before fixation. Otherwise they can be treated electively in the posttrauma period. Extraction should be considered on (1) those teeth that sustained sufficient injury to the tooth, periodontium, and alveolus to preclude a reasonable prognosis for retention (see Chapter 31) or (2) teeth with significant preexisting periodontal disease, periapical pathoses, and/or invasive caries; if left in place, such teeth could later become septic and may compromise the healing of soft tissue lacerations, alveolar fractures, and fractures of the jaws themselves.

Occasionally there is a question of salvageability. If this question arises in teeth that are in or very proximal to a fracture line, they should be removed. The caveats relating to jaw fracture stabilization and prosthetic retention must be carefully considered when planning these extractions.

The successful removal of a tooth or teeth depends on the skill of the operator, the availability of a proper armamentarium, and the presentation of the teeth slated for extraction. In some patients, extraction followed by a period of healing and subsequent dental implant can be considered.

PROCEDURES

An atraumatic technique when removing teeth is of paramount importance. The retrieval of a retained, fractured cuspid root from dense alveolar bone will most often require significantly more force (and concomitant trauma) than the rather simple exercise of removing multiple periodontally compromised, mobile teeth. Before attempting dental extractions, a presurgical radiograph of the extraction site should be available. The radiograph will disclose the height and character of the supporting alveolar bone and root morphology, the knowledge of which should materially aid in the extraction. In cases of embedded molars or large or hypercementosed roots, or when the alveolar bone is dense or without appreciable loss of height, the use of rotary (drill) instruments should be seriously considered.

Elevation

A The judicious use of tooth elevation prior to application of an extraction forceps will usually facilitate luxation from the socket and prevent mucosal tearing. A periosteal elevator should first be used to separate the attached gingiva from the root surface of the tooth. Then a pointed straight-grooved elevator should be interposed between (1) the tooth and the alveolar bone (when a defect is present) and (2) the tooth to be removed and the teeth immediately adjacent. Careful instrumentation allows levering of the offending tooth without harming the adjacent one. This type of instrumentation can also prevent unwanted root fractures at the time of forceps delivery. In cases where repeated attempts at elevation fail to produce tooth movement, reduction of the investing alveolar bone should be considered. Also, teeth with multiple roots that exhibit compound angles to the crown should be removed with longitudinal sectioning. A dental drill or a roto-osteotome is necessary for these maneuvers, and the bone should be irrigated with physiologic solution during the use of one of these instruments.

Forceps Removal

Once the teeth are mobilized as a result of the elevation or are loose from preexisting periodontal disease or trauma, a special forceps should be used for the extraction. The application of the beaks of the forceps and the vectors of force applied to the forceps are important considerations.

UPPER ANTERIOR EXTRACTION

B The forceps used for the removal of maxillary incisors, canines, and premolars are all essentially the same. The beaks are straight projections of the handles without angulation. The beaks should be placed buccolingually. The forces employed should be apical, and for the removal of incisors and canines, an evenly applied rotational component will usually safely luxate the tooth. Sharp or jerky motions should be avoided, as these invite root fracture. For the premolars, the use of rotational forces should be discarded, as these teeth are often birooted. Once the beaks are securely placed, apical and controlled buccolingual forces should be steadily applied. Short buccolingual "rocking" excursions, rather than flamboyant movements, will reduce the incidence of unwanted fractures.

UPPER MOLAR EXTRACTION

C Maxillary molars usually have one lingual root and two buccal roots. In instances where the roots coalesce, are short, or are periodontally compromised, the use of a universal wide-beaked forceps is indicated. The forces for removal should be directed apically and buccolingually. Often the path of least resistance will be readily apparent (pulling coupled with rocking) and this is the path to follow for easy removal. If the roots are well formed and divergent, the use of an anatomic forceps is indicated. This type of forceps comes in both right- and left-sided models. The buccal beak is tapered and pointed and is designed to slide up between the two buccal roots. The lingual beak is wide and engages the lingual root at the neck of the tooth. Careful contraction of the handles of the forcep will expand the investing bone, and the buccolingual forces applied will usually luxate the tooth.

LOWER ANTERIOR EXTRACTION

D The forceps used for removing mandibular incisors, canines, and premolars are quite similar and can be readily interchanged. The beaks are moderately wide and bend down from the handles at about a 45° angle. The application of apical-rotatory forces will easily luxate a tooth with a nonangled root. For canines and premolars, the use of a buccolingual component along with the rotational force may be necessary.

LOWER MOLAR EXTRACTION

E,F The extraction of lower molars can pose significant problems. The root volume is impressive, and the tongue, floor of the mouth, and buccal tissues can obscure the field. The investing bone of the posterior mandible is unusually dense. The forceps used for removal of these teeth have both a buccal and a lingual beak of large proportion. These beaks are placed over the tooth so that their pointed tips engage the tooth at its root bifurcation. With the usual apical pressure, the forces are evenly and strongly applied in a buccolingual, rocking manner. In younger people, the use of a cow horn forceps can expand the alveolar bone to aid in the luxation of the tooth. In some adults, the tooth morphology often mandates sectioning of the crown to the root bifurcation before extraction.

Postextraction Care

Once the extractions are completed, hemostasis should be achieved by pressure and/or cauterization of small vessels. Thin interseptal bone should be removed and the socket periphery smoothed with rongeurs and bone files. The mucosa should be advanced and, if possible, loosely closed over the defect with 3-0 chromic sutures. Prophylactic antibiotics are administered for 5 days. Oral hygiene is maintained with daily chlorhexidine or saline mouthwashes three times a day.

PITFALLS

1. Inappropriate use of force can fracture the tooth, making it difficult to extract pieces of retained fragments. Such forces can also cause fractures of the alveolus and additional fractures to the bone of the jaw.

2. Remove all teeth that can adversely affect bone union. Retention of mobile, infected, or fractured nonsalvageable teeth in an area proximal to the jaw fracture may compromise the healing of the soft tissue and bone.

TOOTH EXTRACTION

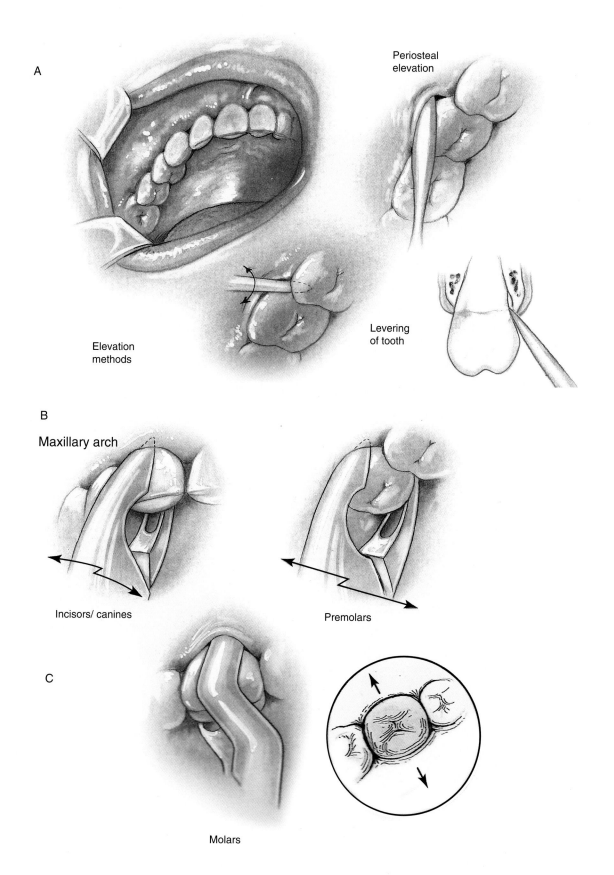

A

Periosteal elevation

Elevation methods

Levering of tooth

B

Maxillary arch

Incisors/ canines

Premolars

C

Molars

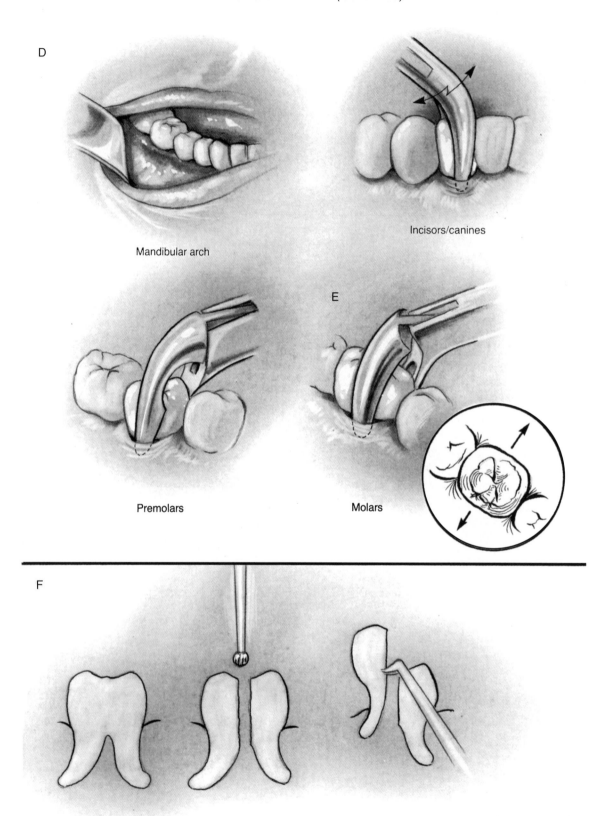

D

Mandibular arch

Incisors/canines

Premolars

E

Molars

F

Sectioning of crown

3. The need for dental extraction should have radiographic corroboration. Radiographs are essential for fully understanding tooth pathology, especially pathosis of the apex region and injuries that involve the alveolus, periodontium, and tooth proper.

COMPLICATIONS

1. Retained roots can be removed with careful use of angled elevators, root picks, and a variety of other specially designed instruments. In most instances, lateral pressure should be used to separate the tooth from the socket walls. Apical pressure should be avoided, except when removing upper anterior teeth, as this vector of force could cause the loss of a root in the antrum, buccal pouch, or compartments inferior to the mandible. Careless instrumentation and loss of the root proximal to the inferior alveolar canal can cause injury to the nerve.

2. Dental or periodontal infection can spread and affect healing of the adjacent fracture. To avoid this problem, extraction should be as atraumatic as possible. All tooth fragments should be removed and the adjacent alveolus adequately debrided. Closure of the mucosa should be loose enough to provide for drainage and healing of the socket from below. Prophylactic antibiotics and antiseptic mouthwashes are helpful adjuncts.

3. Extraction of the tooth (or teeth) can lead to instability of fixation. Postoperatively the patient should have radiographs taken to determine the position of the jaw fragments. If there is displacement of the fracture, an alternative fixation technique will have to be applied.

Closed Reduction of Alveolar Fractures

INDICATIONS

The alveolus is an important structure, and fractures of this area should not be taken lightly. The alveolus provides the neurovascular supply and structural support necessary for the health of the dentition, and in the edentulous patient, it produces a prominent ridge for stabilization of a denture.

Fractures of the alveolar process are common, especially in active teenagers and may be associated with fractures of the body and subcondylar processes of the mandible; rarely it is observed in the edentulous patient. Decisions regarding treatment of the alveolar fracture must be coupled with management strategy for the dental injury.

PROCEDURES

There are two objectives in management of alveolar arch fractures. First is maintenance and restoration of the dentition and second, when the dentition is not preservable, is the maintenance of bone and gingiva. Nonsalvageable teeth are removed, bits of bone attached to periosteum are preserved, and the gingiva is repaired. Sharp bone edges are smoothed with rongeurs or bone files.

For alveolar fractures associated with injured teeth that are important and will be retained, the teeth should be repaired according to procedures described in Chapters 31 and 32. These teeth probably should be treated after the alveolus has been reduced and fixed to the rest of the mandible.

A In the dentate patient, the teeth are the key to restoration. Monoarch stabilization with an arch bar or Essig wire after manual reduction of the fracture is usually sufficient. In the complex, comminuted fracture bimaxillary stabilization with upper and lower arch bars may be required. Manual reduction of the alveolar fragment using finger pressure may require significant force. The interdigitation of the teeth and rigidity of the bar will stabilize the fragment in a position that should be optimal for healing. The arch bar techniques are described in Chapter 19.

B,C In patients who have severe tooth injuries requiring extraction or in patients who are essentially edentulous, other methods must be considered. Often, small fragments of bone can be debrided and the gingiva or mucosa closed over the area of injury. Alternatively, dentures, an acrylic covering, or a lingual acrylic splint with a soft liner can be used in combination with circummandibular wires. If the patient has an incomplete dentition, then a combination of arch bars and acrylic splints (see Chapter 29) attached to the bars can be used to stabilize the intervening fragments.

Alveolar ridge fractures should be immobilized for at least 4 to 6 weeks. Oral health should be maintained with regular brushing and irrigations with a mixture of dilute salt water and hydrogen peroxide

TREATMENT OF ALVEOLAR FRACTURES

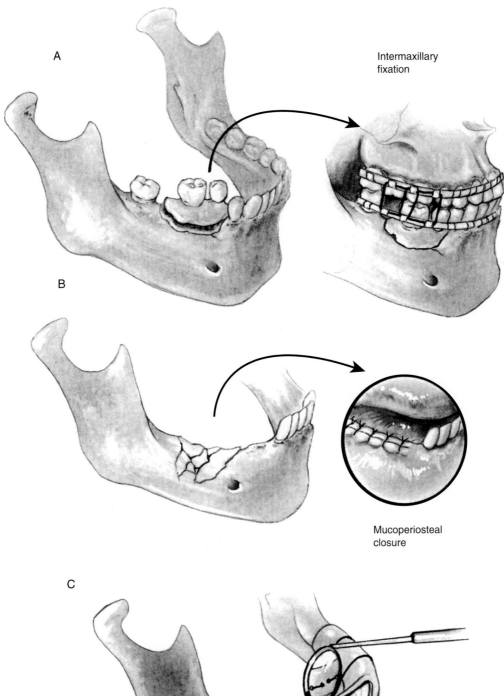

A

Intermaxillary
fixation

B

Mucoperiosteal
closure

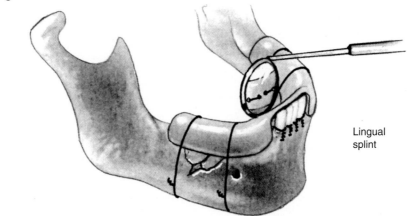

C

Lingual
splint

and twice daily rinses with chlorhexidine. Antibiotics should be provided for 5 to 6 days.

PITFALLS

1. For the most part, treatment of the alveolus should consist of debridement, closure of the gingiva and alveolar mucosa, and closed reduction with or without maxillomandibular fixation. Attempts to open the fracture will further devitalize the fragments and predispose them to infection.

2. Every attempt should be made to retain the alveolar bone and the teeth. However, there are situations in which it may be better to remove the involved ridge of the mandible. This condition often develops following gunshot wounds in which there are multiple pieces of foreign material and devitalized bone. When this occurs, the alveolar mucosa is loosely closed over the area of debridement.

3. Interosseous wires and plates applied to the alveolus should be avoided, as these materials often become exposed and act as foreign bodies. Moreover, an application of poorly fitting dentures can cause delayed complications of erosion and osteomyelitis.

4. Alveolar fractures require meticulous oral care. Lacerations and exposed sockets tend to harbor bacteria and debris. If the wounds are not kept clean, infection can develop in the underlying bone.

5. Remember to repair the alveolar fracture first and then repair the perioral and intraoral lacerations.

COMPLICATIONS

1. If infection should develop in the alveolar ridge, cultures should be obtained and the extent of the infection determined. Devitalized tissues should be removed; this may include the entire alveolar segment. Appropriate antibiotics should be administered for at least 10 days.

2. Displacement of the alveolus, especially in the patient who has teeth, can cause problems with occlusion. Correct occlusion should be achieved at the time of treatment. Oral and maxillofacial surgical or dental consultation might be required. If displacement of the alveolar segment is severe and correct occlusion cannot be achieved, later orthognathic surgery or orthodontic treatment will be required. When it is not necessary to retain the dentition of the alveolar segment, extraction may be the most prudent course of action.

3. Injury to the alveolus can ultimately cause devitalized teeth. In addition to direct trauma to the pulp, the tooth is often subjected to indirect injury caused by disruption of the neurovascular supply to the alveolar segment. Evaluation by pulp testing may be indicated. If the tooth should become nonvital, endodontic therapy is indicated. If the dentition is associated with severe caries or periodontal disease, extraction should be performed.

Nonunion of the Mandible

CHAPTER

34

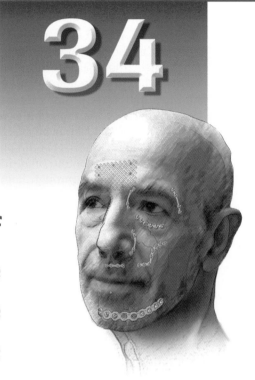

Early Treatment of Nonunion of the Mandible With Reconstruction Plate
Alternative Technique Using External Pin Fixation (Biphase)

INDICATIONS

Nonunion of the mandible is often the result of infection and is usually associated with pain and abnormal mobility of the jaw. The infection can be caused by contamination, retained foreign bodies, or failure to immobilize and reduce the fracture. Other contributing factors include an impaired blood supply and malnourishment, conditions that ultimately affect the healing of bone. All, or at least some, of the factors should be considered preliminarily before proceeding with the repair processes.

A stepwise progression of medical and surgical treatment is necessary. The goal is to obtain a clean, vascularized, and immobilized jaw.

PROCEDURE

Occlusal relationships must be obtained. If there are sets of opposing teeth, they can be aligned with several Ivy loops, intermaxillary fixation screws, or arch bars. In the edentulous patient, stents or splints can be applied, but because the maxillary mandibular relationships can be readjusted at a later time with dentures, simple manipulations to approximate relationships of the jaws are all that are necessary.

A Exposure of the mandibular area of nonunion will depend on the site of nonunion. Standard approaches are described in Chapters 24, 26, and 28. Longer incisions should be planned to accommodate the reconstruction plate.

B Periosteum should be elevated from all surfaces of the involved mandible, carefully avoiding entry into the oral cavity. If torn, the oral mucosa should be repaired immediately and the wound irrigated copiously with normal saline. Devitalized bone and foreign material should be removed from the wound and the area debrided as necessary.

C–E After adequate exposure, the proximal and distal mandibular segments should be reduced and held in position with bone forceps. The remaining bone fragments in the area of nonunion, if any, should be manipulated into anatomic position. The reconstruction plate should be designed so that at least two screws (but preferably three or four) can be placed into each stable segment of the mandible across the nonunion area. A cutter should be available to cut the plate to the desired length. Special bending forceps are used to bend the plate to the contour of the recipient site. Screw holes are then drilled through both cortices and the holes probed with a depth gauge to determine screw length. Screws are then placed through the holes in the proximal and distal segments. The area of nonunion should either have a close approximation of proximal and distal segments or at least bone fragments to fill the gap. If this is not possible because of missing bone then the mandible should be fixated in a position that maintains occlusal relationships with plans to return at a later time for a bone graft repair (Chapter 35).

The wound is closed by advancing the periosteum over the plate site with 2-0 chromic sutures. Dead space must be obliterated. This can be accomplished by freeing up the platysma and subcutaneous layers and inverting these soft tissues into the wound with 2-0 or 3-0 chromic vertical mattress sutures. Penrose drains should be used for 24 to 48 hours or longer if drainage persists. The skin is approximated with 5-0 nylon sutures.

Postoperatively the patient is maintained on intravenous antibiotics for at least 5 days and continued on oral antibiotics for an additional several weeks. The patient can be started and maintained on a full liquid diet; chewing of food should be avoided for at least 2 weeks. The mouth should be washed several times a day with 3% hydrogen peroxide. The wound should be inspected weekly and radiographs obtained after surgery and at 6 to 8 weeks to evaluate adequacy of healing.

PITFALLS

1. Do not reconstruct the jaw if there is any evidence of infection. The mandible must be treated and prepared with appropriate antibiotics and a period of immobilization for at least 4 to 6 months prior to bone grafting (see Chapter 35).

2. Pretrauma occlusal relationships should be obtained prior to fixation. Excessive bite forces can distract the fragments from the fracture site; these forces must be minimized by ensuring normal occlusion in the postoperative period.

3. Intraoral exposure will contaminate the wound. Lacerations created during the elevation of the periosteum should be closed immediately with 3-0 chromic sutures and the wound washed copiously with normal saline.

4. Debride devitalized bone and soft tissue from the wound. Remove foreign material before application of the plate.

5. Dead space should be avoided and/or obliterated. Proper use of drains, rotation and/or advancement of subcutaneous tissues, and pressure dressings will help close the space and provide some prophylaxis against hematoma and infection.

6. The reconstruction plate must be rigidly fixed. Screws must be tight fitting, and this can only be achieved by placing the screw in a hole that is slightly smaller than the screw. Also remember that at least two screws, and preferably three, are required to stabilize the proximal and distal mandibular segments. If one chooses to use a locking reconstruction plate remember to hold the plate firmly against the mandibular cortex while applying screws.

COMPLICATIONS

1. Infection can be prevented by avoiding intraoral contamination, dead space within the wound, insufficient debridement, and less than optimal fixation. If the wound becomes further infected, the infection should be drained and cultures obtained for the selection of appropriate intravenous antibiotics. Dead pieces of bone should be debrided. Sometimes the infection will come under control and the plate can be saved. However, if the amount of purulent drainage does not cease, and the plate is involved (i.e., the screw holes show evidence of osteomyelitis), then the plate and screws should be removed. Further immobilization can be achieved with other previously described techniques (i.e., intermaxillary fixation, splints, stents, and biphase). A period of 4 to 6 months is again necessary before proceeding with reconstruction.

2. Facial deformity from loss of bone and/or soft tissue is common following a nonunion. In these cases, the mandible can be grafted later when there are no longer signs of infection (Chapter 35). Scar revision must also be considered.

3. Nonunion of the mandible is almost always associated with loss of sensation of the inferior alveolar nerve and from repeated surgery, loss of motion of those muscles innervated by the marginal mandibular

EARLY TREATMENT OF NONUNION

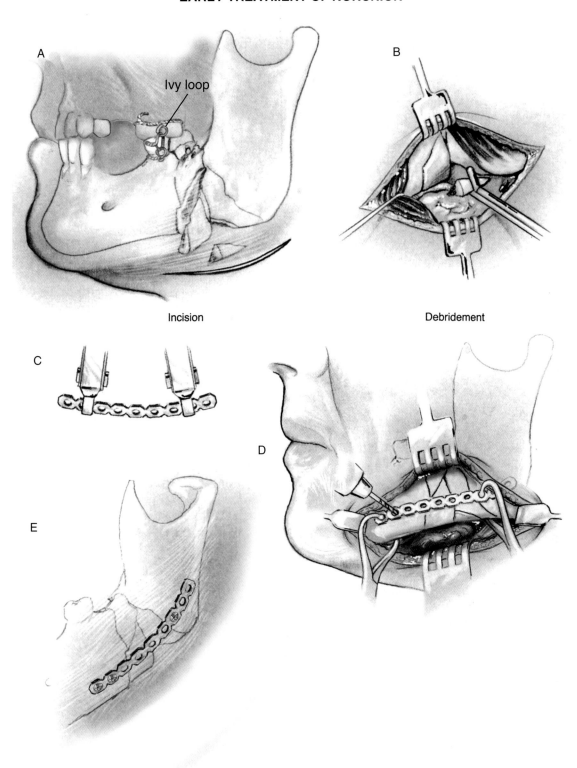

Incision

Debridement

nerve. Attempts at nerve graft are usually not successful and probably should not be attempted. Other methods for minimizing the cosmetic effects are neurotomy of the opposite side and/or muscle transposition to the involved.

ALTERNATIVE TECHNIQUE USING EXTERNAL PIN FIXATION (BIPHASE)

The biphase technique is ideal, as bicortical pins can be placed away from the fracture site and provide for an opportunity to treat the wound locally with debridement and irrigation. Moreover, the mandible can be completely immobilized during the "cleanup" period, which may allow for new bone to bridge the gap. The biphase is also an excellent method to stabilize the jaw during a bone graft procedure (see Chapter 35).

a,b In the patient with teeth, occlusal relationships should be established with Ivy Loops, intermaxillary fixation screws, or arch bars. The area of infection involving the mandible must be opened, drained, and debrided. Any devitalized bone noted previously on radiographs, visually during the procedure or on palpation should be removed. Distal and proximal segments should be reduced and aligned anatomically. Pin holes are subsequently mapped out along the mandible so that at least two pin holes are placed in solid bone proximal and distal to the area of nonunion.

c A small stab incision is made in a crease line over the planned placement of each pin. Using a headlight and a medium, narrow-bladed Cottle speculum for visualization, the deeper tissues are spread with a hemostat in the direction of the facial nerve. On exposure of the cortex of the mandible, the periosteum is elevated with a Joseph elevator, and using a minidriver with a drill bit for a 5/64-inch screw, a hole is made through both cortices. Irrigation with normal saline avoids excessive heating of the bone.

While maintaining visualization of the hole, a special 5/64-inch pin/screw with a hexagonal head and machine screw end is applied to the hole. Different lengths are available. The screw will encounter some resistance at the outer cortical bone, some loosening in the cancellous bone, and then resistance again as it becomes secure in the inner cortex.

The same procedure is carried out for placement of each pin. In most cases, bleeding from the cortex will stop after a few minutes. The pins should always be oriented perpendicular to the cortex of the mandible and at least 2 to 3 cm apart to obtain maximal stability.

d The pins are secured to each other with metal bars and universal joints. As the fragments are realigned, the bars are adjusted and stabilized in a desired position.

e The acrylic bar that will replace the metal bar is fabricated with autopolymerizing denture acrylic (5 to 10 minutes setting time) or with the slower-setting cranioplasty material (10 to 20 minutes). The acrylic is made by mixing appropriate amounts of powder and liquid. It is then poured into a form bar treated with petrolatum to prevent sticking and allowed to "cure." Usually a small piece of acrylic held in the hand and rolled into a ball will, at some point in time, begin to harden. This is a cue for removal of the bar and application to the pins. The acrylic is best removed from the tray by lifting the band beneath the acrylic or cutting it free with a large (No. 12) knife blade.

f In this semisoft condition, the acrylic is positioned over the outer machine threads of the pins. Washer nuts are then secured to the end of the screws and twisted down so that they are flush with the surface of the acrylic. The acrylic gets hot during the self-curing process, and to avoid injury to the bone and/or soft tissues, the pins should be covered with several turns of petrolatum gauze. When the acrylic is completely hardened, the metal bars can be removed.

The wound is closed in layers. Patients are treated prophylactically with antibiotics, and the acrylic bar is maintained until healing is complete (usually in 6 to 8 weeks). The area around the pin is kept clean with 3% hydrogen peroxide and daily application of antibiotic ointment. At 6 to 8 weeks following control of infection, radiographs are obtained, and if there is evidence of union without infection, the bar can be removed. Segments of the bar are cut with a Gigli saw, and each segment is rotated counterclockwise (with the screw) for removal from the bone. Bacitracin ointment is applied to the wound.

g A more rapid, optional method for reconstruction uses a polyvinyl tube. For this procedure, a No. 8 endotracheal tube is cut to size and placed over the end of the pins. Using a No. 15 knife blade, holes are then made where the pins come in contact with the tube and also directly on the opposite side of the tube. The tube is then placed over the screws so that the first hole goes over the pin and the second penetrates the free machine end of the pin. The acrylic is pushed through the tube with a large-bore syringe. Usually the acrylic flows through some of the small holes and through the other end, but the dripping can be controlled with a piece of gauze and finger pressure. When the acrylic stops flowing, the surgeon can attend to other portions of the procedure.

It is often difficult to differentiate devitalized bone from healing bone. Because there is a tendency to try to retain as much bone as possible, there is also a tendency to keep any questionable bone, and if this bone is devitalized, infection will persist. Thus if drainage

ALTERNATIVE TREATMENT USING EXTERNAL FIXATION (BIPHASE)

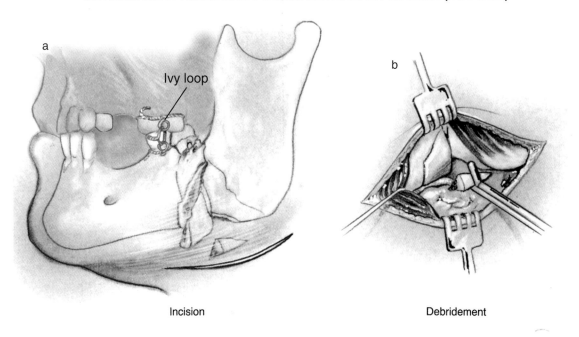

a

Ivy loop

Incision

b

Debridement

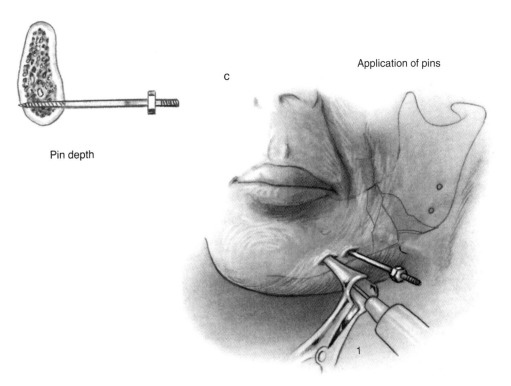

Pin depth

Application of pins

c

1

Wm. Loechel

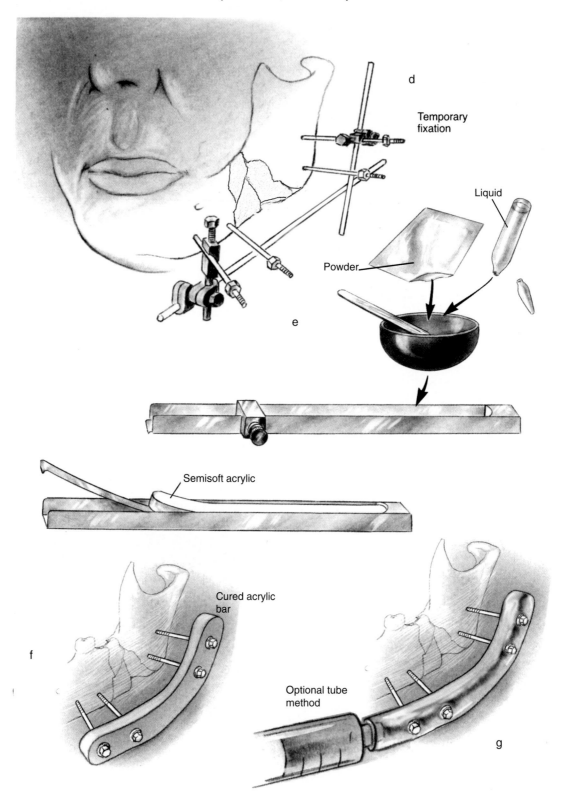

d

Temporary fixation

Liquid

Powder

e

Semisoft acrylic

Cured acrylic bar

f

Optional tube method

g

does not cease, the physician should be alerted to the possibility of reexploration and further debridement. Continuation of infection suggests an underlying cause preventing bone healing. The patient should be thoroughly evaluated for immunologic and hematologic status. Vitamin and mineral deficiencies should be investigated. New cultures should be obtained and appropriate antibiotics (usually intravenous) administered. Also, remember that infections will delay healing for 2 to 4 weeks, and this time must be added to the healing process. Thus the patient should be in fixation for at least 6 to 8 weeks after infection has been controlled before removal of the Biphase or further reconstructive surgery.

CHAPTER 35

Repair of (Late) Nonunion of the Mandible With Iliac Crest Grafts and Reconstruction Plate
Alternative Technique Using External Pin Fixation (Biphase)

INDICATIONS

Nonunion of the mandible can occur in a variety of locations but is often found in an unfavorable angle or parasymphyseal fracture or in a fracture of an area of an edentulous atrophic body. Nonunion of the ramus, condyle, or coronoid process can also develop, but in these locations it does not usually pose a functional problem.

Jaw instability associated with a defect usually requires correction with rigid fixation, but if this fails, and there continues to be a defect at the fracture site, a bone graft technique is indicated. To optimize conditions for surgery, the infection should be brought under control, and there should be a period of 4 to 6 months in which there is no evidence of soft tissue infection or osteomyelitis. Further immobilization is often necessary as described in Chapter 34.

There are many methods for bone grafting and stabilization, but the reconstruction plate has become the most popular. This technique has the advantage of rigid fixation with early mobility and function of the jaw. Bone grafts can be harvested from a variety of sites, but the ileum is preferred. Iliac bone is easy to obtain and easy to shape and fit into the nonunion defect.

PROCEDURE

Harvest of Iliac Crest

To avoid confusion with an appendectomy scar, the left iliac crest should be selected as the donor site. Exposure is obtained by propping the left buttock with rolled towels or sandbags. The skin is prepared and draped as a sterile field. The incision is planned lateral to the crest to avoid a scar on the prominent part of the crest. This helps reduce discomfort that can be caused by pressure of a belt or waistband in this area.

A,B While pulling the skin medially, a 6- to 8-cm incision is made through the skin and subcutaneous fat. The anterior superior iliac spine is identified, and a cut is made through the periosteum from the spine to the flare of the ileum. Using heavy elevators, the periosteum is elevated off the crest. Laterally the elevation is more difficult because of the attachment of gluteus muscles, and these tendons must be incised with scissors or knife. Bleeding will be brisk, and hemostasis should be controlled with an electrocautery. The degree of elevation of the periosteum will depend on the amount of bone required for grafting, but a laterally directed subperiosteal pocket of about 6 × 10 cm can be safely developed without adversely affecting the hip joint.

C,D The graft is harvested with sharp, straight, and curved 8- to 10-mm osteotomes. Using a straight osteotome, the bone is cut in a plane parallel to the outer table, taking a thickness from several millimeters to almost the entire crest. The medial cortex should preferably be left intact. Inferiorly, the cut is developed along the anterior superior iliac spine. Superiorly, the limit is defined by the size of the bone required for the graft. The posterior cuts require a heavy retractor on the muscles, and usually a curved osteotome is necessary to obtain the appropriate direction and force. All bone cuts are then deepened, and when the osteotome tends to bind, it should be freed with a rocking action. Eventually the lateral plate bone becomes loose, and additional pieces of cancellous bone can then be removed with an osteotome and saved for the filling of small defects. The graft should be placed in a basin of blood until it is ready for implantation.

Hemostasis is achieved by applying bone wax to the external surface of the freshly cut ileum. Excess wax should be removed by forcefully wiping the wax with a sponge. Two medium-sized suction drains are placed through stab incisions and secured with 2-0 silk purse string sutures. The periosteum is closed with 2-0 chromic sutures. The fat and subcutaneous tissues are brought together with 3-0 chromic sutures, and the skin is approximated with 5-0 nylon sutures.

Repair of Defect

Occlusal relationships must be obtained. If there are sets of opposing teeth, they can be aligned with several Ivy loops, intermaxillary fixation screws, or arch bars. In the edentulous patient, stents or splints can be applied, but because the maxillary mandibular relationships can be readjusted at a later time with dentures, simple manipulations to approximate relationships of the jaws are all that are necessary. If the patient has a biphase apparatus in position, this can be quite helpful in stabilizing the fragments.

E Exposure of the mandibular defect will depend on the site of nonunion. Standard external approaches are described in Chapters 24, 26, and 28. Longer incisions should be planned to accommodate the reconstruction plate.

F Periosteum should be elevated from all surfaces of the involved mandible, carefully avoiding entry into the oral cavity. If torn, the oral mucosa should be repaired immediately and the wound irrigated copiously with normal saline. The bone edges are often quite smooth and relatively avascular, and these edges must be freshened with bone rongeurs to at least a point at which fresh bleeding occurs.

G After adequate exposure of the outer surface of the mandible and approximation of the position of the mandibular fragments with bone forceps, the bone graft should be cut and placed into the defect. A wedging of the bone into position is desirable.

H In planning for the reconstruction plate, the surgeon should place the plate so that at least two screws (but preferably three or four) can be placed into each segment of the mandible and at least one screw hole through the graft. A cutter should be available to cut the plate to the desired length. Special bending forceps are used to bend the plate to the contour of the recipient site.

I–J Screw holes are then drilled through both cortices and the screw length determined with a depth gauge placed through the holes of the plate. Screws are then placed through these holes proximal and distal to the fragmented area. Another hole or preferably two are drilled into the graft and appropriate size screws placed to secure the graft. If there are any defects at the ends where the graft and mandible join, these can be filled with pieces of cancellous bone. Additional pieces of bone can be used to adjust levels of the graft.

The wound is closed by pulling the periosteum over the plate with 2-0 chromic sutures. Dead space must be obliterated. This can be accomplished by freeing up the platysma and subcutaneous layers and inverting these soft tissues into the wound with 2-0 or 3-0 chromic vertical mattress sutures. Penrose drains may be used for 24 to 48 hours, but if the wound is dry, they should be avoided. The skin is approximated with 5-0 nylon sutures.

Extra pieces of iliac crest can be stored in a hospital bone bank, but if this is not available, the use of a "belly bank" should be considered. Usually the preparation of the hip includes the lower abdomen, which can be used for the bank. A small horizontal incision is then made just beneath the belt or waistline. A subcutaneous pocket is developed and the remainder of the graft inserted. The wound is then closed with subcuticular 4-0 chromic sutures and skin sutures of 5-0 nylon.

Postoperatively the patient is maintained on intravenous antibiotics for at least 5 days and continued on oral antibiotics for an additional 10 to 14 days. The patient can be started and maintained on a full liquid diet; chewing of food should be avoided for at least 2 weeks. The mouth should be washed several times

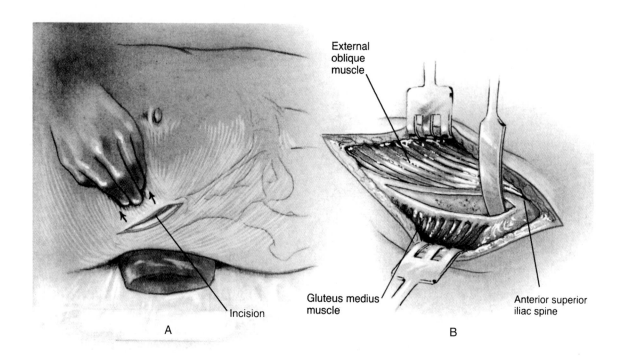

Incision

A

External
oblique
muscle

Gluteus medius
muscle

Anterior superior
iliac spine

B

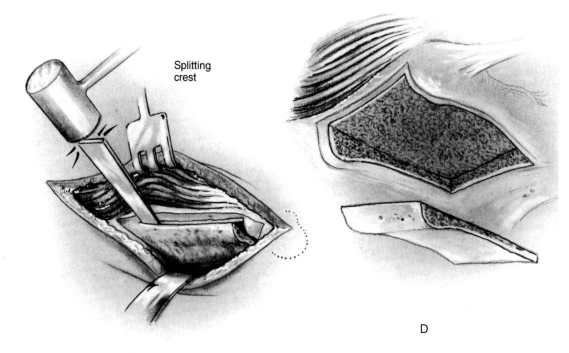

Splitting
crest

C

D

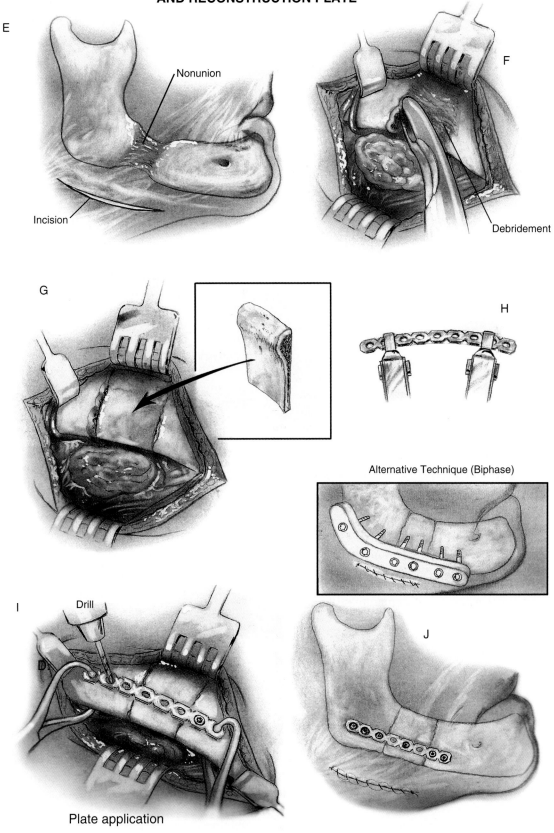

E

Nonunion

Incision

F

Debridement

G

H

Alternative Technique (Biphase)

I

Drill

Plate application

J

a day with 3% hydrogen peroxide. The wound should be inspected weekly and radiographs obtained after surgery and at 6 to 8 weeks to evaluate adequacy of healing.

With regard to the hip, ambulation should begin as soon as possible. Drains are removed when the drainage is <20 to 25 mL/d. Sutures are removed at 7 days.

PITFALLS

1. Understanding the amount of bone necessary to fill the defect is occasionally a problem. To avoid this situation, remove 25% to 50% more bone than is thought necessary to fill the defect.

2. Avoid hematomas of the hip, as they can lead to infection and pain. Hematoma can be prevented by fastidious hemostasis and also by checking for obstruction of the drainage tubes. The drains should not be removed until drainage is <25 mL/d.

3. Sponges can inadvertently be left in the depths of the hip wound. A sponge count while closing can be extremely helpful.

4. In preparing the graft, it is necessary to try to provide a physiologic environment. Keep the graft bathed in a basin layered with blood. The surgeon should irrigate with lactated Ringer's solution while cutting and contouring the bone.

5. Do not reconstruct the jaw if there is any evidence of infection. The mandible must be treated and prepared with appropriate antibiotics and a period of immobilization for at least 4 to 6 months prior to bone grafting. Large contaminated areas of nonunion with an associated defect are best treated with vascular free flap techniques (see Chapter 36).

6. Pretrauma occlusal relationships should be obtained prior to grafting and fixation. Excessive bite forces can distract the fragments from the fracture site; these forces must be minimized by ensuring normal occlusion in the postoperative period.

7. Intraoral exposure will contaminate the wound. Lacerations created during the elevation of the periosteum should be closed immediately with 3-0 chromic sutures and the wound washed copiously with normal saline.

8. Dead space should be avoided and/or obliterated. Proper use of drains, rotation and/or advancement of subcutaneous tissues, and pressure dressings will help close the space and provide some prophylaxis against hematoma and infection.

9. The reconstruction plate must be rigidly fixed. Screws must be tight fitting, and this can only be achieved by placing the screw in a hole that is slightly smaller than the screw. Also remember that at least two screws, and preferably three, are required to stabilize the proximal and distal mandibular segments.

COMPLICATIONS

1. Iliac crest grafts are often associated with hip pain. Early mobilization of the joint is helpful and will prevent guarding and stiffness. Active rehabilitation is advisable.

2. Infection can be prevented by avoiding intraoral contamination, dead space within the wound, and less than optimal fixation. If the wound becomes infected, the infection should be drained and cultures obtained for the selection of appropriate intravenous antibiotics. Dead pieces of bone should be debrided. Sometimes the infection will come under control and the graft can be saved. However, if the amount of purulent drainage does not cease, the graft will have to be removed. If the plate is involved (i.e., the screw holes show evidence of osteomyelitis), then it should also be removed. Further immobilization can be achieved with other previously described techniques (i.e., intermaxillary fixation, splints, stents, and biphase). A period of 4 to 6 months is again necessary before proceeding with reconstruction.

3. Oral rehabilitation is often a problem following a bone graft procedure. Obliteration of the gingivolabial or gingivobuccal sulcus will require a vestibuloplasty. If a large bone graft is used, the osseous integrated implant technique may be necessary for stability of the denture.

4. Facial deformity is common following an iliac crest implant. The bone plate and screws often show through the skin and must be removed. Resorption of the graft may be spotty, and irregularities of the bone will require a smoothing with cutting burs.

5. Bone grafting of the mandible is almost always associated with loss of sensation of the inferior alveolar nerve and loss of motion of those muscles innervated by the marginal mandibular nerve. Attempts at nerve graft are usually not successful and probably should not be attempted. Other methods for minimizing the cosmetic effects are neurotomy of the opposite side and/or muscle transposition to the involved site.

ALTERNATIVE TECHNIQUE USING EXTERNAL PIN FIXATION (BIPHASE)

External pin fixation has the advantage of immobilizing the mandible while treating the nonunion with debridement and antibiotics. The same method used for immobilization is employed for stabilizing the grafts that are used in the repair of the mandibular defect. The disadvantages of the technique are that the fixation apparatus must be taken apart to perform the surgery, it does not provide a fixation as rigid as that obtained with the plate, and it is clumsy to wear in the postoperative period.

The procedure requires setting the jaws into occlusal relationships. The biphase pins are then applied and held in position with universal joints and external bars (see Chapter 34). The hip graft is harvested and the recipient bed prepared as discussed previously. The hip graft is then fitted into place, the acrylic is applied across the pins, and the wound closed in layers.

Postoperative care requires intravenous antibiotics (5 to 7 days), followed by oral antibiotics for another week. Periodic radiographs should be obtained to ensure adequate healing. Pin holes must be kept clean with 3% hydrogen peroxide and daily applications of an antibiotic ointment. The acrylic bar is cut at about 8 weeks and the wound tested for stability. If there is any motion, the acrylic is reapplied; otherwise, the pins can be removed.

36

Repair of Mandible Defect With Fibula Free Flap Technique

In Consultation With George Yoo, MD

INDICATIONS

Composite defects of the mandible associated with loss of significant amounts of skin and mucosa are often the result of gunshots and other severe trauma. The reconstructive goals are to restore function and appearance. The strategy for reconstruction of the mandible is to replace the continuity of the bone and soft tissue. Since the defect is frequently contaminated with oral secretions and the viability of adjacent tissues may be compromised, bone grafts often will not survive. Thus, a more predictable method is accomplished with a vascularized free flap. These same techniques can be used to treat nonunion following failed medical and/or surgical management (see Chapter 35).

Our preferred technique for reconstruction of the mandibular defect is the fibular free flap. The benefits of the fibula flap are the length of bone and the availability of soft tissue and skin. The length of available bone is 25 cm. A robust skin paddle allows for the reconstruction of intraoral and cutaneous defects.

PROCEDURE

The approach to managing a severe ballistic wound to the face and neck requires exposure of all fractured fragmented segments, debridement of soft tissue and a freshening of the bone edges, precise anatomical rigid fixation, and definitive soft tissue coverage. When possible, fractures should be treated with rigid internal fixation. In the preoperative evaluation of the mandibular defect, the length of defect, the number of wedge osteotomies, available donor vessels, and soft tissue requirements should be determined.

A,B To perform the fibular free flap procedure, the surgeon must have an understanding of the basic musculoskeletal and neurovascular anatomy of the leg:

The fibula bone lies between the knee and ankle joints. The fibula is not weight bearing, whereas the tibia is weight bearing. Therefore, the leg function, ankle, and knee joints are not affected if 5 cm of proximal and distal bone are left intact.

The femoral artery divides into the peroneal, anterior tibial, and posterior tibial arteries to supply the lower leg. The peroneal artery provides blood supply to the fibula bone and skin paddle. The skin paddle receives its blood supply from the septocutaneous perforators of the peroneal vessels. These perforators run behind the lateral septum within the soleus muscle.

C In harvesting the fibula flap, the external landmarks, such as the head of the fibula, lateral malleolus, and the skin paddle, should be identified. The size of the skin paddle needed for internal and external defects should be overestimated since the short (1- to 2-cm) lateral intermuscular septum does not allow for significant mobility of the fibular flap skin. The fibular head, lateral intermuscular septum, and lateral malleolus are identified and marked on the skin of the leg. A skin paddle is marked on the leg over the lateral intermuscular septum. The tourniquet is placed around the thigh and inflated to approximately 350 or 200 mm Hg over systolic blood pressure.

REPAIR OF MANDIBULAR DEFECT WITH FIBULA FREE FLAP TECHNIQUE

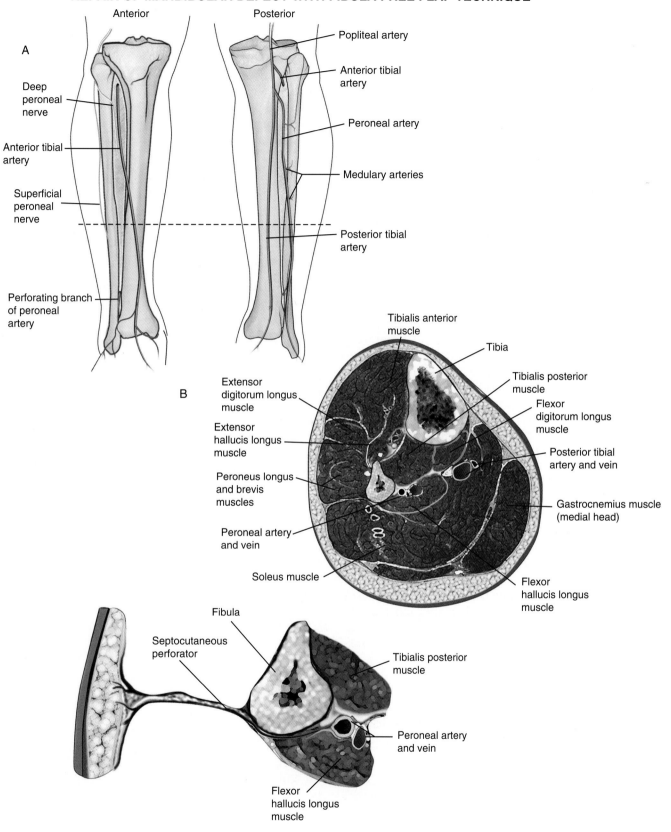

A

Anterior

Posterior

Deep peroneal nerve

Anterior tibial artery

Superficial peroneal nerve

Perforating branch of peroneal artery

Popliteal artery

Anterior tibial artery

Peroneal artery

Medulary arteries

Posterior tibial artery

B

Tibialis anterior muscle

Tibia

Tibialis posterior muscle

Flexor digitorum longus muscle

Posterior tibial artery and vein

Gastrocnemius muscle (medial head)

Flexor hallucis longus muscle

Extensor digitorum longus muscle

Extensor hallucis longus muscle

Peroneus longus and brevis muscles

Peroneal artery and vein

Soleus muscle

Fibula

Septocutaneous perforator

Tibialis posterior muscle

Peroneal artery and vein

Flexor hallucis longus muscle

D Incisions are made through the skin, subcutaneous tissue, and fascia of the peroneal and soleus muscles leaving a skin paddle and 5 cm of bone at the fibular head and lateral malleolus. The muscle fascia and lateral intermuscular septum muscle are carefully excised off of the peroneal muscles until the periosteum of the fibular bone is encountered. The peroneal muscle is dissected off of the periosteum of the fibular bone leaving a 1-mm cuff of muscle while care is taken not to injure the periosteum. The anterior intermuscular septum is incised leaving a 1-mm cuff next to the fibula. The anterior compartment vessels, nerves, and muscles are retracted anteriorly. The anterior tibial nerve, artery, and vein are identified and left intact. The peroneal nerve is left intact. The lateral portion of the extensor hallucis longus muscle is dissected off of the interosseous septum. The interosseous septum is incised leaving a 1-mm cuff next to the fibula.

E The fibular osteotomies are made leaving a 5 cm next to the fibular head and 5 cm next to the lateral malleolus. The distal peroneal artery and veins are identified, clamped, cut, and ligated separately. The tibialis posterior muscle is divided while visualizing the peroneal artery and veins. The posterior tibial vessels and nerve are identified and left intact. Careful dissection of the proximal pedicle of the peroneal artery and veins is performed. Muscle perforating branches are identified, clamped, cut, and ligated at least 1 cm from the pedicle of the peroneal artery and veins. The flexor hallucis longus muscle is identified and divided while visualizing the peroneal artery and veins. The soleus muscle is incised leaving a 1-cm cuff of muscle attached to the lateral intermuscular septum in order not to injure septal cutaneous perforators. The cuff is released for half an hour and blood is allowed to reflow. Palpable pulses are felt in both anterior and posterior tibial arteries along with the dorsalis pedis and posterior tibial area of the foot. Palpable pulses are felt in the peroneal artery. Then after reperfusion, the peroneal artery and veins are clamped, cut, and ligated. The osteocutaneous fibular free flap is transferred to the neck area.

In the leg, minor bleeding is stopped. The drain is placed. The peroneal and soleus muscles are sutured together. The skin is closed primarily proximally and distally. Where skin paddle is taken, a split thickness skin graft is taken from the thigh. A volar splint is placed for 7 days.

F The carotid artery exploration is performed by dissection around the common, external, and internal carotid artery. The internal and external jugular veins are also carefully dissected. Adventitia is cleaned off the external carotid artery, and the best donor artery from the external carotid artery is identified.

G The donor artery is carefully dissected. A microvascular clamp is placed on the proximal donor artery and the distal donor artery is clamped, cut, and ligated. Then, the microvascular clamp is released to determine if there is immediate pulsatile blood flow. The microvascular clamp is reapplied, and the vessel is irrigated with heparinized saline solution. Mechanical dilation is performed with a microdilator and heparinized saline irrigation. This prevents vascular spasm by paralysis of the smooth muscle.

H The mandibular reconstruction is performed by placing the bent reconstruction plate back onto the native mandible using already drilled holes and screws. The length of the mandibular defect is measured. The periosteum is elevated off of the proximal fibular bone leaving enough periosteum on bone to match the mandibular defect.

I Wedge osteotomies are made depending on the location of the defect and angle of the mandible that needs to be replicated.

J Fixation is usually by mandibular reconstruction plates or miniplates. The fibular bone is set into the defect and locked into place with reconstruction plate and screws. Holes are drilled using a drill and irrigation. Screws are placed in the standard fashion. The flap does not need to be completely set into the mandible. However, the orientation of the flap should be stable in order to insure that the vessel geometry is not changed after microvascular anastomosis.

K Under the microscope, vessels are irrigated with copious amounts of heparinized saline solution and dilated using microvascular dilator. The vessel should be handled gently without grasping the intima, that is, no full-thickness forceps grabbing. After the adventitia is cleaned off of each vessel, fresh transverse cuts are made, and clean cuts are noted. Then, the vessels are again dilated using microvascular dilator and irrigated with copious amounts of heparinized saline solution using a blunt needle tip irrigator. Inspection for intimal flaps, intraluminal clots, and intraluminal adventitia is performed.

L Under the microscope, the arterial vessels are placed in the cage approximating clamp. Excellent approximation and size match are desired. No adventitia is allowed in the lumen. Vascular suturing with 9-0 nylon is performed by piercing perpendicularly the full thickness of the vessels. The vessel lumen can be better visualized or stabilized by placing microforceps in lumen or retracting the adventitia. The needle is pulled through in circular motion to avoid vessel injury. Simple suturing by tying with an initial surgeon's knot is then performed. The first two anchoring

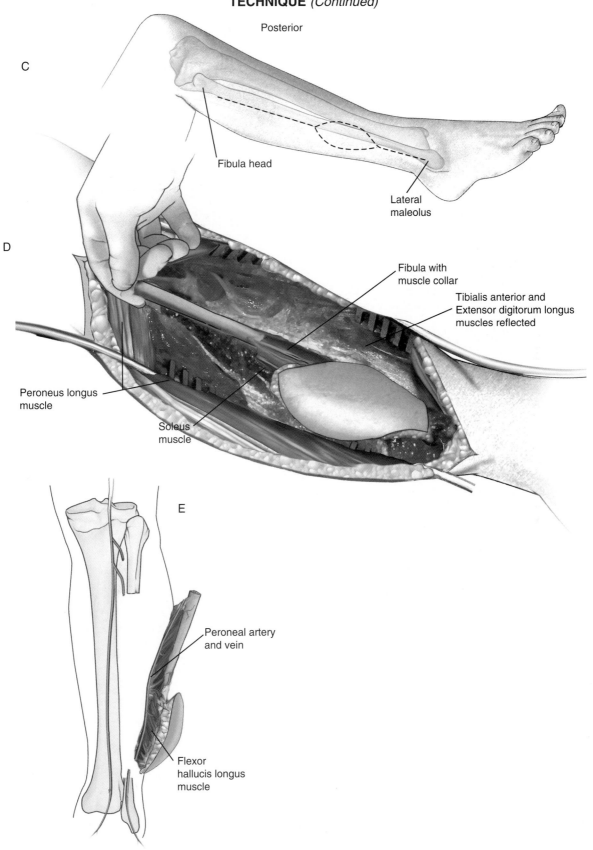

C

Posterior

Fibula head

Lateral maleolus

D

Fibula with muscle collar

Tibialis anterior and Extensor digitorum longus muscles reflected

Peroneus longus muscle

Soleus muscle

E

Peroneal artery and vein

Flexor hallucis longus muscle

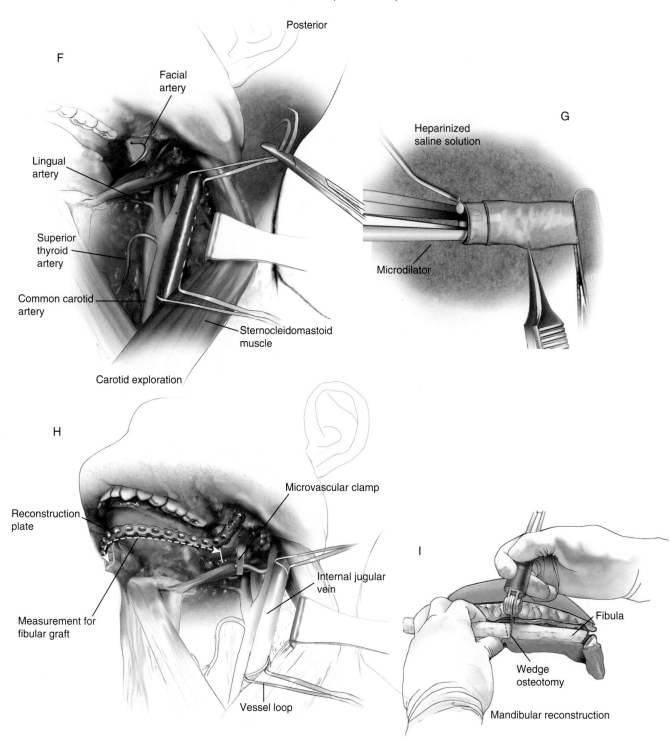

Posterior

F

Facial
artery

Lingual
artery

Superior
thyroid
artery

Common carotid
artery

Sternocleidomastoid
muscle

Carotid exploration

G

Heparinized
saline solution

Microdilator

H

Reconstruction
plate

Microvascular clamp

Internal jugular
vein

Measurement for
fibular graft

Vessel loop

I

Fibula

Wedge
osteotomy

Mandibular reconstruction

sutures are placed and fastened to opposite ended cleats using 9-0 nylon. The anterior wall is anastomosed with interrupted 9-0 nylon sutures. The cage clamp is flipped, and the anterior anastomosis should be completely visualized internally in order to ensure that no suture went through the back wall. The posterior anastomosis is performed by using interrupted 9-0 nylon sutures. The anchoring sutures are cut. The cage clamp is flipped back and then removed.

M Under the microscope, an end-to-side anastomosis of the veins is performed using a running technique. The internal jugular vein is isolated, and vessel loops are tightened to interrupt venous blood flow. An anterior venotomy is made in the internal jugular vein using the curved microvascular scissors. The adventitia is cleaned off. No adventitia is allowed in the lumen. Using microvascular instruments, anchoring sutures are placed using 9-0 nylon proximally and distally. The medial anastomosis is performed using the proximal suture in a running technique and tied to the distal suture with interrupted 9-0 nylon sutures. The anterior anastomosis should be completely visualized internally in order to assure that no suture went through the back wall. The lateral anastomosis is performed using the distal suture in a running technique and tied to the proximal suture with interrupted 9-0 nylon sutures. The anchoring sutures are cut.

N After the microvascular arterial and venous anastomoses are performed, microvascular clamps and vessels loops are removed. There should be immediate good transverse pulsatile blood flow. The muscle, skin, and bone should bleed throughout the closure of the case. Arterial and venous Doppler signals should be observed throughout the closure of the case.

O Final closure in the head and neck area is completed by oral and neck-face skin suturing. If no skin paddle is used, primary closure or skin grafting onto muscle can be completed. The use of a fibular skin paddle usually necessitates removal of part of the cutaneous epithelium.

P Dental reconstruction with possible further bone grafting, vestibuloplasty and osseointegrated implants can be performed at a later time. This allows for improved mastication. Many times there is a scar revision and flap debulking that needs to take place in order to obtain improved cosmetic results. Care has to be taken not to impair the viability of flap.

PITFALLS

1. An experienced microvascular surgeon with expertise in microvascular free flap anastomosis and flap harvest is required to reduce complications and achieve the best functional and aesthetic results. Since the need for a fibular free flap for mandibular reconstruction is not common, the experience of microvascular surgeons is typically gained with reconstruction of head and neck cancer ablative defects.

2. The fibula flap skin paddle is usually robust and we have lost <1% of the skin paddles. On the other hand, the short (1- to 2-cm) lateral intermuscular septum does not allow for significant mobility of the fibular flap skin and thus the skin paddle size needed for internal and external defects should be overestimated for the size of the defect. In these cases excess skin can be removed if necessary to fit the defect.

3. The fibular free flap is not considered to be a bulky flap; however, for just bone reconstruction, such as in cases of osteoradionecrosis, retaining the skin paddle produces too much tissue and a difficult closure. Therefore, for small defects we prefer skin grafts over the muscle. To decrease the bulk of the flap further, the posterior tibia and soleus muscles can be carefully excised.

4. When creating wedge osteotomies, the length of bone required to have a nutrient vessel in a segment of bone is 3 cm. A segment of bone <3 cm places the bone at risk of having only periosteal blood supply. On the postoperative bone scan, a segment of bone may have decreased or no radioactive tracer uptake as a result of no nutrient vessel blood supply even though the flap vascularization is adequate.

5. Preoperative evaluation should include examination of pulses (dorsalis pedis, posterior tibial, and anterior tibial), ankle-brachial index (ABI), and vascular studies. The pulse should be 2+ (normal). Any pulse less than normal requires that a patient undergoes a formal arteriogram. The ABI should be >1.0. If the ABI is <1.0 an arteriogram is required. For an ABI of <0.9 another reconstruction flap should be considered. The gold standard vascular study is an arteriogram of the lower extremity to rule out significant arthrosclerosis and aberrant vascular anatomy. We prefer to use a duplex & Doppler study as a screening test. If the ABI > 1.0, and TBI > 0.7, the vascularity is considered to be adequate. Otherwise, an arteriogram is ordered. An alternative vascular evaluation is an MRI arteriogram.

COMPLICATIONS

1. The most serious complications of fibula free flap reconstruction of the mandible are vascular thrombosis and neurovascular injury to the leg. The expected incidence of vascular thrombosis is between 3% and 5%. Postoperative care requires stringent evaluation for venous thrombosis. Typically, arterial thrombosis will be detected intraoperatively within 15 minutes after the completion of clamp release.

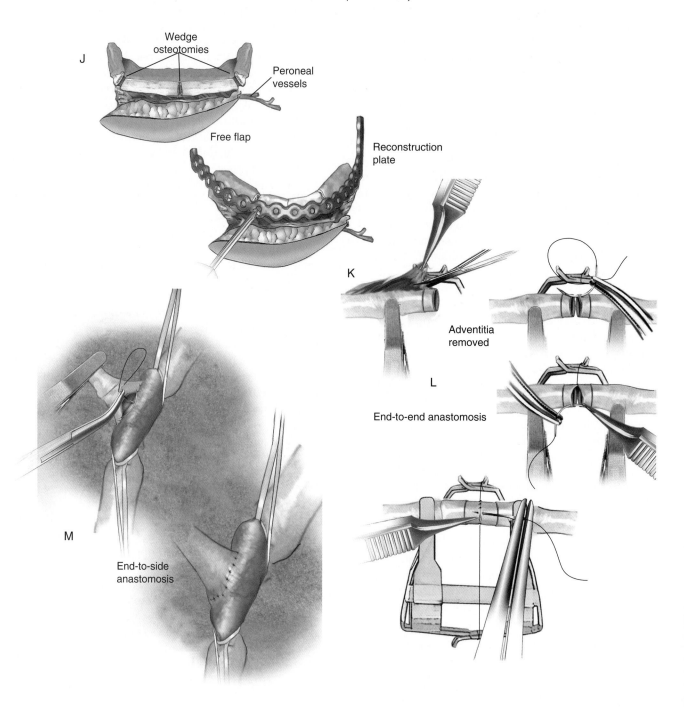

J

Wedge
osteotomies

Peroneal
vessels

Free flap

Reconstruction
plate

K

Adventitia
removed

L

End-to-end anastomosis

M

End-to-side
anastomosis

N

Arterial end-to-end
anastomosis – facial artery

Venous end-to-end
anastomosis – external
jugular vein

Venous end-to-side
anastomosis – internal
jugular vein

Free flap

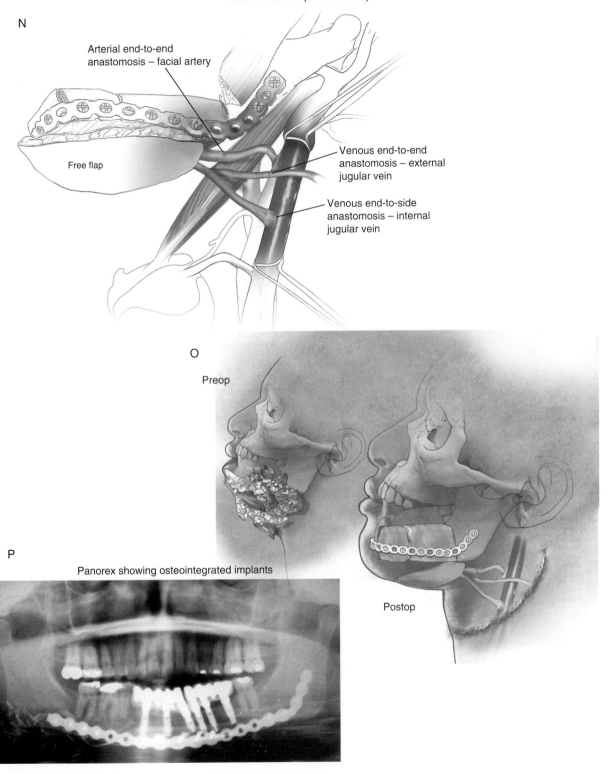

O

Preop

Postop

P

Panorex showing osteointegrated implants

Venous thrombosis is usually detected within 24 to 48 hours. Venous thrombosis can only be salvaged in the early stages. Venous thrombosis is extreme fullness, erythema, and firmness of the flap. Fifty percent of these can be salvaged by reexploration.

2. The donor site complications are ischemia, cold intolerance edema, weakness of dorsiflexion of the great toe. Rarely common peroneal nerve injury can result in equinovarus deformity and numbness along the leg. The loss of the skin paddle has been reported in 5% to 10% of cases. In this case, a backup plan can be to skin graft the muscle of the fibula flap. The other complications in the head and neck site are fistula, malunion, poor dentition, osteomyelitis, infection, and cosmetic deformity.

CHAPTER

37

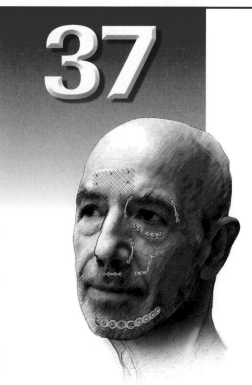

Osteotomy Techniques for Malunion of the Mandible
Alternative Technique Using Onlay Grafts or Bone Cement

In Consultation With Mark T. Marunick, DDS

INDICATIONS

Malunion of the mandible can occur following a mandible fracture when there is imperfect reduction, inadequate fixation and stabilization, and periods of infection and resorption of the bone. The degree of malalignment usually dictates the degree of deformity and dysfunction. Correction should be considered for patients with malocclusion, temporomandibular joint disorders, and facial asymmetry. However, tolerances are variable, and the physician must evaluate the patient for individualized plans of management.

If the patient is edentulous, it is possible to correct many discrepancies of the mandible by denture modification. To some extent, dentures can be fabricated so that differences in the anteroposterior or horizontal plane can be adjusted. Compensation can also be carried out for open bite problems. However, severe interarch distance relationships that preclude denture fabrication may require osteotomies.

In patients with teeth, different techniques must be considered. For minor premature contacts, a conservative occlusal adjustment of the involved teeth may be needed. For moderate occlusal discrepancies, tooth reduction or endodontic therapy with crown fabrication and/or orthodontic treatment will generally resolve the problem. When a single tooth or several teeth provide a major discrepancy, extraction may be a simple and effective approach, especially when prosthodontic treatment will restore the dental arches and function.

For more serious malunions, the physician must consider strategic osteotomies to correct the maxillary and mandibular relationships. If the deformity is caused by malalignment of the fracture, an osteotomy is preferred, either in the fracture line or in a strategic site that will compensate for the problem. If the patient has a deformity and a dysfunction associated with a preexisting malocclusion, then it is more prudent to refer the patient for classic orthognathic surgery. If deformity is the only problem and function is adequate, onlay grafts or bone cement substitutes can be used over the area of deficiency.

PROCEDURE

Presurgical Considerations

To plan for osteotomy sites and methods of stabilization, it is important to study the fractures (i.e., their effects on malocclusion and/or deformity and the cause of the malunion). For this purpose, the surgeon should obtain the patient's previous records (including operative reports and radiographs), and a new set of radiographs and dental casts. Impressions, casts, facebow registrations, jaw relationships, and surgical modification of casts are described in Chapters 20 and 29. Once the plaster boat is fabricated, it is indexed, a registration taken, and the cast placed back into the plaster boat and mounted on the articulator. The lines of fracture are marked out, and cuts are made through these lines. The fractured segments are then placed into anatomic and functional relationships with each other and with the opposing dental arch on the articulator and are held together with dental wax. Bone defects that would occur with repositioning of the fragments will have to be corrected with sliding osteotomies or with autogenous bone grafts. The operative dental casts are also useful in developing a lingual or interocclusal splint, which serves as a guide during the surgical procedure for the correct placement of the fragments (see Chapter 29).

Surgery

The incision and approach will depend on the site of the fracture. In general, the exposure is identical to that used for the external and open treatment of a mandible fracture. To obtain accurate relationships of the intermaxillary occlusion, nasotracheal intubation is preferred.

A–C After exposure of the osteotomy site, the periosteum should be stripped from the bone. Care must be taken not to open into the mouth, but if this does occur, the mucosa should be repaired immediately with 3-0 chromic sutures. Malleable retractors can be placed between the bone and periosteum so that the cuts will not injure the adjoining soft tissues.

The osteotomy can be performed with Lindeman burs, oscillating saws, or with fine, sharp osteotomes. However, the surgeon should recognize that the thicker the osteotomy line, the more chance there is for instability and the need for bone grafting. If the bone has healed completely, a stepwise cut or an oblique sagittal split will provide more surface area for postoperative stability. If the neurovascular bundle is intact, the surgeon should avoid injury to this structure.

D–F The site of osteotomy and the need for stability will determine the appropriate fixation technique. The lingual or interocclusal splint should be applied and will provide the relationships for the approximation of the segments (see Chapter 29). If the bones are in good contact, the surgeon can proceed with intermaxillary fixation with arch bars or Ivy loops and rigid fixation plates (see Chapters 19, 24, 26, and 28). If there is a deficiency, then a bone graft technique with reconstruction plate must be used (see Chapter 35).

Postoperatively the patient should be held in fixation for at least 6 to 8 weeks. Prophylactic antibiotics should be administered for 5 to 7 days, or longer if bone grafts are used. Oral hygiene should be maintained with gentle brushings and/or the use of a water irrigation device.

PITFALLS

1. An understanding of the pathophysiology is essential for obtaining good results. Occlusion can be observed on the casts, and additionally, one surgical hypothesis can be checked against another. An inadequate diagnostic workup is an invitation for problems.

2. Do not overoperate. If the patient's malocclusion can be corrected by occlusal adjustments or other dental treatment, then this is preferred to osteotomy and refixation. Moreover, most edentulous patients can be better treated with adjustments of their denture. If the problem is purely cosmetic, then the physician can even consider onlay grafts or bone cement (see later). Consultation with appropriate dental colleagues is important in making these management decisions.

3. Avoid unnecessary contamination of the operative site. If a dental extraction is necessary, it is probably more prudent to delay a week or two before the definitive surgery. Try to avoid intraoral exposure, but if there is a tear, close the mucosa immediately with sutures.

4. Malunion of the condyle can be associated with temporomandibular joint ankylosis. If this occurs, the surgeon should consider creating a pseudarthrosis or even a condylectomy. Condylar reconstruction following condylectomy can also be considered as an option (see Chapter 38).

5. If malunion of the condyle is associated with satisfactory joint movement (as in subcondylar injuries), but also with shortening of the mandible and premature contact of the molars, it is probably better treated with a ramus osteotomy or a lower sagittal split osteotomy. In such cases, operative intervention of the condyle can cause more damage and should be avoided.

TREATMENT OF MALUNION WITH OSTEOTOMIES

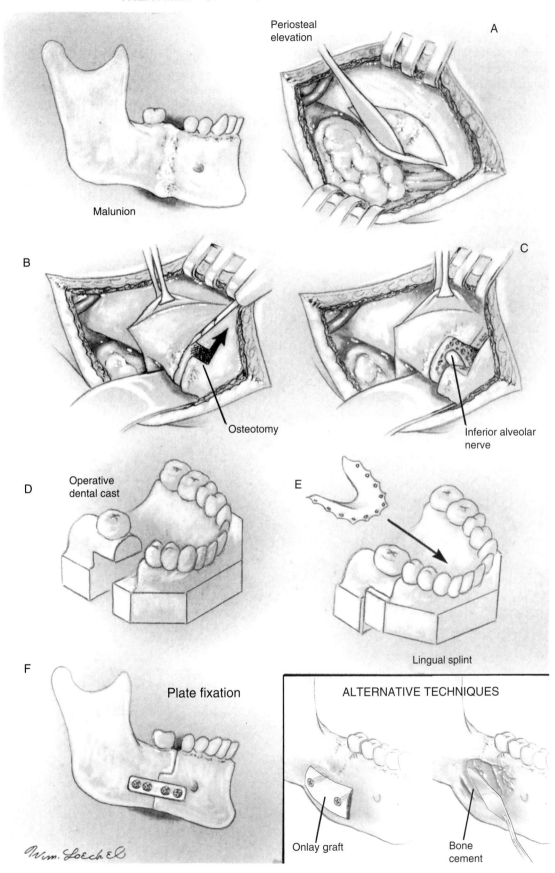

Malunion

Periosteal elevation

A

B

Osteotomy

C

Inferior alveolar nerve

D

Operative dental cast

E

Lingual splint

F

Plate fixation

ALTERNATIVE TECHNIQUES

Onlay graft

Bone cement

Wm. Loechel

COMPLICATIONS

1. As in all mandibular injuries, infection and nonunion are possible sequelae. To prevent these problems, the surgeon should avoid intraoral contamination, drain hematomas and dead space, obtain exact reduction, and maintain a solid fixation during the healing process. Prophylactic antibiotics are also used, and if infection occurs, appropriate specific antibiotic treatment should be applied. Surgical management is discussed in Chapters 34 through 37.

2. Recurrence of malunion should be prevented by proper planning and execution of the surgical technique. If malunion should again develop, then the surgeon will again have to decide on the severity and significance of the malalignment of the fragments and on the appropriate measures for rehabilitation.

ALTERNATIVE TECHNIQUE USING ONLAY GRAFTS OR BONE CEMENT

Occasionally the malunion does not cause dysfunction and is only associated with deformity. If this is the case, the malunion can be corrected with onlay cement or grafting techniques, rather than with an osteotomy. Using the onlay graft does not subject the patient to potential nonunion or dysfunction. However, morbidity will be associated with the donor site, and there may be subsequent irregularities of the graft that will require revisional surgery.

Adequate exposure for the repair will depend on the site of the deficiency. Care must be taken to avoid additional injury to the soft tissues—especially the muscles of mastication and the cranial nerves that supply these regions. The periosteum of the mandible should be elevated to create a pocket over the defect, and bone harvested from the hip or cranium is then contoured and placed into the pocket. Lag screw fixation is desirable (see Chapters 24 and 59). Alternatively, one can apply bone cement (Chapter 82) or an alloplastic implant to the area of deficiency, but these techniques have their own set of complications (i.e., infection, displacement, absorption, and deformity). The periosteum is tied snug around the graft with 2-0 chromic sutures. Postoperative care is similar to that described for other grafting techniques (see Chapter 35).

CHAPTER

38

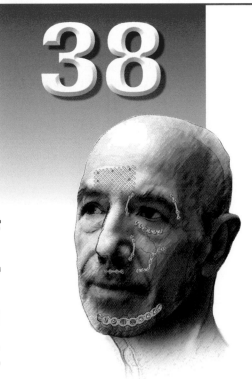

Treatment of Temporomandibular Ankylosis With Resection and Autogenous Rib Graft
Alternative Technique of Prosthetic Replacement

In Consultation With Lewis Clayman, DMD, MD

INDICATIONS

Ankylosis of the temporomandibular joint (TMJ), although infrequent, most often occurs as a consequence of an untreated fracture of the mandibular condyle or subcondylar process. The limitation in mouth opening may result from a direct osseous or fibro-osseous fusion between the condyle and the skull base, from a fibrous union within the joint, or from extra-articular scar formation. The diagnostic image of choice is the CT scan.

If the dysfunction is primarily caused by scarring, steroid injections, forced dilatation of the mouth, and jaw opening exercises are warranted. If an intra-articular fibrous union is present, simple release followed by aggressive physical therapy (PT) is indicated. If, on the other hand, there is a bony fusion, a more aggressive approach consisting of osteotomy or resection coupled with reconstruction should be considered.

For the child who has already developed a growth asymmetry, resection of the bony ankylosis is combined with maxillary and mandibular osteotomies for a one-stage correction of the deformity. In the nongrowing patient, depending upon available surgical resources, treatment ranges from gap arthroplasty to resection/reconstruction with a costochondral graft, and lining of the glenoid fossa with soft tissue grafts. Frequently simultaneous coronoidectomy is required. In the older patient, particularly one with prior arthroplasty, an alloplastic endoprosthesis is suitable. In general, the costochondral graft (CCG) is preferred since the cartilage is well adapted to joint function and the height of the mandibular ramus is restored at the same time.

PROCEDURE

The field is prepared aseptically for an intra- and extraoral approach to the TMJ including the preauricular and submandibular areas. First the ankylosis is released; arch bars are then placed and the occlusion is reestablished. Then the CCG can be adapted, positioned, and fixated.

A–E The incision and approach to the TMJ is similar to that described in Chapter 21. If the joint capsule is still present, soft tissues should be incised and elevated subperiosteally to expose the affected area. The dissection needs to be wide enough to expose the condylar neck, glenoid fossa, articular eminentia, and coronoid processes. If possible malleable retractors should then be inserted deep to the condylar head and neck to protect against injury to branches of the internal maxillary artery. The condylar head or its remnants can be removed with cutting burs and rongeurs. In cases of dense bony fusion, there are no identifiable normal structures. Parallel osteotomies are made at the approximate level of the condylar neck that extend medially about 15 mm. Bone is then removed and the procedure is repeated a bit at a time until the medial side of the ankylotic block is reached. Now the excision is expanded until at least 15 mm of bone in a superoinferior direction is removed. The mouth is now forced open with side action mouth props, being careful not to dislodge the teeth. If a maximum interincisal opening of more than 30 mm is not achieved, an ipsilateral coronoidectomy is performed (see Chapter 18). If 30 mm still cannot be achieved then the contralateral coronoid process is removed.

F,G Another incision is made below the angle of the mandible to expose the angle and ramus region. This technique is similar to the one described in Chapter 24. The masticatory muscles are elevated subperiosteally to completely expose the residual condyle. A subperiosteal pocket is thus created close to the jaw and deep to the facial nerve structures. The ascending ramus of the mandible is contoured with a bur to receive the attachment of the CCG.

H,I The contralateral fourth or sixth rib is harvested from an inframammary incision using the technique described in Chapter 27. The cartilage portion of the rib should be retained. This means that the rib must be handled gently, or the junction between the cartilage and bone will break. The length of the rib is determined according to the requirement for reconstruction of the ramus. The cartilage portion is rounded with a knife or bur, and limited to 5 mm of thickness especially in the growing child, and the total length of the rib adjusted to accommodate firm contact to the new glenoid fossa and ramus of the mandible. The rib is then inserted from below into the newly formed glenoid fossa, and the bony portion of the rib is secured to the mandible with several 25-gauge wires or a combination of 2.0-mm screws and miniplates. No attempt is made to reattach the muscles of mastication, as they will attach to the grafted area during the healing process. The wounds are closed in layers.

Intermaxillary fixation should be maintained for 2 to 4 weeks (or 2 weeks in children) depending upon whether plates or wires were used. Antibiotics are continued for 5 days postoperatively. Opening and closing exercises are initiated as soon as the intermaxillary wires or elastic bands are removed and are continued for 6 months.

PITFALLS

1. The diagnosis of ankylosis must be accurate if the surgeon is to choose the appropriate procedure. Soft tissue scarring can be treated by conservative measures, whereas fibro-osseous union requires a surgical release. Beware, however, of extracapsular ankylosis caused by fusion of the coronoid to the zygoma (usually following zygomatic fractures) or fusion of the lateral pterygoid plate to the ramus of the mandible (occasionally following Le Fort III fractures), as these conditions require alternative methods for correction involving wide surgical exposure and release of the ankylosis.

2. Ankylosis in the child is a serious problem since growth arrest will cause a significant facial deformity. Early diagnosis and treatment are important to minimize these effects. CCG with its potential for growth is the preferred method of reconstruction. Limiting the cartilage to 5 mm of thickness reduces the chance for overgrowth during the pubertal growth spurt.

3. Occasionally ankylosis is associated with infection of the mandible, infratemporal space, and/or external auditory canal and mastoid process. If this occurs, the infection must be brought under control before planning reconstructive surgery. Long-term intravenous antibiotics must be administered, foreign bodies and necrotic bone removed, and the area adequately debrided and drained. Reconstructive surgery should not be started until all signs of infection have been absent for several months.

4. Dental rehabilitation is an important part of the treatment process. As soon as is practical after surgery

RECONSTRUCTION AFTER ANKYLOSIS USING RIB GRAFT

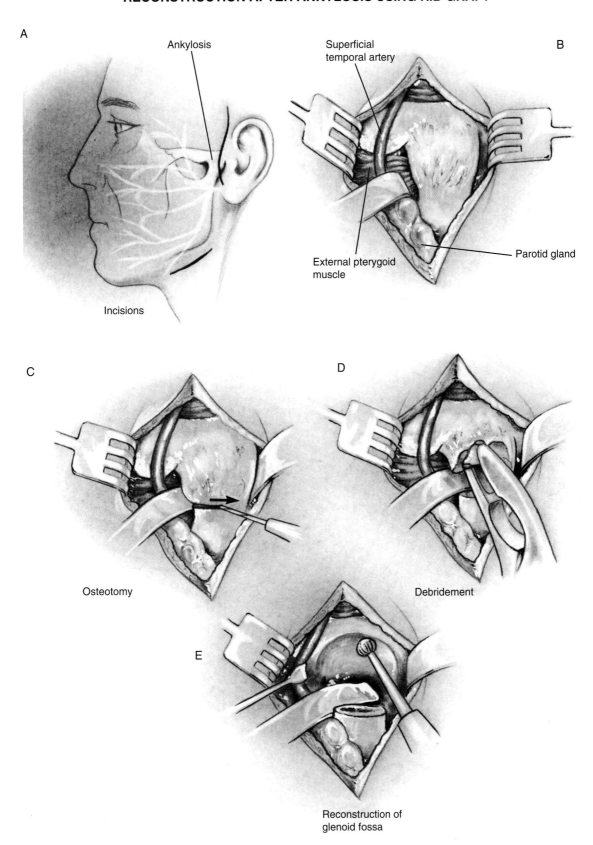

A

Ankylosis

Incisions

B

Superficial
temporal artery

External pterygoid
muscle

Parotid gland

C

Osteotomy

D

Debridement

E

Reconstruction of
glenoid fossa

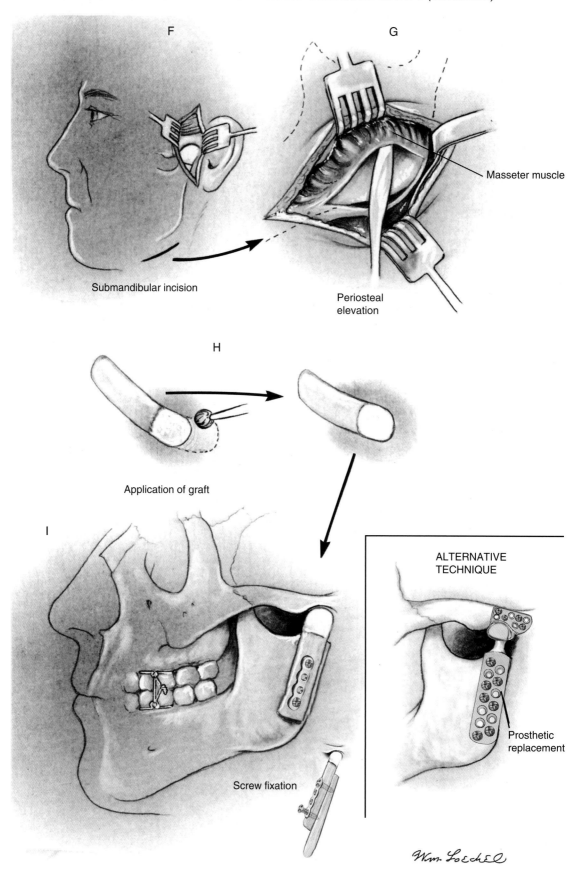

F

Submandibular incision

G

Masseter muscle

Periosteal
elevation

H

Application of graft

I

ALTERNATIVE
TECHNIQUE

Prosthetic
replacement

Screw fixation

Wm Loechel

an active exercise/PT program should be begun. Occasionally these maneuvers must be combined with steroid injections to obtain relaxation of the adjoining tissues.

COMPLICATIONS

1. Bleeding from branches of the internal maxillary artery can be troublesome during the surgical procedure. To avoid this intraoperative complication, the dissection should be close to the surface of the bone and carried out with blunt elevation and spreading clamp techniques. The deep tissues should be protected with a malleable retractor.

2. The temporal branch of the seventh nerve is at risk during surgery but this complication can usually be avoided by keeping the dissection subperiosteal over the zygomatic arch. Also, retractors should be used judiciously on the soft tissues that cover the parotid and facial nerve area. Cauterization of the vessels should be avoided and bleeders clamped and tied. Any injury to the nerve should be recognized immediately and the condition of this injury determined by appropriate electrodiagnostic tests. If there are indications of anatomic interruption of the nerve, exploration and repair should be performed immediately (see Chapter 14).

3. Reankylosis is possible and can occur from infection, failure to remove bone spicules from the operative site, inadequate bone removal, or loss of grafts or inadequate postoperative PT. Early function is encouraged to prevent the development of fusion at the TMJ. Steroid injections may help in the treatment of contracting scar tissues.

ALTERNATIVE TECHNIQUE OF PROSTHETIC REPLACEMENT

Following resective surgery, the condyle, glenoid fossa, and ramus, can be reconstructed with alloplastic materials. Many types of prostheses are available, but experience is limited. Promising data is available for the TMJ Concept and Christensen endoprostheses. The advantages of the condylar prosthesis are its relative ease of insertion and avoidance of a donor site. On the other hand, there is a risk of infection and loosening and displacement of the implant. Removal of a failed prosthesis is tedious and difficult.

The prosthesis is placed through the same incisions as those used in positioning the rib graft. The glenoid component is placed first and then the condyle-ramus unit. The ramus is then grooved to receive the shank of the prosthesis, and to secure the implant, three or four screws are placed through the inner and outer cortices of the ramus. The periosteum is closed over the prosthesis with 2-0 chromic sutures, and the wound is closed in layers. Intravenous antibiotics are used for 5 days and oral antibiotics for at least 2 weeks following the procedure. Rehabilitation is similar to that discussed for the CCG.

PART FOUR

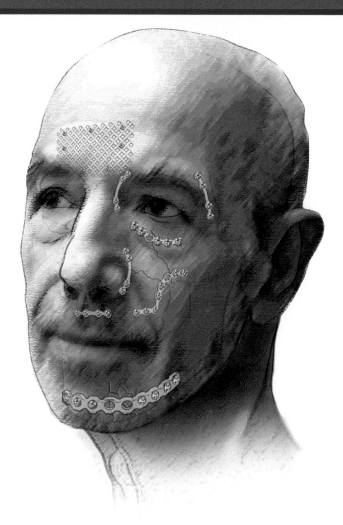

Maxillary Fractures

Classification and Pathophysiology of Maxillary Fractures

CHAPTER

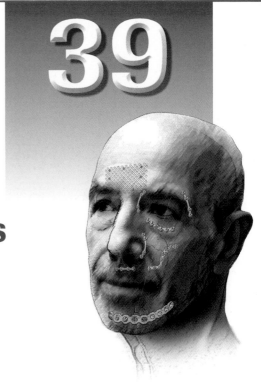

39

General Considerations

Maxillary fractures account for approximately 10% to 20% of all facial fractures. These midfacial injuries can be isolated or can occur in combination with fractures of adjacent structures such as the mandible, nasofrontoethmoid complex, orbit, zygoma, or cranium.

Many maxillary fractures are the result of violent blunt force to the facial skeleton. The displacement of the fracture will depend upon the degree and direction and point of impact of the external force. Muscles that insert into the facial skeleton are believed to play only a minor role in the final position of the fragments.

A–D If the impact occurs primarily at the nasal bridge, the maxilla will be displaced downward along the sloping base of the skull, resulting in a lengthening of the face, retrognathia, and an open bite deformity. The maxilla may become impacted or hang loosely, floating from the cranium. Lateral blows to the facial skeleton can cause a lateral displacement associated with a crossbite dysfunction. Forces directed to the lower front of the midface can produce a pyramidal

fracture involving just the anterior maxilla and naso-ethmoid complex. This same type of fracture can also occur in patients receiving a blow from beneath the chin, in which case the maxilla is often shortened and the fracture associated with zygomatic and hemipalatal fractures.

E–G Other forces to the maxilla can cause different types of injuries. Blows directed anteroposteriorly to the upper alveolus (or lower portion of the maxilla) can also separate the premaxilla and the alveolus from the nose and floor of the maxillary sinus. Limited sharp blows, usually from small objects, can produce isolated segmental fractures.

H For the most part, maxillary fractures are complex and difficult to define. A traditional classification, originally described by Le Fort, is useful, and most fractures fall into one of the Le Fort types. According to this system, a Le Fort III fracture (or craniofacial dysjunction) starts at the nasofrontal suture line and

MAXILLARY FRACTURES

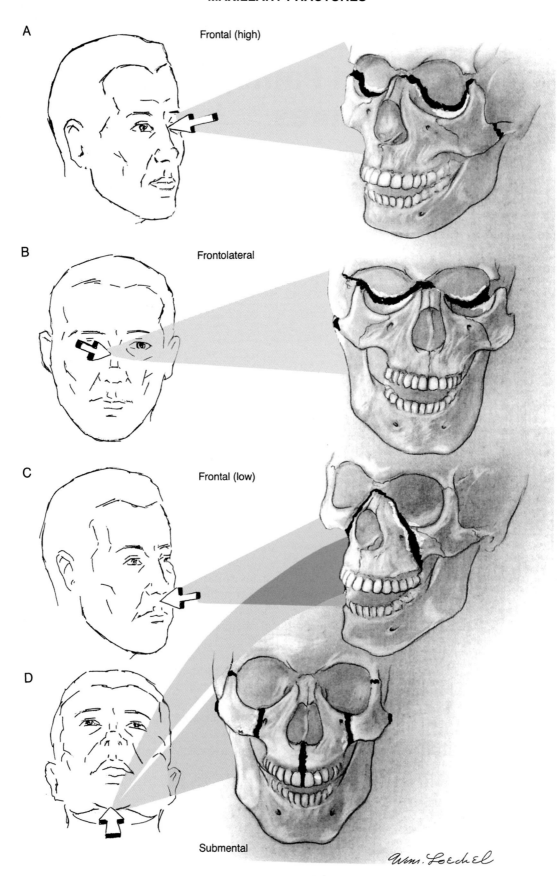

A   Frontal (high)

B   Frontolateral

C   Frontal (low)

D

Submental

Wm. Loechel

extends along the medial wall and floor of the orbit to pass through the inferior orbital fissure, lateral orbital wall, and zygomaticofrontal suture. The fracture line extends across the temporal surface of the zygoma and zygomatic arch, while a branch continues across the maxilla to separate the pterygoid plates from the basisphenoid. The Le Fort II (or pyramidal) fracture starts out at about the same level as a Le Fort III injury but passes more anteriorly to involve the lacrimal bones, the inferior orbital rim, and the anterolateral wall of the maxilla. The pterygoid plates may or may not be fractured. The Le Fort I fracture (Guerin type) crosses the nasal septum, the lower portion of the piriform apertures, the canine fossae, and the zygomaticomaxillary buttresses. The fracture then passes above the maxillary tuberosity to separate the maxilla from the pterygoid plates or, alternatively, to disrupt the lower from the upper two thirds of the plates. In most Le Fort fractures, the bony and cartilaginous portions of the nasal septum are also injured.

Other variations of the maxillary fracture are the medial maxillary, the split palate, and the segmental (partial maxillary or alveolar) fracture. These can occur alone or in combination with other midfacial injuries. The medial maxillary fractures commonly present with a skeletal depression between the nose and maxilla. A split palate often occurs with Le Fort II or III fractures or with fractures involving the malar bone. Alveolar or segmental maxillary fractures commonly are associated with Le Fort I fractures.

There can also be many combinations of injury. Le Fort I, II, and III fractures can occur on one side of the face (hemi-Le Fort), or there can be mixed fractures in which there are different fracture patterns appearing on opposite sides. Le Fort fractures can also be combined with medial maxillary, split palate, and segmental injuries.

The most important clinical aspect of the Le Fort classification is that these fractures involve buttresses and beams that maintain the height, width, and projection of the face. The main vertical supports are paired and are called *nasomaxillary, zygomaticomaxillary*, and *pterygomaxillary* buttresses. There is also an unpaired frontoethmoid-vomerine buttress. The medially positioned nasomaxillary buttress extends upward along the frontal process of the maxilla (nasofrontal section of buttress) to attach to the base of the skull. The lateral zygomaticomaxillary buttress has two cranially directed components (zygomaticofrontal and zygomaticotemporal) that extend along the frontal and temporal processes of the zygomatic bone. The posterior pterygomaxillary buttress essentially attaches the maxilla to the pterygoid plates and the sphenoid bone. The median frontoethmoid-vomerine buttress connects the frontal bone to the surface of the palate.

There are also two main horizontal beams. One has two components, the superior and inferior orbital rims, and extends laterally across the zygomatic arch. The other traverses the maxillary alveolus to stabilize the palate and upper dental arch

I It should also be recognize that one of the more recent classifications (attributed to Manson, PN) uses energy as the differentiating factor. According to this concept, low energy is associated with no or minimal displacement of fractured segments. Middle energy is associated with further displacement and segmentation and high energy with comminution and involvement of adjoining structures.

The goals in treatment of maxillary fractures are to (1) secure pretraumatic occlusion and (2) stabilize one of several buttresses and/or beams that will restore the 3-D of the face. In general, mandibular fractures occurring with the maxillary fracture should be treated first. The Le Fort III fracture should be stabilized at the zygomaticofrontal extension of the zygomaticomaxillary buttress and/or at the nasofrontal extension of the nasomaxillary buttress. The Le Fort II fracture needs fixation across the nasomaxillary, zygomaticomaxillary, and/or horizontal beams of the orbital rims. The Le Fort I fracture requires some type of stabilization across the lower part of the zygomaticomaxillary buttress and/or nasomaxillary buttress.

Treatment in children must be modified to account for more rapid healing and remodeling of the facial skeleton (see Chapter 110). The usual approach is conservative, and intermaxillary fixation with Ivy loops is often satisfactory. Fabrication of palatal splints with suspension can also be considered. For the high maxillary fractures, management generally parallels that in adults.

MAXILLARY FRACTURES *(Continued)*

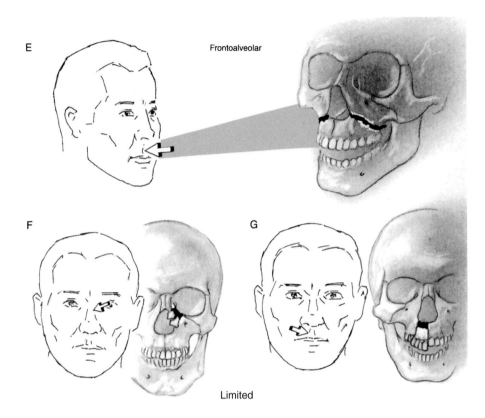

E   Frontoalveolar

F

G

Limited

LE FORT CLASSIFICATION AND MAJOR BEAMS AND BUTTRESSES

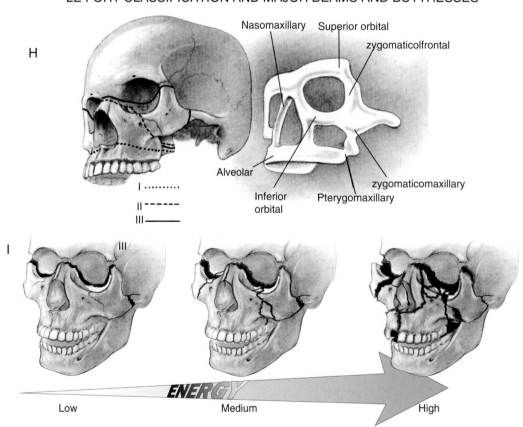

H

Nasomaxillary   Superior orbital

zygomaticolfrontal

Alveolar

Inferior orbital

Pterygomaxillary

zygomaticomaxillary

I ....
II -------
III ———

I   III

ENERGY

Low   Medium   High

CHAPTER

40

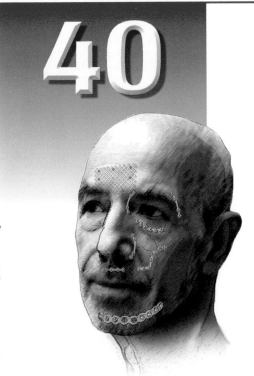

Repair of Maxillary Segmental Fractures
Alternative Technique Using Miniplate Fixation

INDICATIONS

Sharp objects striking the midface can cause abrasions, lacerations, or partial avulsions involving the cheeks, lips, or adjacent gum tissues. Sufficient force, however, will also result in punched-out segmental fractures involving the dentition, alveolus, and lower portion of the maxilla.

Segmental fractures in patients with teeth generally can be reduced with digital pressure and stabilized with either a single arch bar or upper and lower arch bars and intermaxillary fixation. In the edentulous patient, dentures (or splints) suspended from stable portions of the skeleton or lag screwed to the palate can be fitted with arch bars, which are then secured to each other with wires or elastic bands (see Chapters 20 and 47). In those edentulous patients with sufficiently large bone fragments, plating may be a more expedient form of management. Intermaxillary fixation screws are contraindicated because of limited fixation of the fractured area.

PROCEDURE

A–C Most segmental fractures can be treated with local anesthesia and sedation. If a general anesthetic is to be employed, nasotracheal intubation is preferred, as this will provide an opportunity to reduce and stabilize the fracture and immediately check for appropriate occlusal relationships.

To help control hemostasis and provide local anesthesia, the area of fracture is first infiltrated with 1% lidocaine containing 1:100,000 epinephrine. The fracture can then be simply reduced with digital pressure. If lacerations are present, the surgeon should use them to evaluate the adequacy of the reduction and then close the wounds with 3-0 chromic sutures. Teeth should always be inspected, and any injuries to the crown portion should be treated accordingly (see Chapter 31). Loose or extirpated teeth should be repositioned and wired to an arch bar or attached to orthodontic brackets, which are subsequently stabilized by the adjacent uninvolved dentition.

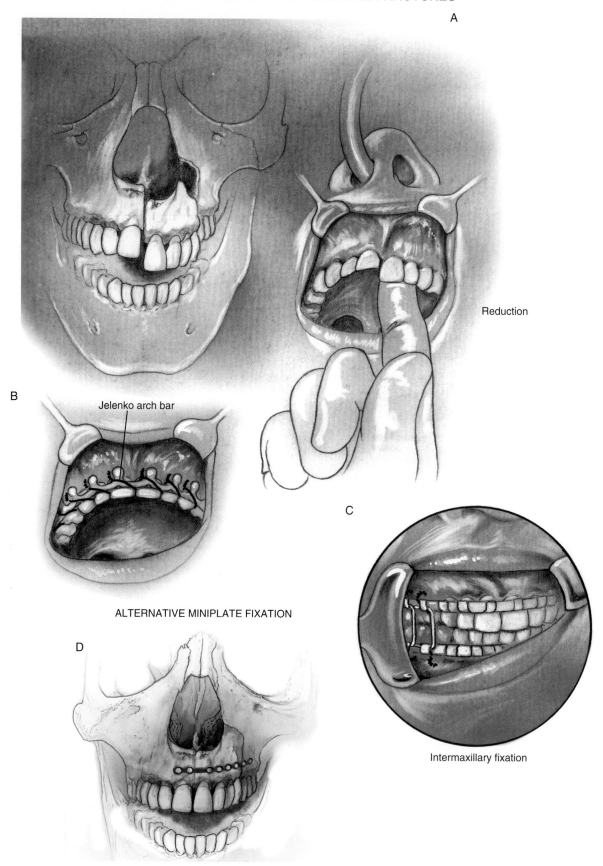

A

Reduction

B

Jelenko arch bar

ALTERNATIVE MINIPLATE FIXATION

D

C

Intermaxillary fixation

Arch bar placement is described in Chapter 19. Wiring of the incisors may be necessary to obtain optimal stability. The surgeon should start with the upper arch, and if the fragments can be held with a rigid bar (i.e., Jelenko), then one arch bar will suffice for the fixation. However, if the fragments tend to move, additional rigidity using a lower arch bar and intermaxillary fixation should be employed.

Postoperatively the patient is treated with prophylactic antibiotics and chlorhexidine mouthwashes. The teeth should be gently brushed or treated with a water irrigation device daily. Most fractures will heal in 4 to 6 weeks, and at that time, the arch bars can be removed. CT Scan evaluation may be helpful, and the patient should be checked for several months thereafter to assure adequacy of healing.

PITFALLS

1. Fixation of segmental fractures often requires a stepwise approach. First, horizontal wiring of the teeth should be attempted. If this does not stabilize the fracture, the surgeon should proceed to arch bar fixation. Alternatively, orthodontic brackets can be applied (see Chapter 31). If instability is still present, intermaxillary fixation should be employed.

2. Careful evaluation of the teeth is important if permanent damage is to be avoided and infection of the alveolar fragments prevented. When there is concern regarding dental injury, dentistry consultation should be obtained.

COMPLICATIONS

1. The segmental fragment can become nonviable if its blood supply is severely compromised and/or infection develops in the area of fracture. This complication can be avoided by applying atraumatic techniques to the soft tissues and by ensuring accurate reduction and fixation. Additionally, the surgeon must be certain that the teeth are viable and will not act as portals of infection or as foreign bodies.

2. If malaligned segments have healed and are causing no deformity or difficulty, then no treatment is necessary. However, if malalignment is affecting appearance or masticatory function, then the complication must be treated. What option to choose will be dictated by the degree and extent of displacement and the need for natural dentition. Orthodontia and/or orthognathic surgery may have to be considered (see Chapter 48).

ALTERNATIVE TECHNIQUE USING MINIPLATE FIXATION

D If the segmental fracture extends beyond the alveolus into the body of the maxilla, the more prudent treatment is to reduce and stabilize the fracture with miniplates. For this approach, a gingival labial/buccal sulcus incision close to the alveolus is performed. Hemostasis can be controlled with injection of 1% Lidocaine containing 1:100,000 epinephrine. If the patient has teeth then the arch bars should be applied to obtain occlusal relationships and correct positioning of the fragments. The periosteum should be elevated to expose the fracture and a miniplate with at least two holes to the side of the fracture bent to accommodate the surface of the bone. Four millimeter long bone screws are applied. The mucoperiosteum is closed over the plate and the patient treated as above in the postoperative period.

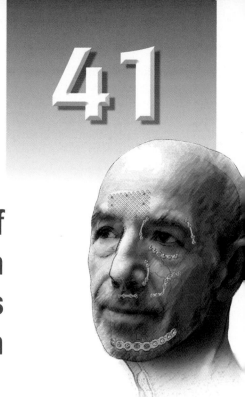

CHAPTER

41

Reduction of Le Fort I Fracture With Disimpaction Forceps and Miniplate Fixation

INDICATIONS

Le Fort I fractures are characterized by a retrodisplacement of the lower portion of the maxilla. Frequently the bone fragments are impacted, and there is premature contact of the molars with an open bite deformity. The maxilla may be shortened or lengthened. The patient may also present with epistaxis, ecchymoses along the gingivobuccal sulcus, and tenderness and crepitus along the fracture line.

The objectives of treatment are threefold: (1) to restore centric occlusion, (2) to reduce and stabilize the palatal segment to the closest rigid maxillary segment, and (3) to replace any septal dislocations. The classic fracture often requires a forceful reduction before the fragments can be manipulated into pretraumatic occlusal relationships. The method of fixation used depends on the postreduction stability of the fracture and the status of the dentition. If the fracture appears reduced and "seems to fit," intermaxillary fixation with arch bars, Ivy loops, or intermaxillary fixation screws can be utilized. If instability is still present or the surgeon prefers not to use intermaxillary fixation, then miniplates can be applied along the medial and/or lateral buttresses. For those Le Fort I fractures associated with higher Le Fort injuries, additional miniplate fixation is the procedure of choice.

Other associated conditions will dictate alternative approaches. If the patient has comminuted fractures and is edentulous, the surgeon can simply treat with application of dentures, suspension wires, and intermaxillary fixation (see Chapters 19 and 20). In patients with associated alveolar segmental fractures, an arch bar with or without intermaxillary fixation should be considered (see Chapter 40). With a split palate fracture, the surgeon can use a special rigid arch bar (Jelenko) or miniplate that is placed across the lower transverse buttress (see Chapters 40 and 46).

PROCEDURE

Disimpaction and Reduction of Le Fort I Fracture

A General anesthesia is usually obtained with nasotracheal intubation or a tracheostomy. The surgeon should then reduce the maxillary fracture with digital pressure or with judicious traction of a tongue retractor or a bone hook behind the palate. If these techniques are not successful, a forceps reduction should be applied.

B The Rowe disimpaction forceps is designed to grasp and rock the lower maxilla symmetrically and to bring it forward. The right- and left-handed forceps have handles that are offset from each other. The straight blade of the forceps is first inserted into the floor of the nose; the curved portion, with its flat end, then fits around the alveolus and hard palate. Standing at the head of the patient, the surgeon grasps the forceps and applies constant pressure in a posterior-to-anterior direction. The forceps are simultaneously squeezed

DISIMPACTION TECHNIQUES

Le Fort I fracture

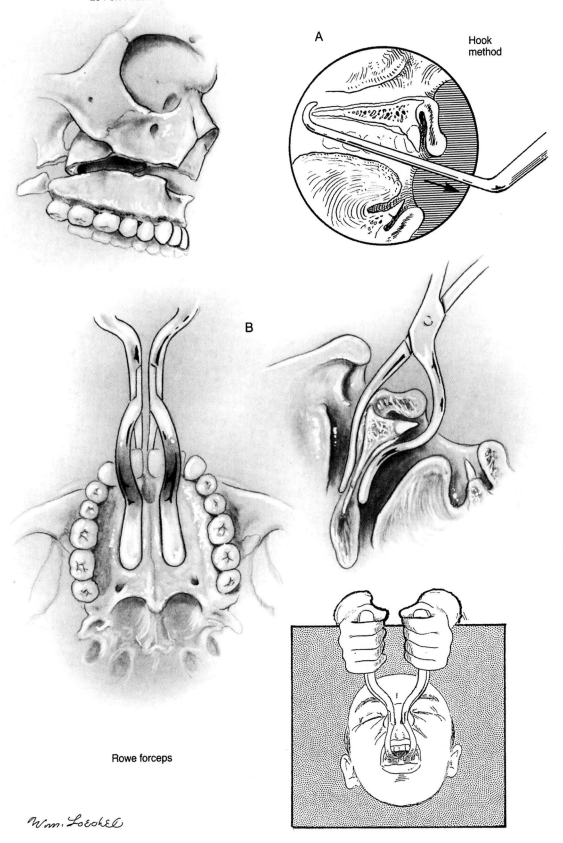

A

Hook method

B

Rowe forceps

Wm. Loechel

and rotated vertically and then horizontally to free and mobilize the segment. The maxillary fracture, when loosened, can then be molded back into a normal position. The patient's nose will bleed profusely during the reduction, but bleeding should stop in approximately 5 minutes.

Miniplate Fixation

C Several strategically placed Ivy loops should be used to secure adequate occlusal relationships. If the fracture extends to areas near the maxillary sinus ostia, the surgeon can, as an option, consider an intranasal antrostomy to better aerate the sinuses in the postoperative period. This small opening can be made by incising the caudal end of the inferior turbinate, infracturing the turbinate, and then, with a Kelly clamp, puncturing through the inferior meatus. The opening is enlarged with Kerrison rongeurs. Preferably the antrostomy should be taken down to the floor of the nose so that there will be a continuity between the nose and antrum. A hole about the size of a dime is desirable. The inferior turbinate is then pushed back into a normal position.

D,E Exposure for application of plates is best achieved through a gingival labial/buccal sulcus incision about 5 to 7 mm above the gingival margin from molar to molar region. The periosteum is elevated along the anterior wall of the maxilla, exposing the zygomaticomaxillary buttresses, canine fossae, nasomaxillary buttresses, piriform apertures, and anterior nasal spine. Care must be taken not to injure the infraorbital nerve and to keep as many fragments as possible attached to their periosteum.

Usually one plate across the zygomaticomaxillary or nasomaxillary buttress provides adequate fixation. The buttress should be stripped of periosteum to expose the area to receive the plate. The fragments should fit together, and any depressed fragments should be elevated into appropriate position.

F–H Miniplates should be used to fit over the area of fracture; this can be facilitated with a malleable template. A rigid straight or L-shaped plate is then selected so that there are at least two holes on each side of the fracture, and with the template as a guide, the rigid plate is bent to an appropriate fit. Holes through the buttress should then be drilled with a drill diameter that is slightly less than the screw diameter.

Drill holes should be measured and 3 or 4 mm screws selected that will penetrate just beyond the bone. These screws are then applied to the holes on each side of the fracture and subsequently to the outer holes for additional support. If the maxilla is still unstable, another plate should be applied to the contralateral side. The incision is closed with interrupted 4-0 chromic sutures.

Postoperatively the patient is maintained for 5 days on antibiotics. As soon as optimal occlusion is ensured, the intermaxillary fixation can be removed and the bite checked for dynamic relationships. Postoperative CT Scans should be obtained to confirm the adequacy of reduction and aeration of the sinuses. Clinical evaluation should be continued for at least 6 months to follow adequacy of treatment.

PITFALLS

1. Reduction of the fracture is probably the most important part of the procedure. Remember that plates are "unforgiving," and the patient will heal in the position in which the maxilla is fixed.

2. Beware of associated alveolar and palatal fractures, as these conditions will complicate the repair. Often the alveolar injury can be stabilized with an arch bar (see Chapter 40). Palatal splits require a plate across the premaxilla and/or placement of a heavy (Jelenko) arch bar (see Chapter 46).

3. The edentulous patient should be treated with the same concern for adequate reduction and immobilization given to the patient with teeth. Although the physician has the option of plate fixation (see *I*), there is also the traditional technique of using dentures with circumzygomatic suspension and intermaxillary fixation (see Chapter 20) or use of palatal lag screws (Chapter 47). The suspension method, however, can shorten the maxilla, and the surgeon must be careful not to overtighten the drop wires.

4. Occasionally there is minimal displacement and a reduction alone of a low maxillary fracture with intermaxiallary fixation will bring about satisfactory stability. If such a situation develops, it is probably more prudent to just place the patient into a short period of intermaxillary fixation and forego an open method.

5. Comminuted fractures of the lower midface can present formidable problems. If the bone fragments are displaced into the adjacent soft tissues, the surgeon should find these fragments and replace them into anatomic position. Stabilization can often be achieved with plate fixation. Sufficient portions of buttress are usually available, and bone grafting techniques should not be necessary.

6. Because the plate has the potential to be palpable or exposed, use only the minimum number of plates required to obtain fixation. Also, avoid plates that are too long, as these will often project beyond the alveolar ridge. Resorbable plates may also be used when there is a sufficient soft tissue covering (Chapter 111).

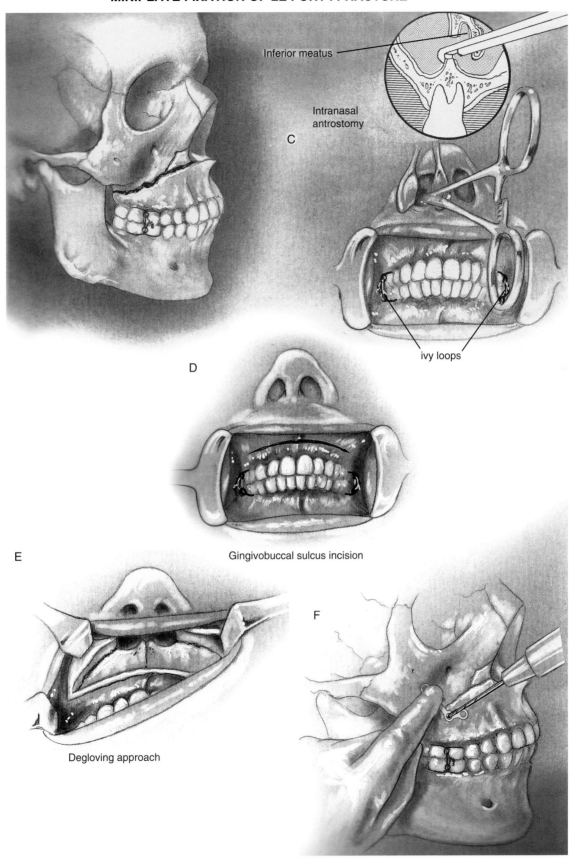

C

Inferior meatus

Intranasal antrostomy

ivy loops

D

Gingivobuccal sulcus incision

E

Degloving approach

F

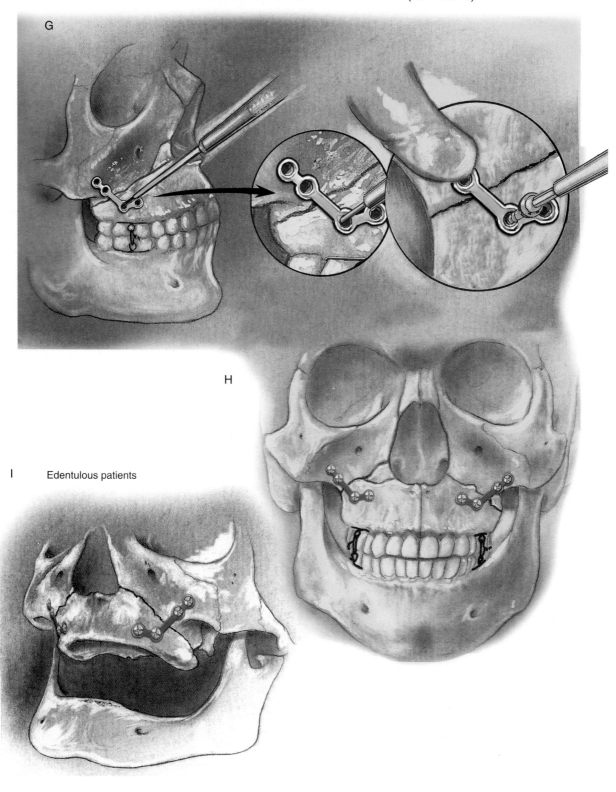

G

H

I   Edentulous patients

7. Make sure that screw placement does not affect the viability of tooth roots. A rule of thumb is that the screw should be placed no closer than the distance described by two times the height of the crown.

8. Treatment in children should be conservative (see Chapters 110 and 111). Remodeling of the maxilla can be expected, and the upper and lower jaws often will adapt to the occlusal plane. Intermaxillary fixation with Ivy loops or arch bars can be used in the mixed dentition; in the younger child, acrylic splints can be fit and secured to the piriform aperture and/or zygomatic arch.

COMPLICATIONS

1. Malunion of the maxilla from a Le Fort I fracture is a complication that can affect appearance and/or function. Generally the patient presents with a retrusion of the upper lip and columella. There is often an open bite and crossbite malocclusion. This problem can be avoided by accurate reduction and appropriate methods of fixation. If retrusion should develop in the early postoperative period, reduction should again be carried out and another method of fixation applied. At a later time, osteotomy and rigid plate fixation with or without bone grafts (see Chapter 48) must be considered. For those patients with minimal deformity and/or dysfunction, treatment may not be necessary.

2. Nonunion of the maxilla is extremely rare. Such a condition can develop from inaccurate reduction and/or poor fixation, but usually there is a history of infection or repeated trauma. The infection should be controlled with debridement and antibiotics. Loss of bone between fragments requires interposition bone grafts.

3. Sinusitis can also develop following midfacial trauma. This can often be avoided by an intranasal antrostomy and prophylactic antibiotic coverage. If the patient complains of pain and swelling of the face, then he or she should be evaluated radiographically. If sinusitis is present, appropriate antibiotics and drainage procedures should be administered.

Le Fort II Fractures

CHAPTER 42

Miniplate Fixation of Le Fort II Fractures
Alternative Technique Using Parietal Cortex Grafts

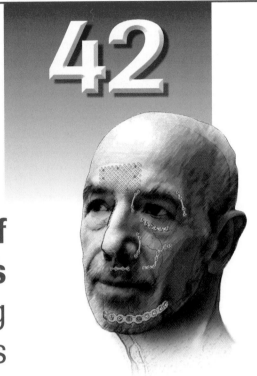

INDICATIONS

The pure Le Fort II injury is characterized by fracture of the nasal bones, the orbital rim (or rims), and the anterolateral walls of the maxilla. The maxilla is usually pushed backward and downward, causing a lengthened scaphoid deformity of the face. Premature contact of the molar teeth causes an open bite malocclusion. Fractures extending into the nasoethmoid complex can be associated with anosmia, cerebrospinal fluid leaks, and loss of consciousness.

An understanding of fracture lines, buttresses, and beams is essential to the planning and repair. Usually the Le Fort II fracture will pass high along the nasomaxillary (frontal) buttresses, through the horizontal beams of the infraorbital rim, and low across the zygomaticomaxillary buttresses. The degloving approach provides an excellent opportunity to evaluate and accomplish the repair. Stabilization of one or several zygomaticomaxillary buttresses will usually provide sufficient fixation to allow healing to take place, but if instability is present, additional fixation across the nasofrontal processes and/or the inferior orbital rims must be considered.

Rigid miniplate fixation is an unforgiving method and should not be employed unless there is complete reduction of the fracture and a return to pretraumatic occlusion. The plates should always be applied to areas of naturally thickened bone. Acute bone grafting is necessary only in rare instances in which the fragments are lost. Suspension techniques (see Chapter 20) generally are to be avoided, because they are inaccurate and can cause compression of the midfacial fragments.

PROCEDURE

General anesthesia is desirable and is preferably administered through a tracheostomy. Nasotracheal intubation makes it difficult to reduce the nasal fractures, and orotracheal intubation interferes with occlusal relationships.

The nose should be anesthetized with 4% cocaine containing epinephrine, and the nose and gingival labial/sulcus should be blocked with 1% lidocaine containing 1:100,000 epinephrine (see Chapter 52). Usually the face and neck are prepared and draped as sterile fields.

The first portion of the procedure requires an application of arch bars intermaxillary fixation screws and/or Ivy loops. The methods are described in Chapter 19. Generally, Ivy loops or intermaxillary fixation screws can be applied, but when many teeth are missing or loose, arch bars are indicated.

A–C To expose the lower maxillary fractures, an incision should be made in the gingival labial sulcus, about 5 mm above the gingiva, from molar to molar region. The incision should be carried through the periosteum, and the periosteum should be elevated off the alveolus superiorly to expose the zygomaticomaxillary buttresses, canine fossae, and piriform apertures. A through-and-through septal-columella incision will facilitate the degloving and provide improved exposure to elevate the periosteum off the lateral walls of the piriform apertures. The surgeon can then also expose the infraorbital nerve and the frontal process of the maxilla.

D–F With the fracture lines visualized, the maxilla is reduced with digital or hook traction or with a Rowe disimpaction forceps (see Chapter 41). The lower maxillary fragments should be loosened and placed into an accurate position in relationship to the more stable upper portions. The nasal fractures, if present, are reduced at this time (see Chapter 52). Intermaxillary fixation is then applied with appropriate techniques.

G,H Once assured that reduction and occlusion are accurate, plates are applied. The plates should be contoured to the buttresses and secured with at least two holes placed over the more stable portions of bone. The initial drill holes are made close to the fracture with a drill bit just smaller than the diameter of the screws. The drilling should be irrigated copiously to prevent heat damage. Hole depths are then measured, and a screw slightly larger than the screw hole is selected and secured to the plate. Other holes are drilled and screws applied to give additional strength. Small fragments of buttress can be skewered with one or two screws. All fragments, however, should be elevated and reduced so that they are stable and in contact with the plate.

The zygomaticomaxillary buttresses are ideal places to achieve fixation, but if the maxilla is not stable, additional plates must be applied to other buttresses. Resorbable plates may also be used to stabilize the fracture(s), but one must be assured of stability and a generous covering of soft tissue over the plate. If there is a need for additional stability or there is still a displacement of associated fractures, the surgeon has the option of exposing the inferior orbital rim through an infraciliary incision or the nasofrontal process through a medial canthal incision and securing the fragments with miniplates (see Chapters 57 and 68). If the fracture line extends near the ostia of the maxillary sinuses, an intranasal antrostomy can be considered (see Chapter 41).

The mucosal incision is closed with interrupted 3-0 chromic sutures. The nose is packed for 24 to 48 hours with gauze or tampons treated with bacitracin ointment. The patient is given prophylactic antibiotics for 5 days. Intermaxillary fixation can be removed in 24 to 48 hours or, alternatively, it can be maintained for a variable period of time. Postoperative CT Scans should be obtained to verify adequate reduction and aeration of the sinuses. Healing should be evaluated weekly for 4 to 6 weeks and then monthly for at least 6 months.

PITFALLS

1. Achieving an accurate reduction and ensuring pretraumatic occlusion are prerequisites for miniplate fixation. Rigid plates are unforgiving, and once they are applied, it is difficult, if not impossible, to change the relationship of the bone fragments.

2. Screws should be applied only through the thicker vertical and/or horizontal buttresses. The length of the screws should be controlled so that they do not penetrate the sinus and act as foreign bodies.

3. Avoid placing screws near or through the roots of teeth. This complication can be avoided by using L, T, or curved plates.

4. Resorbable screws may be applied to the zygomaticomaxillary buttress(es), but make sure that the fixation is stable and that the plates are covered with sufficient soft tissues.

5. Additional stabilization of the Le Fort II fracture may be required at the infraorbital rim and/or nasofrontal processes. Plates can be used, but in thin-skinned individuals, they may be palpable and seen through the skin. The techniques are similar to those used for repair of nasal fractures (see Chapter 53) or zygoma fractures (see Chapter 57).

6. Le Fort II fractures rarely occur alone, and the surgeon must be prepared to reduce and fix other fractures associated with the injury. If the nose is fractured, the nasal fracture is reduced and treated as described in Chapter 52. Zygomatic, orbital, and alveolar fractures must also be treated with appropriate techniques. Mandible fractures can complicate occlusal relationships and for this reason should probably be repaired before the reduction and fixation of the maxillary fracture.

MINIPLATE FIXATION OF LE FORT II FRACTURE

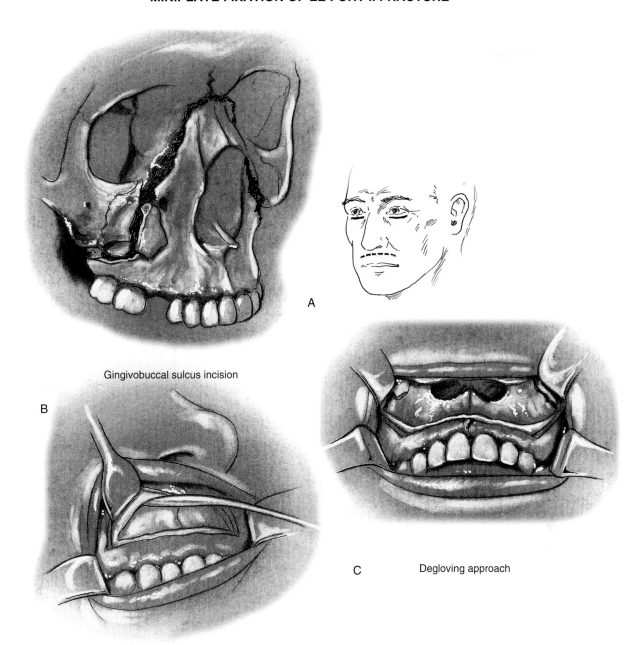

A

B

Gingivobuccal sulcus incision

C   Degloving approach

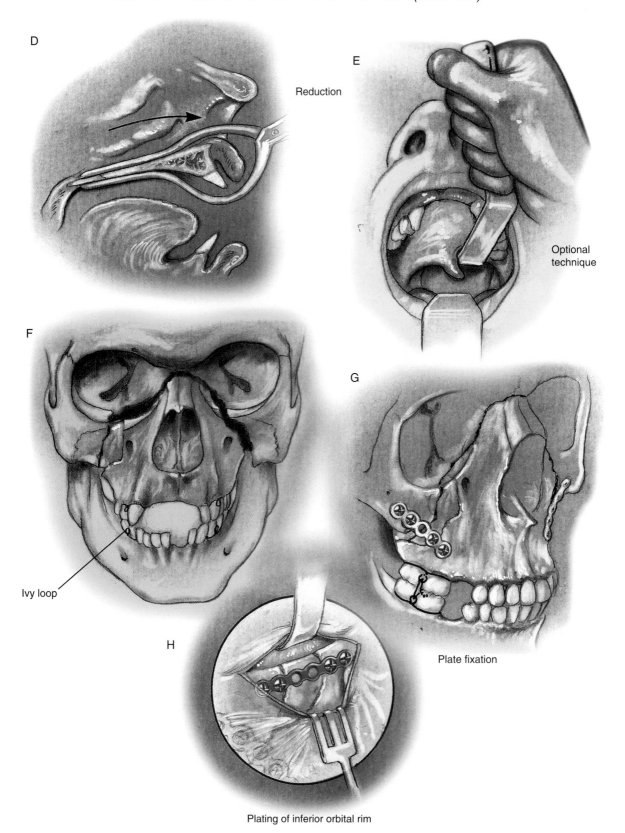

D

Reduction

E

Optional technique

F

Ivy loop

G

Plate fixation

H

Plating of inferior orbital rim

7. Occasionally the midface is so comminuted that there are few, if any, bones of sufficient size to hold the plate, or the fragments of bone are so scattered that they are not readily available. In such a situation, the surgeon should consider harvesting a split parietal cranial bone graft and applying this graft across the remnants of the zygomaticomaxillary and nasomaxillary buttresses. Wires or plates can be used to hold the grafts in place (see later).

COMPLICATIONS

1. Malocclusion can occur following miniplate fixation, especially if the plates are applied when there is an imperfect reduction. To avoid this complication, the fractures should be aligned in exact interdigitation; the maxillary fragments must fit like a puzzle. The plates should be bent and applied in such a way that tightening of the screws does not distract the fragments. However, if malocclusion develops, the surgeon has the option of orthodontia, extraction of involved teeth, and/or osteotomies with refixation of the fragments (see Chapter 49).

2. Facial deformity associated with malunion of the maxilla is unlikely, especially if the reduction and occlusion are accurate. Also, plate fixation is rigid and there should be no postoperative slippage. However, if a deformity develops, orthognathic osteotomy techniques should be considered (see Chapter 49). For minimal deformity and/or dysfunction, no treatment may be necessary.

3. Infection of the maxilla and/or sinuses is a rare complication. Some limited reaction may be observed with resorbable plates but this will usually resolve over time. Rigid and accurate fixation, intranasal antrostomy, and prophylactic antibiotics will usually prevent infection from occurring. If an infection develops, sequestered bone and foreign bodies will have to be removed. The infection should be cultured and appropriate intravenous antibiotics applied. The physician should also ensure that the antrostomy is open and aerating the sinuses.

4. Plate exposure can be a problem, but when it is properly treated, healing of the fractures should still occur. Usually the exposed plate area is treated with 3% hydrogen peroxide and local application of antibiotic ointment. Prophylactic antibiotics are administered. If the mucosa does not close over the plate, the plate should be retained as long as possible. If the wound is kept clean, the plate can be removed at the completion of healing.

5. Palpable or observable plates will eventually require removal. However, the plate should be left in place until all fractures have healed. Usually it can be removed through the original incision. The newer low profile miniplates may obviate this type of complication.

6. Tooth injury is possible, especially if a screw is placed too low and strikes the apex of the tooth. One way to avoid this complication is to make sure that the drill hole is placed in a position on the maxilla at least twice the height of the exposed crown of the tooth. If a tooth becomes injured, the plate will have to be removed and the tooth extracted or treated with appropriate endodontic therapy.

ALTERNATIVE TECHNIQUE USING PARIETAL CORTEX GRAFTS

a Split cranial grafts are indicated when the buttresses are comminuted, and there is little, if any, bone left to secure the plate. Sometimes small pieces of bone are difficult to find, and even when found, they are too small to secure to a screw or wire. The bone graft is preferably harvested from the outer cortex of the parietal skull (see Chapter 64).

b,c The graft is applied through a degloving, infraciliary, or frontoethmoid approach. The graft should be contoured to the zygomaticomaxillary buttress and/or nasofrontal process and secured superiorly and inferiorly to the remaining fragments with plates, or lag screws (Chapter 27). Postoperative care requires a combination of intravenous and oral antibiotic treatment for at least 2 weeks.

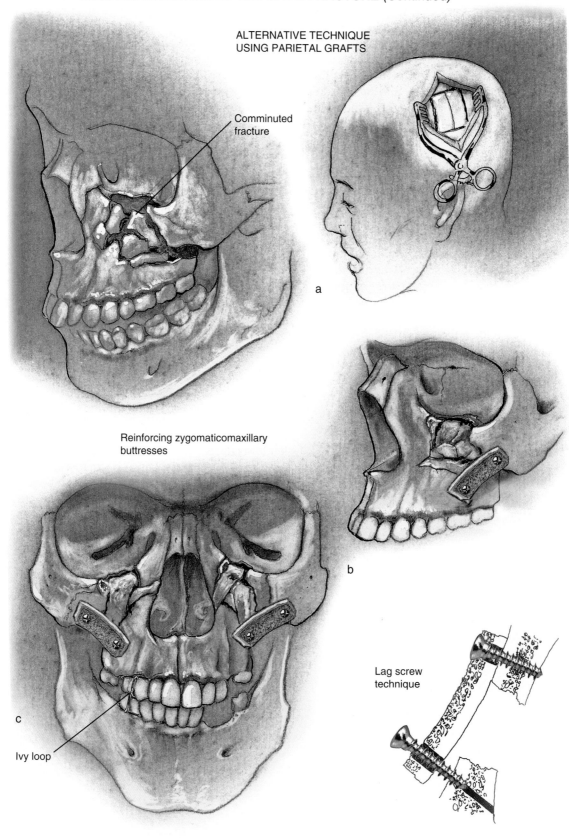

ALTERNATIVE TECHNIQUE
USING PARIETAL GRAFTS

Comminuted
fracture

a

Reinforcing zygomaticomaxillary
buttresses

b

c

Ivy loop

Lag screw
technique

Le Fort III Fractures

CHAPTER 43

Repair of Le Fort III Fracture With Coronal Flap and Miniplate Fixation

INDICATIONS

Le Fort III fracture lines classically cross a series of horizontal beams and vertical buttresses of the face, separating the face from the base of the skull. The main fracture line extends from the bridge of the nose through the nasofrontal processes, the floor of the orbits, the zygomaticofrontal processes, and zygomatic arches. The nasal septum is also fractured, and the maxilla is separated from the pterygoid plates.

Exposure from above, coupled with additional incisions from below, provides an excellent opportunity to explore, evaluate, and repair the fractures. The coronal incision and approach expose the upper part of the vertical buttresses, and if the forehead flap is extended, the zygomatic arches can be repaired. Transconjunctival or infraciliary and gingival labial sulcus incisions can be used to expose fractures of both the orbital rim and floor and the lower maxilla, respectively.

A relative contraindication to the coronal flap is a balding hairline. An absolute contraindication is a need to retain soft tissue flaps that are based on the posterior branches of the superficial temporal arteries. Alternatively, traditional periorbital approaches can be used (see Chapters 56 and 62 through 65).

For Le Fort III injuries that are complicated by additional fractures through the cranium, orbit, lower maxilla, and/or mandible, certain precautions must be considered. Cranial and orbital damage requires a consultation with a neurosurgeon and ophthalmologist. As a general rule, mandibular repair should be performed first. In the case of a condylar fracture, the surgeon may have to consider open reduction and fixation.

Most Le Fort III fractures can be reduced and placed into occlusion with Ivy loops, or alternatively, with intermaxillary fixation screws, and then stabilized with rigid miniplates across major buttresses. Small fragments of bone can be molded into position and held with a basketing effect from the plate. If comminution of bone is extensive, bone grafts may be required (see Chapter 42). Rarely is there a need for an internal or external suspension without rigid fixation, as these techniques can create abnormal forces that affect a shortening and retrusion of the midface.

PROCEDURE

Le Fort III fractures are best managed with a tracheostomy and general anesthesia. This method provides an excellent field for the surgeon, a separate field for the anesthesiologist, and an opportunity to check occlusion during and after the procedure. Nasal fractures can also be reduced without interference from the anesthetic tube.

A–C The coronal incision should extend from the preauricular creases above the pinnae and across the temples to form a gentle curve behind the hairline. A small area of hair should be shaved and the tissues injected with 1% lidocaine containing 1:100,000 epinephrine to help control bleeding.

The face is prepared and draped as a sterile field. Hair is held out of the way with elastic bands covered with towels and attached to the scalp. The incision is beveled along hair follicles and carried through the subcuticular and galeal tissues. Branches of the superficial temporal artery are clamped and ligated with 3-0 silk. A plane is then developed between the galea and periosteum, and the forehead tissues are elevated and rolled over the projection of the superior orbital rims. The periosteum should not be incised until the surgeon is close to the orbital rims, and the surgeon should attempt to preserve the supratrochlea and supraorbital vessels that enter the flap. Laterally, the dissection should be in a plane in the fat just superior to the temporalis fascia, but to be safe and avoid injury to the facial nerve, it is prudent to separate the layers of fascia or, even better, develop a plane beneath the fascia layers all the way to the zygomatic arch. Gentle retraction should avoid injury to the frontal branch of the facial nerve.

D–G With the flap rotated and held with fish hooks, the periosteum is incised along the frontal bone and zygomaticofrontal buttress. If the zygomatic arch needs to be exposed, the supraorbital arteries and nerves are released from their foramina with a small, sharp osteotome and the temporalis fascia, which may already be incised, elevated off the arch. The nasal bridge fracture can be exposed by retraction and additional periosteal elevation off the frontal process of the maxilla and nasal bones.

H To expose the infraorbital rims and lower maxilla, incisions can be made along the lower eyelid (infraciliary) and the gingival labial sulcus (Chapters 41 and 42).

I–J Once all fracture lines are exposed, the maxillary fractures should be reduced with a Rowe disimpaction forceps (see Chapter 41). The fracture sites should be reevaluated, and the surgeon should ensure that the fragments are aligned. The relationships of the jaws should be examined and pretraumatic occlusion

obtained with strategically placed Ivy loops, intermaxillary fixation screws, and arch bars (see Chapter 19).

K–N Miniplates are selected so that they will fit across the zygomaticofrontal fractures. Two screw holes should be available for solid bone fixation on each side of the fracture. The plates should be bent to the exact contour of the reduced fragments, and as the screws are placed, the surgeon should ensure that the bone fragments are retained in a reduced position. Screw holes are made with a drill bit that comes with the plating set. The depth of the drill should be controlled with a malleable retractor or, alternatively, the drill bit can be recessed so that it will not penetrate beyond the bone. Constant irrigation with saline should reduce the heat caused by the drilling and prevent further injury to the bone and soft tissues of the area. Drill holes should be measured so that the screws will pass through the bone but not project into the sinus (or soft tissues). The screws are applied first to holes located directly to the sides of the fracture and then to the outer holes for additional fixation.

For the classic Le Fort III fracture, zygomaticofrontal fixation should suffice. If the arch is severely comminuted and depressed, even after elevation, it may require plate fixation. If the nasofrontal process is unstable, the surgeon can place fine plates to approximate the fragments. If the inferior orbital rim needs repair, a separate eyelid exposure and plate fixation are indicated (see Chapter 57). The zygomaticomaxillary buttress(es) can be repaired with miniplates as described in Chapter 42. As a general rule, the surgeon should use a minimum number of plates to obtain stability.

The coronal flap is returned to its original position over flat suction drains and closed in layers. We prefer 3-0 chromic sutures to approximate the galea and several additional 3-0 chromic sutures in the subcuticular/subcutaneous tissues to coapt the skin edges. The skin is then closed with a running 5-0 nylon suture. Other incisions are treated with a layered closure.

To prevent swelling in the postoperative period, a light compression dressing of fluffs and expandable bandages is applied to the forehead, scalp, and ear areas. The patient should be treated with prophylactic antibiotics for at least 5 days. Dressings are changed as needed and maintained for at least 5 to 7 days. Sutures are removed on the seventh day. Dental hygiene is achieved with a water irrigation device. Intermaxillary elastic bands or wires are removed when correct intermaxillary relationships are ensured. Postoperative CT Scans should be used to verify the relationship of the bone fragments and subsequent aeration of sinuses. The patient should be evaluated every 2 weeks during the first month and then monthly until there is assurance that the injury has healed properly.

CORONAL FLAP AND MINIPLATE FIXATION FOR LE FORT III FRACTURES

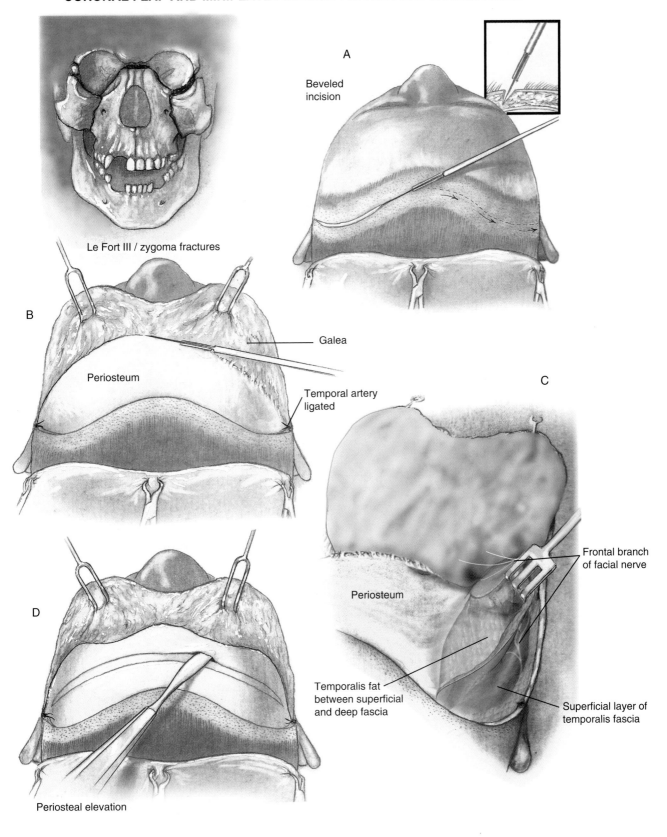

Le Fort III / zygoma fractures

A

Beveled incision

B

Galea

Periosteum

Temporal artery ligated

C

Frontal branch of facial nerve

Periosteum

Temporalis fat between superficial and deep fascia

Superficial layer of temporalis fascia

D

Periosteal elevation

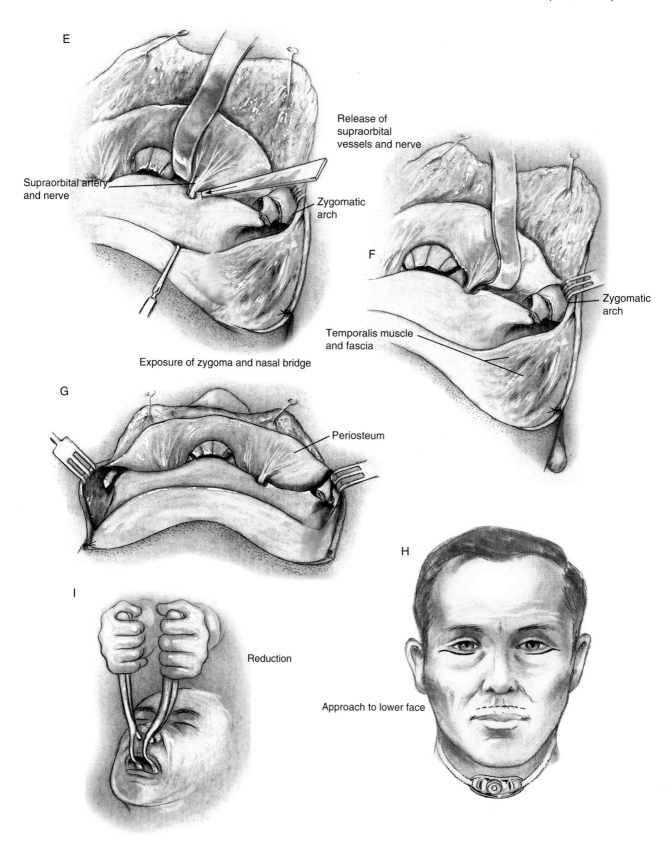

E

Release of supraorbital vessels and nerve

Supraorbital artery and nerve

Zygomatic arch

Exposure of zygoma and nasal bridge

F

Zygomatic arch

Temporalis muscle and fascia

G

Periosteum

H

Approach to lower face

I

Reduction

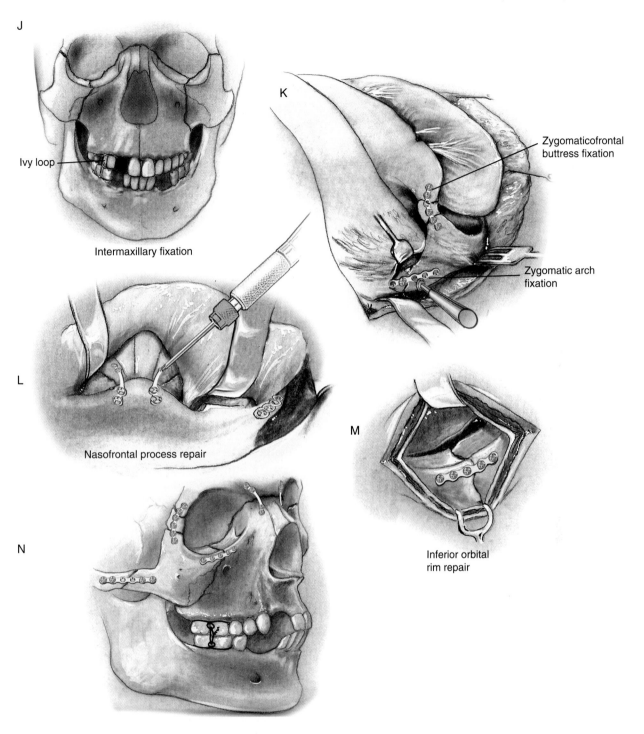

J

Ivy loop

Intermaxillary fixation

K

Zygomaticofrontal buttress fixation

Zygomatic arch fixation

L

Nasofrontal process repair

M

Inferior orbital rim repair

N

PITFALLS

1. Reduction of the Le Fort III fracture may require a forceful disimpaction. If there is a question of impending visual loss, the surgeon must carefully evaluate the site and the extent of the fractures in relationship to the orbit and retrobulbar tissues. Ophthalmologic consultation is advised. In experienced hands, a judicious application of force will reduce the fracture without untoward sequelae.

2. The coronal incision is ideal for exposure but should probably not be used in the patient who is bald (or balding) or in one who will need flaps based on the posterior branch of the superficial temporal vessel. Other alternatives are to use the infraciliary, eyebrow, and medial canthal incisions. The extended subbrow incision can also be employed (see Chapter 75).

3. An accurate reduction of fragments to pretraumatic occlusion must be obtained prior to placement of the miniplates. The rigid plates are unforgiving, and healing will occur in the positions dictated by the plates.

4. Use gentle retraction on the flaps. Excessive pressure can cause injury to the supraorbital and frontal branch of the facial nerve, resulting in paresthesias and weakness of the forehead.

5. The supraorbital artery and nerve should be preserved, but if there is an orbital rim fracture that requires reduction and/or stabilization and the nerve and artery are in the way, then the vessel and/or nerve may have to be sacrificed. The patient should be warned prior to surgery that he or she may have some numbness of the forehead and periorbital region.

6. Although the zygomatic arch can be plated, the procedure can cause potential problems. The retraction necessary for plating places the facial nerve at risk. Moreover, the skin over the arch is very thin and the plate will often be palpable or observable and require later removal. The plate also is not easily removed without again performing a coronal incision. For these reasons, we prefer a reduction of the arch and a check for stability without fixation.

7. Use only a sufficient number of plates to achieve fixation of buttresses or beams. One or two plates applied across the zygomaticofrontal buttresses often provide sufficient stability. If the maxilla is still unstable, additional plates can be added to other fracture sites. There is also the option of intermaxillary fixation for an extended period of time.

8. Plating should go from stable to unstable parts and thus in the direction of the frontal bone to the lower maxilla. In complicated cases in which fractures occur across the lower maxilla and mandible, the surgeon will have to first set the height of the mandible (i.e., repair condyle, ramus, and angle fractures), reduce the maxilla, and establish pretraumatic occlusion before aligning fragments with rigid plate fixation (see Chapter 112).

9. Avoid suspension wire techniques. Internal "drop-wire" suspension can cause a compression of the maxilla between the upper dentition and cranium. Retrusion can also occur. External suspension with a halo tends to pull the fragments up and out and can potentially create an overprojection of the midface.

10. Comminuted bone fragments can often be treated by basketing techniques. Most fragments can be found and manipulated into appropriate position and held with plates secured to the adjacent stable structures. However, when there is an avulsion of tissue, as is often found with gunshot wounds, the bone deficit may require additional methods of support. Split cranial or rib grafts for either stabilization or reinforcement should be considered.

COMPLICATIONS

1. Infections are prone to develop in patients who have soft tissue injuries and/or contaminated wounds. Bone grafts are at risk, and plate exposure can occur. Most infections can be treated with appropriate antibiotics, debridement, and drainage; if necessary, the plate and/or grafts will have to be removed.

2. Sinusitis is rare following Le Fort III fixation. Most fractures pass above the maxillary ostea and below the nasofrontal duct ostea and do not affect drainage of the sinuses. Intranasal antrostomies are not necessary, but if sinusitis develops, the patient should be started on decongestants and antibiotics. Persistent sinusitis may require a surgical drainage procedure.

3. Weakness of the forehead can occur as a result of injury to the frontal branch of the facial nerve. To avoid this complication, the surgeon should apply gentle traction to the forehead flap and stay in the fat plane either between the layers of the temporalis fascia or beneath the fascia. Extensive flaps should be avoided, especially if the zygomatic arch need not be repaired.

4. If there is injury to the supraorbital nerve, the patient can expect anesthesia and/or paresthesia of the forehead. The nerve is particularly at risk during maximal retraction of orbital tissues and with reduction and fixation of the superior and medial orbital rims. Loss of sensation is often transient, and some return of function is expected.

5. Nonunion of the maxilla is very rare. Some looseness of the maxilla can be tolerated, and with time, the maxilla will "tighten up" and require no additional surgical intervention. However, if maxillary movement continues to be a problem, the fracture site will need to be explored, the bone edges freshened, and the fractures treated with interposition bone grafts. Plate fixation can also be applied.

6. Malunion and malocclusion will develop if the reduction is not accurate or there is a slippage of the fragments following the procedure. Occasionally there is a resorption of bone and, in children, the possibility of impaired growth of the maxilla. Malunion, resulting in deformity and/or dysfunction, will require osteotomy and/or bone graft techniques as described in Chapter 50.

7. Plates can be visible or palpable, especially in thin-skinned individuals when the plates are placed over the frontozygomatic buttress, the nasofrontal process, or zygomatic arch. The complication can be avoided by using low-profile miniplates. If the plate causes a deformity, removal may be required.

CHAPTER 44

Repair of Le Fort III Fracture in the Edentulous Patient With Miniplate Fixation and Denture Suspension
Alternative Technique of Denture Fixation With Lag Screws

INDICATIONS

Le Fort III fractures in the edentulous patient are usually treated by reduction, rigid miniplate fixation, and approximation of occlusion, leaving any deficiencies to be corrected later with new dentures. In general, suspension techniques should be avoided. However, if the surgeon is not certain about the adequacy of the occlusion or reduction, then dentures or splints secured by a suspension method should be considered. This technique (also described in Chapter 20) is also useful when there is a need for the suspension wires and denture to cradle small fragments of the alveolus and/or palate in anatomic position.

PROCEDURE

The Le Fort III fracture is exposed through a coronal incision, or alternatively, through medial canthal, eyebrow, and/or infraciliary approaches described in Chapter 43. A degloving gingival labial sulcus incision will expose the lower maxilla (see Chapter 41).

The denture usually is modified to accommodate arch bars or other methods of intermaxillary fixation.

A,B The Le Fort III fracture is then reduced and the fragments placed in anatomic position. A lower denture is secured to the mandible with circummandibular wires. A long (26 to 30 cm) 24-gauge wire is subsequently placed through the drill hole of the zygomatic process of the frontal bone, and the ends of the wire are passed with an awl or trocar behind the zygomatic arch into the gingival labial/buccal sulcus. The wire is pulled tightly and then twisted into a loop that is just exposed in the sulcus.

To form a safety loop, a second loop of 28-gauge wire is applied between the 24-gauge wire loop and the denture near the region of the first molar. The denture is seated and secured into position by tightening the secondary loop. The upper and lower dentures are secured to each other with intermaxillary wires or rubber bands.

C–E A pullout wire should also be fashioned. For this, a 26-gauge wire is passed through the first wire

REPAIR OF LE FORT III FRACTURE IN THE EDENTULOUS PATIENT

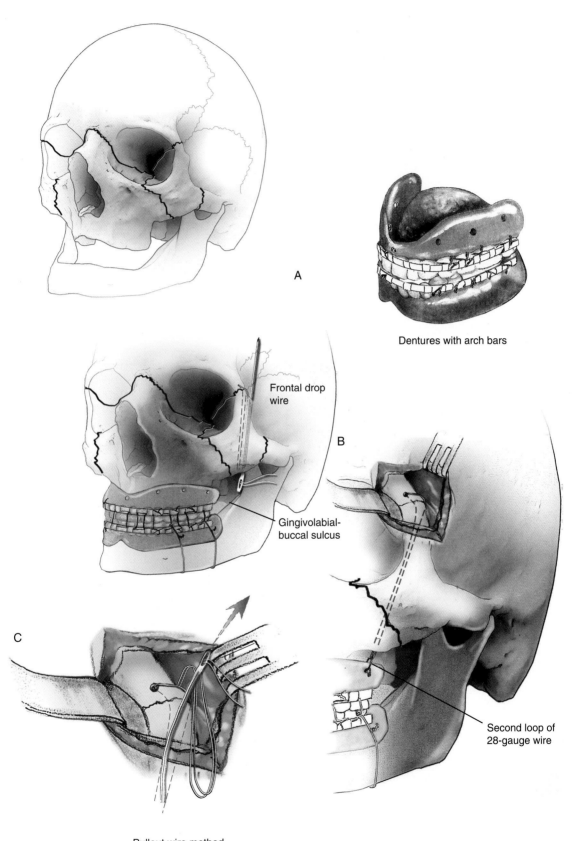

A

Dentures with arch bars

Frontal drop wire

B

Gingivolabial-buccal sulcus

C

Second loop of 28-gauge wire

Pullout wire method

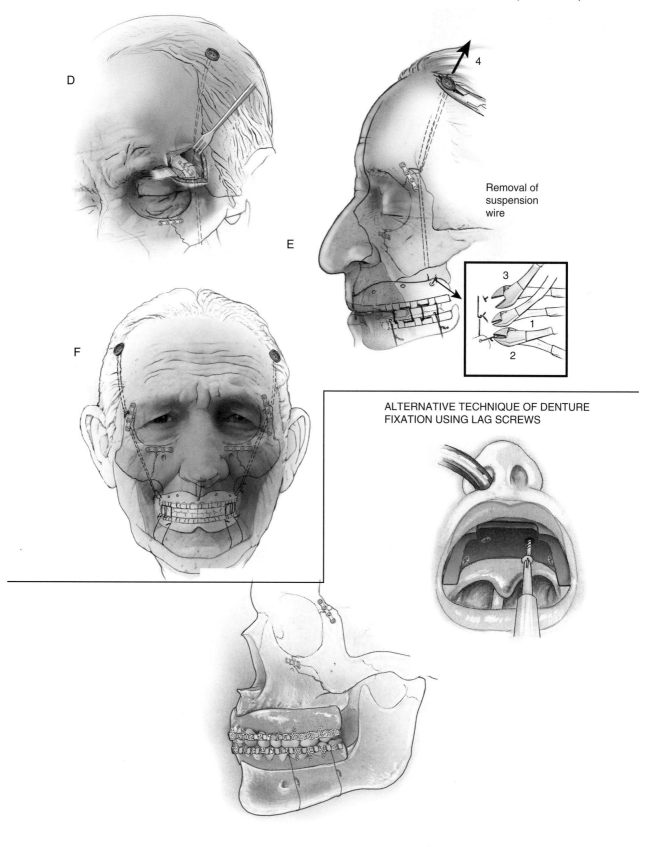

D

E

4

Removal of
suspension
wire

3

1

2

F

ALTERNATIVE TECHNIQUE OF DENTURE
FIXATION USING LAG SCREWS

loop, just beneath its attachment to the frontal bone. The wire is bent back on itself and both ends passed with an awl or needle through the deep subcutaneous tissues to exit from the scalp at a point just beyond the hairline. The wire is secured to a button on the surface of the skin. When the fixation apparatus is to be removed, the long transmaxillary wire loop is cut, and the accessory scalp wire loop is used to pull it out. If there is difficulty in removing the suspension wire, a small incision can be made on the lateral orbital rim and the wire removed directly.

F The suspension procedure is usually performed bilaterally and the wires adjusted so that there is a vertical pull on the denture. If the upper denture should rock, the surgeon should also consider a drop wire from the anterior nasal spine. Placement of this wire, the holes in the denture, and the intermaxillary fixation are described in Chapters 19 and 20. With the patient in intermaxillary fixation, the fractures are stabilized with miniplates as described in Chapter 43. Strategic buttresses and beams should be plated to obtain rigid fixation.

Postoperatively the patient is treated as described in Chapter 43. In about 4 to 6 weeks, suspension wires and loops around the dentures are cut, and the suspension wires are removed with the pullout wire. The wire from the anterior nasal spine can be cut and removed directly.

ALTERNATIVE TECHNIQUE OF DENTURE FIXATION WITH LAG SCREWS

Denture suspension as described above can be tedious and compromised by a loosening of wires. The denture is also difficult to remove and it can be painful to the patient on removal. A more expedient and direct method is to lag screw the denture (or splint) to the palate. The denture can be fitted with arch bars and secured to a lower denture or teeth with intermaxillary fixation.

The lag screw technique requires the placement of holes to be made through the denture or splint directed to the bony part of the palate and/or alveolus (see also Chapters 20 and 43). Smaller holes are subsequently drilled through the denture holes into the bone of the palate and/or alveolus. Screws of at least 10 to 12 mm lengths are then selected to engage the smaller drill holes and with a screw head larger than the palatal holes, the denture is secured to the palate. Intermaxillary wires or bands are subsequently placed for intermaxillary fixation.

Patient care requires CT scan analysis, postoperative antibiotics, and antiseptic mouthwashes. The denture can be removed at the end of the period needed for fixation by evaluating the maxilla for any abnormal movement.

CHAPTER

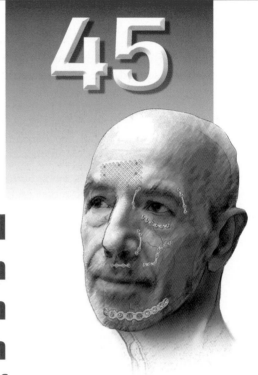

Repair of Medial Maxillary Fracture With Degloving Approach and Miniplate Fixation
Alternative Technique of Closed Reduction
Alternative Technique of Late Reconstruction With Osteotomies and/or Onlay Bone Grafts

INDICATIONS

Medial maxillary fractures present with a characteristic deformity: a C-shaped deviation of the dorsum of the nose, with the tip and root of the nose maintained in a fairly normal position. The deformity can be confused with a simple nasal fracture, except the medial maxillary fracture is associated with an obvious depression of the medial maxillary wall and, in some cases, an extension of the depression to involve the frontal process of the maxilla and inferior orbital wall. The displacement of the medial maxillary wall usually causes nasal obstruction and potentially a disruption and twisting of the lacrimal collecting system. An accurate early diagnosis is essential, and once the injury is defined, reduction and fixation must be considered. Miniplates fixation is effective in stabilizing the repositioned bones.

PROCEDURE

Oral intubation is preferred. The face and neck are prepared with antiseptic solution and draped as a sterile field. The nasal mucous membranes are treated with pledgets soaked in 8 mL of 4% cocaine, to which is added five drops of 1:10,000 epinephrine. The nose is then blocked in a standard fashion with 1% lidocaine containing 1:100,000 epinephrine (see Chapter 52). Additional amounts of anesthesia are infiltrated into the gingival labial/buccal sulcus.

A–C An incision is made 5 mm above the gingival margin from the first molar on the side of exploration to the canine of the opposite side. Hemostasis is achieved with electric cautery. The periosteum is elevated off the alveolus and onto the anterior face of the maxilla. The dissection is continued upward, exposing the anterior nasal spine, piriform aperture, infraorbital canal, and neurovascular bundle. Additional exposure is obtained by making a through-and-through septal-columella incision and extending these cuts along the floor of the nose and the piriform aperture to expose the nasomaxillary buttresses.

D–G Further elevation of the periosteum will expose the frontal process of the maxilla, the nasal bones, and the inferior orbital rim. As an option an additional incision along the frontal process of the maxilla will give exposure to the superior part of the fracture. The thicker portions of the fracture are reduced with a Boies elevator and the smaller fragments with either a Cottle graduated elevator or single skin hooks. The fragments are secured by adopting a straight or slightly curved miniplate along the nasomaxillary buttress. Resorbable plates may also be considered. Screw holes are placed into the stable inferior and superior parts of the buttress. Additional holes and screws are placed in the fractured fragments.

Closure is accomplished by suturing the gingival mucosa with 3-0 chromic sutures. The septum is secured to the columella with several 3-0 chromic mattress sutures, usually placed with a straight needle. The nose should be packed for 3 to 5 days with either a bacitracin-soaked nasal tampon or layered 1/2-inch, bacitracin-impregnated gauze. If the nasal bones are comminuted, a tape and splint are applied to the dorsum of the nose after appropriate reduction (see Chapter 52).

Antibiotics are prescribed for the duration of the packing. Following removal of the packing, the internal nose is kept moist and clean with sprays of normal saline several times a day. The patient should be evaluated every 2 weeks during the first month and then monthly until there is assurance that the injury has healed properly.

PITFALLS

1. The diagnosis is critical for an accurate and early treatment. The degloving approach is not necessary for simple nasal fractures, as these can be easily treated with a closed reduction technique (see Chapter 52). Moreover, the degloving exposure is not sufficient to treat a displaced inferior orbital rim or a fracture of the floor or medial wall of the orbit. These injuries require additional approaches (see G and Chapters 57 and 63).

2. Enophthalmos, hypophthalmos, and diplopia associated with the medial maxillary fracture suggest an orbital injury. When these signs and symptoms occur, an infraciliary incision and floor exposure are necessary (see Chapters 57 and 63).

3. Occasionally there will be cases in which it is more prudent to carry on a simple closed reduction of nasal bones and the medial maxilla (see later). This is indicated in a debilitated individual, especially one who cannot tolerate general anesthesia or the length of time required for the open procedure.

4. Although rare, the medial maxillary fracture can be associated with telecanthus and epiphora. If this occurs, a separate medial canthal incision should be carried out and the medial wall and rim of the orbit explored for injuries. The techniques for repair are discussed in Chapters 67 through 69.

5. The medial maxillary fracture will heal rapidly, and if the diagnosis is not made early, there is a possibility of permanent deformity and dysfunction. If the bones are healed (and this usually occurs after 4 weeks), then the fracture must be reestablished with osteotomies and treated as in an early injury. To make the osteotomies, it is necessary to expose the orbit and nasal bones through a degloving, infraciliary and medial canthal approach. If there is resorption of bone, split parietal cranial grafts may be layered over the defect (see later).

COMPLICATIONS

1. Malunion of the maxillary and nasal bones can be corrected in the first few months with osteotomies, refracture of the segments, and reapproximation with wire or plates. At a later time, there is usually too much resorption of bone, and in such a case, it is more prudent to employ split cranial grafts as an onlay to the area of deficit (see later).

DEGLOVING APPROACH FOR MEDIAL MAXILLARY FRACTURE

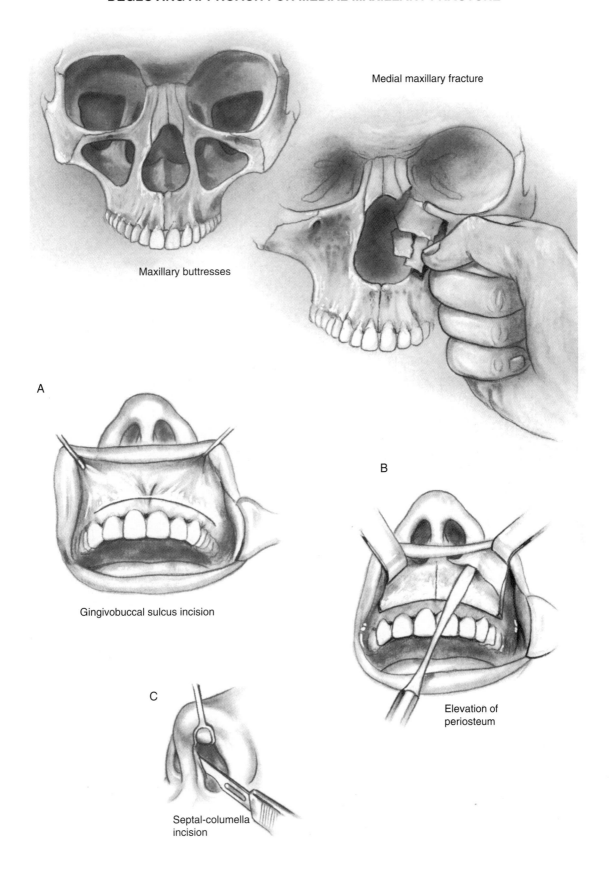

Maxillary buttresses

Medial maxillary fracture

A

Gingivobuccal sulcus incision

B

Elevation of periosteum

C

Septal-columella incision

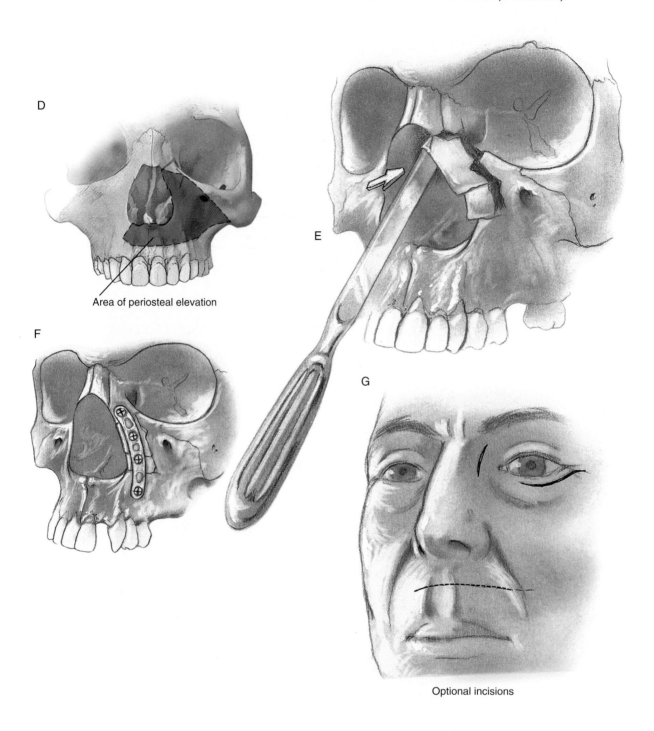

Area of periosteal elevation

Optional incisions

2. Early orbital complications such as enophthalmos, hypophthalmos, and diplopia can be treated early with reexploration, osteotomy (if necessary), and repositioning of the fragments. For late complications, the patient must be evaluated for a complete reconstruction of the orbit (see Chapters 64 and 65).

3. Dacryocystitis is a potential problem, especially if the lacrimal drainage system is obstructed. The lacrimal system should be evaluated with appropriate dye tests. For obstruction at the canaliculus and/or outflow of the sac, conjunctivorhinostomy or dacryocystorhinostomy must be considered (see Chapters 71 and 72). However, the surgeon should make sure that a deviated septum or turbinate is not causing the obstruction, and if these conditions exist, they should be corrected before lacrimal collection system surgery.

4. Deformities confined to the nasal bones can be treated with standard rhinoplasty procedures (see Chapter 54). Usually the physician waits 4 to 6 months so that the bones become solid and the osteotomies can be controlled. If the bones are not healed, the osteotomies potentially can cause further instability of the nasal pyramid.

ALTERNATIVE TECHNIQUE OF CLOSED REDUCTION

A closed method of treatment is indicated for those individuals who are severely debilitated and cannot tolerate the general anesthetic usually given with an open procedure. For such a case, the nose is anesthetized with cocaine-soaked pledgets, and the nose is blocked with 2% lidocaine. Using a Boies elevator, the nasal bones, and medial wall of the maxilla are elevated into position (see *E*). The nose is then packed bilaterally with a tampon or gauze dressing (see Chapter 52). External tapes and plaster may be applied. The disadvantage of this particular procedure is that reduction may not be stable, and there can be a relapse of the fracture.

ALTERNATIVE TECHNIQUE OF LATE RECONSTRUCTION WITH OSTEOTOMIES AND/OR ONLAY BONE GRAFTS

Osteotomy is a valuable adjunctive technique for the late deformity and dysfunction following medial maxillary fracture. The degloving approach provides exposure to the inferior portion of the fracture, but for the superior portion of the fracture that often extends to the frontal process of the maxilla and inferior orbital rim, additional periorbital incisions are necessary. The infraciliary incision, with a skin-muscle flap, provides excellent exposure of the inferior orbital rim. This direct approach also avoids injury to the infraorbital nerve. For the frontal process of the maxilla, a medial canthal incision one-half the distance between the dorsum of the nose and inner caruncle is helpful. Elevation of the periosteum on the frontal process of the maxilla will demonstrate the fracture of the nasal bones and extension of the fracture toward the medial wall of the orbit.

a The osteotomies should be performed with a 3-mm osteotome (hand surgery type), directing the cuts along the fracture lines. With small elevators, the bones are reduced and repositioned into their anatomic relationships. If there happens to be some coexisting resorption, the surgeon can set small gaps and secure the bones with miniplates. Once significant resorption has occurred, interposed bone grafts will be required.

b,c In those cases of medial maxillary fracture in which resorption of bone is significant, the surgeon is advised to proceed directly with onlay grafts. Usually the objective is to fill the concavity caused by the depression of the medial maxillary buttress, but if these deformities extend to the frontal process of the maxilla or infraorbital rim, these areas also must be corrected.

Depending on the requirements to fill the defect, several pieces of split cranial bone graft are harvested from the ipsilateral parietal bone. The medial maxilla is exposed by a degloving, infraciliary and/or medial canthal approach, and the periosteum is elevated off the involved area. The cranial bones are carved to fit the defect, secured with lag screw technique (Chapters 27, 42, 59, and 64) and covered with periosteum using 3-0 chromic sutures.

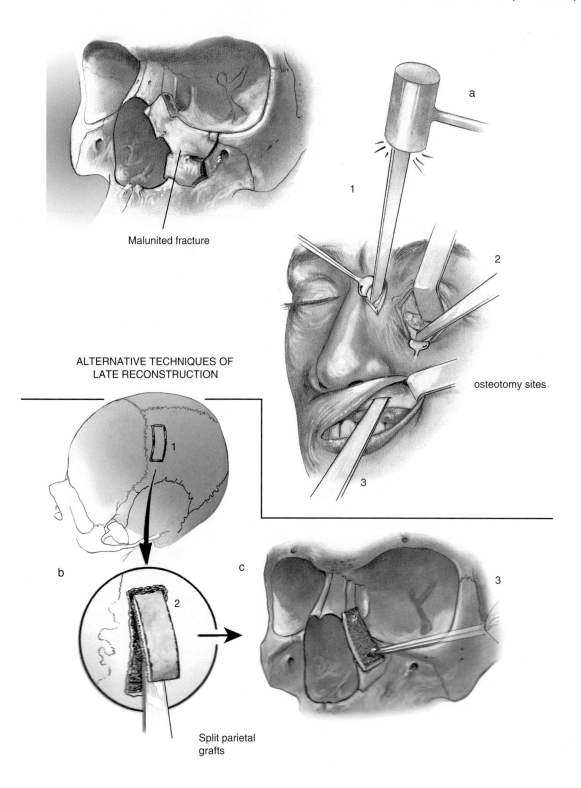

Malunited fracture

ALTERNATIVE TECHNIQUES OF
LATE RECONSTRUCTION

osteotomy sites

Split parietal
grafts

CHAPTER

46

Repair of Split Palate With Arch Bar Fixation
Alternative Technique Using a Heavy Arch Bar (Jelenko) Alternative Technique of Miniplate Fixation

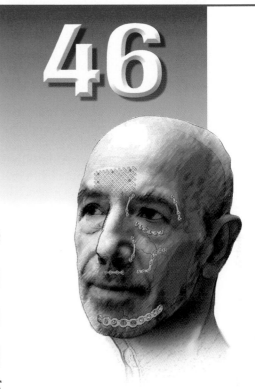

INDICATIONS

A split palate in a patient with teeth is probably best treated with intermaxillary fixation. Setting the upper and lower jaws into occlusion and using the lower jaw to stabilize the upper jaw secure and stabilize the dental arch. The teeth of the lower jaw also serve to stop inward and outward rotation of the hemipalates. The obvious disadvantage of intermaxillary fixation is that the patient's mouth is closed for 4 to 6 weeks and oral and masticatory functions are impaired for this period of time.

PROCEDURE

A Nasotracheal intubation or tracheostomy is performed. The maxillae should be mobilized as

described in Chapter 41 so that the hemipalates are placed into anatomic position. Other facial fractures should also be reduced appropriately.

B,C An Erich arch bar is first attached to the lower dentition (see Chapter 19). The upper dental arch is then manipulated into approximate occlusion and the arch bar attached to the upper dentition to stabilize the midline split. If there is a large cleft, the surgeon can split the arch bar at the fracture and repair the arch bar later with horizontally placed 26-gauge wire loops. Alternatively, the surgeon can use a temporary 26-gauge transdental loop wire across the incisors. The upper and lower arch bars are subsequently secured to each other with elastic bands or 28-gauge wire loops. Reduction and fixation are evaluated, and occlusion is checked to ensure pretraumatic relationships. The associated facial fractures are wired or plated.

Postoperatively the patient is placed on oral antibiotics. Reduction of fractures is confirmed by CT Scans and/or routine facial radiographs. Cleaning of the teeth and arch bars with chlorhexidine mouthwashes and a water irrigation device is important. Intermaxillary fixation is kept in place and adjusted when necessary for approximately 6 weeks. The patient should be followed monthly for at least 6 months. Puréed and soft diets are used to maintain nutritional status.

PITFALLS

1. Complete mobilization of the hemipalates is essential for the reduction and fixation. If the reduction is not accurate, the tension can be adjusted with the elastic bands or wires until the desired results are achieved. If this does not obtain pretraumatic relationships, then a formal open procedure with reduction should be performed.

2. In patients who are partially edentulous, Erich arch bars may not provide sufficient stability. For improved fixation, the surgeon should consider the heavier (Jelenko) arch bars, miniplates (see later), or palatal splints (see Chapter 47).

3. When approximating the fracture anteriorly, be careful not to distract the posterior segments of the palate. The arch bar should be tightened just until intermaxillary fixation and interdigitation of molars are complete. This sequence will prevent lateralization of the hemipalates.

COMPLICATIONS

1. Nonunion following a palatal split is frequently associated with malocclusion and problems with mastication. It usually becomes evident after removal of the arch bars, but if there is infection or soft tissue necrosis, it can be suspected at an earlier time. The complication can be avoided by accurate reduction and fixation, maintenance of local hygiene, and prophylactic antibiotics. Postoperative infection should be treated with cultures and specific antibiotic therapy. Initially the mobile maxilla can be treated as a delayed union with additional fixation, but if movement is still present after 8 to 10 weeks, the surgeon will have to consider alternative methods. As with other nonhealed fractures, it will be necessary to freshen the edges of the fracture, reduce the fragments, and apply rigid plates. Whether bone grafts are necessary will depend on the loss of bone and the malocclusion created by the loss of the bone fragments.

2. Malunion caused by a palatal split should be handled in the same way as malunion resulting from upper alveolar fractures. Occlusal readjustment, limited extractions, and orthognathic methods should be considered.

3. When the palatal fracture is associated with comminution and infection, it is possible for the patient to later develop an oroantral or oronasal fistula. Our preference is to first control the infection and then perform intranasal antrostomies (if the sinus is involved) and allow the wound to close by secondary intention. Contraction of the tissues will make for a smaller fistula and provide for an easier repair. We then consider a three-layer closure: (1) a trap door rotation of the superficial layers of palatal tissue; (2) insertion of a free piece of temporalis fascia between the palate and nasal flaps; and (3) a rotation of palatal flaps based on the greater palatine artery. Bilobed flaps can also be used.

ALTERNATIVE TECHNIQUE USING A HEAVY ARCH BAR (JELENKO)

If the reduction of the palatal split seems to proceed easily and the hemipalates seem to assume an anatomic position, the surgeon can employ the technique using a single heavy (Jelenko) bar. The heavy bar can act as a splint, and if it is applied accurately, it will immobilize the fragments in the desired position. The technique is particularly useful in patients with a partially edentulous jaw and in whom there is a need for stable support across the edentulous areas. However, the procedure should be abandoned if there is any instability and other methods of immobilization (i.e., intermaxillary, rigid plate, or prosthetic fixation) should be used.

For the heavy bar technique, the fractures should be reduced and occlusion ensured by an interdigitation of the teeth without premature contact. A Jelenko arch bar is then attached to the upper dentition with circumdental wires. If the occlusal relationships are questionable, the surgeon should apply an Erich arch bar to the lower dentition and use intermaxillary fixation as a guide.

Postoperatively the patient should maintain oral hygiene with chlorhexidine mouthwashes and water irrigation of the dentition. Prophylactic antibiotics should be used for 5 days and fixation maintained for approximately 6 weeks.

ALTERNATIVE TECHNIQUE OF MINIPLATE FIXATION

In many patients a single rigid miniplate across the premaxilla is sufficient for fixation. The technique is particularly suitable for the split palate in the edentulous patient, as the plate often provides sufficient

REPAIR OF PALATAL SPLIT

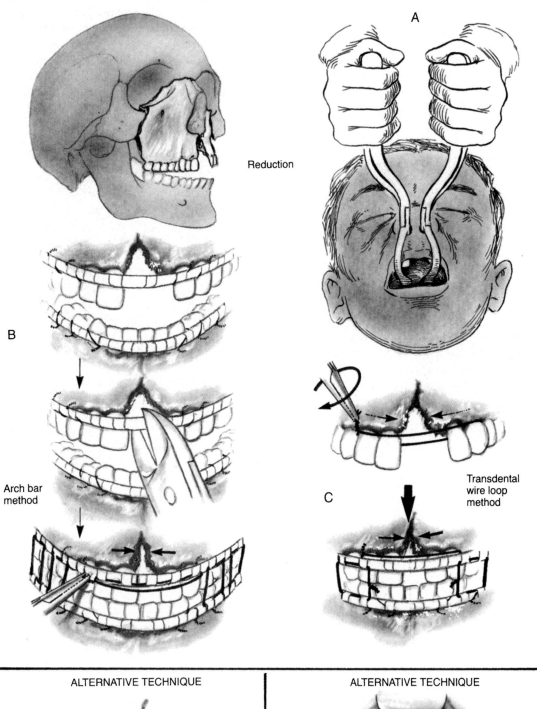

Reduction

A

B

Arch bar method

Transdental wire loop method

C

ALTERNATIVE TECHNIQUE

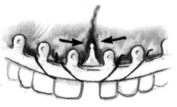

Heavy arch bar

ALTERNATIVE TECHNIQUE

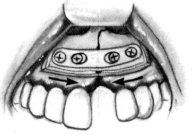

Miniplate fixation

immobilization for the fracture to heal. The disadvantage is that the anterior nasal spine and premaxillary crest can make it difficult to place the plate flat against the premaxilla; also, the plate can sometimes be felt, thus annoying the patient.

The rigid plate technique requires an accurate reduction of the dental arch to pretraumatic occlusion. The premaxilla is approached by a gingival labial sulcus incision 5 mm above the margin of the gingiva. The periosteum is elevated to the level of the piriform apertures, and the fracture is exposed. If the fracture reduction and occlusal relationships are anatomic, the plate can be applied. If there is a pronounced ridge inferior to the anterior, spine, this can be flattened with a cutting bur.

We prefer the miniplate or better a minicompression plate. For compression, the procedure requires that the holes closest to the fracture be drilled first; other screws are then placed through the outer holes to give added support. Preliminary bending of the plate to an accurate contour prevents extraction of the fragments during application of the screws.

The incision is closed with interrupted 4-0 chromic sutures, and the patient is maintained on antibiotics for 5 days. A soft diet should be utilized throughout the fixation period (6 to 8 weeks).

Reduction and Fixation of Split Palate With Prosthesis and Lag Screws

INDICATIONS

In the edentulous patient who has dentures, the surgeon has the option of reducing the split palate and applying the patient's upper denture directly to the upper dental arch and palate. If there is some concern about the reduction, it is also possible to apply arch bars to the dentures, fix the dentures to the upper and lower jaws, and secure the dentures to each other with intermaxillary fixation. This technique provides the best opportunity to restore pretraumatic occlusion. Alternatively, if the surgeon does not want to use the patient's dentures or dentures are not available, a prefabricated splint can be used or occlusion can be approximated and a rigid fixation plate applied across the premaxilla (see Chapters 20 and 46).

PROCEDURE

A–E Using general anesthesia administered through nasotracheal intubation or tracheostomy, the maxillary fractures are reduced as discussed in Chapter 41. Pretraumatic occlusion is approximated, and the upper denture is placed tightly against the reduced palate. Holes are made with a bur on each side of the denture, and with appropriate drill bits (i.e., smaller than the screws), deeper holes are then drilled through the bony palate. Screws, measured so that they

just pass through the bone, are then used to secure the denture to the palate. The screw head should catch the prosthesis and pull the prosthesis tightly against the palate bone. If the maxilla is also unstable, additional fixation techniques must be applied (see Chapters 40 through 45).

Postoperatively the reduction is assured by radiographic evaluation. The patient is treated with prophylactic antibiotics and oral hygiene maintained with chlorhexidine mouthwashes. Healing should occur by about 6 weeks, and at that time, the denture can be removed.

PITFALLS

1. Although the prosthetic technique can be rapidly applied, it is a closed method and there can be problems with the reduction and fixation. Clinical and CT scan/radiographic verification must be obtained in the postoperative period.

2. If there is any question regarding occlusion and/or fixation, alternatively the surgeon can apply arch bars to the upper and lower dentures and secure the upper denture to the zygoma with circumzygomatic wires and the lower denture to the mandible with circummandibular wires. The dentures are then placed into occlusal relationships and held with intermaxillary fixation (see Chapters 20 and 44).

PROSTHETIC STABILIZATION OF SPLIT PALATE

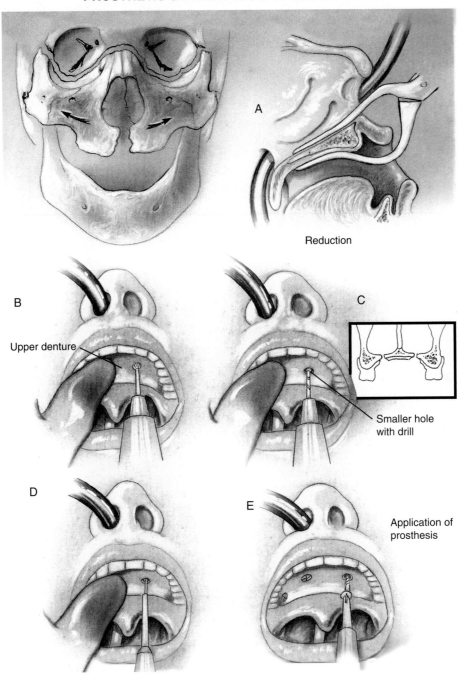

A

Reduction

B

Upper denture

C

Smaller hole
with drill

D

Depth measurement

E

Application of
prosthesis

COMPLICATIONS

1. Erosion beneath the denture is always a possibility. Unfortunately, until the denture is removed, there will be little evidence that this has occurred. Preventive measures are to secure a firm fit and cushion the denture on the alveolus with a soft liner. Prophylactic antibiotics and oral hygiene are helpful. Once erosion is noted, the denture should be removed and the area treated with ointment and local debridement and irrigations. If the damage is severe (i.e., oronasal or oroantral fistula), then flap closures may be necessary.

2. All of the complications associated with denture techniques can develop when using this method for repair of a palatal split. These conditions are discussed in Chapter 20.

Malunion of the Maxilla

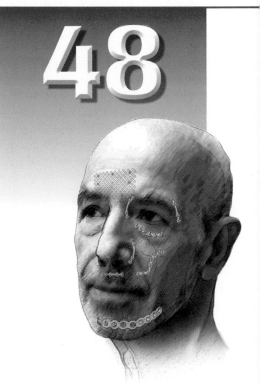

CHAPTER 48

Correction of Low Maxillary Retrusion or Lengthening With Le Fort I Osteotomies
Alternative Technique Using Onlay Grafts

In Consultation With Lewis Clayman, DMD, MD

INDICATIONS

Malposition of maxillary fractures can impose functional and esthetic burdens on the trauma patient. Facial deformity and masticatory, temporomandibular joint, and speech dysfunctions are often presenting complaints. When they are severe, they evoke significant psychological distress.

The objectives for surgical treatment are restoration of proper occlusion and a normal 3-D appearance of the face (i.e., in height, width, and projection) effected by osteotomy. Abnormal findings to correct include retrusion of the upper lip, reduced projection

of the anterior nasal spine, retraction of the columella, submalar flatness, and an open bite deformity (apertognathia).

Pretreatment evaluation should include photographs, radiographs, and study models to assess functional and esthetic deficits. Lateral and frontal cephalometric radiographs utilizing both bone and soft tissue densities will define the skeletal and soft tissue imbalances. Dental films, facial bone plain films, and computed tomographic scans (3-D, when practicable) are also important parts of the evaluation. Dental occlusal relationships should be recorded, and wax bite registration and dental models should be obtained.

Careful review of all these diagnostic aids defines the indications for care and the particular procedures to be employed. Photographs taken in repose and in dynamic facial expression define the frontal, oblique, and lateral facial deformities; intraoral photographs record the functional imbalances of the dental occlusion. Radiographs show lines of fracture and aeration of the sinuses. Cephalometric films define the skeletal deficiency and suggest the degree of movement necessary to establish skeletal norms and effect changes in soft tissue contour. Dental models should be appropriately sectioned and manipulated to define the movements necessary to restore proper occlusal relationships; interocclusal acrylic splints made on the sectioned models are usually necessary to guide and stabilize the occlusion during the surgical procedure. Orthodontic and prosthodontic consultations are advisable to determine the final treatment plan.

PROCEDURE

Nasotracheal intubation is customary in the management of these problems, but if the patient has had a tracheostomy, this provides an ideal method for airway control during anesthesia. The face and neck are surgically scrubbed and draped as sterile fields. Arch bars or Ivy loops are applied to the dentition if the patient does not have the advantage of orthodontic appliances (see Chapter 19). The nasal mucous membranes are treated with 4% cocaine containing epinephrine, and the buccal sulci are infiltrated with 0.5% lidocaine containing 1:200,000 epinephrine. If palatal incisions are to be utilized, the same solution is deposited over the greater palatine and nasopalatine foramina.

A–D There are two commonly employed approaches through the soft tissue to the bone of the maxilla. One entails a horizontal incision made in the gingivolabial buccal sulcus from the mesial of the first molar to its opposite number. Subsequently the periosteum of the nose is elevated along the floor and lateral walls with Cottle or Freer elevators. Medially the mucoperichondrium and mucoperiosteum of the nasal septum are elevated in continuity with the mucosa of the floor of the nose (see Chapter 54). Through the gingivolabial buccal sulcus incision, the periosteum is elevated from the maxilla, exposing the anterior nasal spine, piriform apertures, infraorbital nerves, zygomas, and the maxillary wall to the pterygoid plates. Great care is expended to avoid perforation of the periosteum to keep the buccal fat pad from interfering with visibility during surgery.

The second soft tissue approach is somewhat more difficult but often provides better mobility and freedom of the mobilized bone. Vertical incisions are made from the height of the gingivolabial sulcus inferiorly to the gingiva, at the midline (overlying the anterior nasal spine), in the bicuspid regions, and in the area of the terminal molars. A subperiosteal reflection through these incisions allows elevation of the tissues, as with the other approach. Additionally, however, the palatal soft tissues are reflected along a line of incision that extends in a horseshoe configuration from one greater palatine foramen to the other, coursing anteriorly in the trough between the alveolar arch and the horizontal palate, and across the midline in the area of the rugae. The elevation of the palatal tissues eliminates their restrictive influence on advancement of the maxilla.

E–G Osteotomies are performed with burs, electric saws, or mallet and chisels. Horizontal cuts are initiated through the lateral rim of the piriform aperture at a level at least 5 mm above the apices of the dental roots. The appropriate level can be estimated by measuring the length of the canine crown and making the osteotomy at a point 5 mm higher than twice the crown length. Ideally, although not usually possible, the sinus mucosa can be protected by carrying the osteotomies just through the thickness of the maxillary bone. The nasal mucosa should be preserved by elevating it from the lateral wall and floor of the nose while the osteotomies are being made at these two sites with the osteotomes. A guarded osteotome reduces the chance of lacerating the mucosa. Using subperiosteal tunnels, the cartilaginous septum, the vomer, and the perpendicular plate of the ethmoid are separated from the palate with the septal chisels. Posteriorly the maxilla is loosened from the pterygoid plates with a curved osteotome directed into the pterygomaxillary groove.

If the maxilla has been approached through the optional lateral vertical incisions and the soft tissues of the palate are reflected distally, additional mobility can be obtained by a posterior sectioning of the maxilla. This is accomplished with a vertical osteotomy made through the maxillary tuberosity anterior to the pterygomaxillary interface and onto the palate to continue as a transverse bone cut across the palatal midline to the same region on the opposite side. Great care must be excercised in order to avoid cutting the nasotracheal tube during this maneuver. Blood loss in the posterior aspect of the wound is quite often less with this approach.

H–J Following completion of the osteotomies, the maxilla is mobilized by applying torque to the bone along the fracture lines with osteotomes or elevators and applying traction to the maxilla with Rowe disimpaction forceps. The operator must be careful, in the down-fracture mobilization, to avoid injury to the descending palatine vessels, which should become

LE FORT I OSTEOTOMIES

A

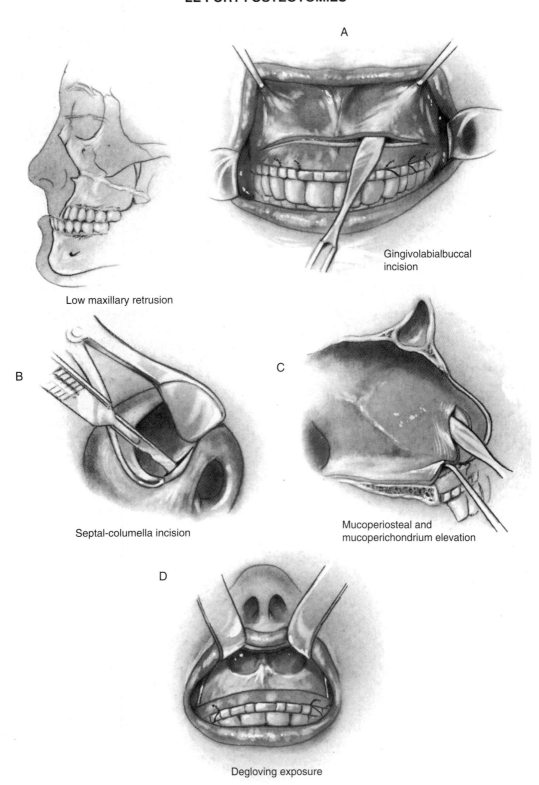

Gingivolabialbuccal
incision

Low maxillary retrusion

B

Septal-columella incision

C

Mucoperiosteal and
mucoperichondrium elevation

D

Degloving exposure

Wm. Loechel

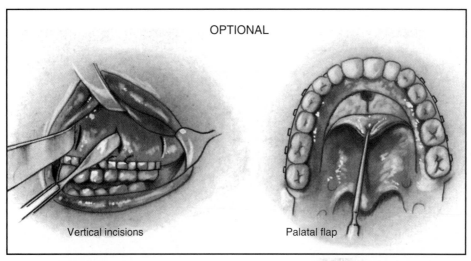

OPTIONAL

Vertical incisions

Palatal flap

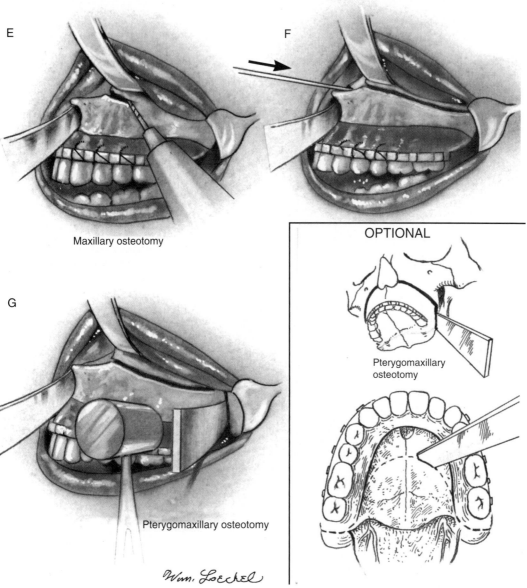

E

Maxillary osteotomy

F

G

Pterygomaxillary osteotomy

OPTIONAL

Pterygomaxillary osteotomy

Wm. Loechel

visualized on the lateroposterior walls of the nose as the maxilla is drawn inferiorly. If the palatal tissues have been reflected and the posterior vertical osteotomies are made anterior to the pterygomaxillary interfaces, the descending palatine arteries will remain intact within the stable posterior bone and the reflected palatal soft tissues and will not be as affected by the mobilization of the maxilla.

K Once the maxilla is fully mobilized and the desired functional relationship with the lower dentition attained with maxillomandibular fixation, preferably using a previously made acrylic splint, it is next stabilized with miniplates. In the edentulous patient, preoperatively prepared acrylic splints are mandatory to provide the appropriate functional relationships of the jaws (see Chapter 20); such splints are first secured to the individual jaws and then to each other with intermaxillary wires. Once fixation is applied, any significant deficits between the bone fragments should be obliterated, depending on size, with grafts from the outer parietal plate, the mandible, or the iliac crest.

Postoperatively antibiotics are administered for an additional 5 to 10 days. Strict adherence to oral hygiene is mandatory and is often best effected with an electric intraoral water spray device after the first 48 hours. Stabilization is maintained for 6 to 8 weeks if maxillomandibular fixation has been required. Monitoring postoperative progress with standard radiographs, cephalometric films, and photographs is very helpful with weekly or biweekly occlusal monitoring.

PITFALLS

1. The tooth roots should be preserved. A point 5 mm above the apex of the canine root should be marked with a small bur hole on the maxillary wall to ensure proper placement of the osteotomy.

2. Avoid unnecessary injury to the blood supply to the mobilized maxilla. When the transverse incision in the vestibule is used, adequate blood supply is derived from the posterior pedicle, but the contribution from the descending palatine arteries should not be ignored and they should be preserved. When vertical vestibular incisions are used and the palatal soft tissues reflected, the palatal blood supply is obviated in the early postoperative stages, and the viability of the maxilla depends on the vessels coursing inferiorly through the lateral soft tissues. The nasal and antral mucosal supply can be important with either technique, and to whatever degree possible, this mucosa should be left intact.

3. Mobilization of the maxilla must be complete to minimize the chance of early relapse. Appropriate traction and torquing with the osteotomes along the lines of osteotomy and careful but firm application of the Rowe disimpaction forceps should be utilized. The advanced maxilla should reach its position with moderate finger pressure.

4. It is important to stabilize the mobilized maxilla in the proper occlusal position. The premade occlusal splint is essential for this purpose.

5. Bone grafts are placed along the anterior and posterior buttresses of the maxilla and pterygoid plates. Miniplate or direct wiring fixation is often required to hold such grafts in their correct anatomic positions.

COMPLICATIONS

1. Brisk intraoperative bleeding may occur during the procedure but will usually stop within 5 to 10 minutes in patients with normal coagulation profiles. When a large vessel has been transected, gauze packing within the mouth and pharynx and nasal packing treated with 4% cocaine containing epinephrine will help to control the bleeding.

2. Postoperative respiratory problems can occur as a result of pharyngeal edema, excessive secretions within the oropharynx, or drowsiness resulting from delayed emergence from anesthesia, significant blood loss, or overmedication with sedatives or analgesics. Extubation thus should not be carried out until the patient is alert and all bleeding has been brought under control.

3. Infection and/or necrosis of the mobilized segment can best be avoided by careful handling of the soft tissues and preservation of the nasal mucosa and soft tissue pedicles. Special attention to preservation of the palatine vessels during manipulation of the maxilla is important. Infection is usually managed with culture guided antibiotic therapy. Healing will often be delayed, with a resultant need for a prolonged period of intermaxillary stabilization that might include return to maxillomandibular fixation. True necrosis may take weeks or even months to run its course, and the degree of debridement necessary will be determined by the extent of tissue death; additional surgery of one type or another is almost always necessary in such cases.

4. The factors that cause regression and/or relapse of the maxillary position are not always clear, but stable fixation with miniplates, maxillomandibular fixation with or without suspension wiring, and maintenance of normal occlusion, with liberal use of bone grafts help to minimize relapse.

5. Postoperative regression or relapse may require prolonged orthodontic treatment and/or reoperation.

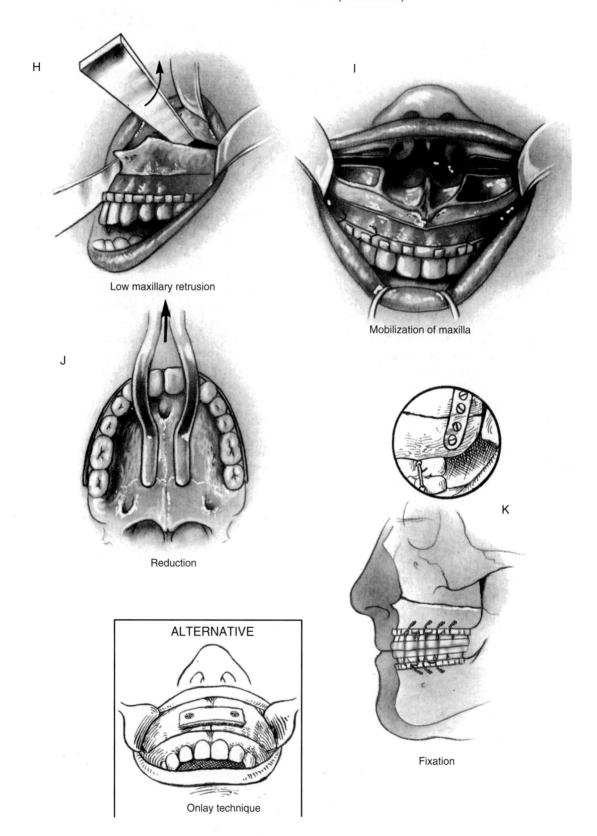

H

Low maxillary retrusion

I

Mobilization of maxilla

J

Reduction

ALTERNATIVE

Onlay technique

K

Fixation

Wm. Loechel

ALTERNATIVE TECHNIQUES USING ONLAY GRAFTS

Upper lip retrusion or accentuation of the nasolabial fold can often be improved with onlay graft techniques. These procedures are useful in those instances in which the occlusion is satisfactory and corrective osteotomies to improve aesthetics would result in unacceptable shifts of the dentition. Onlay procedures are also indicated for small secondary corrections for those patients in whom orthognathic surgical procedures produce incomplete esthetic change. Autogenous onlay grafts harvested from the cranium (see Chapter 59), rib (see Chapter 27), or iliac crest (see Chapter 35) are helpful and alloplasts offer the advantage of not being subject to resorptive remodeling of the graft itself. Their disadvantages include potential mobility and greater chance of infection. Some allografts have also been shown to evoke significant foreign body reactions.

Graft materials consist of autogenous bone, allogeneic bone, or allografts. The areas to be grafted are exposed through small gingivolabial buccal sulcus incisions and subperiosteal dissections sufficient to create pockets just large enough for insertion of the grafts. The graft is appropriately trimmed and inserted and the periosteum closed tightly with chromic sutures. If the graft proves too mobile, it can be secured to the underlying bone with lag screws applied gently to avoid fracturing the graft. Screws may later require removal if they become palpable as the bone graft remodels.

Antibiotics should be continued postoperatively for 5 to 10 days depending on graft material. Chlorhexidine along with normal oral hygiene measures should be employed and a light compression dressing applied.

CHAPTER 49

Correction of Maxillary Retrusion or Lengthening With Le Fort II Osteotomies

In Consultation With Lewis Clayman, DMD, MD

INDICATIONS

Deformity and dysfunction following Le Fort II maxillary trauma can present a formidable problem to the reconstructive surgeon. The patient often has a retrusion of the midface and changes in the length of the face. Apertognathia (open bite) and other imbalances in the occlusion are common. In addition, the fracture is often associated with nasal obstruction, telecanthus, epiphora, and displacement of the medial wall of the maxilla. The surgeon should secure information regarding anosmia, cerebrospinal fluid leaks, loss of vision, diplopia, epistaxis, loss of facial sensation, and nasal obstruction. The surgeon should analyze the degree of flattening of the face in the anteroposterior direction, projection of the nose, and depression of the orbital rims and malar bones. Changes in the positions of the globes and intercanthal distances and in height and width of the palpebral fissures should be noted. Lateral and frontal cephalometric radiographs utilizing both bone and soft tissue densities will define the skeletal and soft tissue imbalances. Like patients with malunions resulting from low maxillary fractures (see Chapter 48), these patients require a sophisticated evaluation of respiration, olfactory and masticatory functions, and esthetic imbalance. Photographic records in both passive repose and dynamic facial muscle function, radiographic imaging (including cephalometry), wax bite registration, and dental models are all pertinent to proper evaluation.

Corrective Le Fort II osteotomies are best applied to those patients with symmetric midface retrusion in which there is symmetry of the nasal bones and normal maxillary height. Malunion resulting from unilateral Le Fort II fracture or from a bilateral but asymmetric fracture is more difficult to correct because of the complexity in planning asymmetric corrective procedures. In any case, corrective Le Fort II osteotomy should be considered when evaluations indicate that both reestablishment of functional dental occlusion and improvement in nasomaxillary aesthetics are required for effective rehabilitation. The preparations for orthognathic surgery of this type are described in Chapter 48.

PROCEDURE

A preexisting tracheostomy is ideal for providing anesthesia. Nasotracheal intubation can be used but makes any required nasal surgery difficult; on the other hand, a nasal-oral "switch" of the endotracheal tube can be performed prior to the nasal surgery. Orotracheal intubation precludes the establishment of good dental occlusion and should be avoided. Tonometric values are recorded preoperatively.

A Exposure is obtained through the gingivolabial buccal, medial canthal, infraciliary or other infraorbital incisions, or transconjunctival incision with or without lateral canthotomy (see Chapter 57).

The gingivolabial buccal incision exposes old fractures on the lateral aspect of the maxilla and provides access for lateral maxillary, retromaxillary, and lower nasal osteotomies. Medial canthal incisions allow exploration of the attachment of the nasal bones to the frontal process of the maxilla and the frontomaxillary buttresses. Infraciliary incisions provide access to the inferior orbital rim and floor of the orbit. These exposures, in combination, provide adequate access for the corrective osteotomies and allow the operator to avoid injury to the medial canthal ligament, the lacrimal sac, the soft tissues of the orbit, and the infraorbital nerve. If extensive nasomaxillary reconstruction is required a bicoronoal flap provides excellent alternative surgical exposure.

B The medial canthal incision is placed in a generally vertical curvilinear direction, one-half the distance between the caruncle of the eyelid and the dorsum of the nose. After cautery or ligation of the angular vessels, the periosteum of the nasal bones and frontal process of the maxilla are elevated, and the trochlea is detached from the orbital rim. By avulsing or clipping the anterior ethmoidal vessels, the surgeon can explore the medial wall of the orbit superiorly and deep to the medial canthal ligament. For visualization of the bridge of the nose, the periosteum should be completely elevated off the nasal bones and lower portion of the frontal bone.

C The infraciliary incision is made about 2 to 3 mm below the cilia and lateral to the puncta of the lower eyelid. A cuff of periosteum is developed inferior to the orbital rim, and the periosteum is then elevated off the rim and floor of the orbit. The periosteal pocket should be connected with the one developed along the medial wall of the orbit.

D–G Using malleable retractors to protect the medial canthal ligament, the lacrimal sac, and orbital soft tissues, Lindeman or other fine burs or saws are used to create an osteotomy across the bridge of the nose, just below the nasofrontal suture. Working on one side at a time, this cut is next extended inferolaterally across the frontal process of the maxilla and along the medial wall of the orbit. Through the medial canthal and/or infraciliary incision, the bone cut is extended across the floor of the orbit with small, sharp osteotomes or fine bone burs. The orbital floor osteotomy is carried laterally to the point for transection of the orbital rim. The bone cut is brought across and through the rim and onto the lateral aspect of the zygoma. The inferior aspect of the osteotomy across the anterior wall of the maxilla can be made at least partially from the superior approach or from below through the intraoral incisions.

Exposure of the maxilla intraorally need not be as extensive as that for the Le Fort I osteotomy. Horizontal incisions in the gingivolabial buccal sulci to ensure full exposure of the zygomaticomaxillary buttresses need only extend from the maxillary tuberosity areas anteriorly to approximately the bicuspid regions. The same exposure can also be obtained through optional vertical incisions made from the height of the sulcus carried inferiorly to the attached gingiva at the bicuspid and tuberosity regions on either side, with the mucoperiosteal tissues between the incisions being elevated creating a subperiosteal tunnel. Use of the vertical incisions allows reflection of the palatal soft tissues; this often eliminates any restrictive tendencies of those tissues to mobilization of the maxilla, while providing direct access to the bone of the palate for placement of an osteotomy (see Chapter 48). No subperiosteal reflection is necessary from the midline to the zygomaticomaxillary buttress, as no osteotomy will be placed in this area. The elevation of periosteum is restricted to the area from the anterior maxilla superiorly to the infraorbital rims, with care being taken to protect the infraorbital nerve with the retractors. The subperiosteal exposure is carried posteriorly to the pterygomaxillary interface.

Using fine burs, saws and/or osteotomes, a bone cut is made inferiorly from the infraorbital rim, either vertically from the lateral aspect of the rim, so as to include the prominence of the zygoma, or obliquely from the rim further medially so as to traverse the anterior maxilla either superiorly or inferiorly to the infraorbital nerve. Again, this cut may be made in part through the infraorbital exposure. In any case, this facial osteotomy will cut through the base of the zygomaticomaxillary buttress at a variable point and then course directly posteriorly above the apices of the teeth to the maxillary tuberosity region.

H The pterygomaxillary osteotomy is carried out through the horizontal or vertical (optional) incisions. If the maxillary osteotomy is carried all the way to the pterygomaxillary junction, it is joined to a vertical separation between the plates and the tuberosity effected with a curved osteotome; if the horizontal osteotomy is terminated in the tuberosity itself, anterior to the pterygomaxillary junction (an optional procedure), it is joined to a vertical bone cut made with the bur vertically through the tuberosity and medially onto the palate. In this latter instance, a bone cut is made transversely across the palate to join the vertical osteotomy coming through the tuberosity on the opposite side. Separating the maxilla through the tuberosity sites avoids some of the bleeding encountered when the maxilla is separated from its junction with the pterygoid plates and provides a more stable posterior surface for support of any interpositional bone grafts.

LE FORT II OSTEOTOMIES

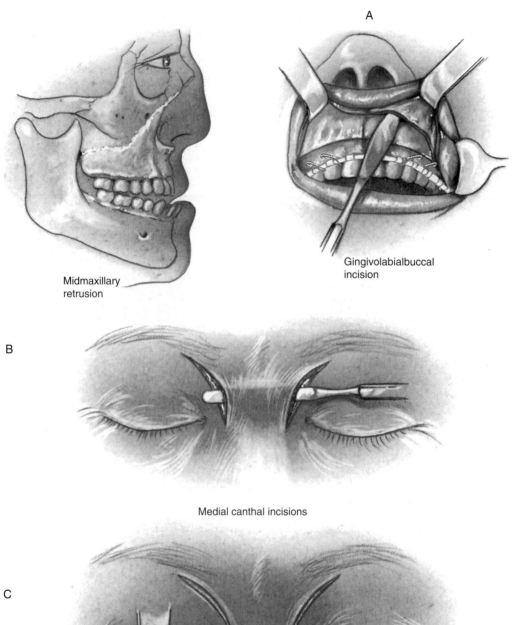

A

Midmaxillary
retrusion

Gingivolabialbuccal
incision

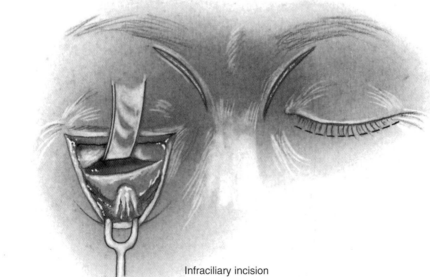

B

Medial canthal incisions

C

Infraciliary incision

Wm. Loechel

D

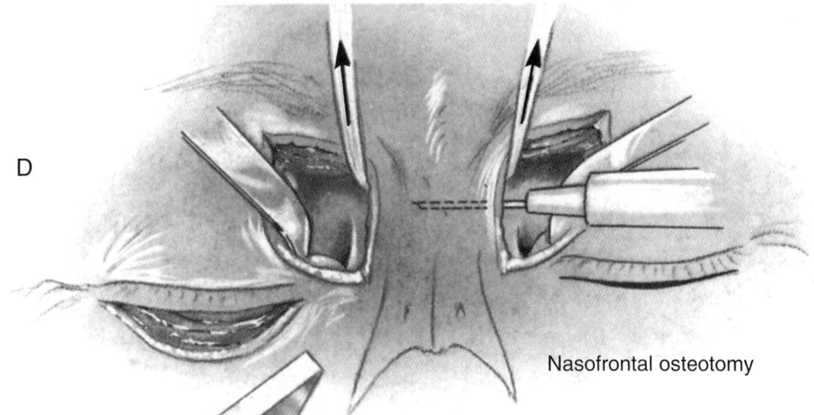

Nasofrontal osteotomy

E

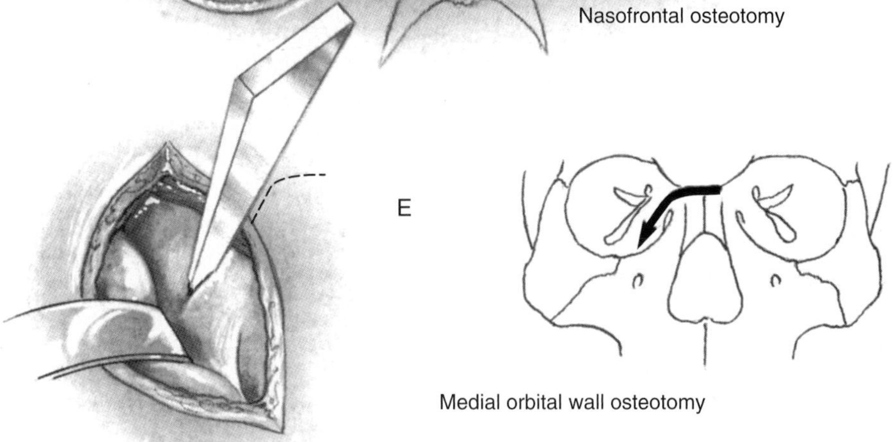

Medial orbital wall osteotomy

F

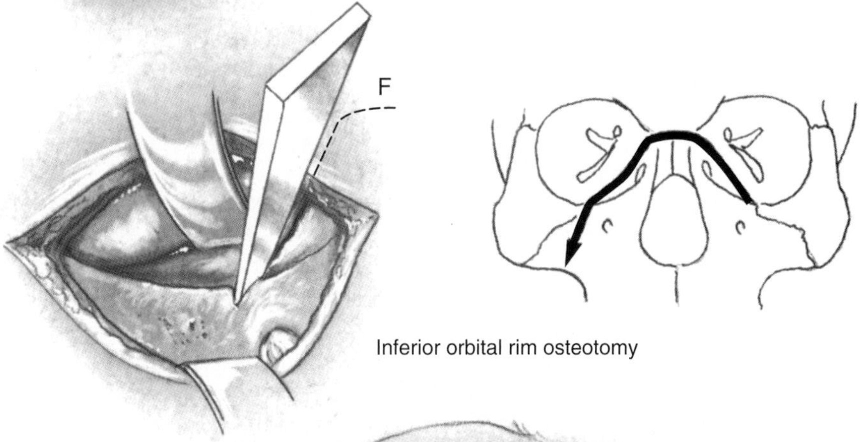

Inferior orbital rim osteotomy

G

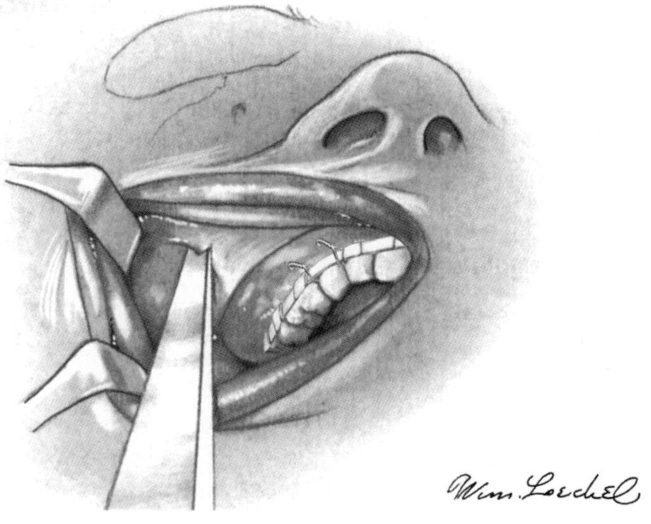

Zygomaticomaxillary
buttress osteotomy

Wm. Loechel

I,J To complete the separation of the maxilla from the skull, the vomer and perpendicular plate of the ethmoid, as well as the lateral wall of the nose, must also be released. These bone cuts are made first by directing a small, sharp osteotome through the osteotomy at the bridge of the nose diagonally downward and backward toward the posterior part of the palate avoiding the cribriform plate and, a second, slightly laterally through the osteotomy at the nasal bridge to transect whatever portion of the lateral nasal wall may be still intact high in the superior portion of the nose. The surgeon can ensure the correct angle of the osteotome as it courses through the septum by placing a finger within the nasopharynx and palpating it as it penetrates the posterior nares. Final mobilization of the maxilla is effected through lifting and torquing with the osteotomes along the osteotomy sites and careful disimpaction with the Rowe or Tessier forceps. Complete mobility of the sectioned midface is necessary to ensure proper adaptation to the mandibular dentition, correct adaptation and stabilization of any grafts, and a reduced tendency toward postsurgical regression.

Bleeding will be brisk during osteotomy and after total mobilization. If the patient has normal coagulation profiles, however, the bleeding should stop in several minutes. The surgeon should wait until all significant bleeding has stopped before proceeding with the fixation portion of the procedure.

K There are several acceptable methods of establishing occlusal relationships and fixation. Usually the occlusion is stabilized with Ivy loops, arch bars or maxillomandibular fixation screws, with or without an interocclusal wafer (splint). The proper occlusal relationships will have been determined preoperatively through study of the dental models and model surgery as described in Chapter 48. In the edentulous patient, proper functional relationships of the maxilla and mandible are determined preoperatively and the mobilized maxilla stabilized with intermaxillary fixation of the patient's preexisting dentures or specially fabricated maxillary and mandibular acrylic splints. The latter are stabilized with either bone screws or wire fixation.

Following establishment of intermaxillary fixation, the fracture lines are inspected and the interosseous defects stabilized with autogenous grafts obtained from the cranium, rib, or iliac crest. Often the grafts can be appropriately morticed and wedged into position so that they do not require fixation. Stabilization of the mobilized midface, however, is mandatory and miniplates offer the best stability.

Tonometric values are again recorded, and all facial incisions are closed in layers. The patient is treated for at least 5 days with intravenous antibiotics. Facial films obtained several days postoperatively are helpful in evaluating the new skeletal relationships. Oral hygiene is best maintained with chlorhexidine or hydrogen peroxide washes, and the dentition is best cleaned with a water irrigation device. Intermaxillary fixation if used is maintained for a 6-week period. With miniplate fixation a liquid diet is maintained for one month followed by a soft diet for two weeks.

PITFALLS

1. The Le Fort II osteotomy is best applied to the patient with a retrusion of the midface and a fairly normal architecture of the nose. The patient with a major nasal deformity is probably better treated with a Le Fort I correction and subsequent independent rhinoplasty.

2. Avoid injury to the soft tissues during osteotomy. The best insurance against this type of complication is adequate exposure of the bony surfaces and judicious use of retractors and sectioning instruments. If the medial canthal ligament or lacrimal sac are injured, they should be repaired during the procedure. Small tears of the periorbita can be left open to heal by secondary intention.

3. Assure proper dental occlusion. This requires a comprehensive preoperative evaluation and osteotomies that gain complete mobility of the maxilla. Appropriate occlusion should be achieved with or without an interocclusal wafer followed by stability of the reconstruction.

COMPLICATIONS

1. Most of the complications related to corrective Le Fort II osteotomies are similar to those related to other midface corrections (see Chapters 48 and 50). Postoperative bleeding, breathing difficulties, infection, and malunion are all possible as a result of the Le Fort II procedure, and the surgeon should become familiar with the methods that are available to prevent and treat these difficulties.

2. Nasal obstruction and deformity is common with the Le Fort II injury and may not be adequately addressed with corrective Le Fort II osteotomies alone. Adjunctive septorhinoplasty procedures may be required. These considerations are discussed in Chapter 54.

3. Residual contour defects following healing of corrective Le Fort II osteotomy sometimes require additional care. Various materials can be used in these efforts, but probably cranial bone or alloplastic grafts offer the best assurance of success. These procedures are usually executed as subsequent revisional operations, but occasionally, when such deficits can be anticipated preoperatively, they can be carried out at the time of the Le Fort II osteotomy.

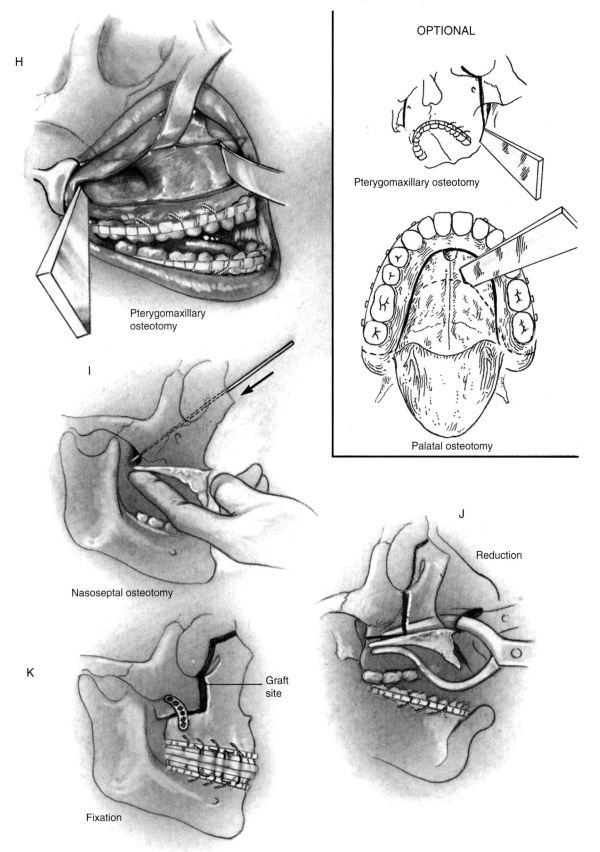

OPTIONAL

H

Pterygomaxillary osteotomy

Pterygomaxillary osteotomy

Palatal osteotomy

I

Nasoseptal osteotomy

J

Reduction

K

Graft site

Fixation

Correction of Midfacial Retrusion or Lengthening With Subcranial Le Fort III Osteotomies

In Consultation With Lewis Clayman, DMD, MD

INDICATIONS

Le Fort III osteotomies are primarily used for midface retrusion associated with inadequate malar and infraorbital rim projection. Such patients usually present with concave facial profiles ("dishface" deformities) and lengthening of the face. A retruded maxillary dentition is characteristic, very often in association with the open bite malocclusion and multiple deformities and dysfunctions found with fractures of the orbits, nose, malar bones, and/or mandible.

Evaluation of the malunited Le Fort III injury mandates assessment of esthetic and functional abnormalities, in skeletal and dental relationships. As in malunion resulting from lower maxillary fractures, these patients require a sophisticated clinical evaluation, photographic records, radiographic imaging, bite registration, and dental models (see Chapter 48). Orthodontic and/or prosthodontic consultation is often helpful in defining the dental and skeletal considerations. Orbital and nasal deformities are particularly important, and ophthalmologic consultation is often mandatory. A neurosurgical opinion is advisable whenever cranial injury is part of the original trauma.

Once all diagnostic criteria have been duly weighed, the surgeon must determine whether Le Fort III refracturing offers a significant advantage over less hazardous lower midfacial repositioning combined with onlay cosmetic procedures.

PROCEDURE

Tracheostomy is the preferred method of providing ventilation and anesthesia and should be carried out as a preliminary procedure either under local anesthesia or following a temporary oral intubation. Arch bars are adapted to the teeth, and the entire face and neck are then surgically scrubbed and draped as sterile fields. Tonometric values are recorded.

A combination of incisions is necessary for adequate access to the maxillofacial skeleton. The more common combinations are coronal and maxillary gingivolabial buccal incisions or frontoethmoid (medial canthal), infraorbital, and gingivolabial buccal sulcus incisions.

A The coronal incision should extend superiorly from just above the preauricular crease on one side to a point just posterior to the recesses of the temporal hairline. It is then placed anterosuperiorly several centimeters behind the hairline in a gentle curving configuration to a similar position on the opposite side (see Chapter 43). Infiltration of the scalp with a vasopressor containing local anesthetic assists hemostasis. The incision is made to the level of the loose fascial layer above the periosteum and the scalp is reflected anteriorly. The flap is progressively rotated anteriorly to a level just above the superior orbital rims, at which point the periosteum is incised throughout the width of the reflection. Branches of the superficial temporal artery are controlled with cautery or suture ligatures. A Periosteal/galeal flap may be developed if necessary to separate the nasal cavity from the frontal sinus or anterior cranial fossa.

B The dissection progresses subperiosteally along the superior orbital ridge and the bridge of the nose. The supraorbital neurovasculature is reflected with the flap; the supraorbital foramina, if present, are opened gently with fine osteotomes to facilitate the maneuver. Progressive subperiosteal reflection allows exposure of the superior and medial walls of the orbit and freeing of the trochlea. An anterioposterior incision in the midline of the periosteum is often helpful in facilitating release of tissue to expose the orbits. Additional relaxation and exposure are obtained by clipping the anterior ethmoidal artery.

Laterally the surgeon should ensure that the dissection avoids injury to the branch of the facial nerve. The attachment of the temporalis muscle at the frontozygomatic process is then elevated. Continuation of the subperiosteal dissection allows release of the lacrimal gland from its fossa. The lateral canthal ligament is also released with its periosteum, and the dissection is continued along the body and arch of the zygoma. To maintain function of the temporal branch of the facial nerve, long periods of forceful retraction on the soft tissues must be avoided.

C The options for exposure of the maxilla intraorally are those used for execution of the Le Fort II osteotomy as described in Chapter 49. One of the approaches entails a circumvestibular (gingivolabial buccal) incision from the mesial of the first molar to the midline bilaterally maintaining the blood supply through the posterior pedicles and the palatal soft tissues. The dissection is continued to include exposure of the pterygomaxillary junction area posteriorly. In this case, vascularity of the posterior maxilla at the alveolar level is maintained through the palatal soft tissues and the posterior lateral buccal pedicles. The second option utilizes vertical incisions made from the height of the sulcus inferiorly to the attached gingiva in the cuspid and third molar regions and a curvilinear reflection of the palatal soft tissues extending from one greater palatine foramen, forward across the rugae, and then posteriorly to the opposite foramen; in this case vascularity to the lower posterior maxilla is maintained through the vertical soft tissue drapes. Subperiosteal reflection exposes the anterior and lateral walls of the maxilla, the zygomaticomaxillary buttresses, the infraorbital nerves, the nasomaxillary junctions, and the piriform aperture. When the palatal reflection is used, direct exposure of the bone of the palate is gained, and the resistance of the palatal tissues to maxillary displacement is obviated.

D Exposure of the orbital rims and floors is accomplished through infraciliary or transconjuctival (Chapter 57) approaches. Access to the nasomaxillary interface through the intraoral exposure and to the orbital floor through the bicoronal flap is limited.

E–G The osteotomies begin at the bridge of the nose, and through the exposure from above, a horizontal cut is made just beneath the nasofrontal suture line. This cut is then brought laterally across the frontal processes of the maxillae and onto the medial walls of the orbit; with appropriate retraction, the osteotomy will not produce injury to the medial canthal ligament or lacrimal sac. With a fine osteotome or fine surgical bur, the osteotomy is carried inferiorly on the medial walls to the floors of the orbits, just behind the lacrimal collecting systems. Once these cuts are completed on both sides, the osteotome is placed into the bone cut at the bridge of the nose and directed inferoposteriorly toward the soft palate through the substance of the septum to free this structure from the base of the skull. The direction and depth of this osteotomy can be wcontrolled by a finger placed in the nasopharynx.

H,I On the lateral walls of the orbits, osteotomies are made at a variable distance below the frontozygomatic suture line, either transversely through the full thickness of the lateral orbital rims or sagittally through the rims for a variable distance inferiorly; the latter cut results in a less abrupt interruption in lateral rim contour and broader contact of bony surfaces. The sagittal osteotomies of the rims should be made with very fine osteotomes or with the fine surgical bur. Through this same exposure, the zygoma (or arch) is osteotomized in a stepwise fashion.

On one side at a time, the orbital contents are retracted medially, and a bone cut is made through the lateral orbital wall inferiorly onto the floor of the orbit anterior to the inferior orbital fissure. The orbital contents are then gently elevated and this bone cut connected in the floor of the orbit to the osteotomy previously made on the medial wall. The bone cut across the floor of the orbit should be made approximately 1 cm dorsal to the inferior orbital rim to avoid trauma to the orbit in the region of the orbital apex. Access to the floor is often limited through the coronal approach, and it is in these instances that access through an infraorbital incision proves beneficial.

J The bodies of the zygomas are next sectioned free of the zygomatic arches. To complete these fractures, the maxilla must be separated at the alveolar arch levels in the region of the pterygoid plates. This may be achieved with an osteotome placed high in the retromaxillary area and directed medially and slightly inferiorly into the pterygomaxillary fissure or

LE FORT III OSTEOTOMIES

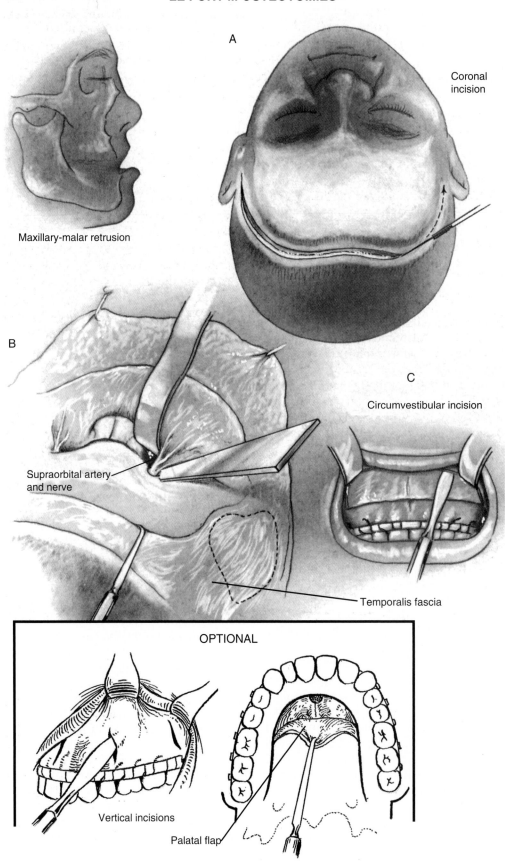

A

Coronal incision

Maxillary-malar retrusion

B

Supraorbital artery and nerve

C

Circumvestibular incision

Temporalis fascia

OPTIONAL

Vertical incisions

Palatal flap

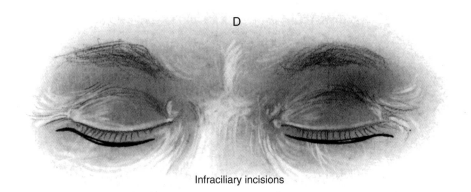

D

Infraciliary incisions

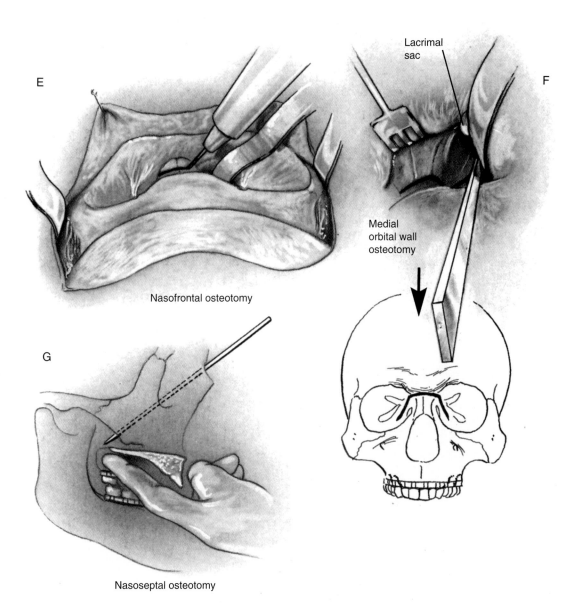

E

Nasofrontal osteotomy

Lacrimal sac

F

Medial orbital wall osteotomy

G

Nasoseptal osteotomy

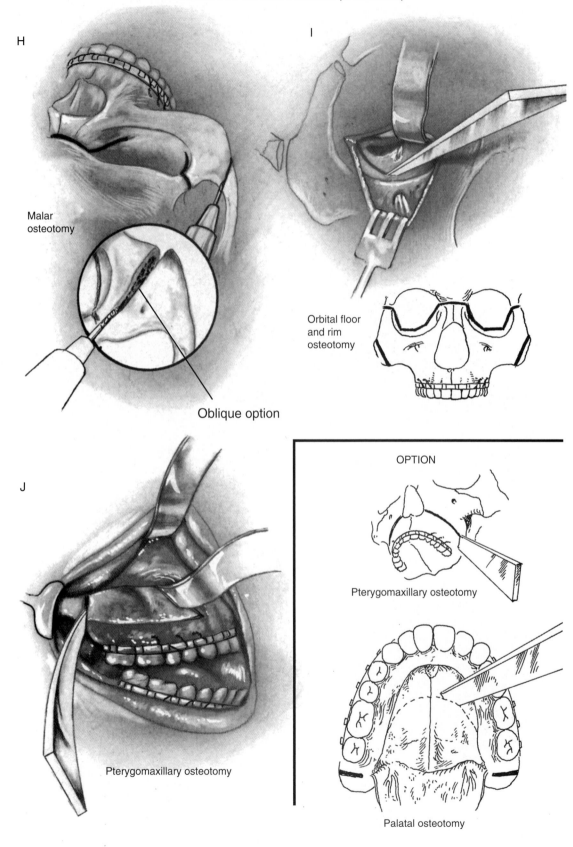

H

Malar
osteotomy

Oblique option

I

Orbital floor
and rim
osteotomy

J

Pterygomaxillary osteotomy

OPTION

Pterygomaxillary osteotomy

Palatal osteotomy

with an osteotomy extending from a point high on the maxillary tuberosity near its junction with the pterygoid plates, inferiorly through the full thickness of the alveolar arch anterior to the pterygomaxillary junction, and across the hard palate to a similar position on the opposite side. This optional osteotomy requires reflection of the palatal soft tissues but lessens the chance of significant bleeding from the descending palatine artery and the pterygoid venous plexus.

K Even careful placement of all osteotomies does not guarantee mobility of the maxilla, and complete separation of the midface commonly requires forcible displacement with the Rowe disimpaction forceps and/or active elevation or torquing with osteotomes placed into the osteotomy sites. Complete mobility must be gained, however, if the surgeon is to ensure proper positioning of any grafts, establishment of correct dental occlusion, and a reduced chance of postoperative regression. Bleeding is usually brisk during these mobilization maneuvers but will come under control spontaneously when mobilization is complete and the maxilla is stabilized.

L Once complete mobilization is gained, preoperatively determined dental occlusion is established using the prepared occlusal acrylic splint and maxillomandibular fixation. Bone grafts, preferably autogenous and taken from the ilium, rib, or parietal cortex, are placed into the osteotomy defects. Careful contouring and wedging often provide sufficient stabilization of these grafts, but the maxilla requires stabilization with miniplates.

The incisions, with the exception of the intraoral, are closed in layers, though it is often impossible to reapproximate the periosteum at every osteotomy site. The temporalis muscle, if detached, must be reattached to prevent an "hourglass" facial deformity from developing postoperatively. Closed suction drains are inserted as needed. A light compression dressing is applied over the scalp flap. Tonometric readings are taken at the completion of the procedure.

Postoperatively the patient is carefully monitored for evidence of hematoma or changes in sensorium and vision; immediate drainage of intraorbital hematomas by lateral canthotomy and aspiration of blood is mandatory. Antibiotics are maintained intravenously for approximately 5 days following surgery. Stability of the dental occlusion is monitored daily in hospital and weekly as an outpatient. Radiographs taken within the first few postoperative days allow evaluation of maxillary and graft positions. The patient should be examined at regular intervals for at least 1 year postoperatively to intercept and treat any observed skeletal regression.

PITFALLS

1. Ensure appropriate indications for the procedure. The Le Fort III osteotomy is a complex operation demanding intimate familiarity with the anatomy and objective evaluation of the gains to be anticipated. The technique should not be used when less extensive osteotomies and/or onlay grafts will suffice. It should be used cautiously in older patients and probably not at all in patients who have sensorium or vision instability.

2. Be prepared for profound bleeding. Brisk bleeding is to be expected during the osteotomy, especially following application of the disimpaction forceps and other final mobilization procedures. Pharyngeal and/or nasal packing may be helpful if blood loss is excessive. Blood transfusion may be necessary.

3. Do not attempt the procedure without a tracheostomy. All anesthetic techniques short of tracheostomy entail significant compromises in access and/or safety and should not be employed. Postoperative respiratory care is also facilitated with the tracheostomy.

4. Adequate mobility of the osteotomized segment must be gained. The pterygomaxillary area is a site of particular resistance, but additional mobility is sometimes achieved by cutting residual pterygoid muscle attachments. The surgeon can also place posterior vertical osteotomies through the tuberosities and anterior to the pterygomaxillary complex. Incomplete sectioning through the septum and through the orbital osteotomies can usually be eliminated with the final disimpaction maneuvers.

5. Appropriate advancement of the facial skeleton should be appreciated. In many patients, reestablishment of the occlusion automatically reestablishes the pretraumatic midfacial proportions. On the other hand, if the original trauma was asymmetric or otherwise erratic, reestablishment of the dental occlusion may not guarantee a satisfactory aesthetic result. If the patient is partially or completely edentulous, determining the proper dental relationships or stabilizing the occlusion intraoperatively can be difficult; in these cases, preoperatively designed interocclusal acrylic stabilization devices can be very helpful.

6. Care must be taken to avoid postsurgical regression. Intermaxillary dental fixation must be maintained for at least 6 weeks, and bone grafts placed at the site of osteotomy must be firmly fixed in position and held with either wedge force or direct plate or wiring fixation. The myriad of interfaces along the osteotomies generally aids in stabilization but does not obviate the need for careful stabilization of the mobilized midface with miniplates.

K

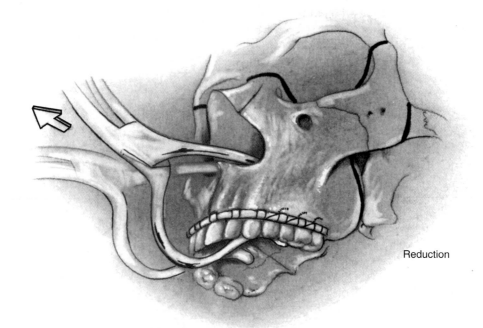

Reduction

L

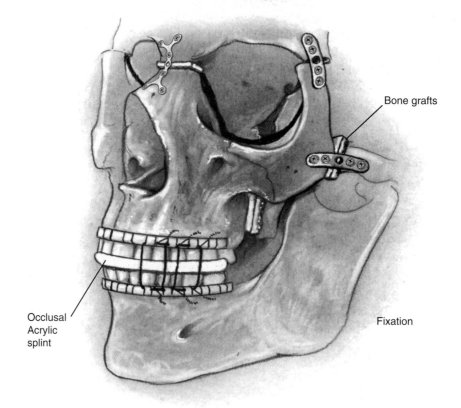

Bone grafts

Occlusal
Acrylic
splint

Fixation

COMPLICATIONS

1. Bleeding and airway obstruction can be life-threatening complications. Intraoperative bleeding generally does not occur as the result of severance of major vessels, and so it can usually be treated with hypotensive anesthesia, a vasopressor containing local anesthetic infiltration, gauze packing, and appropriately administered blood or blood product transfusion. A Le Fort III osteotomy should not be executed without a tracheostomy, as damage or kinking of the endotracheal tube, irritation of the vocal cords during the long procedure, or leakage of blood around the cuff can all lead to significant ventilatory problems. The tracheostomy puts control of respiration both intraoperatively and postoperatively out of the surgical field, and the anesthesiologist and surgeon can work independently of one another. Postoperatively the tracheostomy affords easy assisted ventilation and tracheal hygiene.

2. Injury to the cribriform plate can result in cerebrospinal fluid leakage. This maloccurrence can generally be avoided by keeping the osteotome strictly in the midline, directing it downward toward the soft palate, and controlling its position with a finger in the nasopharynx. If a cerebrospinal fluid leak fails to stop, antibiotics should continue beyond the projected time, and the surgeon should consider repair of the dura using either an endoscopic, frontoethmoid, or intracranial approach (see Chapters 85, 90, and 91).

3. Enophthalmos, hypophthalmos, and/or diplopia may also occur. Small diastases in the orbital floor can be managed with Gelfilm or Marlex mesh, but larger defects are best treated with autogenous bone grafts. Major displacements of an orbital wall are also best managed with appropriate grafting techniques (see Chapters 59 and 64).

4. Visual compromise, including blindness, is best avoided by placing the osteotomy in the floor of the orbit, no more than 1 cm dorsal to the inferior orbital rim, and limiting the vigor of dissection and retraction. The dissection along the medial wall of the orbit should be restricted to the area anterior to the posterior ethmoidal artery. Retractors should be intermittently relaxed, and impingement of the retractors on the retrobulbar tissues must be avoided. Persistent bleeders in the area of orbital dissection should be treated with bipolar cautery or vascular clips. Any decrease in visual acuity should prompt an early ophthalmologic consultation, and hematoma of the orbit must be evacuated as soon as it is recognized. Tonometry at the completion of the procedure often provides an early indication of increasing intraorbital pressure.

5. Residual facial imbalances or occlusal disharmonies can occur following healing of the reparative Le Fort III osteotomy. Such imperfections can often be improved with onlay grafts, preferably of autogenous cranial bone or alloplastic material. Minor occlusal disharmonies can be accommodated with orthodontic or dental restorative measures, but major imbalances resulting from malposition or unacceptable regression may require additional osteotomies. Rarely is it necessary to recreate the entire Le Fort III sectioning.

PART FIVE

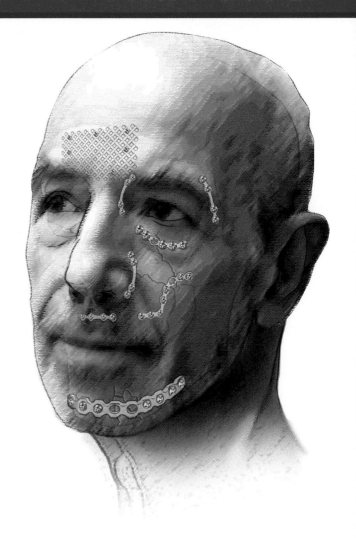

Nasal Fractures

Classification and Pathophysiology of Nasal Fractures

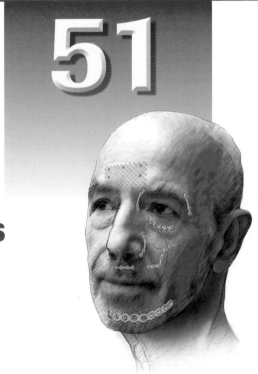

CHAPTER 51

General Considerations

A Nasal fractures are the most common facial fractures. They occur frequently in children and are more often seen in men than in women. The projection of the nose from the face predisposes to injury; the midline septum offers little support, and there are additional weaknesses along the grooves created by the anterior ethmoidal veins. Because there is a greater cartilage-to-bone ratio in children compared with adults, fractures in children usually involve cartilage, whereas in adults the bone is usually broken and displaced, and the cartilage is involved secondarily.

A classification of nasal fractures is difficult because there are many variations. If the impact is from a frontal direction, the fracture will involve, in order, the nasal tip; the nasal dorsum, septum, and anterior nasal spine; and the frontal processes of the maxilla, lacrimal, and ethmoid bones. With a lateral oblique force, fractures will involve, in order, the ipsilateral nasal bone; the contralateral nasal bone and septum; and the frontal processes of the maxilla and

the lacrimal bone. On the basis of this pathophysiology, several syndromes can be defined; these are discussed in the text that follows.

TIP FRACTURE

B1 As a result of frontal impact, the nasal tip alone can be fractured and malpositioned. Usually the lower (caudal) portion of the fracture rotates inward and downward, while the upper (cephalic) portion rotates upward and outward. This rotation causes the development of a small hump and supertip depression.

FLATTENING OF THE NASAL DORSUM WITH SPLAYING OF NASAL BONES

B2 With more force from the anterior direction, the nasal bones are prone to fracture at a higher level and will be pushed inward. The lateral part of the nasal bones at the same time will be splayed outward. The cartilaginous septum will buckle, the anterior nasal spine may fracture, and the nose will have a flattened appearance.

FLATTENING OF THE NASAL DORSUM WITH SPLAYING OF THE FRONTAL PROCESS OF THE MAXILLA

B3 In this condition, the anterior force is powerful enough to fracture the nasal bones, the frontal process of the maxilla, and the anterior nasal spine. Usually fractures are comminuted and tend to lateralize. The nose becomes markedly depressed, the columella becomes retracted, and the medial canthal ligaments are frequently relaxed, creating a telecanthus.

DEPRESSION OF THE LATERAL NASAL BONE

C1 A force from the lateral oblique direction often causes a depression of the nasal bone on one side of the nose. Simultaneously there is a raising of the nasal bone on the opposite side. The septum may buckle. Typically, the patient displays a C- or S-shaped deformity of dorsum of the nose.

DEPRESSION OF IPSILATERAL NASAL BONE AND FRONTAL PROCESS OF THE MAXILLA

C2,C3 If the lateral oblique forces are excessive, the fracture can extend to the frontal process of the maxilla. Usually the dorsum and septum are markedly displaced (more so than the ipsilateral nasal bone depression), and there is a depression of the medial wall of the maxilla. This fracture is a variant of a medial maxillary fracture and is described in Chapter 45.

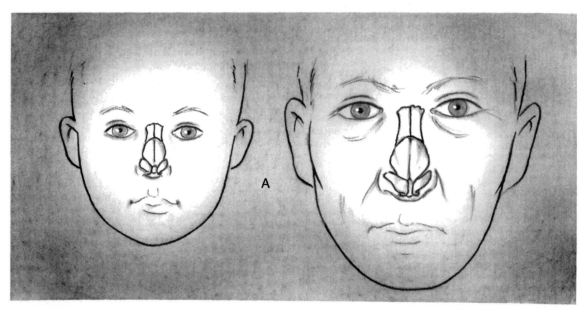

B   Frontal forces

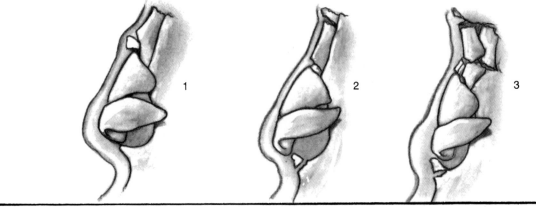

1   2   3

C   Lateral oblique forces

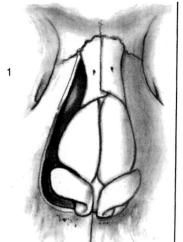
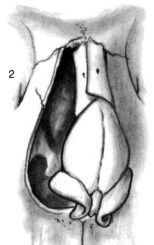
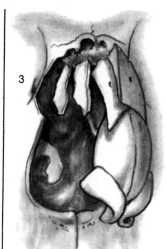

1   2   3

Management Strategies

CHAPTER

52

Closed Reduction of Nasal Fracture by Manipulation

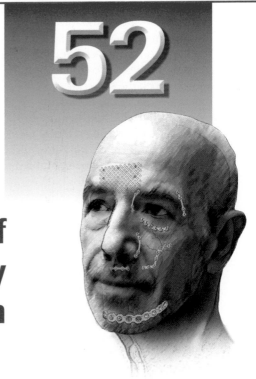

INDICATIONS

Closed reduction usually provides satisfactory results in most types of nasal fractures. It should at least be given a trial, and if it is not successful, the surgeon can still treat the fracture by open reduction and/or elective rhinoplasty. The closed technique is also associated with minor morbidity. It is characterized by a short, easy-to-perform operation and rapid recovery.

The ideal patient for the closed technique is an individual who had a straight, nonobstructed nose prior to the injury and who sustained a tip or depressed ipsilateral nasal bone fracture. The technique is also effective in treating the acutely displaced septum and associated hematoma. The procedure will be limited if there is a frontal bone and/or lacrimal bone fracture or if the fracture also involves the medial wall of the maxilla. Nasal fractures associated with cribriform plate and cerebrospinal fluid leaks are probably better treated with techniques that avoid obstructive nasal packing. Although evaluation of the fracture can be assisted by CT scan and/or routine nasal bone radiographs, the physical examination is more important in making the diagnosis and determining the degree of injury. Timing of the surgery is also important and the procedure is best applied when most swelling has subsided (after about 5 days). After 10 to 14 days, some healing will have occurred, and in these situations, other (open) methods should be considered.

PROCEDURE

A–C Sedation and anesthesia are an important part of the technique. If the surgeon chooses local anesthesia with sedation, the patient should be given sufficient medication for relaxation, cooperation, and amnesia. The nasal mucous membranes are then sprayed with 1/4% oxymetazoline hydrochloride (Neo-Synephrine) followed by several sprays of 4% lidocaine. Additional levels of topical anesthesia should be obtained by strategic placement of cotton pledgets, moistened in a solution of 8 mL of 4% cocaine containing five drops of 1:10,000 epinephrine. This solution will provide sufficient vasoconstriction for the duration of the procedure. The pledgets are usually placed for about 10 minutes beneath the nasal dorsum, at the posterior edge of the middle turbinates, on the floors with extension into the inferior meati, and on the septum.

D,E After application of topical anesthesia, the surgeon should also block the nose with a local anesthetic. A 2% solution of lidocaine containing 1:100,000 epinephrine should be injected along the dorsum, the anterior maxilla, and the base of the septum to anesthetize the infratrochlear, infraorbital, and greater palatine nerves. Additional infiltration of the tip area should block the superior alveolar nerve and branches of sensory nerves to the skin.

If the patient chooses a general anesthetic, the same application of topical and local medications is advised, as these will provide for better visualization and control of bleeding. Moreover, in the postoperative period there will be less need for pain control and sedation.

F,G Manipulation should be carried out with the head slightly elevated so that the surgeon's light will illuminate most of the nasal cavity. Standard operating room lighting should be adjusted to minimize distortions and shadows. If the vibrissae of the nose are blocking visualization of the internal nose, they should be trimmed with scissors. For the simple depressed unilateral nasal bone fracture, a Boies elevator can be used, but before elevation, the surgeon must make sure that the elevator is placed just beneath the depressed bone and not into the cribriform plate area. The depth of insertion is thus controlled by measuring externally the distance from the angle of the glabella to the tip of the nose and then applying the elevator just short of that depth. With a slowly increasing force, the depressed nasal bone is elevated. The degree of elevation is controlled with external pressure exerted by the other hand, molding the fragments into appropriate position. Often the side opposite the depressed nasal fracture is also displaced laterally, and in such a situation, the contralateral bones should be pushed inward to develop the ideal pyramid. For comminuted nasal bone fractures, the bones should be pressed toward each other to create a narrow dorsum, elevating the fragments with a Boies elevator should they be displaced downward. For the nasal tip fracture, the elevation should be directed to the front part of the septum under the dorsum, and with the other hand, the dorsum should be molded into appropriate position.

H The septum should next be inspected. Often elevation of the dorsum will return the septum to the midline, but if this has not occurred, the surgeon can apply Ashe forceps to simultaneously elevate the dorsum and replace the septum to the midline. The septum should then be inspected to make sure there are no mucosal tears and a hematoma has not developed.

I,J Fractures of the nose and septum should be stabilized by external and internal splints. For a severely disrupted septum that has been repositioned in the midline, internal splints made of polyethylene can be trimmed and secured to the columella with a broadly based 3-0 nylon mattress suture. If the septum holds the midline and also has not been severely lacerated, the nasal openings can be packed with bacitracin-treated gauze. Alternatively, a nasal tampon (with or without the polyethylene plates) can be used to control pressure and prevent bleeding. Injection of a local anesthetic with a vasoconstrictive agent into the tampon may assist in postoperative pain management and control of bleeding.

K–P Thermal splints are subsequently used to stabilize the nose after the application of a steristrip tape dressing. The skin of the nose is first treated with an adhesive solution and the skin covered with pieces of steristrip applied to hold the nose in a normal anatomic position. The thermal splint is then placed into a hot water bath and when it softens, applied to the nose with the adhesive part facing the steristrips. The sides of the splint are then compressed to narrow the dorsum. The splint will harden as it cools. A drip pad over the nares is subsequently applied and secured to the cheeks.

The patient should be treated with antibiotics for the duration of the packing. Sufficient stability is usually obtained at 5 days, and at that time, internal and external splints can be removed. Crusts that subsequently develop on the mucous membrane should be actively and prophylactically treated with normal saline douches.

PITFALLS

1. Timing of the surgery is important. If the surgeon operates too early, the anatomy of the nasal structures can be obscured by swelling and ecchymoses. If operation occurs too late, the nasal bones will have united, and reduction will be difficult, if not impossible, to carry out. Ideally nasal fractures in children should be treated in 5 to 7 days. In adults, it is possible to obtain reduction up to 10 to 12 days after injury.

2. Results can be compromised by associated injuries. Radiographs of the nose can miss fractures of the facial bones, and the surgeon should not rely only on the patient's nasal appearance and examination of the nose. If there is any suspicion of additional injuries, the patient should be evaluated by computed tomographic (CT) scans in the horizontal and frontal planes. If additional fractures are found, appropriate techniques should be used to specifically address those fractures.

CLOSED REDUCTION OF NASAL FRACTURE

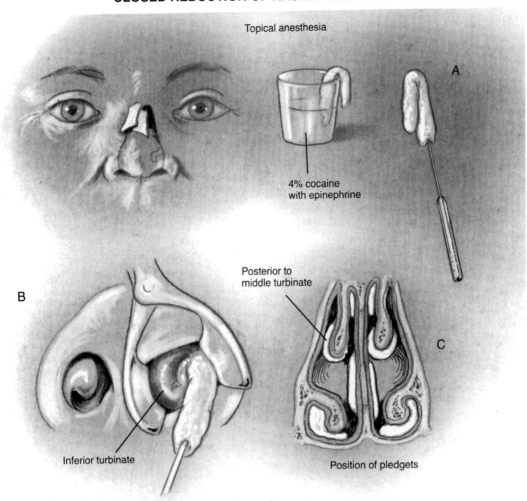

Topical anesthesia

A

4% cocaine
with epinephrine

B

Inferior turbinate

Posterior to
middle turbinate

C

Position of pledgets

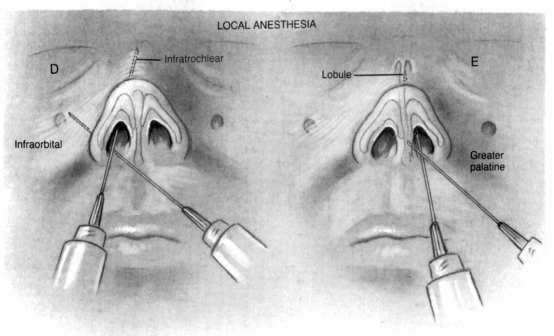

LOCAL ANESTHESIA

D

Infratrochlear

Infraorbital

E

Lobule

Greater
palatine

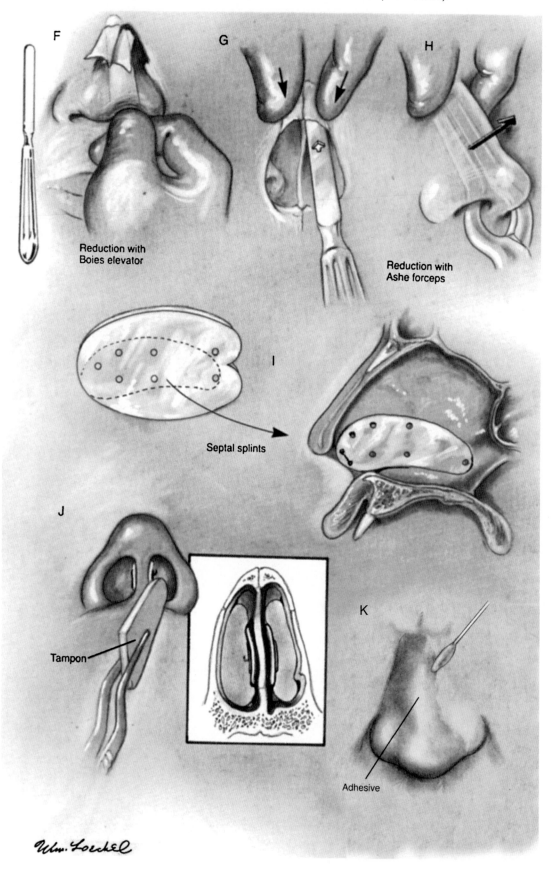

F

Reduction with
Boies elevator

G

H

Reduction with
Ashe forceps

I

Septal splints

J

Tampon

K

Adhesive

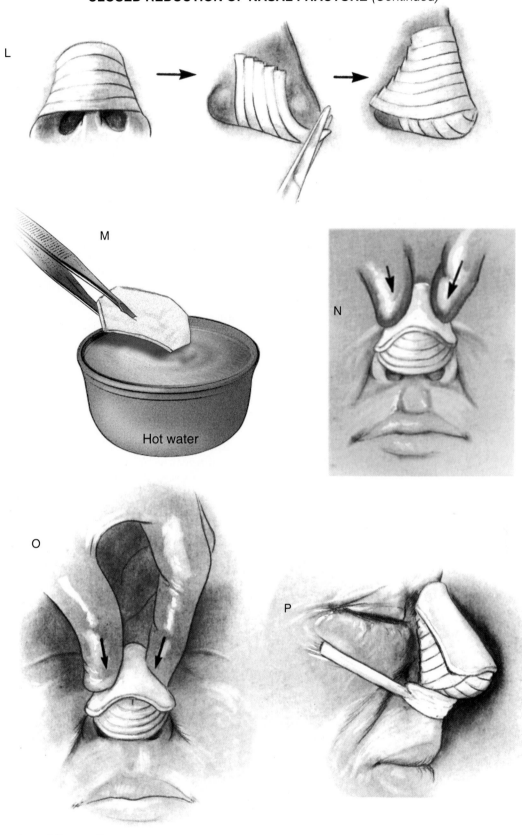

Hot water

3. Adequate sedation and/or anesthesia are important to get good results. The uncooperative patient will often move about in the operating room and cause bleeding. Moreover, postoperative restlessness and confusion can cause reinjury and should be avoided. Using the internal and external splints should at least prevent some of the postoperative traumatic sequelae from occurring.

4. Although the closed method is successful in most cases, the surgeon must be prepared for a semiclosed approach. Occasionally the septal fracture will leaf onto itself, or the nasal bones will not be reduced or held in the desired position. If such a situation develops, the septum can be exposed by a limited Killian incision and the fracture treated by removal of projecting bone and/or cartilage. The nasal bones can be reduced by making a cartilage-splitting or intercartilaginous incision and then manipulating the bones with small, needle-nosed rongeurs (seeChapter 49).

5. Some severely comminuted nasal fractures are just too unstable to be corrected by splint fixation and will require external approaches including cantilevered techniques (Chapter 53).

6. Packing should not be used for the reduction. It should be applied secondarily only after manipulation of bone and cartilage. The packing should support the structures in their anatomic position.

7. Improper application of septal splints can cause necrosis and perforation. To avoid this complication, the septum must have no evidence of hematoma. The suture that holds the splints must be placed into the fleshy part of the columella, not the intermembranous part, and the tie should be through a wide (3- to 4-mm) mattress suture. This approach will avoid excessive pressure and necrosis of intervening tissues.

8. External splints must also be placed properly to avoid deformity and necrosis of soft tissues. The surgeon should check the splints so that there is symmetry of the nasal openings and side walls of the nose.

COMPLICATIONS

1. Failure to reduce the fracture can lead to deformity and/or nasal obstruction. Although a rhinoplasty may be performed, the multiple relatively loose fragments will make control of the osteotomies difficult. Our preferred approach is to wait until the nose is healed (i.e., 3 to 6 months) and then proceed with a rhinoplasty to correct the specific postinjury deformities.

2. Septal hematoma must be recognized and treated appropriately. Failure to do so predisposes to necrosis of septal cartilage, saddle deformity, and retraction of the columella. If a septal hematoma develops, the area should be drained by a small vertical incision through the septal mucosa. The blood must be evacuated by suction. The mucosa should be placed back into normal position, which is then maintained by intranasal packing.

3. Infection following nasal injury is rare, but if it occurs, it can cause significant problems to the support of the nose. There can also be scarring of the overlying skin. Infection can be avoided, for the most part, with proper surgical techniques and prophylactic antibiotics. If an infection should develop, the external splint will have to be removed and the soft tissues treated with appropriate debridement and antibiotic therapy determined by culture.

Open Reduction and Fixation of Nasal Fractures
Alternative Technique Using Coronal Approach and Cantilevered Bone Grafts

INDICATIONS

Because most nasal fractures can be adequately treated with closed reduction techniques (see Chapter 52), the indications for open reduction are controversial. Most of the time, the nasal bones, including the septum, can be reduced and stabilized with internal nasal packs and external splints. However, a case can be made for opening and reducing (1) fractures that have started to heal in malposition and (2) fractures that extend to the frontal process of the maxilla and frontal bones. Alternatively, if any of the closed methods fail, one of the open techniques should be considered.

PROCEDURE

The nose is treated with local and topical vasoconstrictive agents as described in Chapter 48 and then prepared and draped as a sterile field. The design of incisions and approaches depends primarily on the pathologic condition that is to be corrected.

A,B For a *septal deflection*, the incision should be placed caudal to the area of leafing or deflection. This means either an intermembranous incision (between the columella and septum) or a Killian incision, 1.5 to 2.0 cm cephalad to the caudal border of the septum. If the deflection is associated with buckling and the buckling creates a spur at the junction of the septum with the maxillary crest, then the incision should be

carried onto the ledge of the nostril and the floor of the nose approached simultaneously.

C,D Through these incisions, the surgeon should carefully raise the mucoperichondrium off the septum and, if indicated, the mucoperiosteum off the nasal floor. The correct subperichondrial plane can often be obtained by scraping along the side of the septum with a sharp elevator until the blue color of the cartilage becomes apparent. The surgeon can then proceed cephalad with a subperiosteal dissection.

E,H The elevation should extend beyond the area of the fracture, but it should also cross over in front of the fracture and raise the mucoperichondrium of the opposite side. With mucoperichondrial flaps elevated off the area of deflection, the deflection can be removed, trimmed, and/or scored to fit into a relaxed anatomic position.

Takahashi rongeurs should be used to cut off pieces of displaced cartilage and/or bone. A twisting action of the rongeurs will avoid inadvertent extraction of the fractured segment and injury to the cribriform plate. Scoring can be accomplished by making partial cuts through the curvature of the cartilage with a Beaver knife. Stability of the cartilage can be reinforced by through-and-through fine chromic sutures. If there is a tendency for leafing to occur, a figure-of-eight suture can be applied; this will prevent sliding of the fragments.

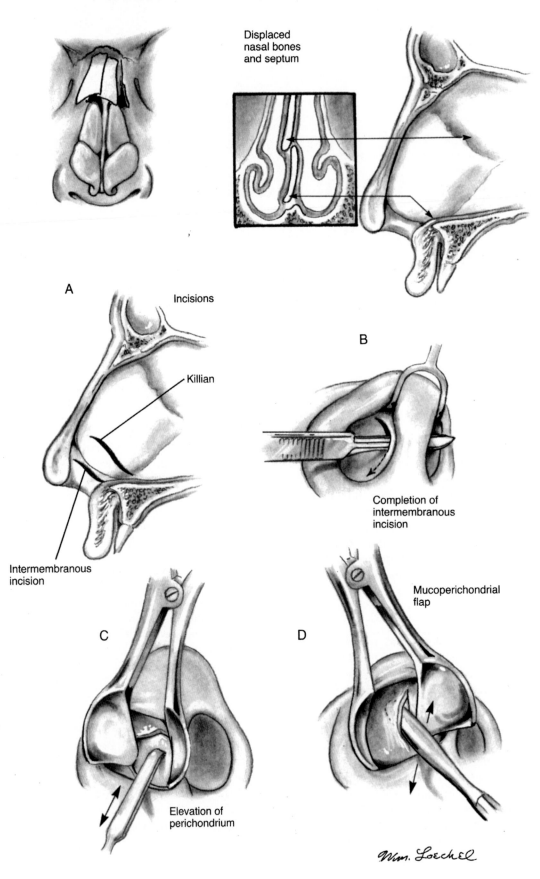

Displaced
nasal bones
and septum

A

Incisions

Killian

B

Completion of
intermembranous
incision

Intermembranous
incision

Mucoperichondrial
flap

C

D

Elevation of
perichondrium

Wm. Loechel

I,J For septal fractures involving the maxillary crest and for fractures in which there is a sharp spur, the surgeon must take special precautions not to tear the mucosa. Approaching the deviation with one of the tunnels described previously will relax the septal mucoperichondrial/mucoperiosteal tissues. The spur, however, may prevent safe elevation and should also be exposed by relaxation of the floor tissues from below. The combined approach will allow the surgeon to tease and cut away the attached mucoperichondrial flaps. The floor tunnel is developed with special Cottle elevators that are narrow, sharp, and curved to fit over the piriform aperture. The floor mucoperiosteum is raised and elevated toward the septum beneath the spur. A special speculum with a more pointed blade (Cottle) is then introduced into both tunnels. When the speculum is opened gently, the spur area will be exposed. The mucoperichondrium/periosteum can then be teased off of the projection.

K,L If the septum is displaced to the side of the crest, reduction will require removal of several millimeters of the cartilage inferiorly. This will allow the septum to swing like a door back into its normal position. A 4-0 chromic suture through the periosteum near the anterior nasal spine and the inferior portion of the cartilaginous septum can be helpful in maintaining the position of the septum. Sometimes a displaced maxillary crest can be repositioned, but if it is unstable, it is probably more prudent to remove it completely.

M Caudally placed incisions through the intramembranous septum can be closed with a 4-0 chromic mattress suture attaching the columella to the caudal septum. More cephalic incisions on the septum can simply be held closed with the nasal packing. Polyethylene splints should be applied to those septums in which instability remains. Nasal packing consisting of tampons or antibiotic-treated gauze is useful in controlling any residual bleeding. The packing also adds support to the septum. These methods and postoperative care are described in Chapter 48.

N For the *early malunited nasal bones* characterized by a limited depression, it is possible to make an intercartilaginous incision, expose the upper lateral cartilage and bone from below, and reduce the bone accordingly. Through this incision, the surgeon should first undermine the skin on the dorsum. A Lempert rongeur can then be inserted with one blade in the pocket and the other in the nasal passageway. The instrument is closed and the bone (including the upper lateral cartilage) rotated into position. The incision should be held closed with packing. An external cast is helpful.

O For *nasal fractures extending to the frontoethmoid region*, additional approaches are necessary for the reduction and fixation. A curvilinear medial canthal incision one-half the distance between the dorsum of the nose and the caruncle of the eye will give satisfactory exposure of the frontal process of the maxilla and the nasal, lacrimal, and parts of the ethmoid bones. The same incision can be used bilaterally, and if additional exposure must be obtained toward the midline, the upper part of the incision can be connected with the horizontal limb (open sky approach). Another possibility is to use the coronal incision and forehead flap described later, but this technique is limited in exposing the medial wall of the orbit. It also requires extensive elevation of periosteum, which can jeopardize viability of comminuted fragments.

P,Q Depressed nasal bone fractures should be exposed by judicious elevation of the periosteum. The fragments should be elevated into position and maintained with strategic placement of low profile miniplates.

The wounds are closed in layers. The periosteum is approximated with 3-0 chromic sutures, the subcutaneous tissues with 4-0 chromic, and the skin with 6-0 nylon. Intranasal packing is used if there is a need to stabilize the septum, but rarely is packing necessary to support the plate fixation. Prophylactic antibiotics are administered for 5 days.

PITFALLS

1. Maintain the supporting structures of the nose as much as possible (i.e., 1.5 cm of caudal septum and 3 to 5 mm of dorsal septum).

2. Splints and packing techniques should be applied in such a way as to prevent hematoma and necrosis of septal tissues. Polyethylene splints should be placed outside the mucosal flaps; pressure exerted by the splints should be appropriate to prevent accumulation of blood beneath the flaps, support the septum in the midline, and avoid necrosis of tissues.

3. Limit incisions and subperiosteal dissections, especially if there is significant comminution of the nasal bones. The open rhinoplasty approach (see Chapter 54) should be avoided, as this method requires an extensive dissection and undermining of tissues. The technique can cause additional trauma. It also will not give sufficient exposure to the lateral part of the nasal bones where they attach to the frontoethmoid region.

4. Plates should not be palpated through the skin. Low profile plates may suffice in thick skinned individuals, but should the plates become noticeable, they may have to be removed.

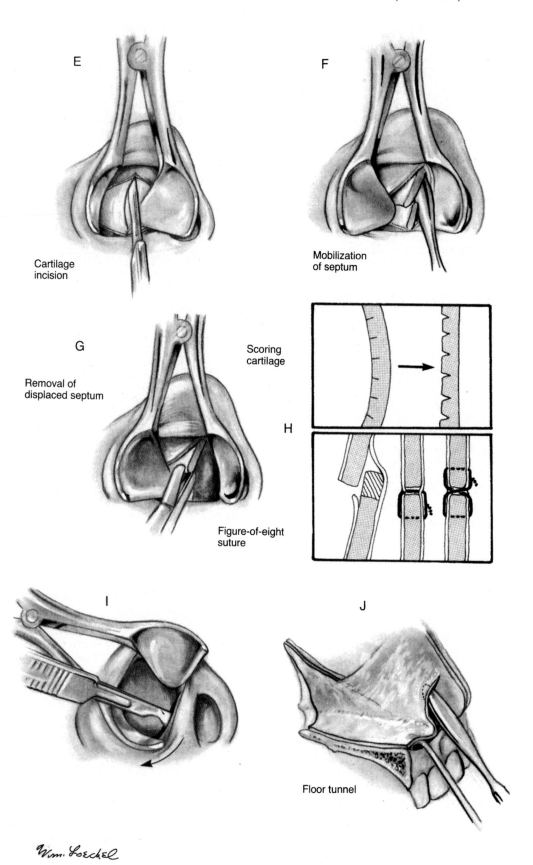

E

Cartilage
incision

F

Mobilization
of septum

G

Removal of
displaced septum

Scoring
cartilage

H

Figure-of-eight
suture

I

J

Floor tunnel

Wm. Loechel

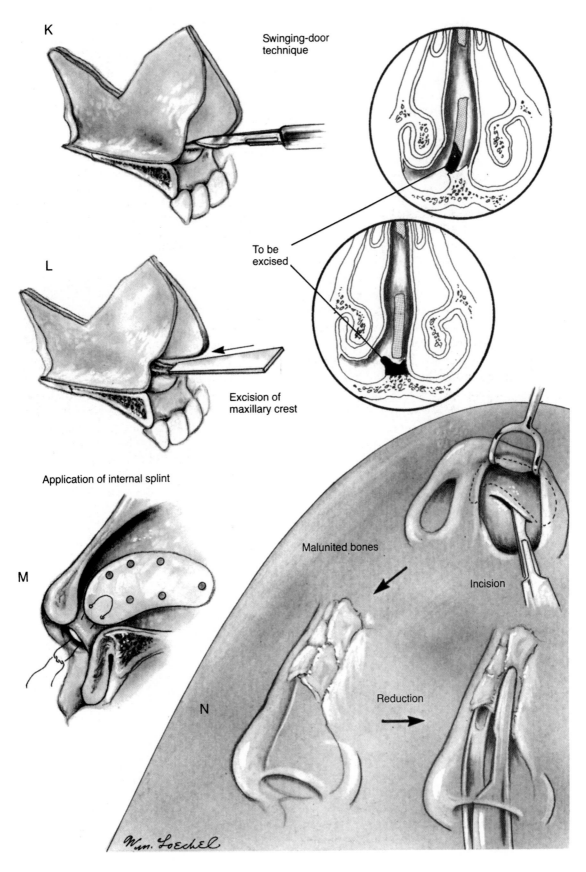

K

Swinging-door technique

To be excised

L

Excision of maxillary crest

Application of internal splint

M

Malunited bones

Incision

N

Reduction

Wm. Loechel

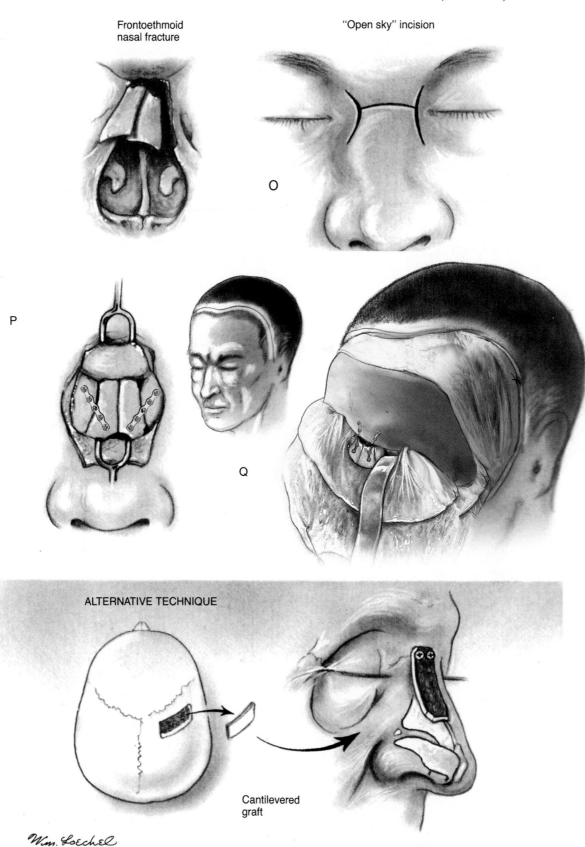

Frontoethmoid
nasal fracture

"Open sky" incision

O

P

Q

ALTERNATIVE TECHNIQUE

Cantilevered
graft

Wm. Loechel

COMPLICATIONS

1. Potential infection can be minimized by atraumatic techniques and prophylactic antibiotics. If infection develops, packing and/or splints should be removed. Cultures should be obtained and the nose irrigated with saline douches.

2. Malunion of the nose with or without obstruction will require a septorhinoplasty. These techniques are described in Chapter 54.

ALTERNATIVE TECHNIQUE USING CANTILEVERED BONE GRAFTS

If comminuted fractures of the nasal bones and septum are associated with fractures of the adjoining buttresses, there may be insufficient support to maintain the projection of the nose. In such cases, internal and external splint techniques methods will fail to establish nasal projection, and cantilever techniques must be considered.

Exposure through the coronal incision and forehead flap is desirable (see Chapter 43). The dissection should extend to the dorsum of the nose so that a subperiosteal and subcutaneous elevation can be achieved at least to the level of the lower lateral cartilages. A 1.5 × 4.5 cm graft is harvested from the outer cortex of the parietal bone (see Chapter 64). The graft is then rotated so that the cortical surface is placed along the frontoethmoid junction and the graft extended over the dorsum of the nasal bones. The graft is secured to the frontal bone by two small bone screws passed through graft into the frontal cortex using lag screw technique (see Chapter 24). The incisions are closed in the standard fashion. External casting is not necessary and probably should be avoided, as it can cause pressure and necrosis of those tissues caught between the graft and cast.

Septorhinoplasty for Nasal Deformity Following Trauma
Alternative Techniques Using Open Rhinoplasty and Cartilage Grafts

INDICATIONS

Probably the most common complication following nasal injury is malunion of the bony cartilaginous framework with or without obstruction. A variety of deformities can be described alone or in combination: dorsal hump; C- or S-shaped deviation of the septum; depression of the dorsum; saddle deformity; deviation of the tip; fallen tip; retracted columella; asymmetry of the nasal bones; asymmetry of the upper lateral cartilages; and asymmetry of the lower lateral cartilages. In addition, the septum can be displaced to one side or another; buckling can occur in the caudal-cephalic or superior-inferior directions. If any of these conditions develop, the patient can be considered for a septorhinoplasty.

Timing of the surgery is important. Ideally the procedure should be performed after the deformities have stabilized; this usually occurs 3 to 6 months after the injury. However, earlier repair can be contemplated if there is (1) obstruction, (2) a simple deformity requiring minimal correction, or (3) severe deformity affecting the patient's well-being.

Before embarking on septorhinoplasty, information should be obtained on the condition of the nose prior to injury and the nature of the new deformities. The patient should have the same expectations as the surgeon and be completely informed about results and complications. CT Scans or sinus radiographs should verify that there is no sinusitis. Photographs are important to document the preoperative status.

PROCEDURE

The surgery can be performed under local anesthesia with sedation or under general anesthesia. Regardless of choice of anesthesia, the nose should be treated with topical 4% cocaine (containing five drops of 1:10,000 epinephrine) and local blocks of 1% or 2% lidocaine containing 1:100,000 epinephrine (see Chapter 52). The face is then prepared with an antiseptic solution and draped as a sterile field.

The surgeon has the option of several approaches. Some are more logical than others, depending on the location and severity of the deformity. The surgeon's experience and techniques will also be factors. For most deformities, a transfixion incision using either an intercartilaginous or intracartilaginous (cartilage-splitting) incision is satisfactory. For those patients requiring low dorsal implants and/or repair of the tip, delivery through a rim incision or open rhinoplasty (see later) is helpful. The transfixion incision also provides an opportunity to do a septoplasty through the same incision.

A Intercartilaginous incisions are made bilaterally, one side at a time. The area to be incised is exposed by placing the blade of the nasal speculum (or double-ball retractor) under the lower lateral cartilage. The cephalic border of the lower lateral cartilage will tend to subluxate over the lower border of the upper lateral cartilage; a groove will develop, and it is this groove where the incision is made. The No. 15 blade should enter the subcutaneous space and not injure the overlying skin.

B As an alternative, the intracartilaginous (cartilage-splitting) incision can be made directly through the lower lateral cartilages. Exposure is obtained by holding the rim with a double-ball hook and pressing downward on the upper border of the lower lateral cartilages with a middle finger so that the cartilages evert into the nasal vestibule. An incision is then made parallel to the rim; the chosen distance from the rim will depend on the desired effect. If there is a need to retain most of the tip support, the incision should be 1 to 1.5 cm cephalad and parallel to the rim. If there is going to be more sculpting, the incision can be made closer to the rim. The incision, while carried through the lateral cartilages, should again avoid injury to the overlying skin.

C The incisions provide entry points for undermining the skin over the cartilaginous and bony dorsum of the nose. Both the cartilage-splitting incision and the intercartilaginous incision can then be extended into a transfixion incision. With the tip of the nose elevated with a double-ball hook and the columella pulled forward with a suture or columella forceps, a button knife is used to incise the tissues over the septum and between the septum and columella to the anterior nasal spine. This frees the lower lateral cartilages and the skin from the upper lateral cartilages and nasal bones.

D,E The rim incision, which is the third alternative, is well suited for cases in which small implants are to be inserted over the cartilages (and/or dorsum) and for tip projection techniques. The incision should be placed in a groove that usually separates the rim of the ala from the hair-bearing skin region. Initially the tips of the scissors are pointed away from the cartilage and then toward the rim. Once around the cartilage, the tips can be rotated and the cartilage separated from the overlying skin. The incision often has to be extended medially along the border of the columella to provide sufficient exposure.

F The septoplasty is usually performed at this stage; details of this procedure are illustrated in Chapter 53. Deviations of the septum often cause deviations to the external nose, and therefore straightening of the septum must take place before the external nose is repaired. The intramembranous incision, which is part of the transfixion incision, can be extended to the nostril sill to gain additional exposure for the floor region. The floor-septum approach is useful in managing sharp spurs and/or dislocation of the quadrilateral plate off the maxillary crest.

With the help of a focused light, a submucosal flap is started at the intramembranous septum. The dissection is continued at a level beneath the perichondrium, and to achieve the appropriate plane, the surgeon should scratch the perichondrial covering over the septum with a sharp elevator or small knife. The correct depth can be appreciated by the appearance of "blue" cartilage. Continued scraping should cause retraction of the edges of the perichondrium, and once this occurs, the dissection should proceed posteriorly with a Freer elevator. The flap should be created only on one side of the septum, as this will protect the soft tissues of the opposite side and prevent problems with necrosis and perforation.

Once the deviation (or leafing) is encountered, an incision can be made through the septal cartilage and the dissection carried out subperichondrially and subperiosteally cephalad on the opposite side. This should expose portions of the remaining quadrilateral plate, perpendicular plate of the ethmoid, and vomer. Deviated parts of cartilage and/or bone can be removed with Takahashi rongeurs. Large segments of cartilage can be harvested with a swivel knife. Twisting motions of the rongeurs will avoid extension of fractures to the cribriform plate.

For spurs in the floor region, it is probably more prudent to use a floor approach in combination with the septal flap. The perichondrial fibers of the septum decussate beneath the septum, and a combined approach allows the fibers to be directly cut. Also, elevation of the septal mucosa over the spur can be made more easily when the surgeon elevates the mucosa from above and below the area of deflection.

Special instruments are usually needed for the floor dissection. First sharp elevators are used to expose the rim of the piriform aperture. Then using a curved Cottle elevator, the mucoperiosteum is elevated off the "blind side." Switching to a more gentle curve of the instrument allows elevation of the periosteum off the remainder of the floor. A thin-bladed Cottle speculum is introduced, with one blade into the floor tunnel and the other into the septal tunnel. The speculum is opened gently, and the junction between the tissues where the fibers decussate is cut with a sharp scissors or knife. The dissection continues cephalad until a complete floor and septal flap is developed. With this exposure, Takahashi rongeurs or a 3-mm chisel are used to resect bony and cartilaginous spurs. Dislocated septal cartilage can often be treated by taking off a 2- to 3-mm section inferiorly and scoring the main concavity. If the septum does not return to the midline, the mucosa on the opposite side may be preventing the rotation and should be elevated accordingly.

SEPTORHINOPLASTY

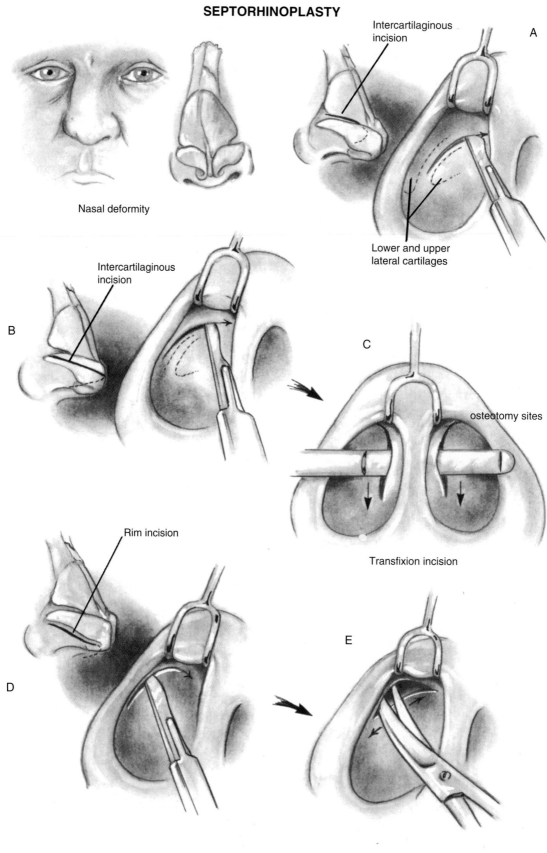

Nasal deformity

Intercartilaginous
incision

A

Lower and upper
lateral cartilages

Intercartilaginous
incision

B

C

osteotomy sites

Transfixion incision

Rim incision

D

E

Wm. Loechel

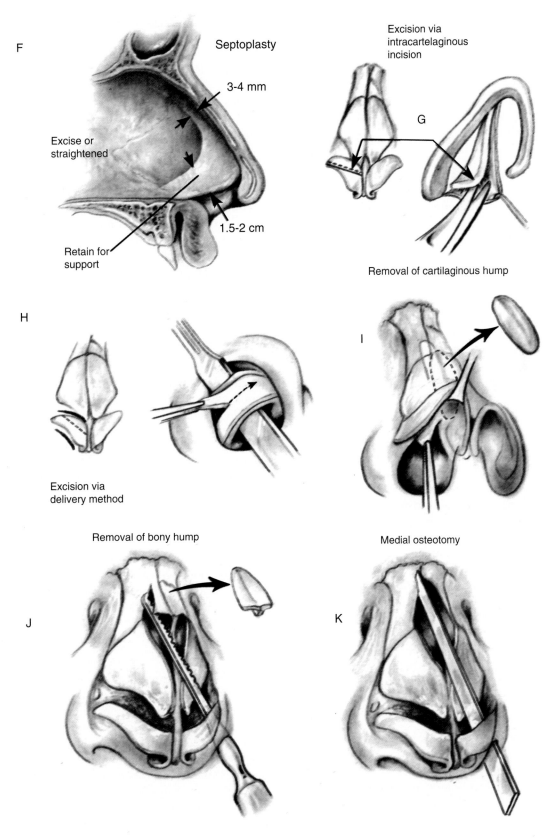

F — Septoplasty

3-4 mm

Excise or straightened

1.5-2 cm

Retain for support

Excision via intracartelaginous incision

G

Removal of cartilaginous hump

I

H — Excision via delivery method

Removal of bony hump

J

Medial osteotomy

K

Wm. Loechel

To retain sufficient support of the nose, the surgeon should maintain at least 1.5 to 2.0 cm of cartilage inferiorly and 0.3 to 0.4 cm of cartilage dorsally. Alternatively, if the surgeon does not want to remove any cartilage, it is possible to move the cartilage back to a midline position by a scoring method. For this technique, multiple parallel cuts should be made on the concave side. The convex surface should be left intact with periosteal attachments. When the deviations are complex, crosshatching may be necessary to achieve desired effects.

G The rhinoplasty part should now be carried out for the other deformities. Assuming that the tip of the nose needs to be rotated upward or made more narrow, the tip area should be exposed. Rotation usually is achieved by removing the cephalic border of the lower lateral cartilage. If the surgeon has chosen the cartilage-splitting incision, then the cephalic flap is pulled downward with a sharp hook and that portion of cartilage cephalad to the incision should be removed. This will leave a strip of lower lateral cartilage caudally. If the dome needs further narrowing, a small wedge of cartilage can be removed retrograde in the region of the dome. This can be accomplished by everting the rim, elevating the perichondrium on both sides of the strip for several millimeters, and making diamond-shaped cuts in the dome with a sharp scissors.

H For those patients requiring more tip work, the lower lateral cartilages should be delivered. Exposure is facilitated by combined rim and intercartilaginous incisions as described previously. The handle of the double-ball retractor is useful in rotating the mucosa and cartilage into view. The surgeon can then design the cephalic border resection and, if necessary, free up the domes for more narrowing, rotation, and projection with a direct suture technique. Usually the cephalic borders are trimmed, leaving a strip inferiorly. The medial crura are then freed up for several millimeters along the columella, and the dome is marked bilaterally with a marking pen. The mucosa beneath the domes is elevated, and the domes are delivered symmetrically into one or the other nostril. They are then held together with a thin-bladed forceps and secured with a 4-0 colorless or white nonabsorbable suture. The knot is buried between the projected domes.

I Tip definition can subsequently be enhanced by removal of the cartilaginous hump. The mucosa beneath the cartilages should be elevated. After exposing the upper lateral cartilages and their attachment to the septum with an Aufricht retractor, the perichondrium is excised. Variable amounts of cartilage from the lower dorsum are removed with a small sharp knife or corrugated nasal scissors.

J,K Following these maneuvers, the surgeon can then appreciate the degree of bony hump deformity that has to be resected. The periosteum should be first elevated. The hump can then be removed with straight saws, and irregularities can later be corrected with a bone rasp. The glabella is deepened, if necessary, with a small chisel and glabellar rasp. If the dorsum needs narrowing, a graduated 6- to 7-mm osteotome is inserted along the sides of the septum, and the bony septum is released (one side at a time) to the glabellar angle.

L–N Lateral osteotomies to narrow the nasal pyramid are performed with offset saws or a 4-mm osteotome. If the bones are thick, the saws can be used to start the cut. Completion of the osteotomy can be accurately accomplished with an osteotome. For the saw technique, incisions are made just in front of the inferior turbinates. The periosteum is elevated off the junction of the frontal process of the maxilla and nasal bones to create a pocket that extends just anterior to the medial canthal ligament. Sawing is facilitated by stabilization of the head by an assistant. Usually the saw cuts are directed along the junction of the nasal bones and frontal process of the maxilla. The cuts are completed with curved, guarded osteotomes. Superiorly the cuts are directed to the glabella angle. As an option, the surgeon can choose just the osteotome technique. For this, the osteotome is directed above the inferior turbinate, along the same path that would be used for the saw. However, the osteotomy ideally should only cut the periosteum and bone on the inner side of the nose, leaving the outer periosteum intact. This technique tends to be less traumatic but can be quite difficult if the nasal bones are thick and in a markedly abnormal position. Narrowing of the nose is completed by exerting finger pressure along the nasal bones and pushing the bones toward each other. A rocking motion often completes the fracture.

At this stage some refinements can be implemented. Additional dorsal irregularities can be removed with appropriate rasps or scissors. More rotation and projection can be achieved by removal of a wedge of the caudal septum.

O The intermembranous incision is closed by attaching the septum to the columella with 4-0 chromic mattress sutures. The rim and intracartilaginous incisions are closed with a single 4-0 chromic suture. The septum can be stabilized with thin polyethylene plates. The nose is packed gently with a tampon or antibiotic-treated gauze, and an external splint and tape dressing as described in Chapter 52 is applied. Antibiotics are prescribed for 5 to 6 days. The packing is removed at 2 days, septal splints are removed at 5 to 7 days, and the external splint and dressings are removed at 7 to 14 days.

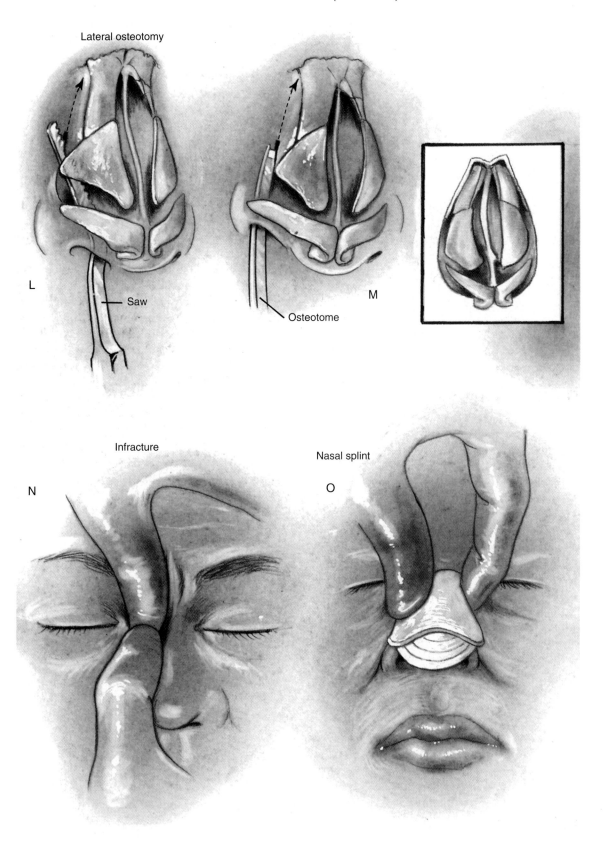

Lateral osteotomy

Saw

Osteotome

L

M

Infracture

N

Nasal splint

O

Wm. Loechel

PITFALLS

1. Careful planning of each step is required for a successful correction of the deformity. Preoperative analysis with photographs and a set of CT Scans or sinus radiographs (to ensure that sinusitis is not present) should be part of the workup.

2. Many deviations of the external nose are caused by deviation of the septum. The septoplasty therefore becomes the foundation of the procedure. It should come first, and following the septoplasty, all deformities should be reevaluated.

3. Exposure and lighting of the septum is important. Avoid excision of septal tissues that cannot be visualized. Ensure that the mucosa has been elevated before removal of any of the fragments.

4. Although the surgeon has the choice of doing the cartilaginous tip before or after the bony skeleton, there are advantages to doing the cartilage work first. Often there is less bleeding than after an osteotomy, and considering that the tip is the "delicate" part of the procedure, optimal exposure is desirable. Moreover, tip projection can be a guide to the level of hump removal.

5. Always ensure symmetry of the procedure. A maneuver performed on one side should be followed immediately by the same maneuver on the opposite side. If pieces of tissue are being removed, they should be placed in front of the surgeon and compared directly to see if they are mirror images of each other.

6. It is always better to make an error in removing too little than in removing too much. Additional amounts of tissue can be removed at any time. However, it is difficult to add tissues and have them restored to normal anatomic contour.

7. Do not remove too much of the lateral portion of the cephalic border of the lower lateral cartilages. This lateral "tail" area is important for maintaining postoperative tip projection. It is also safer to keep the domes and rims intact, although incisions and some trimmings may be necessary in the more difficult cases.

8. When bringing the domes together, remember that it is possible to obliterate the tip highlights. To prevent this from occurring, place the mattress suture on the medial crura side of the dome. The higher placement certainly provides more projection, but the lower placement is better in creating the natural splaying that occurs in the tip region.

9. The level of the lateral osteotomy depends on the desired correction. If more projection of the dorsum is needed, the osteotomy should be placed close to the maxilla. For those patients who just need a narrowing of the dorsum, an osteotomy can be placed in a more intermediate position.

10. Postoperatively swelling can be reduced with elevation of the head and cold compresses. Another option is to administer steroids that will reduce the swelling and inflammatory response.

COMPLICATIONS

1. Epistaxis can occur in the immediate postoperative period. This can sometimes be avoided by making sure that all bleeding has stopped before terminating the procedure. However, if the patient bleeds following the surgery, the surgeon should (1) reduce the blood pressure with analgesics, sedation, and/or blood pressure-lowering agents; (2) apply cold compresses to the face; and (3) adjust and tighten packing. If these maneuvers are unsuccessful, the packing will have to be removed and the bleeding corrected with cauterization and/or repacking. Sometimes more pressure is needed on the bleeding sites.

2. Occasionally the nasal deformity cannot be completely corrected, or a new one may develop. Soft tissue swelling such as that seen with a "polybeak" can sometimes be treated with a direct injection of 20 mg/mL of triamcinolone. Cartilaginous depressions can later be filled with cartilage implants (see later). Repeat septorhinoplasty, in part or as a whole, must sometimes be considered.

3. Nasal obstruction can occur as a result of the procedure. If the problem is caused by deformity (i.e., spurs, displacement of the septum, and/or deviated nasal bones), another septoplasty and/or rhinoplasty must be considered. Some of the more serious problems, such as a collapsing valve, are difficult to treat, and the reader is referred to a more appropriate text or journal.

4. Infections in the postoperative period are rare, but if they do occur, they can cause loss of skin with scarring and loss of skeletal support, later showing as a saddle deformity and retracted columella. These dreaded complications can sometimes be avoided by ensuring that there is no infection such as acne or sinusitis before starting surgery. The surgeon should also ensure that there is no intraoperative hematoma formation. Prophylactic antibiotics should be used throughout the period of packing or stabilization. If infection develops, cultures should be obtained and the appropriate antibiotic administered. Infectious disease consultation is desirable.

ALTERNATIVE TECHNIQUE USING OPEN RHINOPLASTY

The open rhinoplasty is another method for approaching nasal deformity following trauma. Exposure of the nasal architecture using this technique is far superior to that with any others, and this procedure is best used when the deformity is complex, when there is any confusion as to what is causing the deformity or in cases where the tip requires much attention. In performing the open procedure, the surgeon must be aware that there will be a small incision across the columella and that there can be more than the expected edema in dependent areas of the nose.

a,b The area is prepared and draped as in the standard septorhinoplasty. An incision is marked at the junction of the lower and middle thirds of the columella with a small V directed superiorly. The lateral portions of the incision are brought just beneath the rim and then along the rim superiorly to create the rim incision as described previously. The dissection proceeds through the skin, just in front of the medial crura and lower lateral cartilages. Curved scissors are directed away from the edge of the cartilages and then rotated on top of the cartilages to start the superiorly directed subcutaneous elevation. Skin flaps are developed to about the midlevel of the nasal bones.

The procedures that are used for correction of the nasal deformities and/or obstruction are the same as those described for a septorhinoplasty. The effects of trimming and/or removal can be appreciated by repeatedly placing the flaps into their original position. After completion of the procedure, the skin over the columella is closed with interrupted 6-0 nylon sutures. The dressings and postoperative care are the same as those for the standard rhinoplasty procedure.

ALTERNATIVE TECHNIQUE USING CARTILAGE GRAFTS

For those patients with a saddle deformity, retracted columella, or upper or lower lateral cartilage defects, implantation of cartilage can be a useful adjunctive procedure. Cartilage can be harvested using a septoplasty technique, but if there is insufficient material, either because of trauma or previous surgery, then the preferred donor site will be the conchal bowl of the ear.

The patient's face and neck should be prepared and draped in the standard fashion, exposing both the ears and the nose region. Vasoconstrictors are applied to the nose, and the ear is blocked with 1% lidocaine containing epinephrine.

a',b' An incision is then made at the lateral edge of the conchal bowl and a subperichondrial flap elevated to the external auditory meatus. Conchal cartilage of desired shape and size is elevated from the deep surface of the perichondrium. Bleeding is controlled with an electric cautery, and a small elastic band drain is secured to the skin. The skin is closed with interrupted 6-0 nylon sutures. A mastoid dressing of fluffs and stretch gauze (applied later) can be removed at 24 to 48 hours.

c' Grafts harvested from the conchal bowl can be applied to the nose in a variety of techniques. For the saddle deformity, the surgeon can use a rim or intracartilaginous incision. The pocket should be just slightly larger than the desired implant. Contact of the implant with the cartilages and/or bone is encouraged. Implants that are too thin can be made larger by layering pieces of cartilage on each other and holding them together with 3-0 chromic ties. The cartilage can be trimmed to appropriate size and shape; a keel design is desirable for the saddle deformity. Closure and postoperative care are the same as those used for a rhinoplasty.

d' For the columella retraction, incisions are made through the medial crura inferiorly and subcutaneous pockets created with a sharp scissors from the anterior nasal spine to the tip of the nose. Slivers of cartilage are then introduced into this pocket. Incisions are closed with a 3-0 nylon mattress suture.

e' For small deformities involving the lower and upper lateral cartilages, isolated rim incisions can be used. The skin is dissected free from the lower and/or upper lateral cartilages and the implant placed into this pocket. This incision should be closed with a single 4-0 nylon suture.

SEPTORHINOPLASTY *(Continued)*

ALTERNATIVE TECHNIQUE USING OPEN RHINOPLASTY

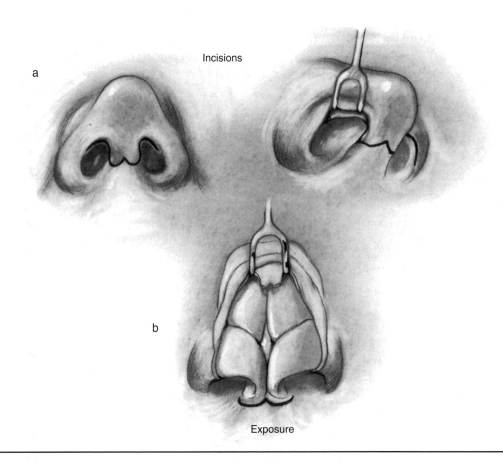

a

Incisions

b

Exposure

ALTERNATIVE TECHNIQUE USING CARTILAGE GRAFTS

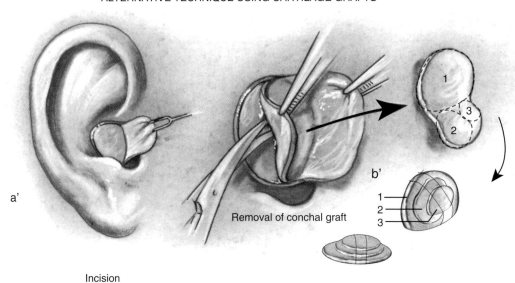

a'

Incision

Removal of conchal graft

b'

ALTERNATIVE TECHNIQUE USING CARTILAGE GRAFTS (CONTINUED)

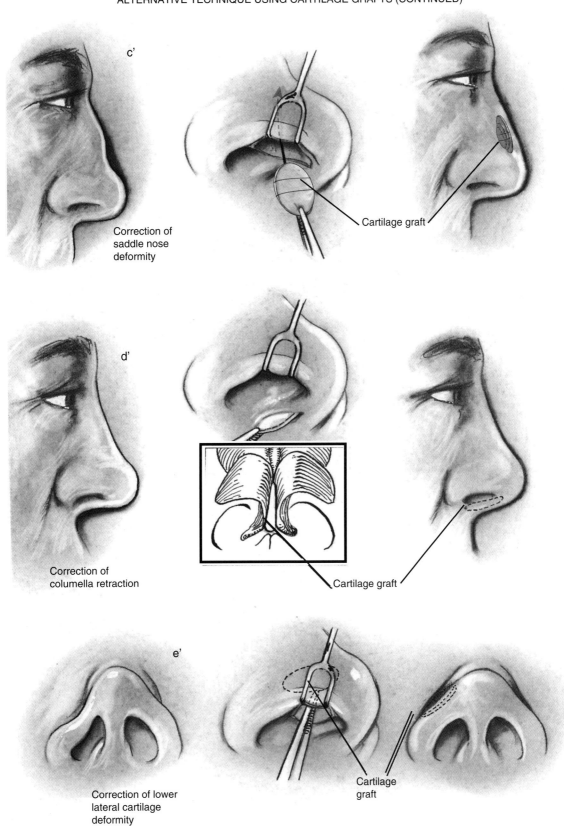

c'

Correction of
saddle nose
deformity

Cartilage graft

d'

Correction of
columella retraction

Cartilage graft

e'

Correction of lower
lateral cartilage
deformity

Cartilage
graft

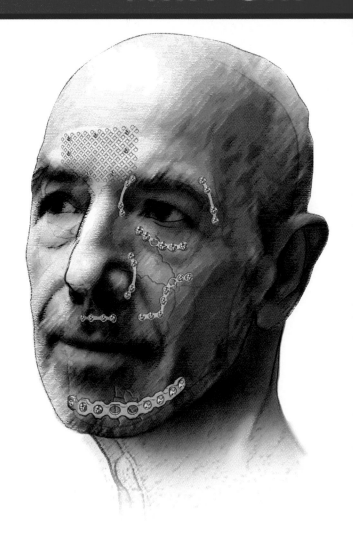

PART SIX

Zygoma Fractures

Classification and Pathophysiology of Zygoma Fractures

CHAPTER

55

General Considerations

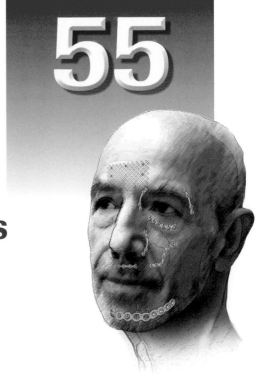

A-C The zygoma attaches to the craniofacial skeleton by frontal, maxillary, and temporal projections, forming a tripod, and by broad suture lines that connect the malar bone with the sphenoid and maxillary bones. The displacement of the bone depends on the direction and magnitude of external forces and the pull of the masseter muscle. The zygoma complex tends to move inward or outward and/or rotate along a vertical or anteroposterior (longitudinal) axis. Sometimes this block of bone is comminuted; at other times, part of the bone, such as the rim or arch, is displaced. A commonly used classification described by Zingg and associates notes the following: A (arch fracture); A_1 (lateral orbital rim fracture); A_2 (inferior orbital rim fracture); B (zygoma as a block); and C (zygoma in addition to frontal and/or maxillary fractures) There are other classification systems, but probably the most important factor is the relationship of the alteration in position of the bone to the development of clinical signs and symptoms.

D–F Rotation and depression of the zygoma fracture often causes abnormalities of the orbit. Typically, when the zygoma is depressed and rotated clockwise, the orbital walls will expand, resulting in enophthalmos and/or hypophthalmos; also, there will be a downward displacement of the lateral canthal ligament. The infraorbital nerve is frequently involved with the fracture, causing hypoesthesia of the cheek and upper dentition. If the bone rotates inward, the orbit is made smaller, and the patient presents with hyperophthalmos and some degree of exophthalmos. Displacement of the zygoma inward and downward can compromise the space occupied by the coronoid process, resulting in trismus and pain on mastication. Unilateral epistaxis, subconjunctival hemorrhage, and periorbital ecchymoses are additional common findings.

ZYGOMA FRACTURES

ZINGG CLASSIFICATION

A

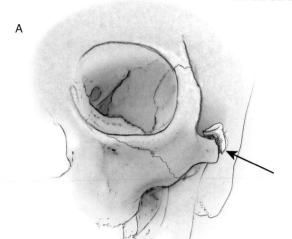

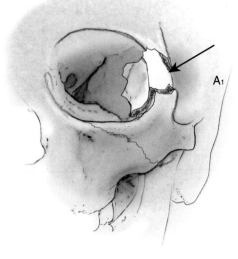

A₁

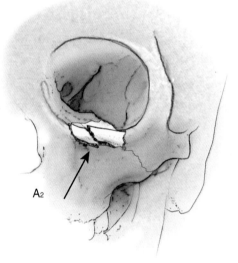

A₂

B

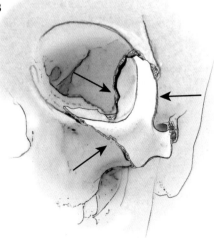

C

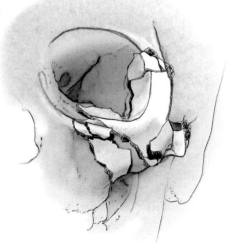

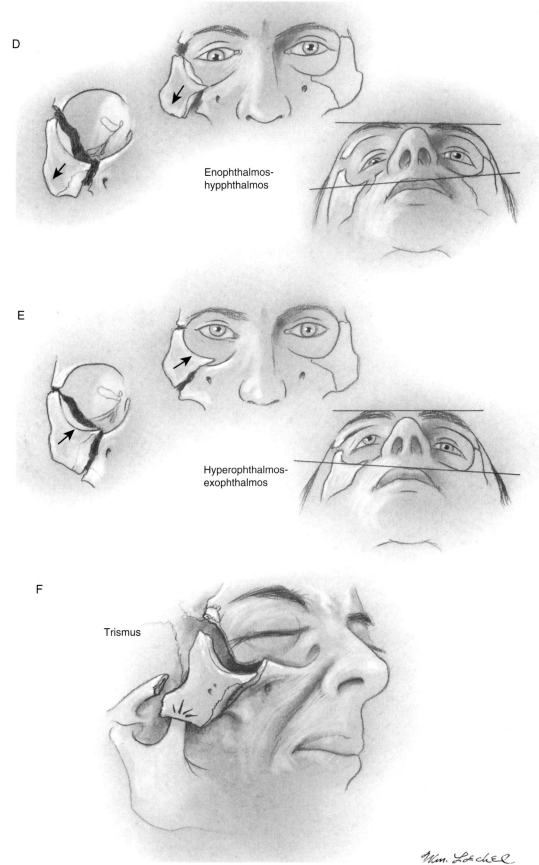

D

Enophthalmos-
hypphthalmos

E

Hyperophthalmos-
exophthalmos

F

Trismus

Wm. Loechel

Management Strategies

CHAPTER

56

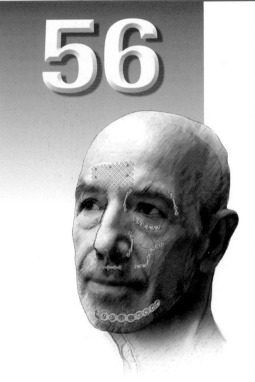

Semiclosed Reduction of Zygomatic Arch Fractures Using Eyebrow, Temporal Hairline, and Intraoral Approaches

INDICATIONS

Fracture and rotation of the zygomatic arch are often associated with a deformity of the lateral cheek. The area of depression may not be appreciated until all swelling has disappeared. Severe displacement of the arch can cause an impingement on the coronoid process and result in trismus and pain on mastication. Injury to the masseter may also cause trismus, but this effect should clear in several days; mechanical obstruction will persist longer. There are many surgical approaches to the arch fracture, but the most popular ones use incisions that are hidden intraorally or in the eyebrow or temporal hairline. Tunnels are then created beneath the arch that can then be used to elevate the arch into correct position. Direct open approaches are avoided because of the potential damage to the frontal branch of the facial nerve. Closed methods using

reduction with a suture or towel clip are described, but they have the disadvantage of being unable to control the rotation. Moreover, the surgeon loses the opportunity to stabilize the fragments by packing beneath the displaced arch.

PROCEDURE

Surgery should be planned when swelling has disappeared and the degree of deformity can be appreciated. The procedure usually is performed under orotracheal anesthesia. The face should be prepared and draped as a sterile field and the area of depression marked on the skin with a marking solution.

A The eyebrow approach (sometimes called the Dingman method) uses an incision through the lateral eyebrow. Some hemostasis can be obtained by infiltration with 1% lidocaine containing epinephrine. The incision is made through the orbicularis oculi and periosteum, exposing the zygomaticofrontal suture line. The periosteum is then elevated laterally and the temporalis muscle retracted from the frontal process of the zygoma. A Joseph elevator is utilized to develop a tunnel along the lateral wall of the orbit beneath the temporalis muscle to the level of the arch. Once the elevator is at the arch, it can then be advanced to the lateral anterior aspect of the maxilla. The Joseph elevator is removed and replaced with a heavy, curved Kelly clamp or Dingman elevator. The clamp/elevator is levered on the prominence of the frontotemporal bone and the arch elevated laterally. The arch is then molded back into position with the other hand. Usually the arch is stable enough that no packing is necessary, but if the arch is unstable, the surgeon can pack beneath it with pieces of Gelfoam. Penrose drains can be used but will cause a widened scar.

B The popular Gillies approach uses an incision just behind the temporal hairline. Usually a small area is shaved, and the incision is made parallel to the hair follicles. The superficial temporal artery may be exposed and either retracted from the wound or ligated. The superficial temporalis fascia is then incised and the elevator used to develop a tunnel beneath the fascia and zygomatic arch. Reduction is carried out with a heavy, curved clamp, Boies or Dingman elevator. As with the eyebrow approach, the arch is overcorrected and then molded back into position with the opposite hand. Gelfoam or Penrose (1/2-inch) drains can be used for packing and brought out through the incision. The temporalis fascia, subcuticular tissues, and skin are closed in layers.

C The buccal (Keen) approach requires an intraoral incision through the gingivobuccal sulcus mucosa. Using a blunt clamp, the tissues are spread and a tunnel developed just lateral to the maxilla and beneath the zygomatic arch. A heavy clamp is introduced through the opening, and the arch is elevated into position. If the arch is unstable, the surgeon can pack Gelfoam beneath the bone; Intraoral contamination precludes the use of Penrose drains. The buccal mucosa should be loosely closed.

Postoperatively the patient is kept from putting pressure on the cheek area. Drains should be removed in 5 to 7 days. Prophylactic antibiotics are administered while the packing is in place. Postoperative CT Scans should be obtained to ensure adequate reduction.

PITFALLS

1. Depression of the zygomatic arch is easily camouflaged by swelling of soft tissues. Thus patients should continue to be evaluated until the arch structure can be seen and palpated. Trismus or pain on mastication are clues that there is a substantial depression of the bone.

2. Make sure that the subtemporalis fascia tunnels lie beneath the arch. Remember that the temporalis fascia inserts into the arch, and for an instrument to achieve reduction, it must be placed deep to this fascial layer.

3. Avoid repeated attempts at reduction, as this will cause instability. One or two forceful attempts at elevation at the appropriate site with sufficient pressure should achieve the reduction. If the fracture becomes unstable, packing should be used to support the fragments.

4. Although packing can be safely used through the hairline incision, packing applied intraorally can potentially cause an infection, and packing through the brow sometimes causes a widened scar. High levels of antibiotics are suggested. Occasionally Gelfoam can suffice as a safe packing medium.

5. Closed techniques may be employed for those patients who are too unstable for anesthesia (see optional method). A towel clip strategically placed around the arch can be used to elevate the arch into approximate position. If the arch is still unstable, a suture can be placed around the arch and attached to a tongue blade, which is secured to the surface of the adjoining facial skeleton.

COMPLICATIONS

1. Unsatisfactory reduction is probably the most common complication of the procedure. Usually in these cases the surgeon has failed to insert the instrument beneath the arch, or the arch is too unstable and falls back to its posttraumatic position. The position of the arch is best evaluated by a postoperative CT Scans, and if the arch is in malposition, reduction and fixation should be repeated.

2. Infection should be avoided with proper postoperative care. Intraoral packing must be removed within several days; packs through the hairline and eyebrow may be left longer but should be inspected daily for evidence of infection. Antibiotic coverage is a very important adjunct. If signs of infection are present, the packing should be removed, cultures obtained, and appropriate antibiotics administered.

3. If the arch heals in malposition and the patient complains of trismus and/or deformity, other procedures must be considered. A coronoidectomy, described in Chapter 22, is a possibility. Deformity of the arch can also be treated with osteotomy and/or onlay grafts (see Chapters 58 and 59).

SEMICLOSED TECHNIQUE FOR ZYGOMATIC ARCH FRACTURES

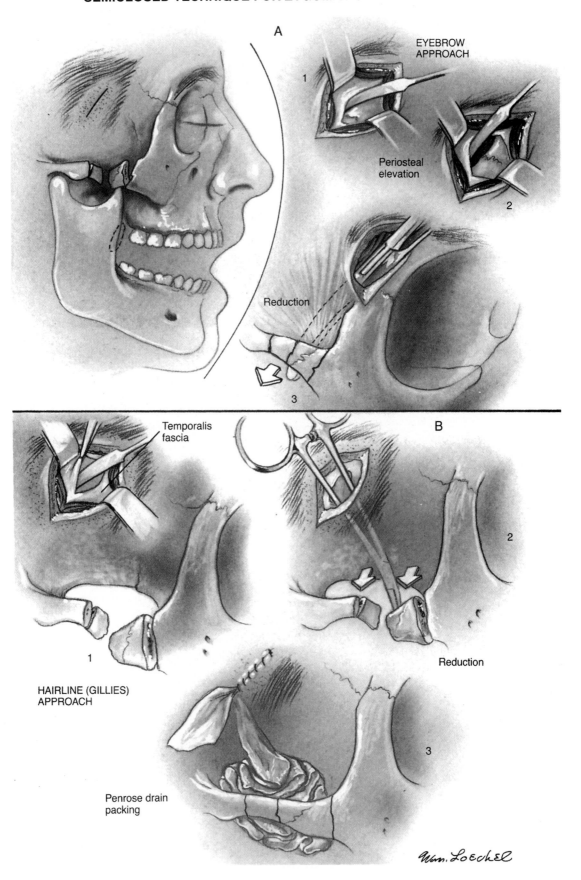

A

EYEBROW
APPROACH

1

Periosteal
elevation

2

Reduction

3

Temporalis
fascia

B

2

Reduction

1

HAIRLINE (GILLIES)
APPROACH

3

Penrose drain
packing

Wm. Loechel

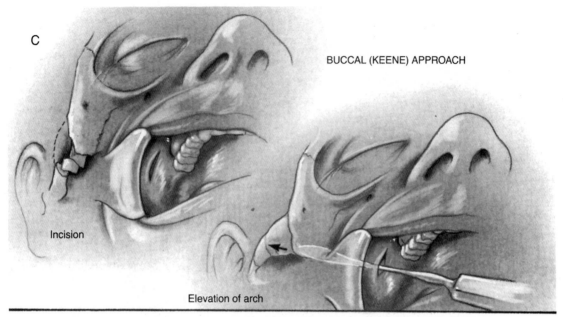

C

BUCCAL (KEENE) APPROACH

Incision

Elevation of arch

OPTIONAL METHOD
USING TOWEL CLIP

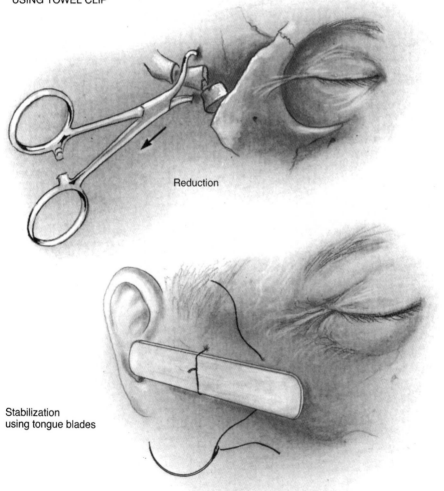

Reduction

Stabilization
using tongue blades

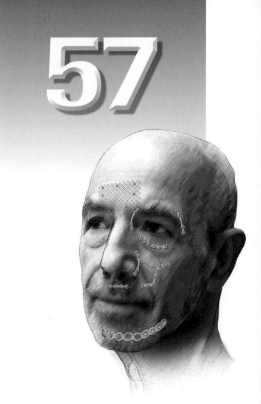

Open Reduction of the Zygoma Fracture With Miniplate Fixation

Alternative Technique Using Transconjunctival Approach and Lateral Canthotomy
Alternative Technique for Repair of Blow-in Fractures

INDICATIONS

Facial asymmetry and trismus, as consequences of a zygoma fracture, are probably the most common indications for open reduction and fixation. Usually the patient presents with a depression of the cheek and an inferior displacement of the lateral canthal ligament. The zygomatic arch can also be displaced laterally to give a widened appearance to the midfacial area. The patient may complain of an inability to open and close the mouth, pain on mastication, and no improvement in jaw function over time.

Other indications for surgery are those associated with the orbital floor component of the fracture (see Chapter 62). If the fracture rotates into the orbit, exophthalmos may be observed. Loss of tissues into the maxillary sinus and/or enlargement of the orbit can cause enophthalmos and/or hypophthalmos. Diplopia secondary to displacement of the inferior rectus muscle is also a concern.

Occasionally the zygoma fracture is only minimally displaced but is associated with a palpable defect of the orbital rim. As posttraumatic swelling disappears, the patient can develop a notable deformity. Surgical correction is desirable.

One controversial indication is hypoesthesia. There is no proof that reduction of the zygoma fracture improves the return of function of the infraorbital nerve, but it is logical to assume that this injury is caused by compression and that decompression with reduction should be effective in treating the sequela. Therefore it is reasonable to explore the canal and remove those fragments of bone that may project into the nerve (see Chapter 60).

PROCEDURE

A Under general orotracheal anesthesia, the face is prepared and draped as a sterile field. The entire face is exposed so that the surgeon can evaluate cheek projection in more than one plane. Infraciliary (or high eyelid) and eyebrow incisions are mapped out with marking solution. The infraciliary incision is made

2 to 3 mm below the cilia and lateral to the puncta; it can be extended into one of the "crow's feet" creases laterally. The high eyelid incision, which can be used as an alternative to the infraciliary incision, can be made in a high crease line below the puncta and lateral to a line drawn perpendicular to the pupil. The eyebrow incision, about 2.5 cm long, is made within the lateral eyebrow, carefully cutting the skin parallel to the orientation of the hairs.

B,C Using the infraciliary or high eyelid incision, the surgeon should separate the orbicularis oculi from the orbital septum and follow the septum to the anterior wall of the maxilla. As described in Chapter 62, the periosteum is incised and a cuff of tissue developed superiorly and elevated from the orbital rim. The fracture should be visualized, and if there is any comminution, the surgeon should attempt to keep the periosteum intact over the fragments. The infraorbital nerve should be identified and these soft tissues protected from further damage. The periosteum should also be elevated from the orbital floor, freeing up any tissues that are caught in the floor part of the fracture.

D,E Using the exposure of the eyebrow incision, the orbicularis oculi muscle fibers are spread, and the periosteum is incised at the level of the zygomaticofrontal suture line. A Joseph elevator is used to elevate the periosteum medially and laterally. With a Freer elevator, the periorbita and lacrimal gland are dissected free from the lacrimal fossa. The fracture line often entraps tissue near the inferior orbital fissure; these displaced tissues should be elevated and freed. The dissection should be continued laterally and posteriorly around the frontal process of the zygoma and then downward to create a pocket beneath the zygomatic arch. This pocket should be extended to the anterior wall of the maxilla, as it will become useful in the reduction of the fracture.

Reduction is carried out through both the eyebrow and infraciliary or high eyelid exposures. A large, curved clamp is inserted through the eyebrow incision and beneath the arch and body of the zygoma to the lateral wall of the maxilla. The zygoma is then lifted laterally and upward and subsequently it is molded back into anatomic position. If the bone does not move with this maneuver, a small elevator or osteotome is inserted between the fragments of the anterior wall of the maxilla. Then, the clamp under the body and the elevator between the maxillary/orbital rim fragments are raised simultaneously. Using steady pressure, the zygoma is elevated anteriorly and laterally. The bone is then manipulated into the desired position. The zygomaticofrontal and inferior rim fractures are evaluated for adequacy of reduction. Confirmation is obtained by palpation of the zygomaticomaxillary buttress and

by ensuring that these fragments are correctly aligned. Cheek projection should be the same on both sides.

F–J Fixation is achieved with low profile miniplates bent to the contour of the frontal process of the zygoma. Depending upon plate design, the length of the plate should incorporate four or five holes with at least two holes provided above and below the fracture. Using drill bits of 3 or 4 mm in length, holes just adjacent to the fracture are first drilled and secured with appropriate size screws. The outer holes are drilled and secured last. The inferior orbital rim is then inspected and if it is not stable, it should be treated with a straight or slightly curved miniplate with at least two screw holes placed to the side of the fracture. Multiple fractures in this area may require a longer plate or several miniplates strategically placed across the fractures. Rarely are plates required at the zygomaticomaxillary buttress, and frequently the entire complex can be stabilized with one miniplate at the zygomaticofrontal buttress. Following reduction and fixation of the zygoma, the orbital floor should be inspected, and if there is a deficit, this condition should be treated with polypropylene mesh as in Chapter 62.

Single 4-0 chromic sutures are used to approximate the periosteum over the inferior and lateral orbital rims. The infraciliary or high eyelid incision is closed with a running 5-0 subcuticular nylon suture. The eyebrow incision is closed with a 4-0 chromic subcuticular suture, followed by a running or interrupted 5-0 nylon suture through the skin. The patient is maintained on antibiotics for 5 days and instructed to keep pressure off the cheek area. A soft diet is recommended for 24 to 48 hours. CT scans are obtained in 2 to 3 days and the cheek projection evaluated at that time. Sutures are removed at 5 to 7 days.

PITFALLS

1. An accurate diagnosis is a prerequisite for appropriate treatment. CT scans should be obtained carefully evaluating the rims of the orbit, floor of the orbit, zygoma and zygomatic arch, sphenoid attachments, and lateral wall of the maxilla. A clinical appraisal should also include palpation of the adjoining facial structures and an analysis of cheek projection. Waiting until all swelling has disappeared will improve the accuracy of the evaluation.

2. The repair process should employ the principle of three-point reduction and stable fixation. Fractures at the zygomaticofrontal suture line and infraorbital rim should be visually reduced, cheek projection should be symmetrical, and there should be no step off or deficit palpated at the zygomaticomaxillary buttress. If there is any suspicion that the zygomaticomaxillary

MINIPLATE FIXATION OF ZYGOMA FRACTURES

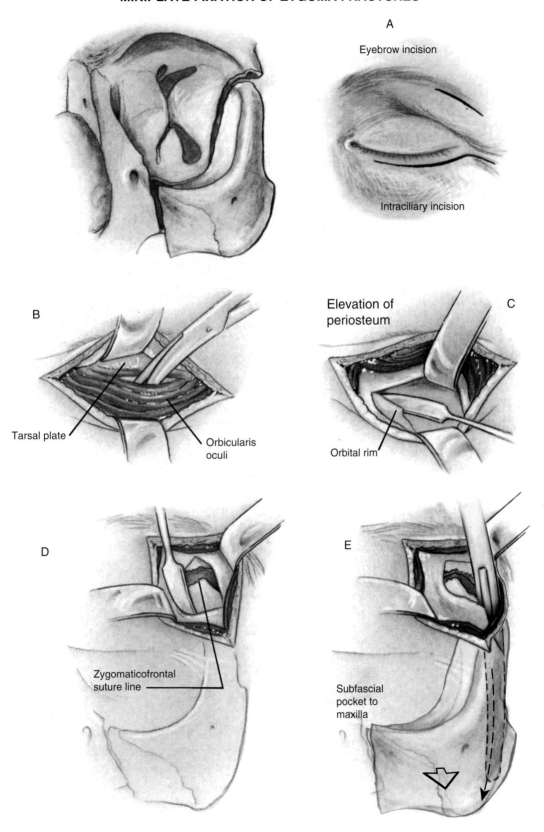

A

Eyebrow incision

Intraciliary incision

B

Tarsal plate

Orbicularis
oculi

Elevation of
periosteum

C

Orbital rim

D

Zygomaticofrontal
suture line

E

Subfascial
pocket to
maxilla

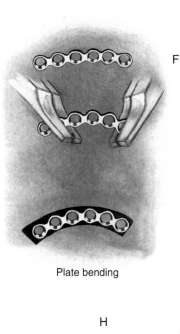

F

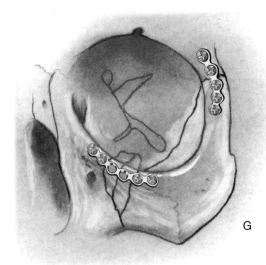

G

Plate bending

H

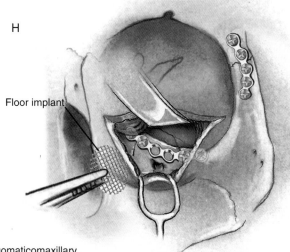

Floor implant

I

Optional zygomaticomaxillary
fixation

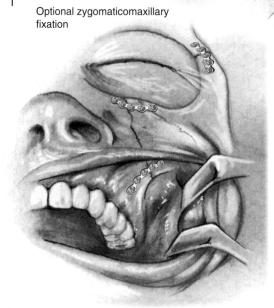

J   Optional miniplate
alone

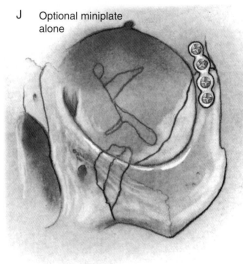

Wm. Loechel

buttress is not in correct alignment or that instability continues, an incision should be placed in the gingival buccal/labial sulcus and this area exposed and evaluated directly. An additional miniplate (resorbable or titanium) can be placed at this fracture site (see I).

3. Be careful not to injure the tarsal plate, as trauma to this structure can later cause ectropion. Leaving some orbicularis oculi fibers attached to the plate will help avoid the development of this complication.

4. While the minidriver is being used to drill holes, the soft tissues should be protected with a malleable retractor. Also, to prevent heat damage, there should be a constant flow of irrigation solution (isotonic saline).

5. Because a zygoma fracture is often associated with injury to the floor of the orbit, the surgeon must ensure that the reduction of the zygoma does not cause additional damage to the floor. To avoid this problem, the floor of the orbit should be initially exposed and then reevaluated prior to closure. Occasionally the floor will need to be repaired, as in a blowout fracture (see Chapter 62).

6. Small fragments of bone that become loose at the inferior orbital rim can contribute to instability, and, if they are not retained, they can cause a step deformity. Every attempt should be made to keep the periosteum on these fragments. Occasionally the fragments can be stabilized with a stenting by the orbital rim miniplate. A more conservative but effective approach is to stabilize the zygoma with a miniplate at the zygomaticofrontal fracture site and "basket" the reduced comminuted fragments with a tight periosteal closure (see J).

7. Delay in treatment can be associated with resorption and malunion of the zygoma. When 4 to 6 weeks have elapsed after injury, osteotomy, refracture, and use of minplate fixation are satisfactory (Chapter 58). If later treatment is required, the surgeon should consider osteotomy (and/or grafts) or onlay grafts alone (Chapter 59).

8. Blow-in fractures are an infrequent variant of zygoma fracture and can be also associated with orbital floor damage. The diagnosis and management of these fractures are discussed later.

COMPLICATIONS

1. Blindness is rare following treatment of the zygoma fracture. However, the surgeon must be aware of the possibility of an intraorbital hematoma, optic nerve compression, and retinal artery occlusion (see Chapter 62). Ophthalmologic evaluation is desirable before surgery especially if there is any indication of changes in vision and/or injury to the muscles, nerves, or globe. To avoid iatrogenic injury, the fracture sites should be exposed before manipulation, and the

forces of reduction should be sufficient to reduce the fragments without causing new fracture lines.

2. Orbital deformity and dysfunction (e.g., enophthalmos, hypophthalmos, and/or diplopia) are common complications. These conditions and methods of treatment are discussed in Chapter 65.

3. Postoperative depression of the zygoma can be avoided by an accurate reduction and adequate fixation. Although it is unlikely that the masseter will pull the zygoma out of position, the patient should be placed on a soft diet for several days. We instruct the patient not to lie on that side and to avoid any activities in which there is potential physical contact. If the cheek becomes displaced, immediate exploration and correction should be considered. If malunion has occurred, osteotomy and onlay bone grafts may be necessary (see Chapters 58 and 59).

4. Trismus following repair of the zygoma fracture may indicate an inadequate reduction and continued impingement of the zygoma (or zygomatic arch) on the coronoid process of the mandible. The patient often complains of pain on opening and/or closing the jaw, and some cheek depression is usually observed. In the early stages (i.e., up to 6 weeks), osteotomy of the zygoma is an option. If the complication is seen later, then coronoidectomy with or without augmentation of the malar eminence should be considered. If there is no significant deformity or displacement of the zygoma, then a coronoidectomy alone is the preferred treatment (see Chapter 22).

5. Ectropion often with epiphora can occur following the infraciliary approach. In the early stages the complication will correct itself and watchful waiting is advised. If after a few weeks the deformity persists, an injection of triamcinolone (20 mg/mL) can be applied to counteract scarring. If this does not correct the problem the incision will need to be reexplored, adhesions severed, and lamellar flaps mobilized into anatomic location. Ophthalmological consultation is desirable.

ALTERNATIVE TECHNIQUE USING TRANSCONJUCTIVAL APPROACH AND LATERAL CANTHOTOMY

The transconjunctival approach combined with a lateral canthotomy provides an alternative exposure for zygoma fractures avoiding the problems of ectropion that sometimes occur with the infraciliary incision.

a After satisfactory anesthesia the lower eyelid is rotated with a cotton tipped applicator and the conjunctiva marked with line just beneath the lower border of the tarsal plate. The lower eyelid is retracted with two 4-0 silk sutures placed on a line lateral to the pupil and deep enough not to cut through the eyelid margin from inadvertent excessive traction. The conjunctiva is then injected with 1% lidocaine containing 1; 100,000 epinephrine.

b At the lateral canthus a 4 to 5 mm horizontal incision line is marked at the lateral commissure. The area is then infiltrated with 1% lidocaine containing 1:100,000 epinephrine. After allowing for vasoconstrictive effects the skin is incised through the orbicularis oculi muscle down to the periosteum of the frontal process of the zygoma. The lateral canthus is subsequently incised and the periosteum elevated off the underlying zygoma.

c The conjunctiva is incised and the upper edge of the mucosa is secured with two 4-0 silk sutures placed in a line lateral to the pupil. These sutures are used as retractors bringing the mucosal flap over the pupil while protecting the eye. Through the conjunctival incision the surgeon gently spreads the tissues with a mosquito clamp establishing a plane above the orbital septum and below the lower eyelid orbicularis oculi muscle. The dissection is continued to the orbital rim and then carried laterally, cutting more conjunctiva until the dissection reaches the lateral canthus.

d,e Using a malleable retractor to hold and protect the orbital septum and orbital fat, and a Senn retractor to retract the lower eyelid downward, an incision is made through the orbital rim periosteum. The periosteum is elevated inferiorly about 1 cm and superiorly along the frontal process of the zygoma to reach the frontal suture line.

f The zygoma fracture is subsequently reduced and stabilized with the technique(s) described above. The periosteum is loosely closed with 3-0 or 4-0 chromic sutures and the conjunctiva with two 6-0 fast-absorbing chromic sutures placed medially and laterally to the pupil. The lateral canthus is closed with repair of the orbicularis oculi muscle and coaptation of the skin with 5-0 nylon sutures.

This technique can be quicker than the infraciliary approach, but it requires finesse and understanding of orbital anatomy. Magnification and use of small instruments are helpful. The procedure has potentially the same complications as the infraciliary approach, except excessive scarring in this case causes entropion rather than ectropion and, if this occurs, consultation with ophthalmology is advisable.

ALTERNATIVE TECHNIQUE FOR REPAIR OF BLOW-IN FRACTURES

Downward and rotatory forces on the zygoma can cause the bone to be displaced into the orbit. Characteristic signs and symptoms are depression of the cheek, hyperophthalmos (elevation of the globe), and exophthalmos. The zygomatic arch may be displaced laterally. A step deformity can be observed or palpated along the inferior orbital rim. There may also be difficulty in opening and closing of the mouth and double vision on upward and downward gaze. A tent-shaped configuration of the floor of the orbit and a medial displacement of the lateral maxilla on CT scan confirm the diagnosis.

a' The blow-in fracture should be explored through the transconjunctival and lateral canthotomy or infraciliary (or high eyelid) and lateral eyebrow incisions. Infiltration of the incision sites with 1% lidocaine containing 1:100,000 epinephrine should be considered for hemostasis.

b',c' Blow-in fractures are explored as described for the laterally displaced zygoma (see earlier). Reduction is accomplished by elevation in an anterior and lateral direction. Fixation is obtained by application of miniplates at fracture sites. Closure of the incision and postoperative care are identical to those used in other zygoma repairs.

TRANSCONJUCTIVAL APPROACH

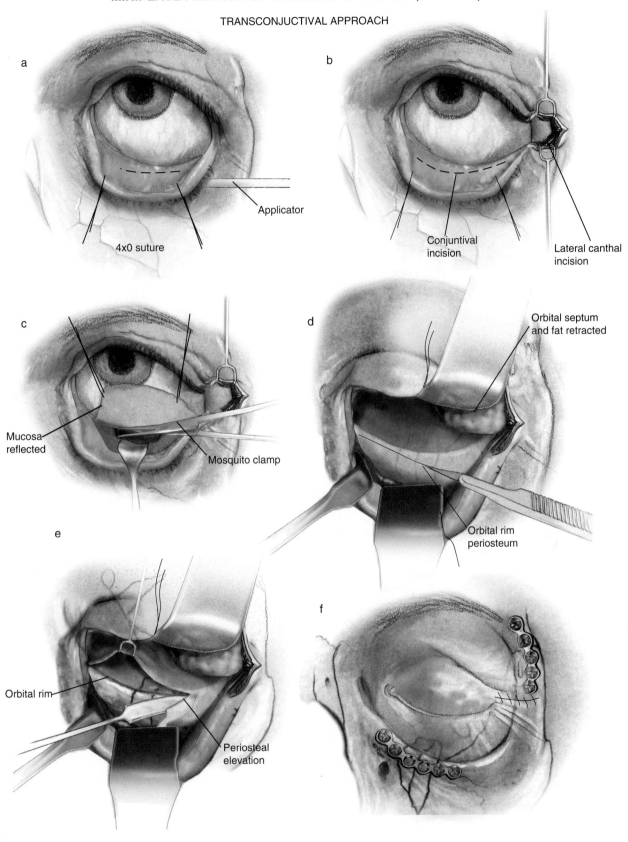

a

4x0 suture

Applicator

b

Conjuntival
incision

Lateral canthal
incision

c

Mucosa
reflected

Mosquito clamp

d

Orbital septum
and fat retracted

Orbital rim
periosteum

e

Orbital rim

Periosteal
elevation

f

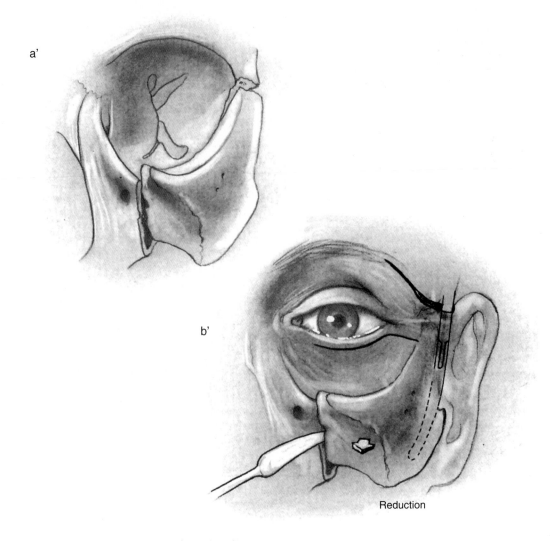

a'

b'

Reduction

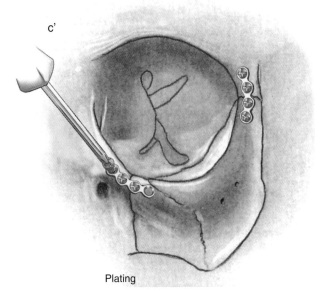

c'

Plating

Repair of Malunited Zygoma Fracture With Osteotomies
Alternative Technique Using a Coronal Approach

INDICATIONS

Residual deformity following zygoma fractures presents a formidable challenge. Depression of the cheek is often associated with enophthalmos, hypophthalmos, and limitations in mastication and conjugate gaze. If some healing has taken place, it is possible to osteotomize the fractured lines and reset the zygoma into proper position with plating techniques. However, if the processes of the zygoma have undergone resorption, then the bone will be unstable following osteotomy and adjunctive bone grafts become important.

PROCEDURE

A Osteotomies can be performed through the standard eyelid, transconjunctival, infraciliary, or high eyelid crease and eyebrow incisions (see Chapter 57). General anesthesia and infiltration of the incision with 1% lidocaine containing epinephrine are desirable to help control hemostasis.

B,C It is important in this procedure to strip the periosteum from the fracture lines. Through the eyebrow incision, the soft tissues of the orbit should be retracted medially and the periosteum elevated along the zygoma-sphenoid suture line to the inferior orbital fissure. The periosteum is also elevated off the posterior wall of the frontal process. A tunnel is developed beneath the zygomatic arch to the lateral maxillary wall. Using the infraciliary approach, the floor of the orbit should be explored and the periosteum elevated posteriorly to the junction of the infraorbital canal and inferior orbital fissure. The periosteum should also be elevated laterally to connect with the dissection that was performed through the eyebrow incision. Additionally, periosteum should be released from the anterior wall of the maxilla and zygoma to expose the zygomaticomaxillary buttress.

D Following these maneuvers, the fractures (or suture lines) should be evaluated. The soft tissues of the cheek should be retracted and osteotomies carried out through the fracture lines with sharp-pointed 3- to 4-mm osteotomes. The initial cut is started at the zygomaticofrontal suture and follows the fracture or suture line to the inferior orbital fissure. The next cut starts at the inferior orbital rim and follows the fracture laterally to the inferior orbital fissure. The osteotome is then turned and directed downward along the lateral face of the maxilla through the zygomaticomaxillary buttress. A heavy clamp (Kelly) is then inserted underneath the zygomatic arch, and with an elevator directed through the inferior orbital rim osteotomy, the zygoma is rocked and lifted into the preferred position (see Chapter 57). The arch or any other parts of the malar bone that were not osteotomized will usually fracture along the natural suture lines.

E The zygoma should be fixed with miniplates applied to the zygomaticofrontal buttress and inferior orbital rim (see Chapter 57). Closure of the wounds and postoperative care are identical to those used in the repair of zygoma fractures.

PITFALLS

1. The osteotomy technique is best applied to fractures that have partially healed and can be opened with a "nudge" of the osteotome. If the bones have healed completely and the fracture sites have undergone resorption, the zygoma will not "fit." Bone grafts will have to be placed behind the osteotomy sites to secure a firm fixation, or alternatively, bone grafts will need to be applied to the outer surface of the zygoma as described in Chapters 59, 64, and 65.

2. To avoid entry into the intracranial cavity while performing the osteotomies, the osteotome should be at or below the suture lines. The osteotome should also just penetrate the bone, so that if there is dura beneath the osteotomy site, it will not be cut. Postoperatively the patient should be observed closely for development of any intracranial signs or symptoms.

3. If the zygoma cannot be reduced following the osteotomies described previously, the surgeon should consider another osteotomy through the junction of the arch and the body of the zygoma. As an alternative to the eyebrow incision, the surgeon can use a coronal approach and expose even more of the arch for the osteotomy (see later and Chapter 50).

4. Avoid using oscillating saws for the osteotomy. The width of the saw determines the width of the cut, and removal of too much bone can affect the fixation. For these reasons, use of the sharp, thin osteotome is preferred. It also provides for irregularities in the bone that can be used to hold the zygoma in its natural position.

COMPLICATIONS

1. The most feared complication of the osteotomy technique is a dural tear, which can be associated with bleeding and cerebrospinal fluid leak. Usually the tear can be avoided by keeping the osteotome shallow and just below the cranium. Should the patient develop or experience any intracranial signs and symptoms, neurosurgical consultation should be immediately obtained.

2. Instability of the fragments following osteotomy can be a problem. This can be somewhat avoided by early diagnosis, narrow osteotomies, and rigid internal fixation with miniplates. Deficits at the osteotomy site should be filled with free bone grafts from the parietal or hip region.

3. Blindness is a possibility, especially if the fracture extends into the retrobulbar and optic nerve regions. Direct compression of the optic nerve, retrobulbar hemorrhage, and retinal artery occlusion are all possible. These complications should be recognized and treated immediately (see Chapter 62); ophthalmologic consultation should be obtained.

4. Exposure of the zygomatic arch places the frontal branches of the facial nerve at risk. Injury can be avoided with judicious use of retraction and limitation of the dissection to a subperiosteal plane over the arch.

ALTERNATIVE TECHNIQUE USING A CORONAL APPROACH

a,b A zygoma osteotomy can also be carried out through a standard coronal approach. The incision is the same as that described in Chapter 43, except that the dissection is continued along the frontal process of the zygoma and superficial temporal fascia to the zygomatic arch. In carrying out the dissection, the surgeon should recognize that the deep temporal artery has a branch that comes through the fascia, and the frontal branch of the facial nerve lies in the soft tissues just superficial to the fascia. Also, the fascia becomes continuous at the superficial musculoaponeurotic layer just above and lateral to the arch. Exposure from above, however, will show most of the arch, the frontal process, and the lateral half of the body, but the floor of the orbit cannot be appreciated. To give this exposure, the surgeon should use a lower eyelid (infraciliary, subtarsal or transconjunctival) approach.

c–e The subperiosteal elevation and osteotomy maneuvers are identical to those used for the direct exposure method described earlier. The surgeon can additionally osteotomize the zygomatic arch. Plate fixation should be applied and the flap replaced and closed in a routine fashion. The patient is placed on prophylactic antibiotics for 5 to 7 days, and the zygoma is clinically and radiographically evaluated for adequacy of reduction and fixation.

OSTEOTOMIES OF THE ZYGOMA

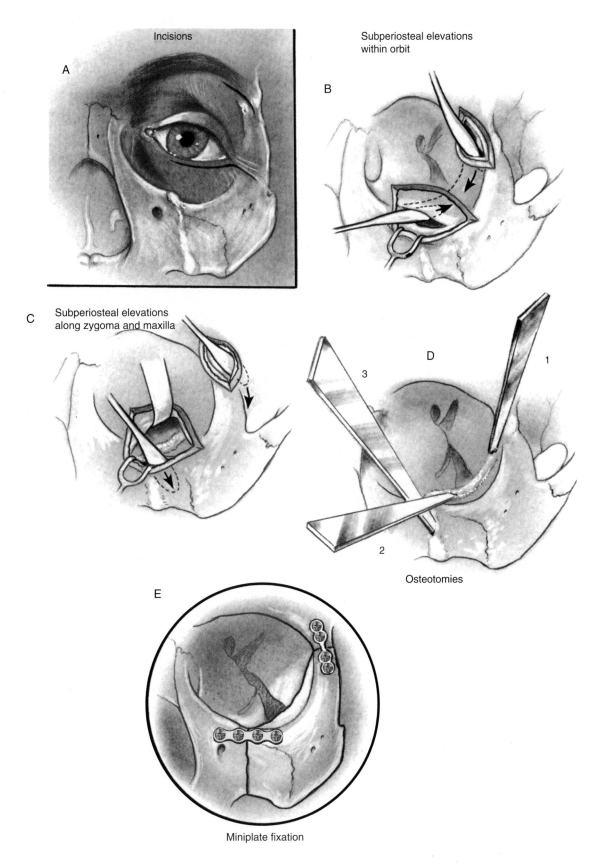

A — Incisions

B — Subperiosteal elevations within orbit

C — Subperiosteal elevations along zygoma and maxilla

D — Osteotomies

E — Miniplate fixation

OSTEOTOMIES OF THE ZYGOMA

ALTERNATIVE TECHNIQUE USING CORONAL APPROACH

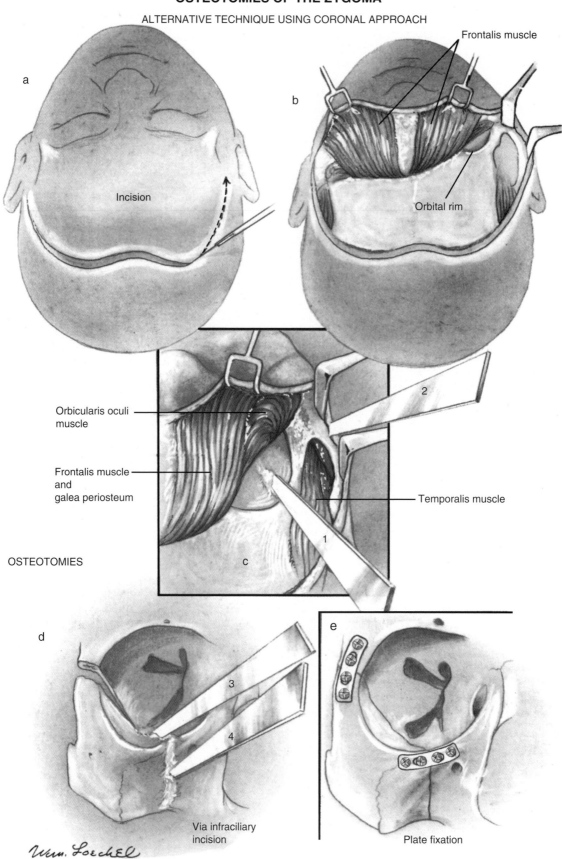

a

Incision

b

Frontalis muscle

Orbital rim

Orbicularis oculi
muscle

Frontalis muscle
and
galea periosteum

Temporalis muscle

OSTEOTOMIES

c

1

2

d

3

4

Via infraciliary
incision

e

Plate fixation

Treatment of Malunited Zygoma Fracture With Onlay Hip Grafts
Alternative Technique Using a Coronal Approach and Cranial Grafts
Alternative Technique Using Rib Grafts

INDICATIONS

The malpositioned, completely healed zygoma fracture is probably best treated with onlay bone grafts. When the zygoma fracture heals, the bony processes are absorbed and sutures and fracture lines obliterated. Under such conditions, osteotomy is difficult to perform, and even with a freeing up of the bone, there will be marked instability and a probable need for adjunctive grafts. The zygoma onlay graft technique is also suitable for those patients in whom the orbit or other parts of the facial skeleton need grafting. The procedure will not help alleviate associated trismus or difficulty in mastication resulting from the zygoma impinging on the coronoid process. For the latter condition, osteotomy and/or intraoral coronoidectomy should be considered (see Chapter 22).

For the augmentation of the zygoma, autogenous grafts are preferred to alloplastic implants. Rejection and infection are rare with the autogenous graft that is eventually incorporated into the adjacent bony skeleton. Disadvantages are the need to harvest the graft through a separate incision and the increased morbidity of a second procedure.

PROCEDURE

The face, neck, and hip should be prepared and draped as a sterile field. The hip graft is obtained as described in Chapters 35 and 64. Either hip can be used, as the graft can be contoured and bent into a variety of shapes. Ideally the graft should have a curvature that corresponds to the cheek, but if the graft needs to be bent further, this can be achieved by partial osteotomies with Lindeman burs through the outer cortical layers. The bone graft can then be bent to the contour of the anterior maxilla and zygomatic processes. Additional contouring can be obtained with cutting burs.

A,B Exposure for onlay grafting is accomplished through an infraciliary incision extended through a "crow's foot" crease. To reduce bleeding, the area should be infiltrated with 1% lidocaine containing epinephrine. The proper plane is easily obtained by incising between the orbicularis oculi and the septum orbitale. The tarsal plate should be protected during these maneuvers by leaving a small strip of muscle on the plate. The dissection should continue to the inferior orbital rim. A periosteal incision is then made over the anterior wall of the maxilla just beneath the rim. A cuff of soft tissue is elevated superiorly, and the floor of the orbit is explored to the junction of the infraorbital canal and inferior orbital fissure. The subperiosteal dissection should continue laterally to free up the periosteal attachments along the frontal process of the zygoma and the outer wall of the orbit. This will relax the lateral canthal ligament. Additionally, periosteum is elevated off the anterior arch and the body of the zygoma. Medially the infraorbital nerve is exposed; if it is in the way of grafting, it should be sacrificed. To obtain appropriate contour, the subperiosteal dissection may often have to be extended to the lateral aspect of the nasal bones.

C–E The bone graft is shaped to fit over the maxilla and zygoma and adjusted to the desired level in relation to the orbital rim. Several additional small pieces of bone are then placed on top of the frontal process of the zygoma and the anterior floor of the orbit. These additional pieces of bone are used to construct a smooth orbital wall. The bone is held firmly with lag screw technique (Chapter 24) and the sides and edges contoured with cutting burs. The periosteum is closed with 2-0 chromic sutures. The infraciliary incision is closed with a running 5-0 nylon subcuticular suture. A light compression dressing is applied to help stabilize the grafts and prevent swelling.

Postoperatively the patient is maintained on intravenous antibiotics. The reconstruction is inspected every 2 to 3 days with appropriate dressing changes. The dressings are maintained for approximately 10 days, and the sutures are removed at 5 to 7 days.

PITFALLS

1. Ideally the zygoma graft should be one piece of bone. This will ensure more stability and a smoother contour of the cheek. Fracture of the graft can be avoided by using sharp, cutting instruments and gentle handling of the bone. Osteotomies performed in preparation for bending of the graft should be strategically placed through the cortex, and bending should be done with just enough force to bend without breaking the bone. If the graft should fracture, each part can be applied to the malar and maxillary bones separately and immobilized with lag screws and tight periosteal closure.

2. Do not rely on remodeling to create a smooth cheek contour. Fill all defects and cracks with pieces of cancellous bone.

3. Dressings are important and must be properly placed if they are to assist in stabilization of the graft. The eye should be treated with an ophthalmic ointment and two eye pads placed over the closed eyelid. Fluff dressings are then built up over the cheek, around the ear, and over the eye and held with wraps of stretch type dressings. A figure-of-eight design around the upper neck and chin is helpful in keeping the dressing in a desired position.

COMPLICATIONS

1. Movement of the graft can result in an irregularity of the cheek and subsequent failure to correct the deformity. This complication can be avoided by securing the grafts with lag screws and heavy chromic sutures through the periosteum and by the dressings described earlier. The patient also should be instructed to avoid any pressure and contact activities that could affect the grafted area.

2. Irregularity of the graft can develop with time. Resorption is unpredictable and occurs in a spotty fashion. A palpable and noticeable irregularity of the cheek can be corrected by exposing the graft through the same incision and smoothing it with cutting burs.

3. Infection can jeopardize the survival of the graft and can be avoided with the use of prophylactic antibiotics, atraumatic techniques, and optimal hemostasis. The patient should also be evaluated for any active infection of the sinus(es) that, unless brought under control, would preclude the bone graft procedure. If infection develops, the wound should be debrided and cultures obtained. Failure to control the infection requires removal of the graft.

ALTERNATIVE TECHNIQUE USING A CORONAL APPROACH AND CRANIAL GRAFTS

The zygoma can also be approached by combining parietal onlay grafts with coronal and infraciliary eyelid incisions. The coronal approach is described in Chapter 58. Harvest of the bone graft is discussed in detail in Chapter 64. The grafts will have a natural curve, but unfortunately they are brittle, and there is little capability to bend the graft further without causing a fracture. Thicker grafts can be obtained by placing grafts on top of one another and securing them with heavy chromic sutures. Also, the sides and edges can be beveled to the appropriate contour. Resorption is believed to be less with cranial grafts than with grafts from the rib or hip region.

ONLAY HIP GRAFTS FOR MALUNION OF THE ZYGOMA

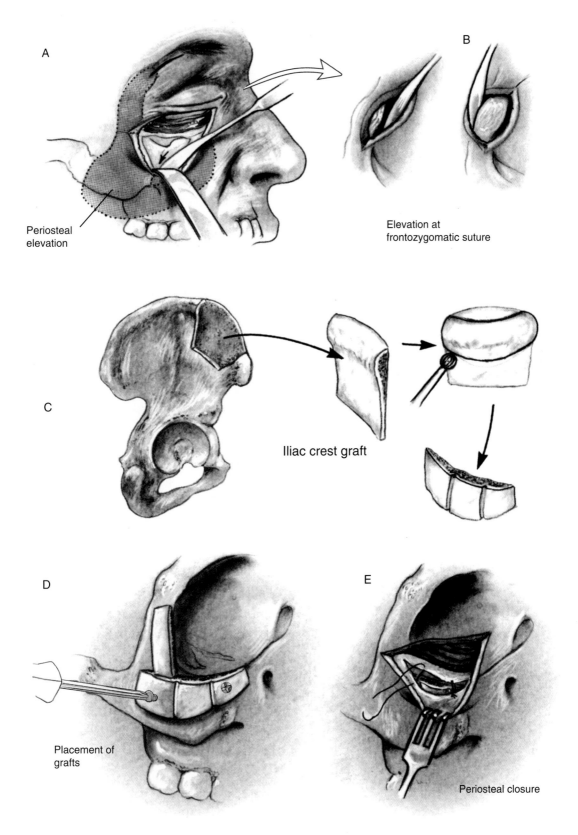

A

Periosteal
elevation

B

Elevation at
frontozygomatic suture

C

Iliac crest graft

D

Placement of
grafts

E

Periosteal closure

Wm. Loechel

ALTERNATIVE TECHNIQUE
USING CRANIAL GRAFTS

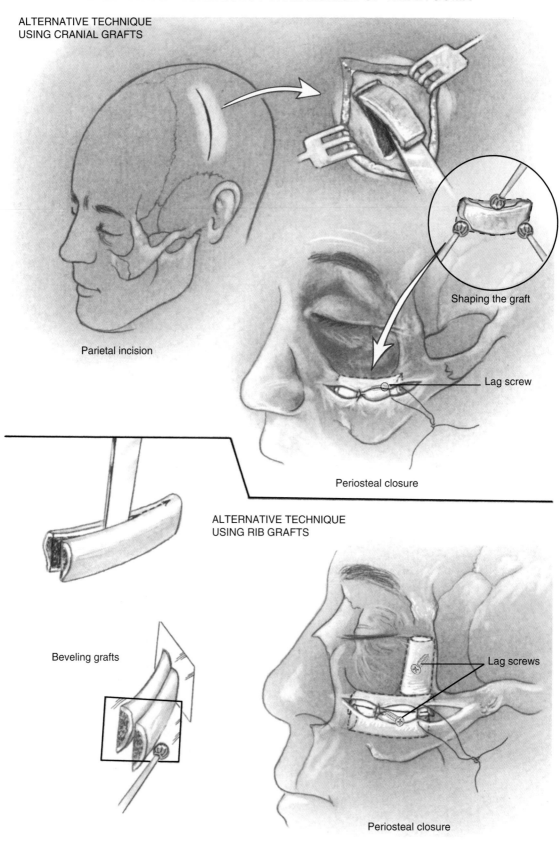

Parietal incision

Shaping the graft

Lag screw

Periosteal closure

ALTERNATIVE TECHNIQUE
USING RIB GRAFTS

Beveling grafts

Lag screws

Periosteal closure

ALTERNATIVE TECHNIQUE USING RIB GRAFTS

Rib grafts are ideal to use as onlay grafts for the malar deformity. Harvesting of the rib graft is described in Chapter 27. When split, the grafts can be bent to exact curvature, and multiple grafts can be placed on top of each other for additional thickness. The grafts are beveled and secured beneath the periosteum with 2-0 chromic sutures. The major disadvantage of the rib graft is that absorption is very unpredictable and often exceeds that observed with other graft methods.

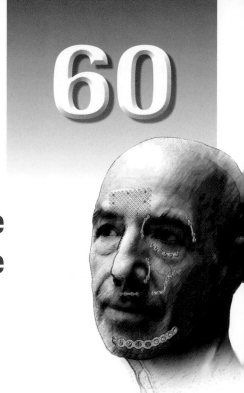

Decompression of the Infraorbital Nerve

INDICATIONS

Fracture of the zygoma is often associated with loss of sensation over the cheek and upper dentition. Return of sensation is variable, and occasionally the patient develops pain and paresthesias. If an injection of 2% lidocaine to the infraorbital foramen alleviates this pain, then the surgeon should consider a decompression of the infraorbital nerve.

PROCEDURE

A–D Under general anesthesia, the face is prepared and draped as a sterile field. Bleeding is partially controlled with a prior injection of 1% lidocaine containing 1:100,000 epinephrine. An infraciliary or transconjunctival incision will provide adequate exposure.

The skin-muscle flap, which is lifted between the orbicularis oculi fibers and the septum orbitale, should be used to gain access to the anterior wall of the maxilla (see Chapter 57). The orbicularis oculi and zygomaticus muscle attachments are cut and the periosteum is incised just beneath the inferior orbital rim. The periosteum is elevated off the superior wall of the maxilla to expose the infraorbital nerve and foramen. Using a sharp elevator (Cottle), the nerve is dissected free from the foramen. The foramen can be enlarged with rongeurs; additional depressed fragments are elevated from the floor of the orbit and either removed or replaced into anatomic position. The wound is then closed in layers.

PITFALLS

1. The results of infraorbital nerve decompression are variable. If the patient does not obtain relief, there is always the option of reoperating and lysing the nerve. However, the surgeon must be aware of the neural supply carried by other branches of the infraorbital nerve through the maxilla and recognize that the decompression is aimed only at the anterior portion of the nerve that innervates the cheek tissues and the anterior upper dentition.

2. The patient must be warned that the procedure may also cause hypoesthesia. Scar tissue at the foramen can make the dissection difficult, and the nerve can be inadvertently injured.

3. Neuromas at the foramen are not easily treated. Decompression will not help in such cases, and it is more practical to lyse the nerve and remove the mass of neural tissues.

COMPLICATIONS

Probably the most common complication of the procedure is the return of hypoesthesia. The patient should be warned of this possibility, and the surgeon should take precautions to prevent it from happening. Scar tissues at the foramen should be gently teased from the nerve. The rongeurs should be directed away from neural tissues, and depressed fragments of bone in the infraorbital canal should be elevated or removed.

DECOMPRESSION OF INFRAORBITAL NERVE

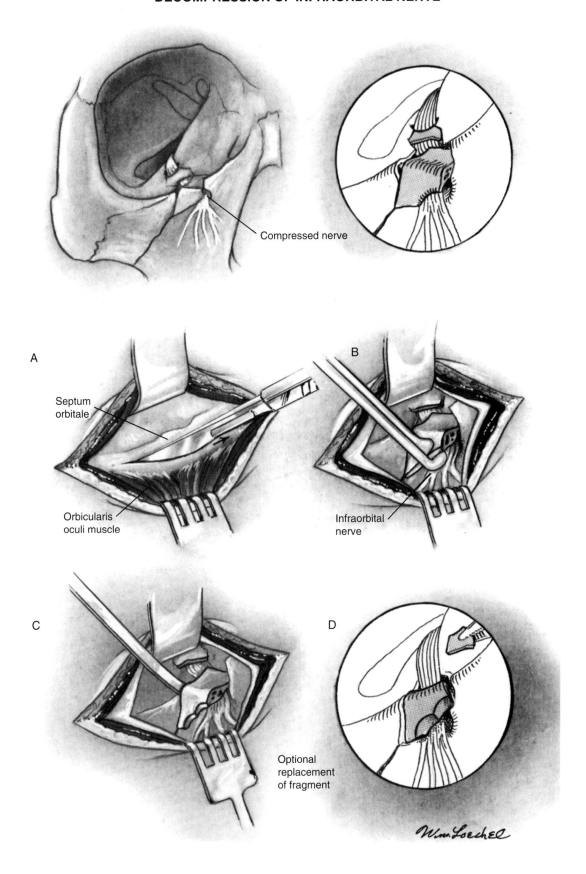

Compressed nerve

A

Septum orbitale

Orbicularis oculi muscle

B

Infraorbital nerve

C

Optional replacement of fragment

D

Wm. Loechel

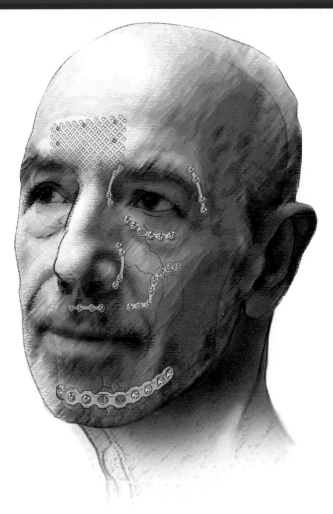

PART SEVEN

Orbital Wall Fractures

Classification and Pathophysiology of Orbital Wall Fractures

CHAPTER

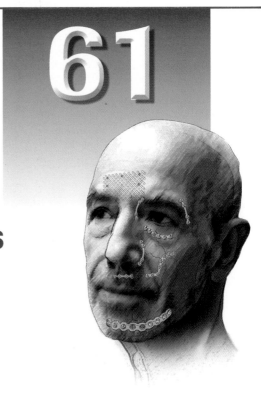

61

General Considerations

A–C The most common site of a blowout fracture is the orbital floor, but similar injuries can be noted, in order of prevalence, on the medial, lateral, and superior walls. The pure blow-out fracture is generally understood as a trap-door rotation of bone fragments involving the central area of a wall. However, if the injury is associated with a fracture line extending to one of the orbital rims, it is then considered an impure type of fracture. The impure fractures are commonly found with malar, maxillary, naso-orbital, and frontal bone fractures.

D–F The defect created by the blow-out fracture is variable in size and often filled with soft tissues of the orbit. Significant defects will translate into an increase in the orbital volume described by the walls and a reduction of intraorbital contents. These events can lead to the clinical appearance of hypophthalmos and/or enophthalmos.

The fat tissues that enter the blow-out contain fibrous septae, which in turn support the position and mechanical activity of the extraocular muscles. In a small defect, the muscles may become trapped, but it is usually the septae that are displaced, and it is this change in position of the septae that causes alterations in muscle performance. Changes in the globe position can also have an impact on the tension and contraction of the muscle. In addition, there is a possibility of direct neural and/or muscular damage. All of these factors, alone or together, can cause a failure in conjugate gaze and produce the symptom of diplopia.

Different sites and sizes of the wall defect produce different clinical pictures. Large defects on the floor often cause hypophthalmos and/or enophthalmos, but because the large opening does not usually trap muscle or fat, extraocular movements can be excellent, and diplopia should not occur. However, small defects of the floor can entrap the fat and/or muscle, restrict muscle activity, and cause diplopia on upward gaze; enophthalmos or hypophthalmos should be a minor complaint. Defects on the medial wall, depending on

BLOWOUT FRACTURES

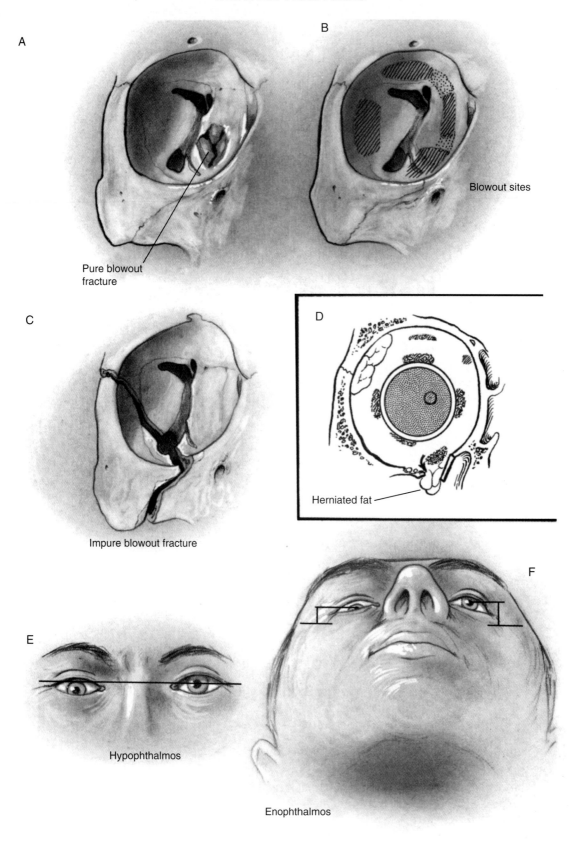

A

B

Pure blowout
fracture

Blowout sites

C

D

Impure blowout fracture

Herniated fat

E

Hypophthalmos

F

Enophthalmos

Wm. Loechel

size, can be associated with enophthalmos; if a muscle is disturbed, it is usually the medial rectus, which in turn can affect medial and lateral gaze. Injuries affecting the junction of the medial and inferior walls are often relatively large, and enophthalmos will usually be apparent. Fractures of the other walls of the orbit can also affect volume/content relationships of the orbit and muscle activities; these effects are generally determined by the size of the wall defect and relationship of the muscle to the injured wall.

CHAPTER

62

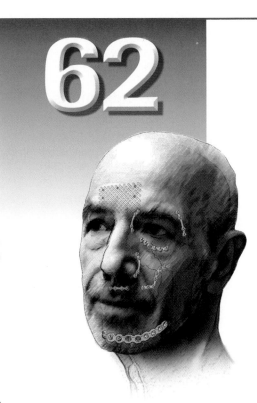

Repair of Blowout Floor Fracture With Polypropylene Mesh
Alternative Techniques Using Parietal Cortex Bone Graft or Titanium Mesh Implant
Alternative Technique Using Transconjuctival Approach
Alternative Technique Using the Antrostomy Approach With Endoscopic Option

INDICATIONS

Most blowout fractures need to be repaired surgically; some can be treated by conservative management. Usually the latter are associated with minimal displacement of an orbital wall and no diplopia. These conditions, however, must be substantiated with CT scans and by repeated examinations; otherwise, what appears to be an unimportant injury becomes associated with a progressive malposition of the globe, neuromuscular imbalance, and persistent deformity and dysfunction. There are both absolute and relative indications for exploration and corrective surgery to avoid these sequelae.

Absolute Indications

1. Acute enophthalmos (>2 to 3 mm) and/or hypophthalmos (>2 to 3 mm)

2. Mechanical restriction of gaze associated with diplopia

Relative Indications

1. Conditions that can later cause enophthalmos and/or hypophthalmos; theoretically, 2 to 3 mm of a 1.5- to 2-cm^2 area of displaced wall or soft tissue noted on CT scan can cause these deformities.

Generally, displacement of a wall can be recognized and evaluated on horizontal and coronal CT scans. Some devices are equipped to perform computer-generated volumes of the orbit, but unfortunately, the variability in the volumes normally between eyes precludes the use of the opposite unaffected eye as a control. Moreover, there are no absolute measurements that determine the degree of volume change.

2. Persistence of diplopia, presumably caused by small defects and mechanical changes that are not perceptible by forced duction tests; such cases should have no evidence of neural injury.

The timing of surgery is important. Surgery performed too early can be associated with an inaccurate diagnosis, swelling that obscures surgical planes and anatomic landmarks, and excessive bleeding that accompanies the inflammatory phase of healing, whereas exploration performed too late may reveal malunion and resorption of bone with contraction of soft tissues by scar. Therefore surgery is best performed at 7 to 10 days. If associated craniofacial fractures are also to be treated, the procedures should be coordinated so that they can be carried out at the same time. In general, children will heal early and should be done early. Adults can be delayed for 10 to 12 days. Additional delays can compromise results, but it is still worthwhile to attempt a repair up to 4 to 6 weeks after injury.

PROCEDURE

A pure blowout fracture of the floor can be approached through an infraciliary, high eyelid (subtarsal) or transconjunctival (see later) incision. The infraciliary incision is designed 2 to 3 mm below the cilia of the lower eyelid, just lateral to the puncta. If injuries of the malar bone must be repaired, the incision can be extended laterally into one of the "crow's foot" creases. The alternative high eyelid (subtarsal) incision is designed about 5 to 7 mm below the cilia in a crease line medial to a line perpendicular to the pupil of the eye. Limiting the length of this incision will help minimize postoperative edema.

B–D The incision should be injected with 1% lidocaine containing 1:100,000 epinephrine to help control hemostasis. Using a sharp knife, the surgeon cuts both skin and the orbicularis oculi muscle fibers. The dissection then proceeds in a plane between the orbicularis oculi muscle and the orbital septum inferiorly, until the surgeon reaches the level of the anterior maxillary wall. Using a malleable retractor to hold and protect the septum orbitale and another retractor to pull the eyelid downward, an incision is made 5 mm below the rim through the orbicularis oculi-zygomaticus muscles and periosteal attachments. This incision should avoid injury to the infraorbital nerve and artery, which lie just medial and inferior to the area of dissection.

E,F The periosteum and attached soft tissues are released with a Joseph elevator. The subperiosteal dissection continues over the orbital rim and onto the floor of the orbit. Lighting and control of bleeding are very important, as the surgeon must be able to see each maneuver and identify the different types of tissue attached to the floor region. Using a Freer elevator, the periosteum is lifted medially and laterally to the defect. The attached or extravasated soft tissues can then be teased out with a smaller Cottle elevator. The dissection proceeds posteriorly and, to ensure completeness of the procedure, the dissection should expose the junction of the infraorbital canal and inferior orbital fissure.

After soft tissues are elevated from the defect, the bony trap-door deformity should be reduced. This can be accomplished by dropping a small, single skin hook beneath the fragment, twisting the hook to engage the fragment, and elevating the fragment into position. Other depressed fragments are treated identically. The area of fracture is then reinforced with a piece of polypropylene (Marlex) mesh so that the mesh covers the defect and adjoining intact floor.

G,H Forced ductions are performed, and if reduction is satisfactory, the periosteum is closed with a single

REPAIR OF BLOWOUT FLOOR FRACTURE

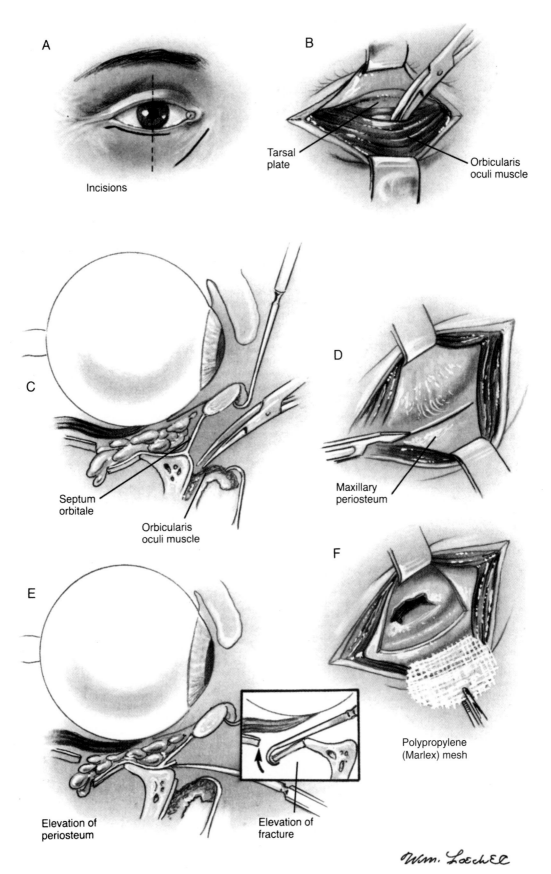

A

Incisions

B

Tarsal plate

Orbicularis oculi muscle

C

Septum orbitale

Orbicularis oculi muscle

D

Maxillary periosteum

E

Elevation of periosteum

Elevation of fracture

F

Polypropylene (Marlex) mesh

Wm. Loechel

G

H

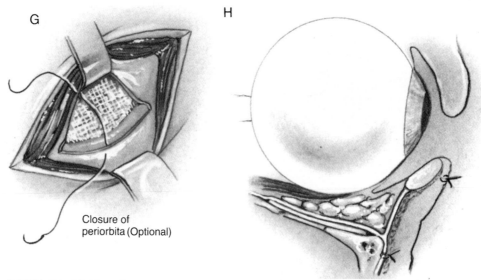

Closure of
periorbita (Optional)

ALTERNATIVE TECHNIQUE USING PARIETAL CORTEX GRAFT or TITANIUM MESH IMPLANT

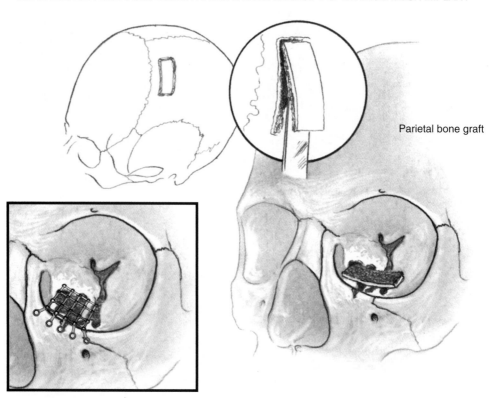

Parietal bone graft

Titanium mesh implant

3-0 chromic suture. The skin is approximated with a 5-0 subcuticular nylon suture. Prophylactic antibiotics are administered for 5 days. The patient should be evaluated at 1 week and monthly thereafter to ensure stability and uneventful healing.

PITFALLS

1. Accurate diagnosis is essential for proper management. Historical and clinical examination should be complemented by CT scans in the horizontal and coronal planes. An ophthalmology consultation is highly recommended.

2. Measurements of enophthalmos and hypophthalmos can be compromised by swelling of the tissues and/or a displacement of the reference point (the lateral wall of the orbit). It is therefore important that a final evaluation be delayed until the swelling has disappeared. If the wall of the orbit is displaced, projection of the globes in relationship to the cheeks and forehead can be estimated by visualizing these structures tangentially from above or below the patient.

3. Restriction of muscle activity should be suspected when there is diplopia and nonconjugate movement. Confirmation should be obtained by forced duction tests and radiographic evidence of disruption of the orbital wall near the affected muscle.

4. Contraindications to repair of the floor are hyphema, retinal tear and detachment, and globe perforation. Traumatic optic neuropathy and retinal artery occlusion are also important considerations. Surgery should also not be performed on an only-seeing eye.

5. Timing of surgery is important. Early exploration and repair coupled with an accurate diagnosis are necessary for successful results. An optimal time for surgery is 7 to 10 days after injury.

6. Avoid damage to the tarsal plate. The orbicularis oculi inserts onto the lower portion of the plate, and to be safe, a cuff of these tissues should be left on the plate. Scarring in and around the tarsal plate can lead to retraction of the lower eyelid.

7. Keep eyelid incisions small. Long eyelid incisions compromise lymphatic drainage and cause postoperative edema.

8. Orbital fat herniating into the sinus must be treated with atraumatic techniques. Avoid direct injury or amputation of fat, as this causes necrosis and/or resorption. Changes in intraorbital contents will ultimately affect the globe position.

9. Injury to the infraorbital artery should be avoided, but if this should occur, gentle pressure will control the bleeding. Bipolar cauterization or vascular clips can be applied to the bleeding vessel.

10. Polypropylene (Marlex) mesh is the preferred implant in the treatment of the blow out fracture that is diagnosed and treated early after injury. It has an excellent record of providing good results without the adverse sequelae reported with other types of alloplastic materials. Silastic tends to extravasate and must be anchored into position. Autogenous bone grafts, if too thin (i.e., from the anterior wall of the maxilla), tend to resorb. Autografts from the cranium tend to be too thick and are difficult to mold to appropriate wall contours. Titanium mesh implants are a reasonable alternative (see later), but they are quite expensive and are very difficult to manage should revision be necessary. On the other hand, the bone graft or, alternatively, the titanium mesh implant may be necessary when there is insufficient bone in the floor to support the polypropylene mesh in anatomic position.

11. When the orbital floor has undergone healing and fusion of malpositioned bone fragments, a more aggressive approach is required. These fractures may require reduction with a strong elevator. Sometimes the entrapped tissues have to be freed by cutting away areas of the depressed wall with Kerrison rongeurs. The defect can be subsequently repaired with the appropriate implant.

12. Fractures that are more posteriorly and medially oriented may require a transantral approach for adequate reduction (see later). The anterior antrostomy should be large enough to allow the surgeon to visualize the floor region and admit a finger for palpation and reduction of the fragments. This approach ideally should be performed in combination with one of the eyelid approaches so that the floor can also be inspected from above and reinforced with polyethylene mesh. Alternatively, the orbital floor can be inspected from below by just an intranasal antrostomy and endoscopic visualization. The repair can be managed with endoscopic instruments. Maxillary packing is rarely indicated. If the floor fragments do not hold in a reduced position, the surgeon should consider a more substantial implant, such as a titanium mesh implant or bone graft (see later).

13. For large floor defects, polypropylene mesh will not provide sufficient support. In these cases, a bone graft or titanium mesh implant must be considered. The outer parietal cortex is the preferred donor site.

COMPLICATIONS

1. Loss of vision is probably the most dreaded complication associated with a blowout fracture. This loss can occur from an injury to the lens or cornea, hyphema, retinal tear, and/or globe perforation. Optic nerve injury and/or retinal artery occlusion can develop primarily from trauma near the optic canal or secondarily from excessive retraction on the globe, retro-orbital hemorrhage, and displacement of an implant. The medical condition of the eye and results of visual tests should be recorded. Surgery should be delayed if there are factors present that would predispose to additional injury. If the heart rate should fall during the procedure, this could mean impending injury to the optic nerve; the dissection should be halted and other approaches considered. If visual loss occurs following surgery, the condition should be recognized and treated immediately. If applicable, the surgeon should remove a displaced implant, control bleeding, remove accumulated clots, and reduce pressure on the retrobulbar area with a canthotomy and lysis of the periorbita. In addition, the surgeon can administer steroids and diuretics to relieve intraorbital and retro-orbital pressures.

2. Persistence of diplopia and/or enophthalmos may indicate an inadequate repair. In the early postoperative period, it is possible to reexplore and reduce the fracture and again reinforce the wall defect. In our experience satisfactory results can be obtained up to 6 weeks following surgery. Beyond that time, other alternatives such as orbital reconstruction with bone grafts should be considered (see Chapter 64).

3. Postoperative hypoesthesia is a common sequela following blowout fractures. The neural deficit may also be associated with paresthesia and pain over the distribution of the infraorbital nerve and its maxillary branches. Theoretically, an early and accurate reduction of the floor should prevent this complication from occurring and allow for regeneration of the nerve. If the complication persists, the surgeon can consider exploration of the nerve for a neuroma. Any compression phenomena can be treated by opening and decompressing the infraorbital canal (see Chapter 60).

4. Ectropion can usually be avoided by careful atraumatic technique. The tarsal plate should be protected and repeated cuts through the orbicularis muscle should be avoided. Reactive scarring can be minimized by closing the periosteum with only one chromic suture. If ectropion should start to develop, steroid injections (20 to 40 mg/mL) of triamcinolone should be started and the eyelid massaged daily. If the ectropion persists, the surgeon must consider lysis of the scar and/or split-thickness grafts applied to the skin.

ALTERNATIVE TECHNIQUE USING PARIETAL CORTEX GRAFT OR TITANIUM MESH IMPLANT

Occasionally the floor fracture extends along the floor to involve the medial wall and is so severely comminuted that polypropylene mesh is not able to provide sufficient support. For such a condition, a bone graft or a titanium mesh implant is desirable.

The bone graft is the preferred technique, and the outer cortex of the parietal bone is a preferred donor site. This area is within the same operative field as the injury and the graft can be harvested with minimal morbidity. Anterior maxillary wall grafts are not as satisfactory, because they tend to resorb. Iliac crest or rib grafts can be used, but they are more difficult to obtain and are often associated with added discomfort during the postoperative period.

The parietal cortex is exposed and the bone removed as described in Chapter 64. The graft is then rotated so that the curve approximates the floor (outer surface down), and the bone is trimmed appropriately with cutting burs and rongeurs. Because the graft will be only slightly resorbed (if at all), the amount of correction must be exact. If the graft tends to raise the floor to a higher level, this will cause hyperophthalmos, and the graft should be thinned accordingly. If the graft lies at a low level, it must be reinforced with other grafts to accommodate the loss of orbital volume. The graft is usually stabilized by closing the periosteum over it with 3-0 chromic sutures. The eyelid skin is approximated with a 5-0 subcuticular nylon suture, and the patient is treated with prophylactic antibiotics for at least 7 to 10 days.

The other alternative implant, titanium mesh, can be used with also effective results. The implant can be expensive, but is readily available. The technique obviously avoids donor site morbidity. The implant comes in many shapes and sizes but still must be bent to the contour of the floor, sometimes difficult to judge in severely damaged orbit. The implant is usually stabilized to the orbital rim with bone screws. The implant is rapidly incorporated into adjoining bony and soft tissues and this can pose a management problem if the patient requires revisional sugary.

ALTERNATIVE TECHNIQUE USING TRANSCONJUCTIVAL APPROACH

a–d The transconjuctival approach is a rapid and direct method to treat blowout fractures and is effective in avoiding ectropion. This technique is detailed in Chapter 57 but for the isolated blowout fracture does not require the canthotomy used for exposure of the lateral orbit. As noted, the procedure requires identification of the inferior border of the tarsal plate, the development of a mucosal flap to cover the pupil, and a careful dissection between the orbital septum and orbicularis oculi to the inferior orbital rim. Exposure of the floor and management of the defect is the same as described earlier. The main, but rare complication is entropion, and should this occur, ophthamology consultation is recommended.

ALTERNATIVE TECHNIQUE USING THE ANTROSTOMY APPROACH WITH ENDOSCOPIC OPTION

In fractures of the floor of the orbit characterized by severe injury, comminution of fragments, and extension of the fracture to the posterior portion of the orbit (ethmoid ledge), a transantral approach may be helpful. The procedure should be carried out in conjunction with the orbital exploration from above, so that as the surgeon reduces the fragments from below, the correct position can be ensured from more than one direction.

a′–d′ The approach is through an incision about 3 to 4 mm above the gingival margin from the first or second molar to the lateral incisor. Hemostasis is achieved with electric cautery. The periosteum is then elevated from the canine fossa superiorly onto the face of the maxilla. The dissection is continued superiorly to the level of the infraorbital canal, posteriorly to the zygomaticomaxillary buttress, and anteriorly to the nasofrontal buttress. An osteotomy is made in the anterior wall of the maxilla, and using Kerrison rongeurs, the opening is enlarged to approximately 2 × 3 cm. Blood is suctioned from the cavity, and the floor of the orbit is visualized from below.

e′ Assuming that the periorbita has already been elevated from the fracture site, the surgeon can then slip a finger through the antrostomy, palpate the fragments, and push the fragments into appropriate position. If the fragments do not stay in that position, the floor can be examined from above and appropriate adjustments carried out.

The surgeon may be tempted to pack the sinus from below, but this should be avoided. Packing of the maxillary sinus often leads to stasis of secretions, localized inflammation, and ultimate absorption of the floor. If the floor is unstable, we prefer instead to reinforce the floor of the orbit with a cranial bone graft.

f′ The maxilla should be drained with a small hole (1.5 cm in diameter) made through the medial wall of the maxilla, below the inferior turbinate, and into the nose. The gingival mucosa is closed with 4-0 chromic sutures. Prophylactic antibiotics are prescribed for 7 to 10 days.

g′ Alternatively, the blowout fracture can be evaluated and managed with endoscopic techniques. For this approach, the patient requires a small intranasal or anterior antrostomy (not both) and insertion of a nasal endoscope into the maxillary cavity. Other endoscopic instruments can be introduced through the antrostomy to push the fat back into the orbit, apply an implant to reinforce the floor and reduce the floor fracture. Instabilty of the repair following this approach requires balloon tamponade and/or further repair through one of the more traditional approaches described earlier. For the intranasal antrostomy, a soft tampon is placed into the inferior meatus. For the anterior antrostomy, the mucosa is closed with a 4-0 chromic suture. The patient is subsequently managed as with the other described techniques.

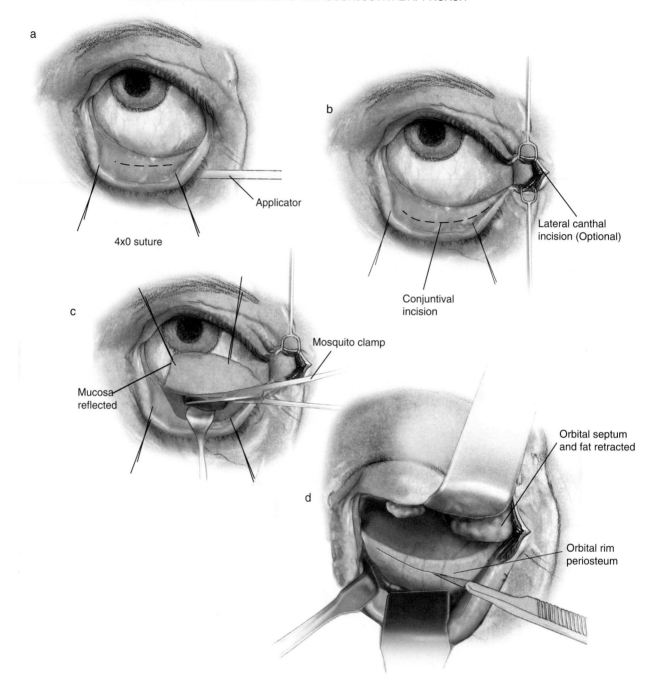

a

Applicator

4x0 suture

b

Lateral canthal
incision (Optional)

Conjuntival
incision

c

Mosquito clamp

Mucosa
reflected

d

Orbital septum
and fat retracted

Orbital rim
periosteum

REPAIR OF BLOWOUT FLOOR FRACTURE *(Continued)*

ALTERNATIVE ANTROSTOMY APPROACH

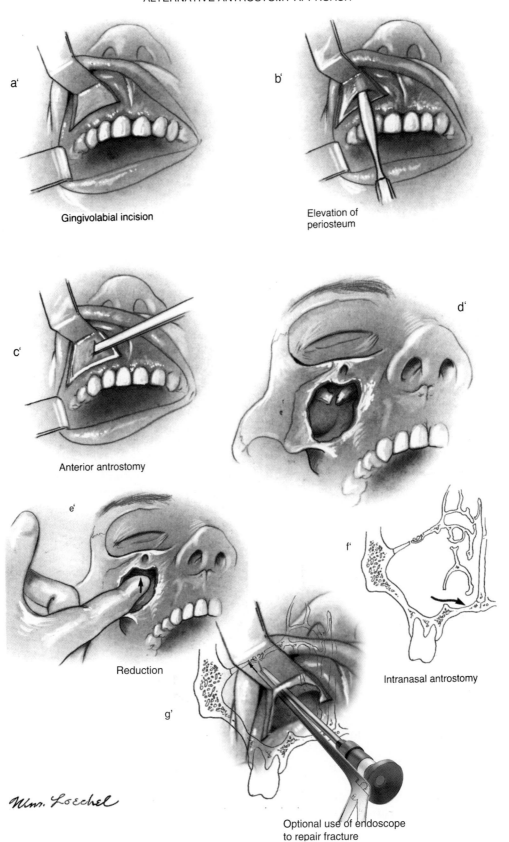

a'

Gingivolabial incision

b'

Elevation of
periosteum

c'

Anterior antrostomy

d'

e'

Reduction

f'

Intranasal antrostomy

g'

Optional use of endoscope
to repair fracture

Wm. Loechel

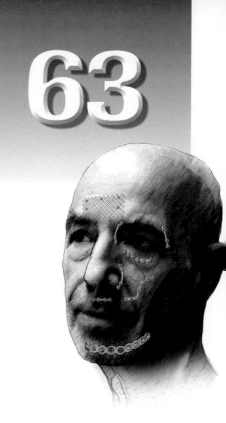

CHAPTER 63

Repair of Medial Wall Fractures of the Orbit With Polypropylene Mesh
Alternative Technique for Repair of Junctional Injuries

INDICATIONS

The same philosophy employed in the treatment of the floor fracture is applied to the management of the medial wall (see Chapter 62). Consequently, if the surgeon has a full understanding of the pathophysiology, uses appropriate indications for surgery, and applies standard surgical techniques, medial orbital wall surgery can provide for an effective repair with minimal or no sequelae.

Pure blow-out fractures of the medial wall often present with enophthalmos and/or diplopia. Defects that extend to the inferior wall (junctional type) produce significant intraorbital volume-to-content discrepancies and thus are often associated with marked retrodisplacement of the globe. Smaller defects occurring near the medial rectus muscle can cause displacement of the muscle and subsequent impairment of movement. Fractures on the deeper aspect of the medial wall can additionally affect inferior rectus functions, and if the injury extends to the optic canal, a loss of vision can occur.

Absolute indications for surgical exploration include the following:

1. Acute enophthalmos (>2 to 3 mm) and/or hypophthalmos (>2 to 3 mm)
2. Restriction of lateral (or medial) gaze associated with diplopia

Relative indications include (1) large defects (an area of 2 to 3 cm²) associated with at least 2 to 3 mm of

wall displacement on CT scan and (2) persistent diplopia on lateral gaze, presumably caused by a small defect, and mechanical changes not perceptible by forced duction tests. Such cases should have no evidence of neural injury.

Ideally the procedure should be performed when swelling has decreased and function can be accurately assessed, usually at 7 to 10 days following the injury. The open approach described later is preferred although it is possible to achieve good reduction with a nasal endoscopic technique. If there are associated fractures that require treatment (i.e., naso-orbital), the procedures should be coordinated to take place at the same time. Surgery performed too late can be compromised by malunion of small fragments of bone and scarring and contraction of soft tissues. Nevertheless, it is still worthwhile to explore and repair medial wall fractures up to 4 to 6 weeks after injury.

PROCEDURE

A The medial wall of the orbit is best approached by a curved incision approximately 2.5 cm in length placed one-half the distance from the lacrimal caruncle to the dorsum of the nose. Prior injection with 1% lidocaine containing 1:100,000 epinephrine will help in hemostasis. The angular vessels should be ligated or cauterized and the periosteum incised along the frontal process of the maxilla.

B Using Joseph and, subsequently, Freer elevators, the periosteum is elevated toward the medial orbital wall. The dissection should be superior to the junction of the anterior and posterior lacrimal crests, thereby avoiding injury to the medial canthal ligament and the lacrimal sac. The trochlea is then detached from the superior orbital rim. Elevation of the periosteum along the medial wall should expose the anterior ethmoidal artery, which is often involved with the fracture. However, if the artery is intact, it should be detached and bleeding controlled with gentle pressure, bipolar cautery, or vascular clips. The extent of the dissection posteriorly should be limited by the posterior ethmoidal artery.

C–E The periorbita should subsequently be teased out of the fragmented lamina papyracea. Often the periorbita is torn, and the surgeon must be careful not to injure the displaced fat. The hook technique, described in Chapter 62, can be useful for elevation of the bone fragments. Most medial orbital wall defects can be repaired by placing an appropriate piece of polypropylene (Marlex) mesh of appropriate size along the defect. If the ethmoid/lacrimal complex is displaced medially, reduction can be facilitated by placing a Boies elevator along the middle turbinate and pushing the wall laterally. Adequate reduction should be confirmed with forced duction tests applied to the insertion of the medial rectus muscle.

The periosteum is closed with a 4-0 chromic suture. The subcutaneous tissues are brought together to relieve tension on the skin with a 4-0 chromic suture. The skin is closed with a 5-0 or 6-0 nylon suture. Prophylactic antibiotics are prescribed for 5 to 7 days. The patient should be evaluated at 1 week and then monthly for 6 months to ensure stability and uneventful healing.

PITFALLS

1. Patients with suspected medial wall injuries should have appropriate imaging studies performed and an accurate evaluation of globe position and eye movements. Size, site, and severity of the injury will dictate the clinical and/or surgical management. Ophthalmologic examination and consultation are highly recommended.

2. Contraindications to surgery are hyphema, retinal tear, and/or globe perforation. Traumatic optic neuropathy and retinal artery occlusion are also important considerations. Surgery should not be performed on an only-seeing eye.

3. Surgery should be timed to a period when inflammatory responses and swelling have subsided.

Ideally exploration should precede bone healing and soft tissue scar contraction. If there are associated fractures that must be treated, surgery should be coordinated with those repairs.

4. Avoid injury to the medial canthal ligament and lacrimal sac. Elevation of the sac should be limited to the fundus region only, and the surgeon should preserve those ligamentous attachments that surround the body of the sac and insert onto the anterior and posterior lacrimal crests.

5. Bleeding of the anterior ethmoidal vessels can make surgery difficult and cause problems later (i.e., retro-orbital hemorrhage). Usually bleeding from the vessel can be controlled with gentle pressure. If bleeding does not stop, bipolar cautery or vascular clips can be judiciously applied.

6. The optic nerve can be damaged by the initial injury or by a too-aggressive dissection on the medial wall of the orbit. The posterior ethmoidal artery is a valuable landmark, and dissection should be anterior to this vessel. The so-called "standard distances" cannot be relied on to determine the exact position of the optic nerve.

7. Large unstable defects of the medial wall probably should be treated with bone grafts. In grafting this area, the surgeon should make sure that the graft is properly contoured to the defect. A graft that is too large can cause pressure on the optic nerve and should be avoided. The nasal mucosa should be kept intact if contamination and resorption of the implant are to be prevented.

8. If the medial wall fracture extends inferiorly and is associated with a floor injury, the fracture is better repaired by an additional exposure from below. The infraciliary, transconjunctival or high eyelid (subtarsal) incision, combined with the medial canthal incision, will provide an excellent approach. Bone grafts or titanium mesh implants are sometimes necessary to reinforce this area of fracture (see later).

COMPLICATIONS

1. The medial wall fracture places the optic nerve at risk at the time of injury and at the time of exploration and repair. Careful preoperative evaluation, coupled with a skillful dissection, should help minimize any injury to the nerve.

Vision disturbances occurring postoperatively must be immediately evaluated. Ophthalmic consultation should be obtained. If indicated, the surgeon can remove the implant or drain a retro-orbital hematoma. Additionally, retro-orbital pressures can be relieved by periosteal incisions and canthotomy. Steroid and diuretic administration may be helpful.

REPAIR OF MEDIAL WALL BLOWOUT FRACTURE

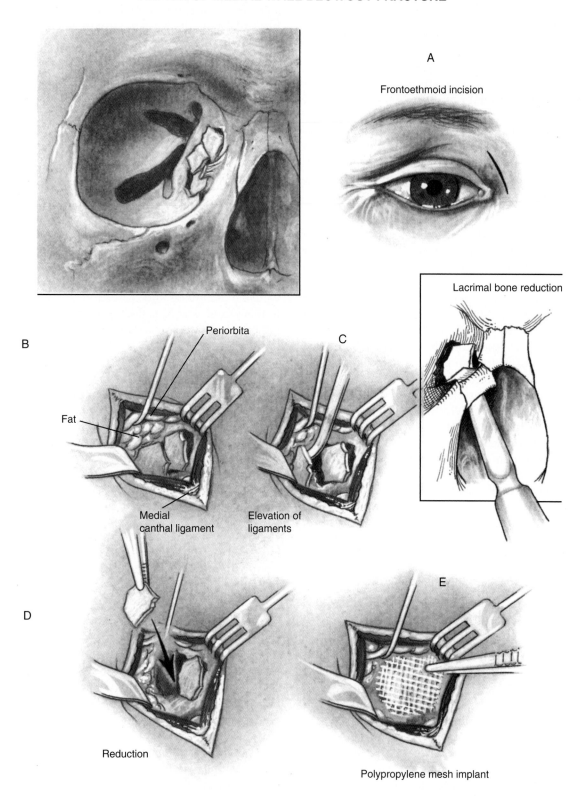

A

Frontoethmoid incision

Lacrimal bone reduction

B

Periorbita

Fat

Medial
canthal ligament

C

Elevation of
ligaments

D

Reduction

E

Polypropylene mesh implant

Wm. Loechel

2. Persistence of diplopia should be evaluated and treated appropriately. If restriction of eye movement is not caused by neural injury, the surgeon should consider reexploration and repair.

3. Postoperative enophthalmos usually indicates an intraorbital volume-to-content discrepancy and suggests a failure in adequately reducing the orbital defect. Reexploration and repair should be considered, but if these complications persist or are noted to develop at a later time, then orbital reconstruction with strategic implantation of bone grafts (see Chapter 64) is preferred.

4. Medial canthal displacement and/or obstruction to the lacrimal system can be prevented by maintaining the anatomic integrity of this area. If telecanthus and/or epiphora develop, appropriate measures (see Chapters 67 through 73) should be taken.

ALTERNATIVE TECHNIQUE FOR REPAIR OF JUNCTIONAL INJURIES

Fractures that extend from the medial wall to the inferior wall create a unique set of problems. The defect tends to be large, there is loss of tissue into the nose and sinuses, and the potential for enophthalmos is high. The injury is not well appreciated by the medial canthal incision, and thus a combined technique becomes advantageous.

a The procedure should utilize infraciliary, transconjunctival and medial canthal incisions. The floor dissection is carried more medially, hopefully avoiding the area anteriorly that contains the lacrimal sac and nasal lacrimal duct. From the medial canthus incision, the dissection is carried above and behind the medial canthal attachment and posterior lacrimal crest. The subperiosteal dissections should then meet at the junction of the medial and inferior walls.

b–e For the reduction of fragments, the surgeon can use the skin hook technique. If the ethmoid complex is displaced, elevation of the lateral wall of the nose with a Boies elevator, as described previously, is helpful. If the reduction cannot be stabilized with one or several pieces of polypropylene mesh, the surgeon must consider the use of bone grafts or Titanium mesh (see Chapter 64). The wounds are closed in standard fashion, and the patient is administered prophylactic antibiotics.

REPAIR OF MEDIAL WALL BLOWOUT FRACTURE *(Continued)*
ALTERNATIVE TECHNIQUES FOR REPAIR OF JUNCTIONAL INJURY

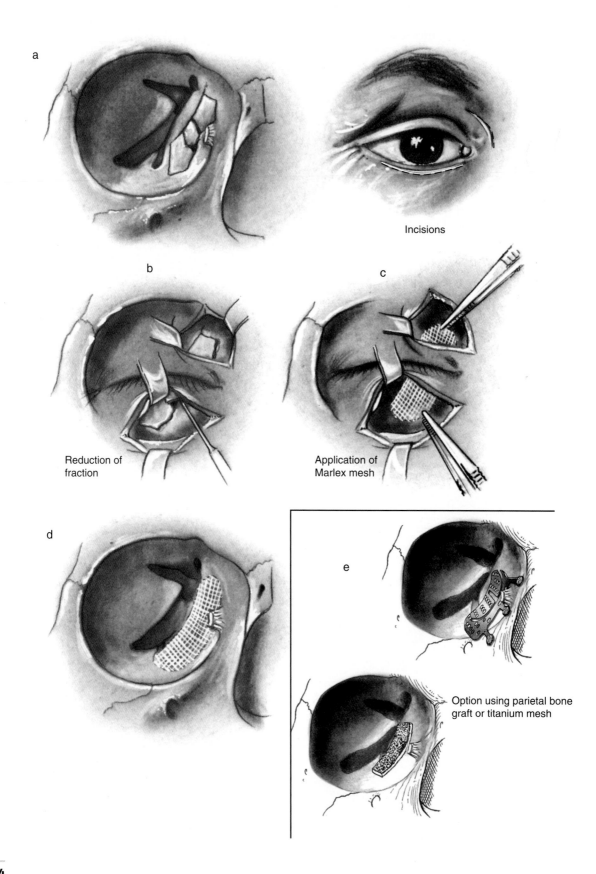

a

Incisions

b

Reduction of
fraction

c

Application of
Marlex mesh

d

e

Option using parietal bone
graft or titanium mesh

64

Reconstruction of the Orbit Using Iliac Crest Grafts

Alternative Techniques Using Cranial Grafts and Osteotomies

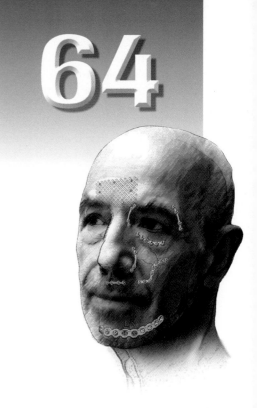

INDICATIONS

Persistent or progressive enophthalmos following injury to a wall of the orbit can occur as a result of an expansion of the orbital wall, reduction in space occupied by intraorbital tissues, or a shift of fat behind the globe to a more peripheral position. Other possible, but less likely, causes are dislocation of the superior oblique muscle, cicatricial contraction of retrobulbar tissues, or rupture of the orbital ligaments or fascial bands.

Enophthalmos is frequently associated with hypophthalmos and/or diplopia. Muscle imbalance occurs as a result of muscle (or fibrous septae) entrapment, neuromuscular injury, or displacement of the axis of the globe. The inferior rectus muscle, close to the inferior wall, and the medial rectus muscle, close to the medial orbital wall, are often involved.

Early after orbital trauma, a displaced globe and restriction of muscle movement can be treated by exploration and repair (see Chapters 62 and 63). However, if these findings are observed later, there is a possibility of malposition or resorption of an orbital wall and/or atrophy and loss of soft tissues. When this occurs, the orbit must be reconstructed. The muscles and their attachments will have to be freed, and the walls will have to be rebuilt by osteotomy or onlay grafts. The soft tissues will have to be replaced or augmented by implant materials.

PROCEDURE

Our reconstructive technique is designed to reduce the size of the orbit and increase intraorbital contents by the strategic implantation of bone grafts. Soft tissue contractions are released by a 280° subperiosteal dissection, carefully sparing injury to the anulus tendineus, the superior orbital fissure, and the medial superior quadrant that contains the optic nerve and ophthalmic artery. The grafts are then placed against the orbital walls, especially along those in which there is a defect. The implants are positioned so that they displace the tissues primarily from behind the equator and along the horizontal-vertical axis of the globe. Bone autografts are preferred over alloplastic implants to reduce the chance of rejection and infection. Moreover autografts fuse rapidly with adjoining bone and thus avoid displacement from any additional trauma. One exception noted previously (Chapters 62and 63) is the thin polypropylene mesh which, when used to reinforce a wall of the orbit, is apparently well-tolerated by the body.

General anesthesia and oral intubation are used, and the patient is placed in a supine position. The left hip is elevated on a pillow or sandbag. The hip and face are then prepared and draped as sterile fields. If two operating teams are available, the harvesting of the graft can be done by one team while the other prepares the orbit.

The bone graft is obtained as described in Chapter 35. The surgeon should harvest sufficient bone, and if the enophthalmos is >3 to 4 mm, the surgeon should anticipate using a block of bone 1 × 3 × 6 cm. The bone should be kept in a basin containing blood until it is carved and implanted. The hip wound should be drained and closed appropriately.

The position of the eye should be remeasured, as the degree of enophthalmos can be affected by anesthesia and by the pull of gravity in the supine position. The opposite eye should be used as a reference for position, forced duction tests, and what would be palpated as "normal" tissues.

A The surgical approach is usually through three incisions: the conjunctiva or the lower eyelid, lateral eyebrow, and medial canthus. The pathologic condition often indicates which incisions are best utilized for the exploration.

B The medial wall of the orbit is explored through a medial canthal incision made one-half the distance between the lacrimal caruncle and the dorsum of the nose. A local anesthetic containing epinephrine is injected for vasoconstriction effects. The angular vessels are ligated or cauterized as described in Chapter 63. The trochlea is released, while the periosteum is elevated to expose the anterior ethmoidal artery. The dissection should avoid injury to the medial canthal ligament and lacrimal sac. The anterior ethmoidal artery can be ligated or avulsed at its entry into the ethmoid bone, and hemostasis can be obtained with gentle pressure, bipolar cautery or application of vascular clips. The posterior ethmoidal vessel limits the dissection posteriorly and serves to protect the optic nerve.

C The approach to the lateral wall is through an eyebrow incision in which the area is infiltrated earlier with 1% lidocaine containing 1:100,000 epinephrine. The incision should not extend beyond the level of the hairs of the lateral eyebrow, and to avoid injury to the hairs, the incision should be beveled in a plane corresponding to the hair follicles. The orbicularis oculi is cut and the periosteum incised at the level of the zygomaticofrontal suture. Using Freer elevators, the periosteum is then elevated off the lateral wall of the orbit, relaxing the attachment of the lateral canthal ligament from the lateral orbital tubercle and elevating the lacrimal gland from its fossa. Small vessels are encountered, and bleeding can be controlled by gentle pressure.

D The lower eyelid incision (infraciliary) is designed 2 to 3 mm below the lash line and extended into a "crow's foot" crease laterally (the transconjunctival incision can be extended via lateral canthotomy). After injection with 1% lidocaine containing 1:100,000 epinephrine to control bleeding, the skin is incised

through the orbicularis oculi to the orbital septum. The septum is then separated from the muscle, and the dissection is continued inferiorly toward the orbital rim. It is at this point, with good visualization of the rim, that the orbicularis oculi and the zygomaticus muscle insertions are released. The incision is then carried through the periosteum to the anterior wall of the maxilla.

Using Joseph elevators initially and Freer elevators later, the periosteum is elevated off the rim and floor of the orbit. By beginning in a nonfractured area, a difficult dissection is made somewhat easier. In places where there are old fractures and adhesions of the periosteum, the surgeon may have to refracture displaced fragments or even enter a plane above the periosteum. In patients treated earlier with floor implants, it is desirable to remove the implant, but in the case of polypropylene mesh, the mesh will be incorporated into the soft tissues and it is better to elevate the mesh with these tissues and leave it in place. In severely injured patients, it is difficult to maintain the integrity of the infraorbital nerve and vessel, and the dissection often requires avulsion or a cutting of these tissues.

Laterally the dissection often encounters adhesions at the inferior orbital fissure. Fat can be observed coming either up through the fissure or downward from the orbital contents. In many cases, the surgeon has to dissect through the fat and adhesions, keeping as close as possible to the imaginary level of the floor.

The dissection should proceed posteriorly to the junction of the infraorbital groove of the maxilla and the inferior orbital fissure. Just medial to this junction, the orbital plate of the ethmoid forms a ledge that limits the posterior dissection and serves as a "guard" to the optic nerve. Entrapment of muscle posterior to this area is not considered surgically and safely accessible, at least from the inferior approach.

E–G The dissections should create pockets along the medial and lateral walls to the floor. The pocket along the medial wall should be posterior to the lacrimal sac and nasolacrimal duct. Superiorly and laterally, the dissection should elevate the periosteum behind the globe to a level of approximately the pupil.

H Following this extensive subperiosteal dissection, the globe should be completely mobile in all directions. The first implant is usually in the shape of a shield and placed along the floor region. As the globe is elevated, pressure will be exerted along the superior wall; this will also tend to project the globe outward. The primary effect, however, will be to elevate the globe and correct a hypophthalmos.

I–K For the most part, projection is obtained by placing a curved, crescent-shaped piece of bone through the eyebrow incision behind the equator of

RECONSTRUCTION OF THE ORBIT WITH ONLAY GRAFTS

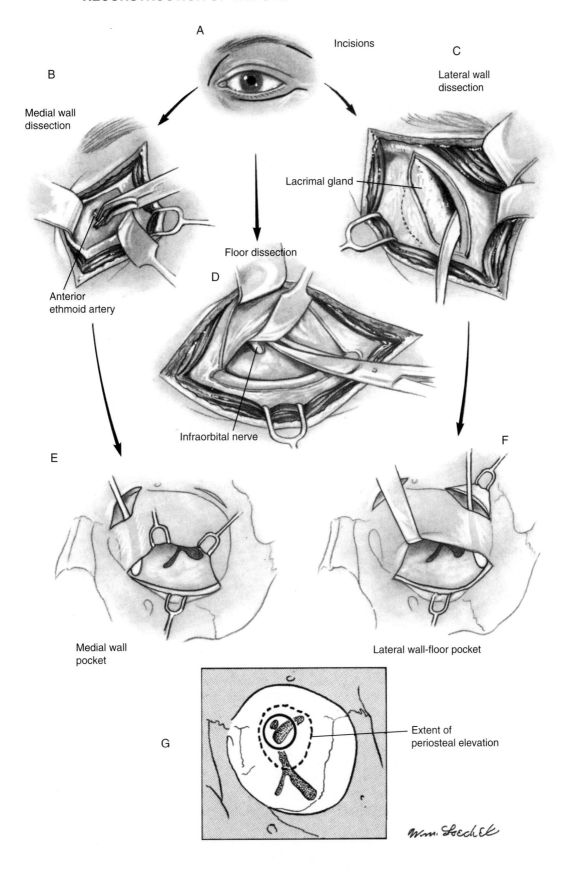

A

Incisions

B

Medial wall
dissection

C

Lateral wall
dissection

Lacrimal gland

Anterior
ethmoid artery

Floor dissection

D

Infraorbital nerve

E

Medial wall
pocket

F

Lateral wall-floor pocket

G

Extent of
periosteal elevation

Wm. Loechel

the globe. This graft will have the effect of pushing the eye outward, but there also will be a tendency to push it medially. The medial displacement must be corrected by placement of a pyramidal piece of bone along the medial wall. This will also add to the intraorbital contents and increase the projection of the globe. Ideally the surgeon will be aiming at an overcorrection of the hypophthalmos and enophthalmos by about 1 to 2 mm; to get these effects, the surgeon will have to either add or trim the implants. Walls with the greatest defects will obviously receive the most volume of graft.

Following placement of the grafts, there will be some tension on the globe; this should be checked by palpation. The contralateral globe is used as a reference. Because the muscles will be stretched, forced duction tests will give false impressions of binding. However, some movement is to be expected.

The periosteum is then closed with one or several interrupted 3-0 chromic sutures. A subcuticular 5-0 nylon suture is used to approximate the infraciliary incision. The other wounds are closed in layers. The eye is washed with a balanced salt solution and treated with an appropriate eye ointment. A light compression dressing of fluffs and stretch gauze is applied for 48 hours to prevent chemosis and swelling of the eyelid. Prophylactic antibiotics are prescribed for 7 to 10 days. Diet and exercise are advanced as tolerated.

PITFALLS

1. Indications for the procedure, alone or in combination, are enophthalmos or hypophthalmos >2 mm and/or diplopia in at least one field of gaze. These conditions can be accurately evaluated by history and physical examination and by forced duction tests used to assess globe mobility. The degree of deformity and dysfunction should be documented and quantified so that the patient and surgeon can appreciate the results of the surgical procedure.

2. An understanding of the pathophysiology is important if the surgeon is to obtain the desired correction. This information is derived from the history and physical findings, along with a complete set of imaging studies. Clues will thus be obtained on where to make the correction. The larger deficits obviously require a larger implant. Restricted muscles need to be adequately freed by the subperiosteal dissection.

3. Avoid surgery on those patients who have evidence of sinusitis. Two most dreaded complications are infection and extrusion of the grafts, and these can often be prevented by successfully treating the sinusitis before embarking on the reconstructive procedure.

4. The surgeon should not operate on an only-seeing eye. Although our experience has shown that there is little risk to vision, the risk far outweighs the benefits. All patients are informed that loss of vision is a possibility.

5. Ophthalmologic evaluation is important for diagnosis and proper treatment of the condition. The ophthalmologist is an important part of the team and should be available throughout the procedure.

6. Relative contraindications to surgery are a small contracted globe and ophthalmoplegia from retrobulbar cicatrization of soft tissues. The small globe is difficult to position. The scarring associated with ophthalmoplegia may sometimes not be completely relaxed and will limit repositioning of the globe and movement of muscles.

7. Limited degrees of dysfunction and/or deformity can often be treated with only one or two of the incisions. If a patient has only a mild to moderate hypophthalmos, a floor implant is all that is needed.

8. The hip graft is probably the best type of graft when the orbital reconstruction is associated with globe displacement >3 to 4 mm. Cranial or rib grafts give only limited amounts of bone, and because they are thin grafts, the surgeon often has to stack several pieces of bone to obtain appropriate size and contour. This can cause problems with instability and proper positioning of the graft.

9. Exposure for the procedure requires exact placement of the head and focused lighting. A surgeon-controlled table and headlight are helpful adjuncts for the procedure.

10. The dissection must be adequate to obtain visualization of all wall deformities and relaxation of all "entrapped" tissues. Failure to achieve this degree of dissection will compromise the results.

11. The patient should be warned about the possibility of hip pain persisting for days to weeks following the procedure. Suction drains in the hip wound are best left in place until drainage is <20 mL/d. Early ambulation and rehabilitation are desirable.

12. Overcorrection of the enophthalmos and hypophthalmos is desirable. A sufficient amount of bone grafts will put increased tension on the globe that must be checked constantly, relating the globe pressure in the operated eye to that on the unoperated eye. Sudden increases in tension may be caused by retrobulbar hemorrhage, and the surgeon must try to distinguish these changes from those that would occur from the placement of the graft. Also, a sudden decrease in heart rate may indicate too much pressure on the optic nerve and, should this occur, graft[s] should be removed immediately.

13. Patients who have associated injuries such as a depressed zygoma often present with a more severe type of enophthalmos than that occurring from the blowout alone. These patients require more intraorbital

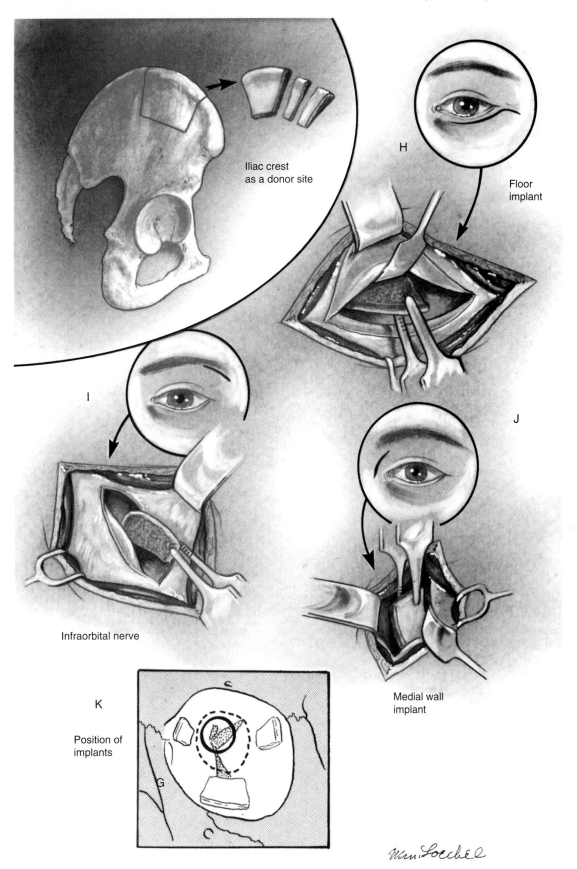

Iliac crest
as a donor site

H

Floor
implant

I

Infraorbital nerve

J

Medial wall
implant

K

Position of
implants

Wm. Loechel

grafting. In addition, the associated malar deformity must also be treated (see Chapter 65).

14. The dressing that is used to control soft tissue swelling can also mask the same conditions that cause loss of vision (i.e., retrobulbar hemorrhage, hyphema, etc.). If the surgeon is concerned that one of these complications may be developing at the time of surgery, the dressing is better left off. If the patient complains of pain in the postoperative period, the dressing should be immediately removed and the eye examined.

In applying the dressing, the eye should be well lubricated and the upper eyelid pulled down over the globe. The dressing must be tight enough to hold the upper eyelid in position. If the eyelid becomes raised, it is possible to develop a corneal abrasion. This will become suspect when the patient complains of pain and mentions that the eyelid is moving under the dressing.

COMPLICATIONS

1. Although loss of vision from this procedure is extremely rare, all patients should be told of this possibility and be prepared to accept the risk. Vision can be compromised by increased intraorbital tension and compression of the optic nerve. This can be associated with displacement of the graft, retrobulbar hemorrhage, or retinal artery occlusion. Proper analysis and treatment should be implemented (see Chapters 62 and 63).

2. Infection of the graft is possible, and when this occurs, the patient should be treated vigorously with intravenous antibiotics. Debridement and removal of the graft may be necessary. This complication can be partially avoided by ensuring aeration of sinuses and healthy soft tissues around the graft. The dissection should also avoid exposure of contaminated areas such as the mucosa of the nose.

3. Although results are generally good with the reconstructive procedure, some degree of enophthalmos and hypophthalmos can return. This problem can occur with the resorption of bone, from infection, or from poor vascularity, but usually the malposition reflects inadequate correction with the implant. In the patient with a small contracted globe or ophthalmoplegia, the surgeon is most likely to have problems properly positioning the globe.

4. Diplopia, although often improved, can persist in some patients. If the surgeon is certain that there has been an adequate dissection and relaxation of tissues and that the globe is in an appropriate anatomic position, then it is logical to assume that there is a neuromuscular deficit or intramuscular contraction phenomenon (i.e., Volkmann's contracture). Eye muscle surgery may be helpful in correcting the problem.

5. Hip pain is to be expected. If this pain persists for more than a few weeks, consultation with an orthopedic surgeon is advisable.

6. Ectropion of the lower eyelid can occur as a result of the initial injury or as a result of surgery in those tissues that surround and support the eyelid. This complication can be somewhat avoided by careful atraumatic technique. However, if ectropion occurs, it can be treated initially with steroid injections (40 mg/mL of triamcinolone) into the contracted tissues. If this is unsatisfactory, the tissues will have to be lysed and the lower eyelid strengthened. Occasionally the tissues will need to be supported by a split-thickness graft.

ALTERNATIVE TECHNIQUE USING CRANIAL GRAFTS

For the most part, the hip graft is quite satisfactory for the reconstruction of the orbit. The donor site provides an adequate amount of bone that can be readily carved to appropriate size and shape. The grafts are stable and viable within the orbit; the main disadvantage is the hip morbidity that accompanies the procedure.

Limited dysfunction and deformity of the eye, however, can be treated satisfactorily with outer cranial cortex grafts. The procedure has minimal morbidity. The graft is well tolerated in the orbit, and in fact, it is believed to be more resistant to resorbtion than the hip graft. Moreover, its curvature fits conveniently along one of the orbital walls. However, the bone is thin, and if thicker pieces are needed, it will be necessary to stack the bone, which can cause instability. If large amounts of bone are needed, the exposure and the dissection must be expanded to include other ipsilateral and contralateral cranial bones.

a The procedure is carried out by first shaving the hair in a vertical line directly above and posterior to the auricle. This incision can be extended into a complete coronal incision if additional bone is desired from the opposite side. Infiltration of the area with 1% lidocaine containing epinephrine will help control some of the bleeding.

The incision is made through the skin, subcutaneous tissues, galea, and periosteum. Branches of the superficial temporal muscle will need to be ligated or cauterized to control bleeding. The periosteum is then elevated off the parietal bone. Self-retaining retractors are used to expose the bone and hold the tissues in position.

The surgeon should map out the location of the temporal, coronal, sagittal, and lamboidal suture lines. The dissection should stay several centimeters lateral to the sagittal suture line if the surgeon is to prevent the brisk bleeding that can occur from penetration of the sagittal sinus. The temporal bone should be avoided, as this bone is thin and extremely brittle.

b,c The harvest of bone is carried out by making parallel troughs about 2.0 cm apart through the outer cortex with cutting burs (3 mm) and saline irrigation and then joining the troughs horizontally at points lateral to the sagittal sinus and above the temporal suture line. This will provide grafts with a length of approximately 4 to 5 cm. The diploë will be more vascular and softer than the outer cortex, and the surgeon should proceed through the diploë until the more compact inner cortex is exposed. The troughs are then widened to accommodate a curved, sharp osteotome that is inserted into the diploë. With the tap of a mallet, the outer cortex is separated from the inner portion of the skull. Alternatively, the surgeon can use an offset oscillating saw. Additional grafts can be harvested as necessary from the frontal and occipital regions, and this can potentially provide grafts totaling 6 × 10 cm from one side of the head. However, it should be realized that females have thinner bone, and their cortical plates and diploë are not as well developed as those in males.

d Bleeding of the diploë can be controlled by application of bone wax. The depression in the donor area can present a deformity later, especially if there is balding in the area, and it is thus better corrected at this time with an application of fast curing bone cement. The wound is closed in layers of 3-0 chromic, first approximating the periosteum and galea and then the subcuticular tissues. A 5-0 nylon suture is used to close the skin.

e The bone is kept in a physiologic solution (or preferably a blood bath) until it is ready for grafting. When the surgeon has an estimate of the size and location of the defect, the bone can be carved and contoured to appropriate size and shape.

Complications from this procedure are cranial fracture, dural tear, and bleeding. If the osteotome is used as a fulcrum, it is possible to create a depressed fracture of the inner table. A small depression is probably inconsequential, but the patient should be followed postoperatively for changes of sensorium and/or other evidence of intracranial damage. Dural tears with cerebral spinal fluid leakage should be repaired. Bleeding of the dura should be brought under control. Injury to the sagittal sinus or to one of the branches of the middle meningeal artery can be quite troublesome, and if this should occur, neurosurgical consultation is immediately indicated.

ALTERNATIVE TECHNIQUE USING OSTEOTOMY

a'–c' Reduction in size of the orbit can also be accomplished with the osteotomy technique. This method is particularly important in the relatively early period when the bones of associated craniofacial fractures (e.g., zygoma or naso-orbital) have just started to heal in malposition. The osteotomy ideally will recreate the fracture and usually provides an excellent opportunity for reduction and fixation with correction of the orbital wall.

It is also possible to perform an osteotomy at a later point in time, but usually the results are compromised by resorption of bone and instability of the reduction. The technique of lateral and inferior wall (zygoma osteotomy) is described in Chapter 58. The medial wall or medial maxillary correction is described in Chapter 45. Further improvement of the enophthalmos can often be obtained by shortening one of the orbital walls prior to repositioning the block of bone. Osteotomy can be also combined with onlay graft techniques.

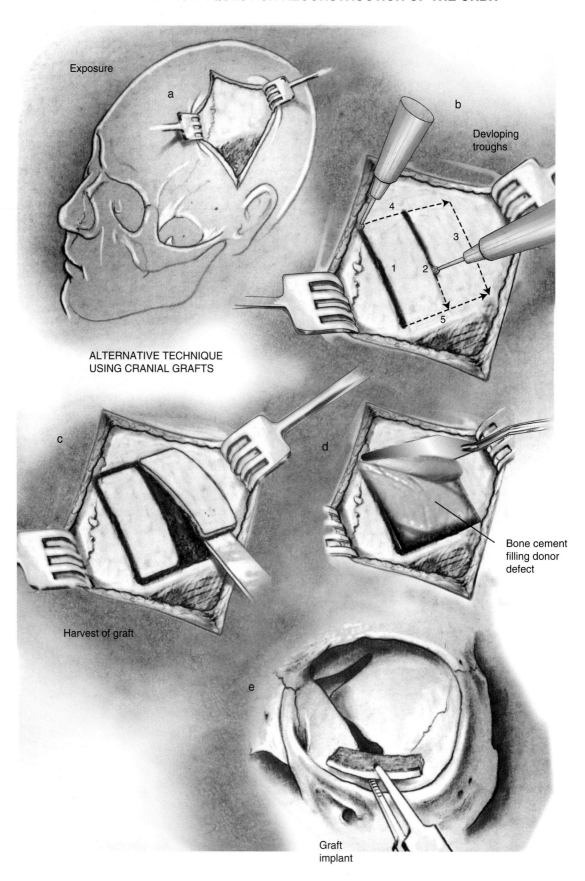

Exposure

a

b

Devloping troughs

4

3

1

2

5

ALTERNATIVE TECHNIQUE
USING CRANIAL GRAFTS

c

d

Bone cement
filling donor
defect

Harvest of graft

e

Graft
implant

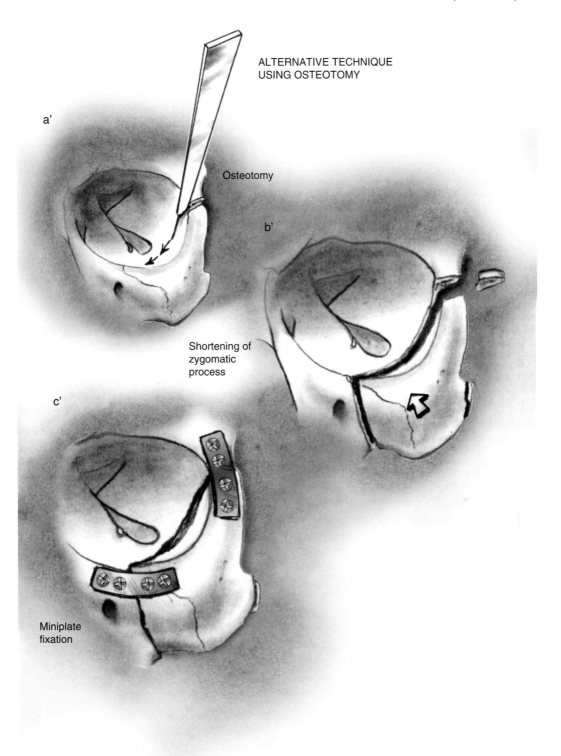

ALTERNATIVE TECHNIQUE
USING OSTEOTOMY

a'

Osteotomy

b'

Shortening of
zygomatic
process

c'

Miniplate
fixation

Reconstruction of the Orbit for Combined Orbital Trauma Syndrome

INDICATIONS

If the floor fracture is associated with a zygoma fracture, the pathologic abnormalities can be additive, causing a more severe degree of deformity and dysfunction. In the floor fracture, the loss of the floor leads to failure in support of the globe and hypophthalmos. In the zygoma fracture, the suspensory ligament of Lockwood is displaced inferiorly, contributing more to the support problem. The floor fracture, when depressed, causes an increase in the volume of the orbit described by the walls, and this may be associated with some atrophy or necrosis of soft tissues; the zygoma fracture presents with an even greater depression and lateralization of the walls, adding to the discrepancy. It is important to recognize these effects, as the design of the procedure should be sufficient to correct them. The early repair (i.e., reduction and fixation) is described in Chapters 56, 57, 62, and 63. The technique described here is for those patients in whom there is moderate to severe enophthalmos and hypophthalmos, with or without diplopia, associated with both a malunited blow-out fracture and a zygoma fracture.

PROCEDURE

Essentially, the patient is prepared as for the orbital reconstruction (see Chapter 64). The graft harvested from the hip should be at least $1 \times 5 \times 8$ cm. The graft should be kept in a physiologic solution (preferably blood) until it is ready for shaping and implantation.

Eyebrow, medial canthal, and infraciliary incisions are useful approaches to the orbit. For the zygoma exposure, the surgeon can extend the infraciliary incision into one of the "crow's feet." The dissection is carried out as in Chapter 64, and the periorbita is elevated in all planes except that quadrant containing the ophthalmic artery and optic nerve. The subperiosteal dissection is also continued along the walls of the zygoma (including the frontal process of the zygoma, the anterior arch, and the zygomaticomaxillary buttress). The anterior wall of the maxilla is also exposed. If the deformity also involves the anterior wall of the maxilla, then it is necessary to extend the subperiosteal pocket to include the nasomaxillary buttress. This extended dissection frequently requires a sacrifice of the infraorbital nerve and vessel.

The bone harvested from the iliac crest must be large enough to accommodate a curved piece of bone to fit the anterior wall of the maxilla and malar eminence (**A** and **C**). Smaller pieces are carved to fit strategically within the orbit (**A** and **B**); the design of these grafts is described elsewhere (see Chapters 59 and 64). Pieces of cancellous bone should also be available and are placed between the floor and zygoma implants to provide a smooth contour to the rim. Additional pieces of graft may be necessary to provide a smooth transition between the malar graft and the adjoining frontal process of the zygoma.

The onlay grafts are usually held in position with lag screws and the grafts within the orbit by securing 2-0 or 3-0 chromic sutures to the overlying periorbita/periosteum. A light compression dressing of fluffs and stretch gauze is desirable for 5 to 7 days. Prophylactic antibiotics should be given intravenously for 5 days and extended orally for an additional week.

PITFALLS

1. The same pitfalls pertain to the combined procedure as pertain to the separate reconstructions described in Chapters 59 and 64.

2. Remember that a reconstruction of the zygomatic eminence will project the inferior wall of the orbit and create a relative enophthalmos. It is thus important that the techniques to project the eye overcompensate sufficiently to place the globe in proper relationship to the zygoma.

3. Avoid deficits that will develop between the planes of the orbital floor and the reconstruction of the zygomatic eminence. A smooth contour should be established with appropriate carved pieces of cancellous bone.

4. To prevent displacement of grafts in the early postoperative period, a light compression dressing should be used. The dressing can be removed in 24 hours. The malar grafts and eye functions should be examined and the dressing applied for an additional 48 hours.

COMPLICATIONS

1. Loss of vision, persistence of enophthalmos and/or diplopia, and hip pain are discussed in Chapter 64. Methods to prevent and treat displacement and/or absorption of a zygoma graft are described in Chapter 59.

2. Ectropion is a common complication, as the surgeon must perform an extensive dissection, and the grafts have a tendency to pull the lower eyelid downward. Measures to prevent retraction of the lower eyelid include relaxation through an extensive subperiosteal dissection and careful placement of periosteal sutures so that the tension is distributed in a natural direction. The surgeon should also provide sufficient tissues to cover the tarsal plate and should try to retain the integrity of the orbicularis oculi muscle. Excessive foreign body reaction should also be avoided by using only necessary suture material. Occasionally a Frost suture that holds the lower eyelid to the forehead superiorly is helpful. If ectropian should develop, the surgeon should first consider the use of steroid injections (triamcinolone, 40 mg/mL) and massage. Persistence of the ectropion may require oculoplastic reconstruction of the lower eyelid.

3. Hypoesthesia will develop, especially if the surgeon has to cut the infraorbital nerve. This is a "trade-off," as a pocket in this area is often necessary to hold the appropriate-sized graft.

RECONSTRUCTION FOR COMBINED ORBITAL TRAUMA

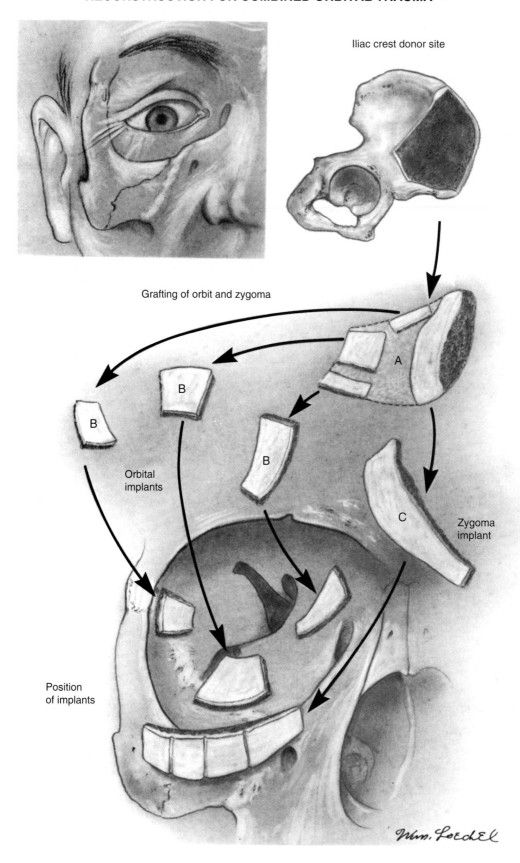

Iliac crest donor site

Grafting of orbit and zygoma

A

B

B

B

C

Orbital
implants

Zygoma
implant

Position
of implants

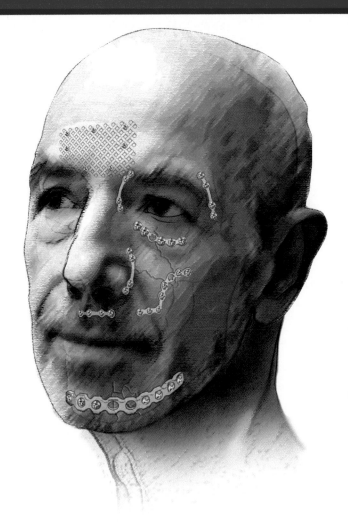

PART EIGHT

Naso-Orbital Fractures

Classification and Pathophysiology of Naso-Orbital Fractures

CHAPTER

66

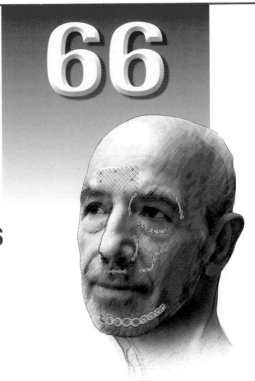

General Considerations

Naso-orbital fractures occur as a result of injury to the anteromedial wall of the orbit. They are commonly associated with multiple deformities and dysfunction. In many cases, there is a change in appearance of the palpebral fissure, accompanied by tearing and failure of the lacrimal collecting system.

A,B The orbit is formed medially by the frontal process of the maxillary bone, the lacrimal bone, and the lamina papyracea of the ethmoid bone. The frontal and maxillary bones define the superior and inferior extent. The lacrimal fossa, in which lies the lacrimal sac, is formed by the posterior portion of the frontal process of the maxilla and the anterior portion of the lacrimal bone. Anterior and posterior crests receive insertions of the anterior and posterior slips of the medial canthal ligament and, additionally, on the posterior crest, an extension of the orbicularis oculi called *Horner's muscle*.

The anatomic relationships of the bone and soft tissues are important in understanding the pathophysiology of fractures in the region. The lacrimal collecting system, consisting of the puncta, canaliculi, sac, and duct, is intimately associated with the medial canthal ligament and orbicularis oculi muscle fibers. Tears normally enter the puncta at the medial free edge of the upper and lower eyelids and are transported through upper and lower canaliculi to a common canaliculus, which enters the sac near the junction of the body and fundus. Exit of tears is through a nasolacrimal duct that runs through the medial maxilla to the inferior meatus. The posterior portion of the orbicularis oculi, which attaches to the posterior crest, pulls the puncta against the globe. The puncta then picks up the tears from the surface of the globe. On closing the eyelids, the orbicularis oculi squeezes the tissues surrounding the lacrimal system. This causes alternating negative and positive pressures that collect and pass the tears. Failure of this pumping action as a result of trauma will result in epiphora.

The medial canthal ligament is also important in defining the palpebral opening. The medial canthal ligament is an extension of the tarsal plates. These plates also connect to the lateral canthal ligament, which attaches to the lateral wall of the orbit. The tarsal plates and ligaments receive insertions of the orbicularis oculi muscles. If the medial canthus becomes displaced or lax, the palpebral fissure becomes narrow, the medial caruncle moves laterally, and the medial aspect of the eye takes on a rounded appearance. Normally the palpebral fissure width equals the intercanthal distance and the palpebral fissure width of the other side, but with lateral displacement of the medial canthal ligament, these relationships are altered. Thus, measurements become an important part of the evaluation.

C–E Injuries to the medial wall can be classified according to the degree of deformity and dysfunction. Surgical repair can then be designed according to this classification system. Type I injury indicates that the medial canthal ligament has been displaced with a small piece of attached lacrimal bone or that the ligament has been severed completely. The patient presents with telecanthus, epiphora, blunting of the inner angle, and narrowing of the palpebral fissure. A type II injury implies that the medial wall of the orbit is comminuted and displaced. In addition to the signs and symptoms associated with the type I injury, there can be entrapment of the medial rectus muscle, cerebrospinal fluid leak, and damage to the optic nerve. In the type III injury, the medial walls of both orbits are fractured. This implies also a fracture of the nasoethmoid complex, including the nasal bones, septum, and portions of the frontal sinus. Patients with this type of injury have a flattening and widening of the nasal dorsum, nasal obstruction and epistaxis, bilateral telecanthus, blunting of the inner angle, narrowing of the palpebral openings, and epiphora. Intracranial damage and a cerebrospinal fluid leak often occur.

F–H Other classification systems use the degree of displacement and comminution of the nasal and lacrimal complex including fractures of the frontal, maxillary, and ethmoid bones. According to the Leipzinger and Manson (1992) classification, in Type I, the medial canthal ligament is displaced with an attached lacrimal bone. In Type II, the medial wall of the orbit is comminuted, but the medial canthal ligament is attached to bone. In Type III, injury to the medial wall is comminuted, but the medial canthal ligament is disrupted or avulsed. The Type III injury may be unilateral or bilateral.

NASO-ORBITAL FRACTURES

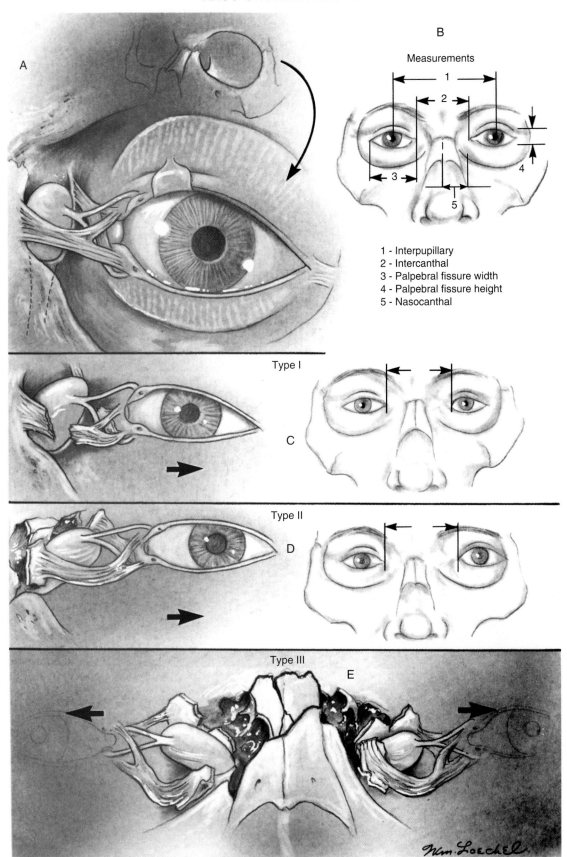

B
Measurements

1 - Interpupillary
2 - Intercanthal
3 - Palpebral fissure width
4 - Palpebral fissure height
5 - Nasocanthal

Type I

C

Type II

D

Type III

E

Wm Loechel.

F

L-M Type I Fracture

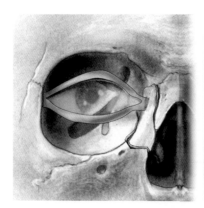
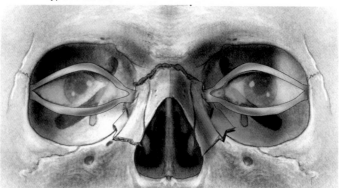

G

L-M Type II Fracture

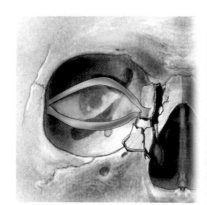
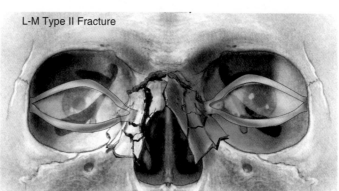

H

L-M Type III Fracture

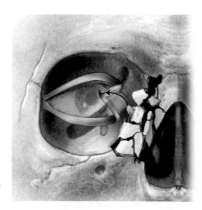
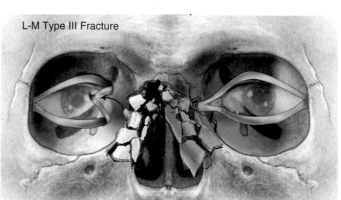

Management Strategies for Naso-Orbital Fractures

CHAPTER

67

Open Repair of Medial Canthal Ligament Injury

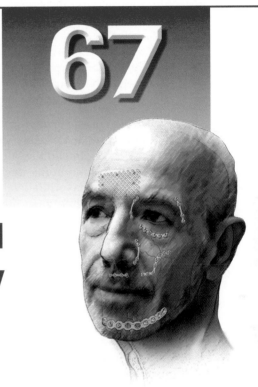

INDICATIONS

Early diagnosis and repair is important in the treatment of medial canthal ligament type of naso-orbital injury. The patient may present with a sharp penetrating wound of the medial canthus or with blunt trauma and a limited fracture of the lacrimal bone. In these patients, the palpebral fissure is narrowed, the inner angle becomes rounded, and tears collect in the lacus lacrimalis. Clinically, there is telecanthus of a variable degree. The eyelids are lax, which is confirmed by pulling one of the eyelids laterally and testing for the presence or absence of tension near the attachment of the medial canthal ligament. The extent of bone involvement should be determined with appropriate imaging studies.

PROCEDURE

A Under general anesthesia, the face is prepared and draped as a sterile field. The palpebral fissure openings and nasocanthal distances are measured and recorded so that the amount of correction can be known before the start of the procedure (see Chapter 66). A curved medial canthal (frontoethmoid) incision halfway between the caruncle and dorsum of the nose is designed with marking solution. Another incision is marked in the lateral eyebrow region. Both areas are infiltrated with 1% lidocaine containing 1:100,000 epinephrine to help with hemostasis.

B,C Through the medial canthal incision, the angular vessels are either cauterized or ligated. The periosteum overlying the frontal process of the maxilla is incised, and with a Joseph elevator, the periosteum is elevated toward the margin of the medial orbital rim. The trochlea is identified, detached, and retracted laterally. The periorbita is elevated inferiorly to identify the lacrimal fossa and both crests. Additional exposure can be obtained by cutting the anterior ethmoidal vessel and retracting the soft tissues of the orbit laterally with malleable retractors. Hemostasis is achieved with gentle pressure, but if bleeding does not stop, bipolar cattery or vascular clips can be applied. The lacrimal collecting system (in particular the sac portion) should be explored and evaluated for damage.

D The repair requires relaxation of the lateral canthal ligament. This will remove the countertraction and provide an opportunity to overcorrect the position of the medial canthal ligament. For this portion of the procedure, the eyebrow incision is used, the orbicularis oculi is separated, and the periosteum of the frontal process of the zygoma is incised. The periosteum is elevated with a Freer elevator along the lateral wall and rim of the orbit. This releases the attached lateral canthal ligament. The wound is closed in layers with 4-0 chromic and 5-0 nylon sutures.

E The point of attachment for the medial canthal ligament is important. If a piece of the lacrimal bone is displaced with the ligament, the bone can be reduced and stabilized with low profile miniplates. However, if the bone of the medial orbital wall is intact and the ligament has been severed, then the ligament should be attached with a strong ligature to the superior portion of the posterior lacrimal crest. The pull of the ligament upward and backward will facilitate improved contact of the puncta with the surface of the globe. The hole through the posterior crest can be made with a fine drill.

F–H The medial canthal ligament is next identified. The lacrimal sac and the inner caruncle are useful landmarks. The ligament can usually be found as a subcutaneous band of firm tissue that covers the lacrimal sac. To isolate the ligament, the subcutaneous tissues should be dissected over the sac for several millimeters until the surgeon meets resistance from the medial canthal ligament. These "tough" tissues can then be grasped with a forceps, and a 30-gauge stainless steel wire attached with a sharp cutting needle. This wire is then secured to the hole made on the superior part of the posterior crest. Assurance that the medial canthal ligament has been corrected can be obtained by repeating the eyelid tension test. Overcorrection is desirable. The periosteal and subcutaneous tissues are closed with 4-0 chromic sutures, and the skin is closed with a 6-0 nylon suture. Antibiotic ointment is applied to the wound.

The patient should be observed for at least 24 hours for any increase in intraorbital tension. Prophylactic antibiotics are prescribed for 5 days. The sutures are removed in 5 to 7 days.

PITFALLS

1. The best results are obtained with early diagnosis and treatment, as these will avoid the sequelae of scarring, chronic obstruction of the lacrimal system, and dacryocystitis. During the first few days, swelling will obscure the degree of injury. As the swelling disappears, the physician should continually evaluate for signs and symptoms. The eyelid tension test should be used to determine dehiscence of the medial canthal ligament.

2. Overcorrection of the medial canthal ligament is desirable and can be obtained by relaxation of the lateral canthal ligament.

3. Make sure that the traction on the ligament is upward and backward. This is best achieved by attaching the wire to the superior part of the posterior lacrimal crest.

4. Avoid the use of lead plates or buttons to hold the medial canthal ligament in position. These materials often cause necrosis of the skin, leave scars, and usually do not exert sufficient posterior pressure to maintain the desired position of the ligament.

COMPLICATIONS

1. Persistent or recurrent telecanthus presents a formidable problem. This complication can be avoided by early exploration and accurate attachment of the ligament. However, if this is not achieved or the wire becomes detached from the tissues, then reexploration must be performed.

2. Telecanthus that is diagnosed and treated late requires a different approach. Because of the scarring and retraction of tissues, the late surgery demands a more extensive dissection of the periorbita. Removal of bone along the medial wall of the orbit, as performed with a late repair (see Chapter 68), may also be required.

3. Injury to the lacrimal collecting system can result in obstruction and epiphora. Any part of the system can be compressed or twisted. Such injuries should be recognized and treated at the time of exploration. Damage to the puncta or canaliculus necessitates a repair, but if this is not successful, the surgeon can later perform a conjunctivodacryocystorhinostomy or conjunctivorhinostomy. If an outlet obstruction or infection develops, a dacryocystorhinostomy is the procedure of choice. These techniques are described in Chapters 71 and 72.

MEDIAL CANTHAL LIGAMENT REPAIR

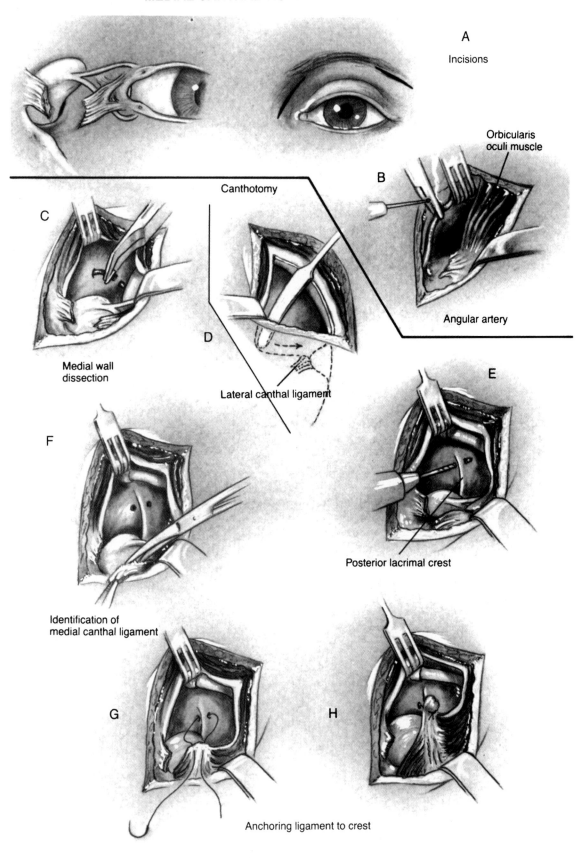

A
Incisions

B
Orbicularis oculi muscle

Angular artery

Canthotomy

C
Medial wall dissection

D
Lateral canthal ligament

E
Posterior lacrimal crest

F
Identification of medial canthal ligament

G
H
Anchoring ligament to crest

Open Repair of Unilateral Naso-Orbital Injury With Transnasal Canthoplasty
Alternative Techniques for Late Repair

INDICATIONS

Naso-orbital injury involving fractures of the nose, frontal process of the maxilla, lacrimal and ethmoid bones should be identified and treated early if a successful result is to be obtained. These fractures may be displaced as a block or comminuted and unable to support the attachment of the medial canthal ligament. In the latter situation, it becomes important to find a more suitable purchase point; this usually requires transnasal wiring to the opposite orbital wall. Patients with this injury present with telecanthus, blunting of the inner angle, narrowing of the palpebral fissure, and epiphora. The medial rectus and superior oblique muscles may be involved. Cerebrospinal fluid leak and compression of the optic nerve are rare but can also occur.

PROCEDURE

A–C The patient is prepared as described in Chapter 67, except that an additional medial canthal incision is marked on the opposite side. These approaches allow exploration of the medial canthal ligament and lacrimal sac on the involved side, a relaxing lateral canthotomy, and exposure of the lacrimal crests on the opposite side.

The angular vessels should be ligated and the trochlea and periosteum elevated from the medial orbital rim. The orbital soft tissues should then be retracted laterally, and with a Freer elevator, the junction of the

anterior and posterior lacrimal crest should be exposed. If more relaxation is necessary, the anterior ethmoidal artery can be ligated and additional periorbita elevated off the medial wall of orbit. Displaced fragments of bone should be replaced and, secured with low profile miniplates; herniated fat and entrapped muscle should be released and the medial orbital wall, if necessary, reinforced with polypropylene mesh (see Chapter 63). Through the lateral brow incision, the perioorbita is elevated to relax the lateral canthus and thus remove tension from the medial canthus.

D,E The medial canthal ligament is identified as described in Chapter 67 and secured with a 30-gauge stainless steel suture. One end of the wire is then attached to a large curved needle, which is passed through the nasal septum and out through the lacrimal bone on the opposite side. The other end of the wire is passed in a similar way, but preferably through the lamina papyracea so that the wires exit on each side of the posterior lacrimal crest. The soft tissues of the orbit must be carefully protected with malleable retractors during these maneuvers.

F The 30-gauge wire is then secured to the opposite lacrimal crest in a way that ensures overcorrection of the displaced ligament. The ends of the wire are twisted flat against the wall of the orbit. The periosteum is closed using 4-0 chromic sutures; 5-0 nylon sutures are used to coapt the skin edges. The patient should be evaluated during the next several days for

TRANSNASAL CANTHOPLASTY

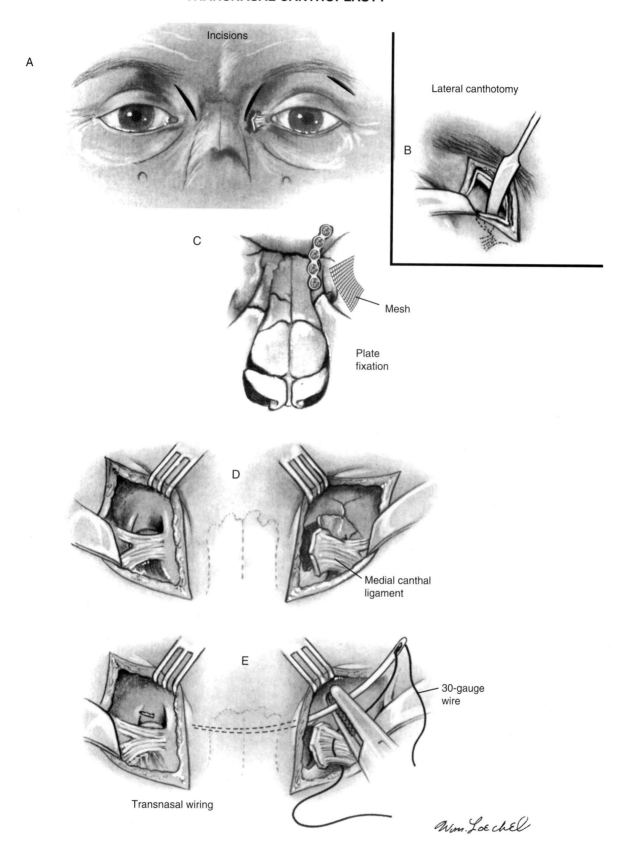

A

Incisions

B

Lateral canthotomy

C

Mesh

Plate
fixation

D

Medial canthal
ligament

E

30-gauge
wire

Transnasal wiring

Wm. Loechel

changes in intraorbital tension. Prophylactic antibiotics are prescribed for 5 days, and sutures are removed in 5 to 7 days.

PITFALLS

1. An accurate diagnosis and fixation of bone fragments is essential for successful treatment. If the surgeon tries to attach the wire to a fragmented piece of bone on the same side that is unstable, the bone will slip, and telecanthus will return.

2. If the surgeon attaches the wire to the nasal or frontal bone, it is possible that the medial canthal ligament will be pulled too far anteriorly, creating a deformity and failure of the puncta to reach the globe. Placement of the wire in the area of the posterior lacrimal crest will give the posterior superior pull to the ligament which will approximate the natural relationships.

3. Some degree of stretch is expected and should be compensated for by a more medial placement of the medial canthal ligament. Relaxation of the lateral canthal ligament will also help in the overcorrection.

4. Carefully inspect the lacrimal collecting system to make sure that there are no kinks or twists. Also, pass the fixation wire superior to the main part of the sac so that the sac is not obstructed by the wire. An ideal position is in the fundus or in the soft tissues that lie just superior to the fundus.

5. The fixation point on the opposite medial wall of the orbit must be intact and strong enough to "hold" the area. If strength is a problem, the wire should be secured to a screw or hole at the edge of the frontal process.

6. Avoid external buttons or plates, as they tend to cause necrosis of the skin and leave permanent scars. Also, it is unlikely that these materials are placed far enough posteriorly to hold the medial canthal ligaments in anatomic position.

7. For late repairs in which scarring and/or dacryocystitis develops, other techniques must be applied. These are discussed later and in Chapter 71.

COMPLICATIONS

1. Inadequate repair will result in residual telecanthus and/or epiphora. Usually this occurs when the postoperative swelling pulls the soft tissues from the wire or the wire loosens from the lacrimal bone. If this occurs, reexploration and repair are necessary. Late correction can be difficult to perform, and results are often compromised.

2. Dacryocystitis can occur from obstruction of the lacrimal collecting system. If this develops, the patient should be treated with appropriate antibiotics and the lacrimal collecting system evaluated with the Jones dye test for the degree and level of obstruction. Persistent dacryocystitis must be treated as described in Chapter 71.

3. If a cerebrospinal fluid leak persists or presents in the postoperative period, the patient should be continued on antibiotic therapy. Most leaks stop in a few days, but if a leak continues beyond 2 to 3 weeks, the site should be determined and preparations made for repair of the leak (see Chapters 84, 85, 90, and 91).

4. The transnasal wire technique can pull soft tissues of the involved orbit into the ethmoid sinus and potentially obstruct the nasofrontal duct. If the patient complains postoperatively of pain and swelling around the eye, appropriate CT scans should be obtained to evaluate the frontal sinus. Obstruction of the nasofrontal duct requires either reconstruction of the duct or obliteration of the frontal sinus with fat (see Chapters 76 through 80).

5. Medial canthal scars can result in web formation and deformity. This problem can be prevented by designing incisions with irregular patterns. If this complication does occur, a zigzagplasty or Z-plasty is indicated (see Chapters 13 and 73). Early injection with 40 mg/mL of triamcinolone may also be helpful.

ALTERNATIVE TECHNIQUES FOR LATE REPAIR

When treatment of the naso-orbital injury is delayed, the walls of the orbit become malunited, the periorbita is pulled into fracture lines, and the soft tissues become fixed with scar formation. Obstruction of the lacrimal collecting system causes epiphora, and longterm stasis leads to dacryocystitis. New bone often forms along the medial wall of the orbit. Under these conditions, alternative techniques must be applied.

a,b The incisions and approaches are the same as in the acute injury. Because scarring will limit the exposure, the surgeon will have to free up large areas of periorbita. This is accomplished by developing subperiosteal pockets that are extended along the floor and superior wall regions. If sufficient laxity of the tissues is not obtained, then an infraciliary incision and a subperiosteal dissection as described in Chapter 64 are carried out.

c–e New bone formation on the medial wall of the orbit requires removal of the bone with cutting burs and Kerrison rongeurs. The resection should accommodate the relocation of the medial canthal ligament. If the growth of scar tissue and bone tissue prevents passage of a large curved needle, the surgeon must use a fine

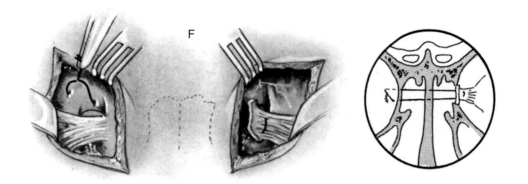

F

ALTERNATIVE TECHNIQUES FOR LATE REPAIR

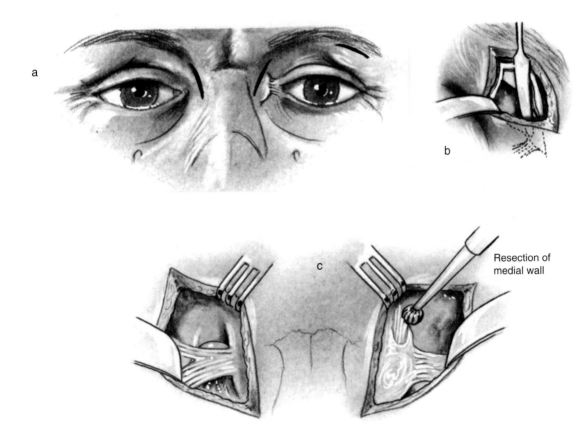

a

b

c

Resection of
medial wall

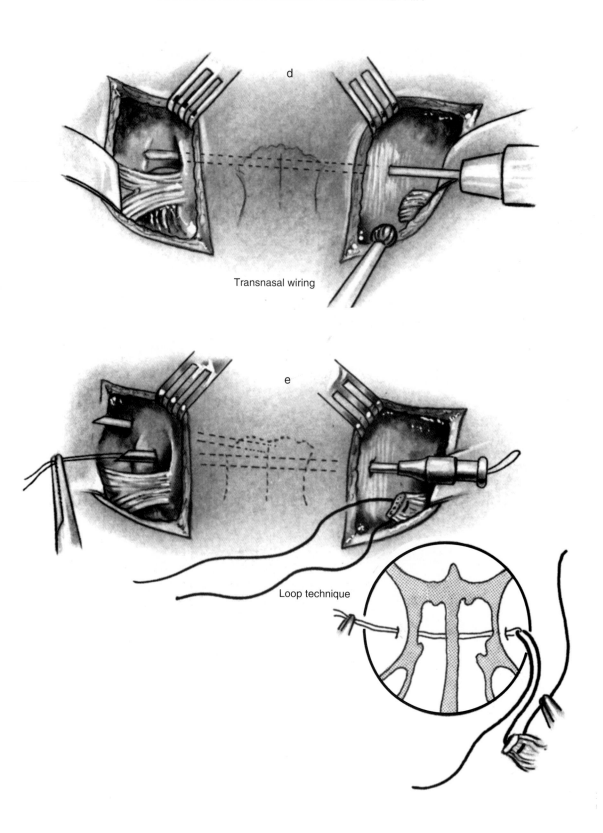

Transnasal wiring

Loop technique

drill or drill holes with a 0.035 inch K wire and minidriver. The holes can be cannulated with a 14-gauge needle, and through the needle, the surgeon can then pass the transnasal wires. The process can be simplified by first passing a loop of 30-gauge wire through the needle, pulling through the end of the medial canthal-attached wire, removing the needle, and leaving the end in place. Another cannulation is then performed with an exit point just beyond the first; again, a 30-gauge wire loop technique is used to pass the other end of the medial canthal wire. The technique requires sufficient exposure of the medial walls of the orbits and retraction and protection of the globes and soft tissues with malleable retractors. Attachment of the medial canthal wire to the lacrimal crest of the opposite side, overcorrection of the medial canthal ligament, and closure of incisions are carried out as in the acute injury.

If the patient has a history of dacryocystitis, a dacryocystorhinostomy, described in Chapter 71, should also be performed. Timing is important. The dacryocystorhinostomy repair should be carried out after the attachment of the wire to the medial canthal ligament, but before the wire is attached to the bone and the medial canthal ligament brought into the corrected position. If the dacryocystorhinostomy is done too early, there is a risk of pulling out the mucosal sutures with the transnasal wiring technique. If the dacryocystorhinostomy is done too late during the procedure, then the exposure will be compromised by the medially displaced orbital tissues.

Open Repair of Bilateral Naso-Orbital Injury With Intercanthal Ligament Fixation

Alternative Technique Using Frontal Process Fixation

INDICATIONS

Bilateral naso-orbital injury is characterized by comminution of the upper midface. The damage involves the medial walls of both orbits. Clinically there is marked bilateral telecanthus, displacement and blunting of the inner angles, narrowing of the palpebral fissures, and epiphora. The nasal bones are usually depressed. There is a history of epistaxis and unconsciousness, and often there is evidence of nasal obstruction and cerebrospinal fluid leak. Recognition of this type of injury is important, as stable bony attachments are not readily available, and the surgeon must find alternatives for attachments of the ligaments.

PROCEDURE

A–C The patient should be in stable medical condition for the procedure. The head and neck are prepared with antiseptic solutions and draped as a sterile field. The incision sites are injected with 1% lidocaine containing 1:100,000 epinephrine to assist in the hemostasis. The surgeon has the option of marking out bilateral lateral eyebrow incisions and standard bilateral medial canthal incisions (as described in Chapters 68 and 69), performing the open sky approach in which the medial canthal incisions are connected with a horizontal limb to each other or, even better, using a coronal

flap approach as described in Chapters 43 and 53. If the coronal flap is used, it will, however, be important to extend exposure along the medial walls of the orbit.

Working on one side at a time, the angular vessels are ligated or cauterized. The periosteum is incised and elevated superiorly off the glabella angle and prominence of the brow. Inferiorly the lacrimal fossa, the lacrimal collecting system, and the medial wall of the orbit are explored. Additional exposure is obtained by releasing the attachment of the trochlea and anterior ethmoidal artery. Hemostasis is carried out with gentle pressure, bipolar cautery, or vascular clips. Bone fragments involving the medial wall of the orbit are reduced, and if necessary, the wall is reinforced with polyepropylene mesh (see Chapter 63). The nasal and frontal bones are reduced and fixed with bone plate techniques (see Chapters 53 and 75). Lateral canthotomies as described in Chapter 67 are performed bilaterally.

D On one side, the medial canthal ligament is secured to a 30-gauge wire with a cutting needle. Both ends of the wire are then attached to a large curved needle, which is passed through the superior portion of the septum to the opposite side. Entrance and exit on the medial walls of the orbit should be through the lacrimal bone region. The globes and soft tissues of the orbit must be protected with malleable retractors during these maneuvers. One free end of the 30-gauge wire

BILATERAL NASO-ORBITAL REPAIR

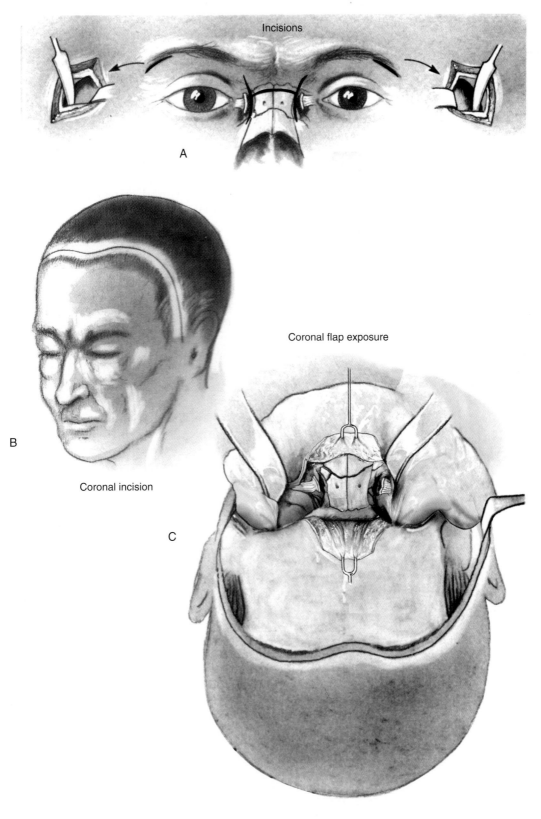

Incisions

A

B

Coronal incision

C

Coronal flap exposure

is then attached to a fine curved needle and the needle passed through the opposite medial canthal ligament. The wire is tightened and the ends pulled together so that the ligaments pull toward each other. The twisted ends of the wire are subsequently bent back against the wall of the orbit.

Closure is in layers. The periosteum is closed with 4-0 chromic sutures. The soft tissues are secured in anatomic position. Antibiotics are prescribed for at least 5 to 7 days, or for a longer time if there is any evidence of a cerebrospinal fluid leak. The sutures are removed at 5 to 7 days. The status of the frontal sinus should be evaluated with CT Scans in the postoperative period.

PITFALLS

1. As described in Chapters 67 through 69, the pull on the medial canthal ligament should be upward and backward, with an overcorrection toward the midline. To achieve these relationships, the transnasal wire must be placed high along the septum. The surgeon must take precautions to avoid entering the anterior cranial fossa. A ligament placed too low will tilt the medial canthal ligaments downward and cause scleral show. Alternatively, the surgeon can place crossed transnasal wires attached to the frontal process of the maxilla (see later).

2. The transnasal wire technique requires protection of the globes during the transfer of the needle and wires from one side to the other. Large, carefully placed malleable retractors and skilled assistants are helpful during these maneuvers.

3. Avoid passing wires through the lacrimal collecting system, as this can cause obstruction. The wires should be passed high above it.

4. For the repair of injuries that have healed with deformity, drill techniques for passage of the wire are required. These methods are similar to those described for the unilateral late repair (see Chapter 68).

5. External plates or buttons should be avoided since they will be of little, if any, assistance in holding the medial canthal ligaments in position. Excessive pressure from plates/buttons can cause necrosis of the skin and should be avoided.

6. Diagnosis of the degree and extent of associated frontal sinus fractures is important if the surgeon is to select and apply appropriate treatment. Anterior wall fractures of the frontal bone can frequently be managed with titanium mesh or thin plate techniques. Fractures extending to the posterior wall or floor of the frontal sinus may cause dural injury and/or obstruction to the nasofrontal duct and need to be treated differently. These conditions are discussed in Chapters 76 through 80.

COMPLICATIONS

1. Residual eyelid deformity and dysfunction of the lacrimal collecting system must be recognized and treated as soon as the complication is recognized. These sequelae can be best treated when the tissues are soft and the bones are mobile. Later, scarring, retraction, and malunion can cause significant problems in the reduction and repair. Techniques to free up the periorbita, relax orbital tissues, remove bone, and perform a transnasal repair are described in Chapter 68.

2. Low placement of the transnasal wire can lead to a downward displacement of the medial canthal ligament and excessive scleral show. If this condition occurs, the wires should be reattached high through the septum. If there is only mild asymmetry of the medial canthal ligaments, this may be managed by VY- and Z-plasty techniques (see Chapters 13 and 73).

3. Obstruction of the lacrimal collecting system, alone or with dacryocystitis, is a common postoperative problem. Epiphora occuring early after the injury may be caused by postoperative swelling that affects the transfer of tears through the lacrimal collecting system. However, if the epiphora persists, the surgeon must seriously consider the possibility of a mechanical obstruction. Confirmation can be obtained by a fluorescein dye test. For lower system obstruction, the surgeon must consider a dacryocystorhinostomy (see Chapter 71). If the injury is confined to the cannaliculi and/or puncta, a conjunctivodacryocystorhinostomy or conjunctivorhinostomy should be performed.

4. Obstruction of a nasofrontal duct can later cause frontal sinusitis. This condition should be recognized by a failure of the frontal sinus to aerate. Occasionally the patient will complain about swelling and pain over the forehead region. If these problems develop, the surgeon has the option of reconstructing the nasofrontal duct or obliterating the frontal sinus (see Chapters 76 through 80).

5. Cerebrospinal fluid leakage can continue following surgery. If this occurs, the patient should be treated with antibiotics, and if the leak persists beyond 2 to 3 weeks, the surgeon should be prepared for evaluation of the site and closure of the area of fistula (see Chapters 83, 84, 85, 90, and 91).

6. Webbing of the medial canthal incision site can initially be treated by injection of 40 mg/mL of triamcinolone. If the scars remain unsightly, Z-plasty or zigzagplasty techniques should be performed (see Chapters 13 and 73). Sometimes making an irregular medial canthal incision at the time of initial surgery will avoid this complication.

ALTERNATIVE TECHNIQUE USING FRONTAL PROCESS FIXATION

a,b The transnasal canthoplasty, attaching one medial canthal ligament to the other, is an excellent method to overcorrect placement of the medial canthal ligament. However, if the medial canthal ligament and inner angle rotates inferiorly, then the surgeon should consider attaching the wires transnasally to the opposite frontal process.

The incisions and approaches are identical to those used above. Following exposure of the medial canthal ligaments and relaxation of the ligaments by way of lateral canthotomies, a wire is passed through the medial canthal ligament transversely to the opposite wall of the orbit in the region of the upper lacrimal fossa. A drill hole is made through the anterior crest on the frontal process of the maxilla, and the wire is then passed through the hole. A similar procedure is carried out with the other end of the wire, but through a passageway several millimeters distant to the first hole. The ends of the wire are then tightened to bring the ligament into proper position. The other medial canthal ligament is secured with a similar transnasal technique. The procedure will thus affect a crossing of wires within the nasal vault. The advantage to this intercanthal wire is that one medial canthal ligament can be adjusted independently of the other. The disadvantage is that there can be asymmetry in the placement of the ligaments. Postoperative care is the same as that following the intercanthal method.

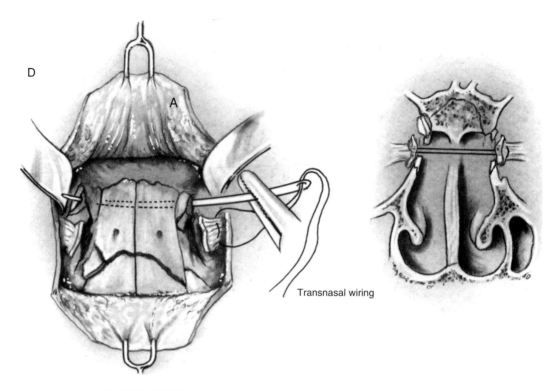

Transnasal wiring

ALTERNATIVE TECHNIQUE USING FRONTAL PROCESS FIXATION

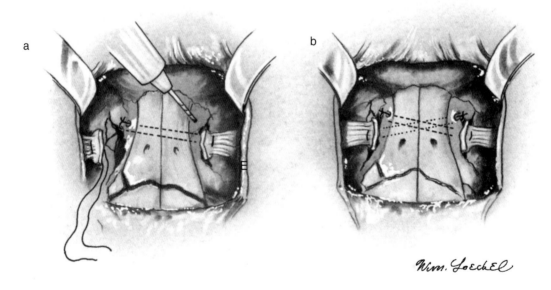

CHAPTER 70

Open Reduction and Repair of Telescoping Naso-Orbital Injury

INDICATIONS

Instead of breaking into small pieces, the naso-orbital fracture can also be driven as a block of bone beneath the frontal bone. The medial walls of the orbit are often involved, and if the fracture extends into the lacrimal bones, the medial canthi will splay laterally. The injury causes a characteristic appearance in which the naso-frontal angle is accentuated. Frontal bone fractures are common. There is often a telecanthus and epiphora involving one or both eyes. Epistaxis, cerebrospinal fluid leakage, and intracranial damage can occur.

PROCEDURE

Under general orotracheal anesthesia, the face is prepared and draped as a sterile field. An open sky or coronal incision (see Chapter 69) is mapped out with marking solution. The operative site should be infiltrated with 1% lidocaine containing epinephrine to help with hemostasis.

The periosteum is elevated from the nasal bones and outer cortex of the frontal bone. The medial walls of the orbits are exposed as in Chapters 68 and 69. Additional exposure can be obtained by releasing the anterior ethmoidal vessels. Bleeding can be controlled by gentle pressure, bipolar cautery, or application of vascular clips.

A–C A forceful reduction is required. A small curved osteotome is inserted through the fracture line, and if the frontal bone is intact, the osteotome can be levered on the face of the frontal bone to elevate the nasoethmoid complex into correct position. If the frontal bone is also fractured or the nasoethmoid depression is severe enough to affect optimal mechanical leverage, then the nasoethmoid complex must be reduced by an anteriorly directed force. This can be accomplished by applying a towel clip to the frontal processes of the maxilla and pulling outward. Care must be taken not to be overly forceful, or the complex will be extracted from the craniofacial skeleton.

D After reduction is accomplished, the medial canthal ligament is restored to anatomic position (see repairs in Chapters 67 through 69). Usually the reduced frontoethmoid block of bone is stable, but if this is not the case, low profile miniplates can be applied to the nasomaxillary buttresses.

The wounds are closed in layers. The periosteum and subcutaneous tissues are approximated with 4-0 chromic sutures, and the skin is closed with 5-0 or 6-0 nylon sutures. Prophylactic antibiotics are prescribed for 5 to 7 days or longer if there is evidence of a cerebrospinal fluid leak. The sutures are removed in 5 to 7 days. Serial CT scans are obtained postoperatively to evaluate the frontal sinuses.

PITFALLS

1. Reduction is the most difficult part of the procedure. If the nasoethmoid block of bone is overcorrected, there will be a tendency for cerebrospinal fluid leakage.

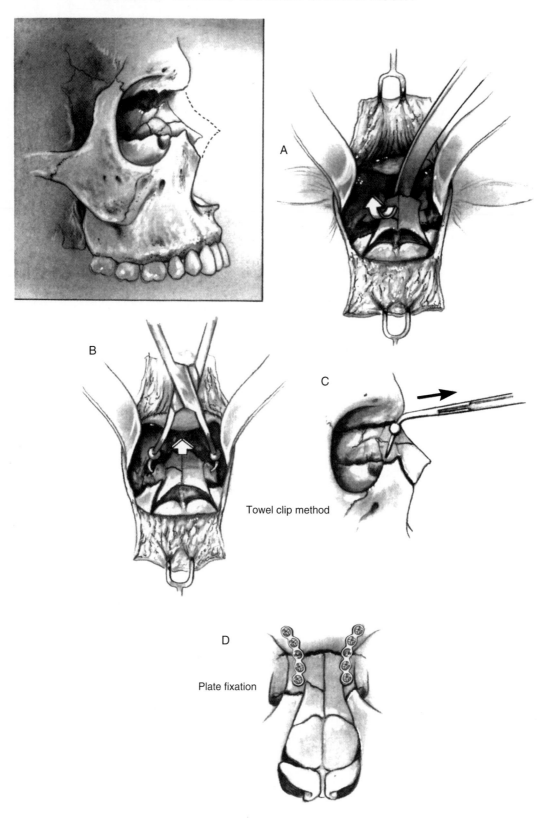

A

B

C

Towel clip method

D

Plate fixation

Wm. Loechel

Extraction of the bone is also possible, especially if the surgeon does not take precautions in the amount of force exerted to effect the reduction. Overcorrection or extraction can sometimes be avoided by keeping pressure on the dorsum of the nose as the lifting is carried out. Gentle rocking can also be effective.

2. Beware of associated injuries. In addition to the telecanthus, there can be fractures extending through the cribriform plate and frontal bone. Accurate reduction of the cribriform plate will usually approximate dural tears and help seal cerebrospinal fluid leaks. However, fractures extending into the frontal bone may interfere with subsequent normal aeration and drainage of the sinus, and if there is evidence of such a fracture, it should be treated accordingly (see Chapters 76 through 80).

3. Nasal septal injury should be managed by one of the closed or open techniques (see Chapters 52 and 53). If cerebrospinal fluid leakage is also noted, packing should be avoided and the septum stabilized with polyethylene plates. Antibiotic coverage is mandatory.

4. Injuries directed to the nasofrontal angle can also transmit forces to the base of the skull and cause injury to the optic nerve. If the patient has a decrease in vision related in time to the fracture, the surgeon should consider the possibility of optic nerve compression and treat the injury as described in Chapters 86 and 87.

COMPLICATIONS

1. Failure to achieve an adequate reduction will cause a depression of the nasofrontal angle. If the bones heal in malposition, it is probably more prudent to correct the deformity by cartilage and/or onlay bone grafts to the dorsum of the nose. Osteotomies are difficult to perform and can be complicated by unstable fragments of bone, cerebrospinal fluid leaks, and damage to the nasofrontal duct.

2. Although rare, it is possible during reduction to extract the nasoethmoid complex. This complication can be avoided with gentle rocking and counter pressure by the opposite hand. If the bone is inadvertently removed, it should be replaced immediately and wired into position. Exposed and torn dura require repair. Neurosurgical consultation should be obtained.

3. Obstruction of the nasofrontal duct can be a complication of naso-orbital injury, and if it is not recognized, it can later cause a life-threatening sinusitis or mucocele. The surgeon should evaluate the extent of the fracture, and if it involves the duct, it can be treated with reconstruction of the duct or obliteration of the frontal sinus with fat (see Chapters 76 through 80). If the surgeon chooses to manage the fracture conservatively, the sinuses must be evaluated for permanent aeration.

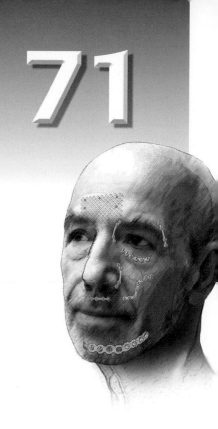

CHAPTER 71

Dacryocystorhinostomy
Alternative Endoscopic Technique

In Consultation With Adam Folbe, MD

INDICATIONS

Injury to the naso-orbital region has the potential to cause problems with many parts of the lacrimal collecting system. If tear collection is inadequate or obstructed, epiphora will occur. Soft tissue injuries can affect the upper collecting system (i.e., canaliculi and/or puncta); this is discussed in Chapter 72. Twisting or kinking to the lower portion of the system (i.e., naso-lacrimal duct and/or sac) will cause stasis of secretions, which potentially can result in dacryocystitis. In the latter condition, there is inflammation of the medial canthus and intermittent mucopurulent discharge through the puncta. Manual pressure on the sac region will cause retrograde discharge of the mucopurulent secretions.

It is important to determine the level and degree of obstruction. In the absence of infection, a simple fluorescein dye test can be applied. The fluorescein is placed in the lower conjunctival sulcus; if the system is functioning normally, the fluorescein, on opening and closing the eyes, will be transmitted to the inferior meatus of the nose. The dye can then be examined on a pledget placed in this area. Failure of the dye to pass indicates that there is a blockage or malfunction somewhere in the system. The puncta and canaliculi should then be irrigated with saline. The appearance of the dye in the inferior meatus indicates that there was some retention of the dye in the lacrimal sac, and more force (not just natural pumping action) was necessary to pass it into the nose. These findings also suggest that the canaliculi and puncta are intact and functioning

normally. For those obstructions distal to the sac, the surgeon should consider a dacryocystorhinostomy. For obstructions proximal to the sac, a conjunctivorhinostomy (or conjunctivodacryocystorhinostomy) is indicated (see Chapter 72).

PROCEDURE

A The nose should be treated preliminarily with 4% cocaine and epinephrine as described in Chapter 54. The face is prepared and draped as a sterile field. An incision is mapped out with marking solution one-half the distance between the caruncle and dorsum of the nose, but instead of the medial canthal incision described for the telecanthus repair, the incision is extended inferiorly along the inferior orbital rim. The angular vessels should be ligated or cauterized. The periosteum is incised over the frontal process of the maxilla and the periosteum released off the anterior lacrimal crest with a Freer elevator.

B–D The elevation should expose the medial or nasal side of the lacrimal sac. Working medial to the sac, the periosteum and sac are elevated from the lacrimal fossa to expose the posterior lacrimal crest. The lacrimal fossa is then fractured, and using Kerrison rongeurs, the opening is enlarged, removing the anterior and inferior portions of the anterior crest. Portions of the frontal process of the maxillary bone are also excised. The mucosa of the nose should be kept intact, and to avoid injury to the mucosa, the mucoperiosteum on the nasal side should be elevated before bone is removed. Dense, thick bone can also be excised by drilling with cutting burs. When the bone becomes thin, the remainder can be removed with Kerrison or Takahashi rongeurs.

E,F With the nasal mucosa and sac exposed, the lower canaliculus and puncta are dilated with a lacrimal probe. A No. 00 probe is then passed into the sac, and where it tents the sac, an incision is made vertically through the sac. Two 4-0 chromic sutures are passed through the posterior flap of the sac and held with a small hemostat.

G,H The nasal mucosa is tented with a clamp inserted intranasally and incised in a superior-to-inferior direction. This will also create posterior and anterior flaps. The posterior flaps of the nasal and sac membranes are subsequently attached by the chromic sutures and held loosely out of the field.

I,J At this point, silastic tubing swaged onto flexible probes is passed through the superior and inferior canaliculi, through the opening in the sac, and into the nose (see Chapter 72). The probe wires are cut free, and the silastic tubing is tied into a loop that lies in the inferior meatus. The two sutures that had been placed through the posterior flaps are then tied securely. Two additional sutures are placed through the corresponding anterior flaps and tied down. The periosteum and subcutaneous tissues are approximated with additional 4-0 chromic sutures, and the skin is closed with a 5-0 nylon suture.

Prophylactic antibiotics are utilized for 5 days, and an ophthalmic antibiotic ointment is applied for several days. The nose is kept clean with saline douches three times a day and then daily until the tube is removed at 3 to 4 weeks.

PITFALLS

1. An incision directly over the sac, as described earlier, is helpful in exposing the lacrimal fossa and the entire sac area. The standard medial canthal incision can also be used but would make the inferior portion of the osteotomy difficult to perform. However, it is useful when combining the dacryocystorhinostomy with a telecanthus repair.

2. If the dacryocystorhinostomy is to be done in conjunction with a telecanthus repair, the surgeon must plan the timing of the procedures. If not done in the proper sequence, one procedure can adversely affect the other. We have found that the medial canthal exploration and repair and the lateral canthotomy should be done first, followed by attachment of the 30-gauge

wire to the medial canthus. The wire is left loose, and preparations are made for the wire to be attached either to the upper posterior lacrimal crest or to the crest or medial canthal ligament of the opposite side. The dacryocystorhinostomy is then performed. The medial canthal ligament is subsequently pulled into position, and the wound is closed in a standard fashion.

3. Before performing a dacryocystorhinostomy, the surgeon must be certain that the puncta and canaliculi are functioning and the eyelid comes in contact with the surface of the globe. Therefore it is important that the lacrimal collecting system be first studied with a dye test and obstruction be evaluated with probe dilatations. Early injuries of the upper (proximal) collecting system can be treated with intubation and repair of the canaliculus, but if this fails, a conjunctivorhinostomy or, alternatively, a conjunctivodacryocystorhinostomy (see Chapter 72) must be considered.

4. Make sure that the nasal passageways are patent and not involved with pathologic processes. Avoid the procedure in patients with sinusitis, nasal masses, or polyps. These conditions should be controlled before performing the dacryocystorhinostomy.

COMPLICATIONS

1. Continuation or return of epiphora will occur if the lacrimal collecting system again becomes obstructed or fails to function properly. Occasionally there is still a problem with the proximal system (canaliculus and puncta), and the surgeon must be certain that these parts are patent and that the puncta is in contact with the surface of the globe. Stenosis occurring at the outlet of the lacrimal sac will cause accumulation of secretions within the sac, stasis, and infection. If this occurs, another dacryocystorhinostomy should be performed. In elderly patients in whom tearing is diminished, a dacryocystectomy can be considered. If there are associated problems with the proximal segment, a conjunctivorhinostomy (see Chapter 72) may be the procedure of choice.

2. Dacryocystitis is a serious infection that occasionally extends from the sac to involve other periorbital tissues. Orbital abscesses and orbital cellulitis can occur. If such conditions develop, the sac should be drained and the patient administered intravenous antibiotics. Cultures should be taken to evaluate microorganism susceptibility. Antibiotics should be administered until there is no longer any sign of inflammation. Subsequently (i.e., several weeks later) the patient should be considered for a repeat dacryocystorhinostomy or dacryocystectomy.

DACRYOCYSTORHINOSTOMY

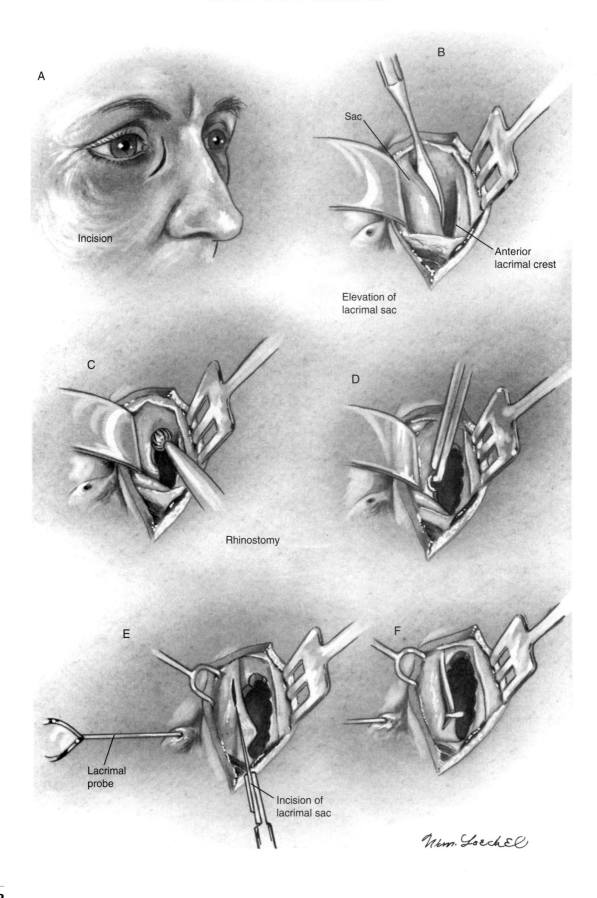

A

Incision

B

Sac

Anterior
lacrimal crest

Elevation of
lacrimal sac

C

Rhinostomy

D

E

Lacrimal
probe

Incision of
lacrimal sac

F

DACRYOCYSTORHINOSTOMY *(Continued)*

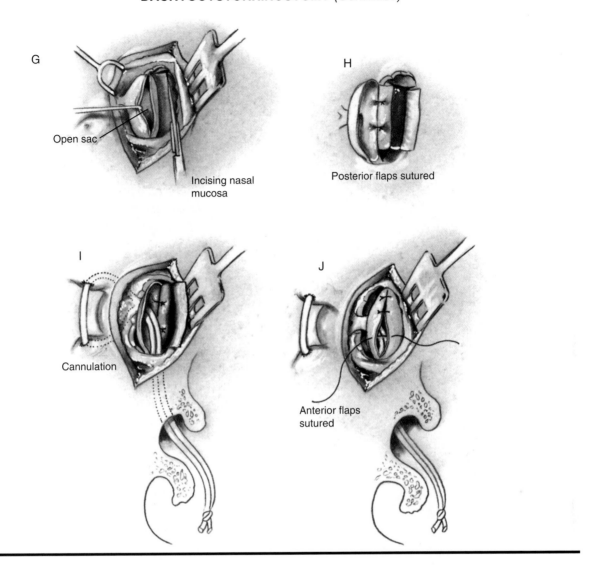

G

Open sac

Incising nasal mucosa

H

Posterior flaps sutured

I

Cannulation

J

Anterior flaps sutured

ALTERNATIVE ENDOSCOPIC TECHNIQUE

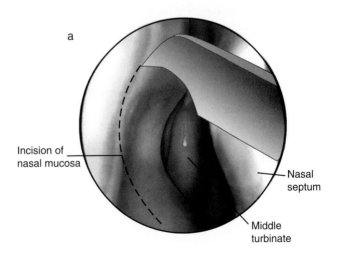

a

Incision of nasal mucosa

Nasal septum

Middle turbinate

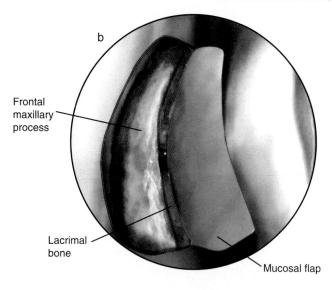

b

Frontal
maxillary
process

Lacrimal
bone

Mucosal flap

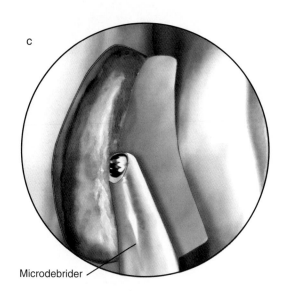

c

Microdebrider

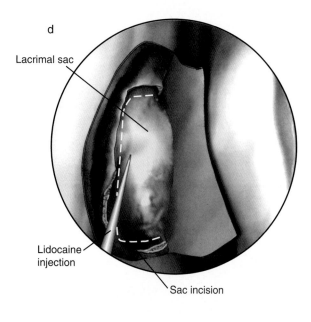

d

Lacrimal sac

Lidocaine
injection

Sac incision

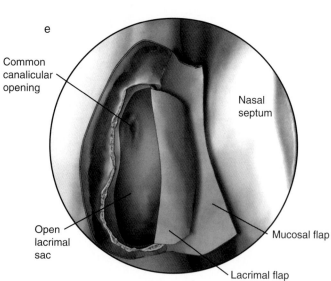

e

Common
canalicular
opening

Nasal
septum

Open
lacrimal
sac

Mucosal flap

Lacrimal flap

ALTERNATIVE ENDOSCOPIC TECHNIQUE

With pledgets containing 4% cocaine and epinephrine as described in Chapter 54 the nasal mucus membranes are prepared to control hemostatsis. The lateral wall of the nose is then injected with 2% lidocaine containing 1:100,000 epinephrine.

a,b The initial incision should start 1 cm above the axilla of the middle turbinate and extend in a C-shaped fashion laterally onto the frontal process of the maxilla toward the insertion of the inferior turbinate. Superiorly the incision should extend to the uncinate process. A mucopereosteal flap is then elevated exposing the frontal process of the maxilla and the lacrimal bone posteriorly.

c A microdebrider or diamond bur is utilized to remove the lacrimal bone over the lacrimal sac and a portion of the frontal process of the maxilla. The technique requires a thinning of the bone and then elevation with a curette or elevator. The osteotomy should be enlarged to expose the extent of the lacrmal sac.

d The sac is then injected with lidocaine containing epinephrine, and an incision is made anteriorly and vertically with two horizontal limbs superiorly and inferiorly directed posteriorly at the upper limits of the osteotomy.

e The flap created on the sac is rotated medially to cover the lateral nasal flap. The flaps are held in place with gelfoam (or merocel which must be removed in 3 days). Stenting is possible with silastic tubing as described in Chapter 72 and is probably indicated when there is a small or atrophic sac. Postoperatively the patient is placed on prophylactic antibiotics and antibiotic eye drops. The nose should be moisturized with saline sprays to prevent clots and mucus plugs and examined and cleaned endoscopically during the next several weeks.

Repair of Canaliculi
Alternative Method of Conjunctivorhinostomy

INDICATIONS

Trauma to the naso-orbital region can be associated with lacerations, which, if extensive, can sever the medial canthal ligament and parts of the lacrimal collecting system. Early recognition of the injury and immediate repair are necessary if the surgeon is to restore normal anatomic relationships and physiologic functions. Damage to the lacrimal collecting system will prevent the collection of tears and, if not treated, can result in chronic epiphora. Most of the flow is through the inferior canaliculus, and it is thus important that damage be recognized and that the canaliculus be repaired early after injury. The superior canaliculus may also be repaired, but a functioning inferior canaliculus will probably suffice. Treatment of injuries to the lower (distal) portion of the lacrimal collection system is discussed in Chapter 71.

PROCEDURE

Under general anesthesia, the face is prepared and draped as a sterile field. To help with hemostasis, the medial canthal region is infiltrated with 1% lidocaine containing 1:100,000 epinephrine.

A The procedure is carried out with the operating microscope. The laceration should be irrigated with normal saline and the edges examined for the ends of the severed canaliculus. The proximal segment (near the puncta) is easy to identify, as the surgeon can dilate the puncta with lacrimal dilators and pass the probe through the canaliculus into the laceration. The probe will then point to the severed canaliculus of the opposite side. If the distal end still cannot be seen, the surgeon can then irrigate the superior canaliculus with normal saline, press on the sac, and force the fluid retrograde through the inferior canaliculus.

B–D Following identification of the ends of the canaliculus, a Silastic tube swaged on a flexible probe is passed through the superior (or inferior) canalicular system into the sac and out through the nasolacrimal duct. The other swaged end is passed through the inferior (or superior) part into the sac to follow the same route as the first tube. The probes are then cut from the tubing, and the tubing is tied into a knot, which is placed on the floor of the nose. The tubing, acting as a stent, provides support while the surgeon approximates the cut ends of the canaliculus with 8-0 nonabsorbable sutures.

E–I The eyelid laceration is closed with a special suture technique. A 5-0 chromic suture is secured and buried near the edge of the tarsal border. A 6-0 silk suture is placed at the level of the meibomian gland orifices at about 1 to 2 mm from the wound margins. A second 6-0 silk suture is placed on the posterior eyelid near the junction of the skin and conjunctiva. A third 6-0 silk suture is placed in front of the first silk suture so that the needle is passed through the lashes. The sutures are then tied down and the ends brought anteriorly to be held by the most anterior suture.

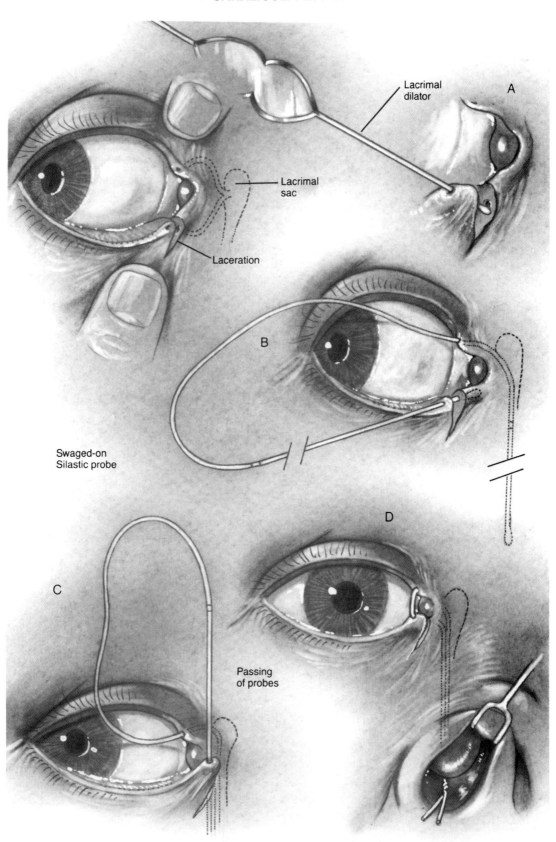

Lacrimal dilator

A

Lacrimal sac

Laceration

B

Swaged-on Silastic probe

D

C

Passing of probes

Wm. Loechel

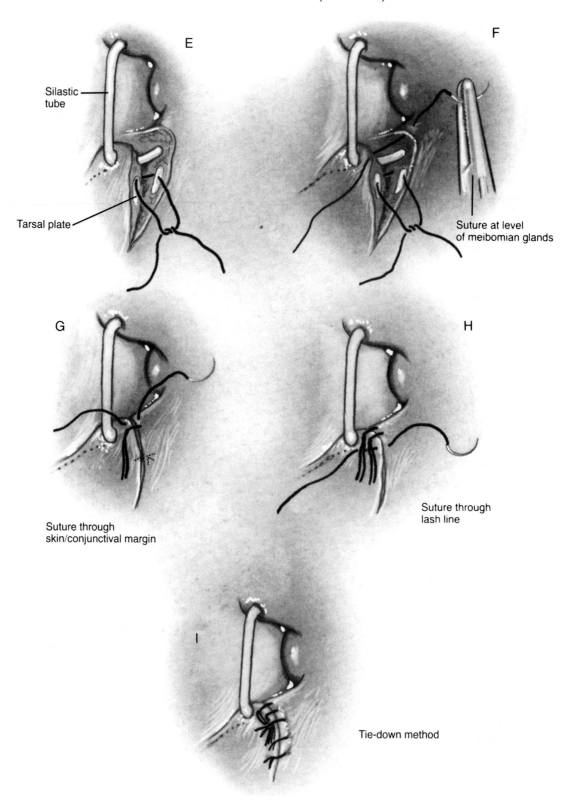

E

Silastic tube

Tarsal plate

F

Suture at level of meibomian glands

G

Suture through skin/conjunctival margin

H

Suture through lash line

I

Tie-down method

Antibiotic eye ointment is applied for several days. The sutures are removed in 3 to 5 days, and stents are retained for 2 to 3 weeks. The nose should be kept clean with normal saline douches.

PITFALLS

1. The lacrimal collecting system should be carefully examined when there are lacerations through or near the medial part of the eyelid. Dehiscences of the canaliculi can be evaluated by cannulation and instillation of saline solution. The wound should also be explored, using the microscope to determine the site and degree of damage.

2. Although the lower eyelid canaliculus carries most of the tears, the surgeon should still attempt to repair the upper canaliculus. The additional function of the upper canaliculus ensures a more efficient excretion mechanism. Moreover, if the lower canaliculus fails, the upper canaliculus can take over and possibly prevent epiphora from occurring.

3. Canaliculus repair should be performed under the most ideal conditions. The procedure should be done within 24 to 48 hours of injury and during a time when equipment and assistants are readily available. Late repairs can be complicated by secondary infection and scarring and should be avoided.

COMPLICATIONS

1. The main complication of the canalicular repair is restenosis and failure to conduct tears. With the Silastic stent in position, function is difficult to evaluate. When the stent is finally removed several weeks later, scarring can develop, which will preclude any simple revision of the collecting system. In such cases, the surgeon should consider a conjunctivorhinostomy or conjunctivodacryocystorhinostomy. In the elderly patient, tear secretion is often reduced, and with sufficient evaporation, conservative management can be considered.

2. Displacement of the tubing can be a problem. The tubing can break and come out or, occasionally, loosen and fall into the palpebral fissure. The tubing can also erode through the canaliculus. To avoid these problems, the patient should be instructed on the correct position of the tubing. If inflammation develops, ophthalmic antibiotic drops should be administered.

3. Ectropion or entropion can be secondary problems related to the repair of the canaliculi and the eyelid laceration. These complications can be difficult to treat and are beyond the scope of this text. Ophthalmologic evaluation and consultation are desirable.

ALTERNATIVE METHOD OF CONJUNCTIVORHINOSTOMY

Failure of the upper (proximal) lacrimal collecting system following repair of the canaliculus should probably be treated with a bypass method. The diagnosis is obtained with standard fluorescein dye (Jones) tests, described in Chapter 71. Conjunctivodacryocystorhinostomy, using a Jones tube, is generally effective, but the technique may be complicated by granulation tissue formation, infection from unopposed mucosal flaps, and inefficient passage of tears through scar as a result of the secondary healing. Caniculodacryocystorhinostomy affords the advantages of physiologic reconstruction but is limited by availability of sufficient canaliculus, requires lengthy tedious dissection, and must be performed using a microscopic approach. Our method is a variant of a conjunctivorhinostomy. It provides a total lacrimal bypass and has the advantages of bipedicled mucosal flaps, optimal temporary stenting, and improvement of epiphora.

a–c Preparation consists of application of a vasoconstrictive agent to the nasal mucosa and infiltration with 1% lidocaine containing 1:100,000 epinephrine. The medial canthal incision (one-half the distance between the medial canthus and the dorsum of the nose) is used for exposure. The angular vessels are ligated, and the periosteum is elevated off the nasal bones and along the medial wall of the orbit to expose the lacrimal crests and fossa. A rhinostomy is created as described in Chapter 71. The mucoperiosteum of the nose is elevated on the nasal side, and a flap is developed along the anterolateral wall of the nose. To obtain satisfactory exposure, the middle turbinate should be fractured medially. Vertical and horizontal incisions can be designed and the flap rotated through the rhinostomy defect.

d,e On the orbital side, an inferiorly based flap of approximately 1 × 2 cm is developed from the medial aspect of the bulbar conjunctiva, just lateral to the limbus. A horizontal incision is made at the inferomedial aspect of the flap in the fornix and deepened to join the original medial canthal incision. The conjunctiva is sutured (end to end) to the mucosa of the nose using 5-0 chromic sutures. As an option, the surgeon can place a Jones tube stent through the fornix into the nose. The medial canthal incision is closed with a subcuticular 4-0 chromic suture and the skin with 6-0 nylon sutures. Prophylactic antibiotics are administered for 5 to 7 days.

REPAIR OF LACRIMAL COLLECTING SYSTEM

ALTERNATIVE TECHNIQUE OF CONJUNCTIVORHINOSTOMY

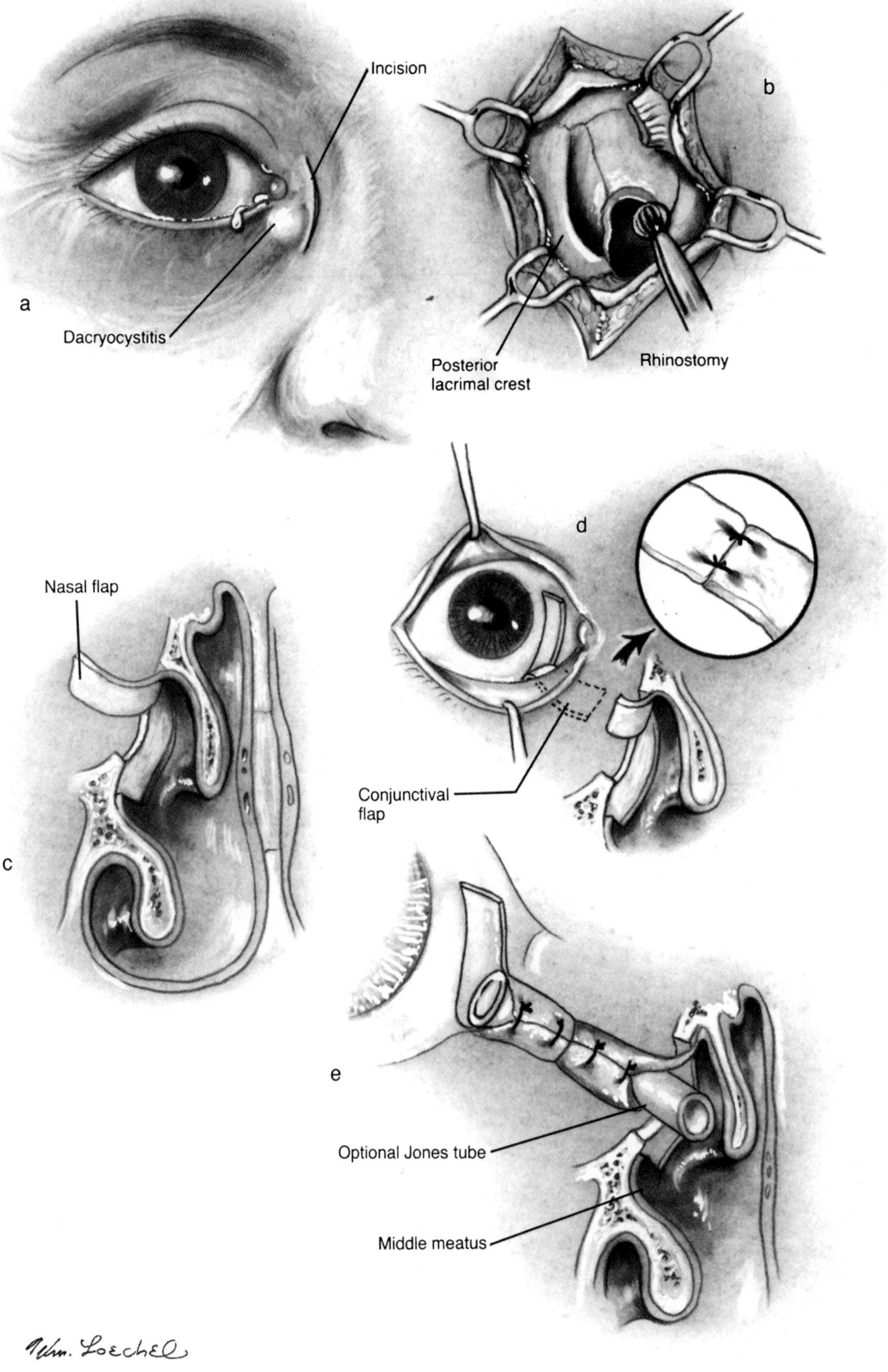

a — Incision / Dacryocystitis

b — Posterior lacrimal crest / Rhinostomy

c — Nasal flap

d — Conjunctival flap

e — Optional Jones tube / Middle meatus

Wm. Loechel

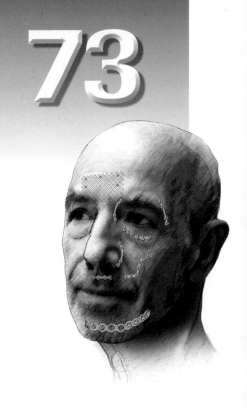

Repair of Widened Scars, Webs, and Displaced Angles of the Medial Canthus

INDICATIONS

Posttraumatic telecanthus can be associated with a variety of deformities that often can be corrected with limited skin surgery. A marked displacement of the inner angle and caruncle requires a formal telecanthus repair (see Chapters 67 through 69), but occasionally the displacement is minimal (i.e., 1 to 2 mm), and an advancement and/or rotation of skin flaps can provide a satisfactory result. Widened scars or web deformities can often be treated by application of zigzag- or Z-plasty techniques. If the angle of the medial canthus is displaced upward or downward, these sequelae can usually be corrected with transposition flaps (Z-plasty). These techniques are also described in Chapter 13.

PROCEDURE

In preparation for the surgery, the palpebral fissure width and height should be measured and compared with the palpebral fissure of the opposite side. The inner angle should be symmetric, and any displacement upward or downward should be appropriately recorded. Photographic documentation should be obtained prior to the repair.

Widened Scars and Web Formation

A Usually the medial canthal incision heals well with minimal scar formation. Occasionally, however, the scar widens or contracts into an unsightly web.

If these sequelae are observed early, it is possible to inject 40 mg/mL of triamcinolone to counteract the pathophysiologic processes. However, if the scar has matured, correctional surgery should be performed.

After preparation and draping of the face, the widened scar is outlined with marking solution. The area of scar is then infiltrated with 2% lidocaine. Sedation is used as necessary. If the inner angle is at the correct level, most scars can be camouflaged with a zigzag plasty. The scar is then excised with a geometric broken line at the level of the dermis. The adjacent tissues are undermined at a subcutaneous level, advanced, and closed in layers using 5-0 colorless or white nonabsorbable suture in the subcuticular tissues and interrupted (or running) 6-0 nylon sutures in the skin.

B If the scar is contracted and appears as a web, the surgeon should consider an excision and Z-plasty technique. The excised scar should correspond to the diagonal of the Z. Arms are then created at 45° to 60° to the diagonal. The flaps are undermined and rotated into position. Closure again should utilize 5-0 nonabsorbable sutures in the subcuticular layer and 6-0 nylon sutures in the skin.

Postoperatively the wound should be kept clean with 3% hydrogen peroxide and application of antibiotic ointment. Sutures are removed at 4 to 5 days.

Displaced Angle

If the inner angle is displaced laterally, inferiorly, or superiorly, it can often be corrected by an advancement

REPAIR OF SKIN DEFORMITIES

A

Widened scar

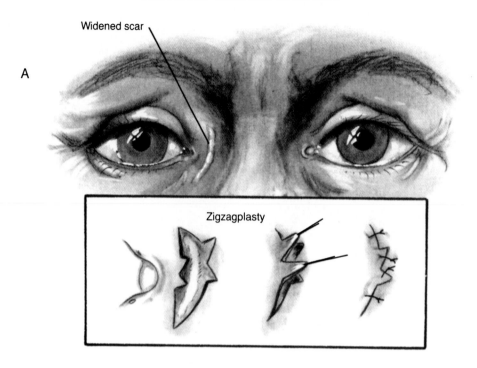

Zigzagplasty

B

Web formation

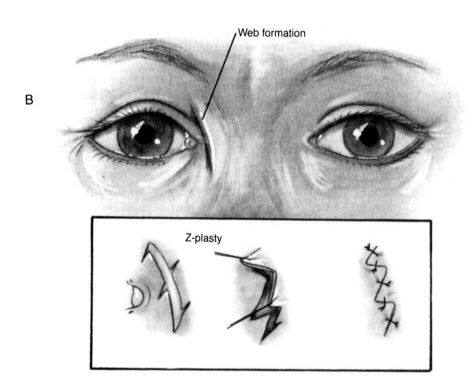

Z-plasty

Wm. Loechel

and/or transposition technique. The patient is usually prepared as for the scar revision described previously. The area is marked according to the design of the correction and infiltrated with 2% lidocaine.

C If the inner angle needs to be advanced medially, then a V-shaped incision is marked on the eyelid with the lines of the V parallel, but 1 to 2 cm below or above the eyelid margins. The point of the V is then extended as a line directed medially to form a Y. The length of this line should approximate the degree of lateral displacement and allow for 1 to 2 mm of overcorrection. The tissues are incised to the subcutaneous level and undermined approximately 0.5 to 1 cm. The flap is then advanced to the end of the Y to form a new medially displaced V, and the flap is secured with 5-0 white or colorless nonabsorbable subcuticular sutures. The skin is closed with interrupted 6-0 nylon sutures.

D If the inner angle is rotated upward or downward, then a Z-plasty should be designed to transpose the angles appropriately. One flap of the Z should contain the inner angle; the other flap should occupy space to which the inner angle will be transposed. Usually one arm of the Z will parallel the eyelid margin; the second arm will be more acutely drawn to the diagonal. The tissues are conservatively undermined and transposed. The wound is closed with 5-0 white or colorless nonabsorbable subcuticular sutures, with 6-0 nylon sutures in the skin. The incision is kept clean with 3% hydrogen peroxide and an antibiotic ointment. Sutures are removed in 4 to 6 days.

PITFALLS

1. Do not use soft tissue techniques if the lateral displacement is >2 mm. For such conditions, it is probably better to perform a telecanthus procedure and reset the medial canthi into a more optimal position (see Chapters 67 through 69).

2. Avoid repeated injections of triamcinolone, as this will cause atrophy and increased vascularity within the scar. Steroid injection should be used only once or twice to alleviate web contraction or widening. If the steroid injection fails to correct the scar, revisional surgery should be carried out.

3. Local infiltration of 1:100,000 epinephrine should be avoided. Small, thin flaps will often not tolerate a reduction in blood supply caused by the vasoconstriction of the agent. For these reasons, plain 2% lidocaine should be administered and the tissues handled with great care.

COMPLICATION

The vitality of the tissues is important if the surgeon is to obtain rapid healing of the wound with minimal scar formation. The surgeon should apply atraumatic techniques and, as described earlier, avoid the use of vasoconstrictive agents. If a scar develops, steroids can be administered. Later, surgical revision should be considered.

C

Laterally displaced angle

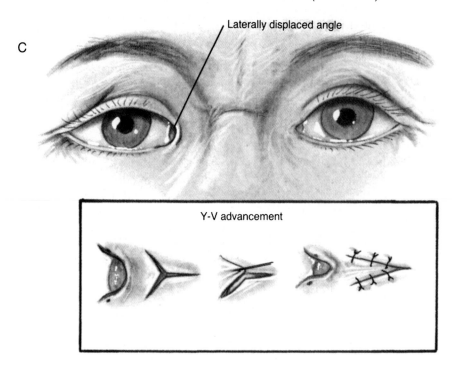

Y-V advancement

D

Inferiorly displaced angle

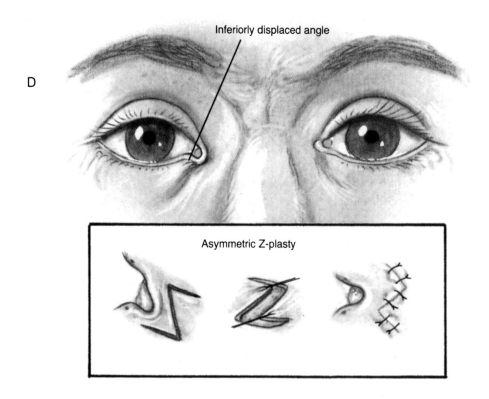

Asymmetric Z-plasty

Wm. Loechel

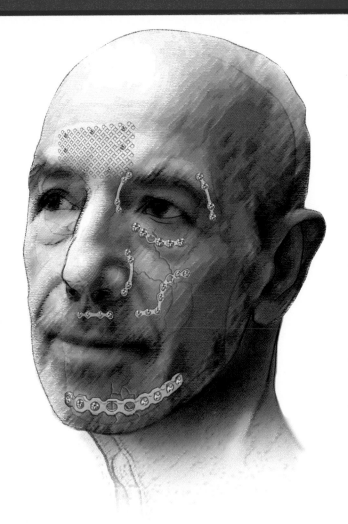

PART NINE

Frontal Sinus
Fractures

Classification and Pathophysiology of Frontal Sinus Fractures

CHAPTER

74

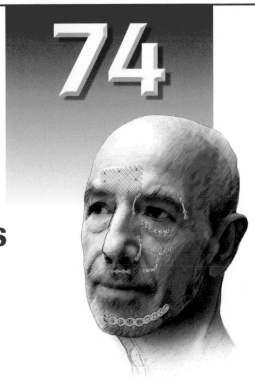

General Considerations

Early recognition and treatment of frontal sinus fractures is important if the surgeon is to restore normal appearance and prevent the sequelae of sinusitis and intranasal infection. Such fractures can alter the contour of the forehead and be associated with cerebrospinal fluid leakage and intracranial damage. Some injuries can cause obstruction of the nasofrontal duct, which in turn can cause stasis of secretions within the frontal sinus and sinusitis and mucocele formation. The adjacent orbital roof can be displaced, resulting in dystopia and possibly in a malfunction of the superior rectus, superior oblique, or levator muscles.

Frontal sinus fractures are classified according to anterior, posterior, or inferior wall injuries. Each takes into consideration the site and extent of the fracture, signs and symptoms, and the potential for complications.

A *Anterior wall fractures* can be linear, depressed, or comminuted. They can occur beneath intact skin, or they can be exposed through open wounds. The fractures are usually associated with deformities involving the forehead but can also extend to the posterior wall and/or floor and present additional signs and symptoms associated with the adjacent sites of injury.

B *Posterior wall fractures* are characterized by damage to the protective shell of the cranium. These fractures may also be linear, depressed, or comminuted. Injuries to the posterior wall are usually associated with dural tears and cerebrospinal fluid leaks. Intracranial damage (i.e., epidural and intracranial hematomas) can also occur. Posterior wall fractures may be observed with the anterior and/or inferior wall injuries, and in these cases, signs and symptoms will reflect the extent and site of the fracture.

C *Inferior wall fractures* are considered primarily fractures of the anterior skull base. They have the potential to cause nasofrontal duct obstruction, stasis of secretions, and sinusitis. These injuries can also

437

FRONTAL SINUS FRACTURES

A

ANTERIOR WALL

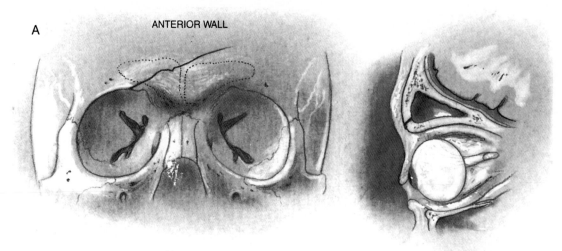

Linear

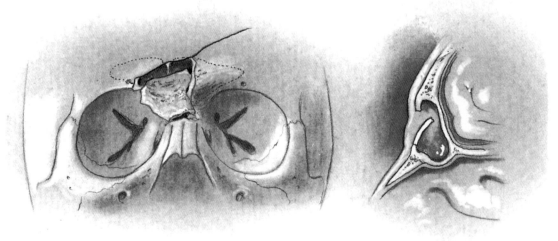

Depressed

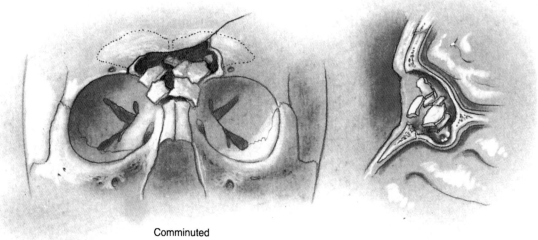

Comminuted

Wm. Loechel

B

POSTERIOR WALL

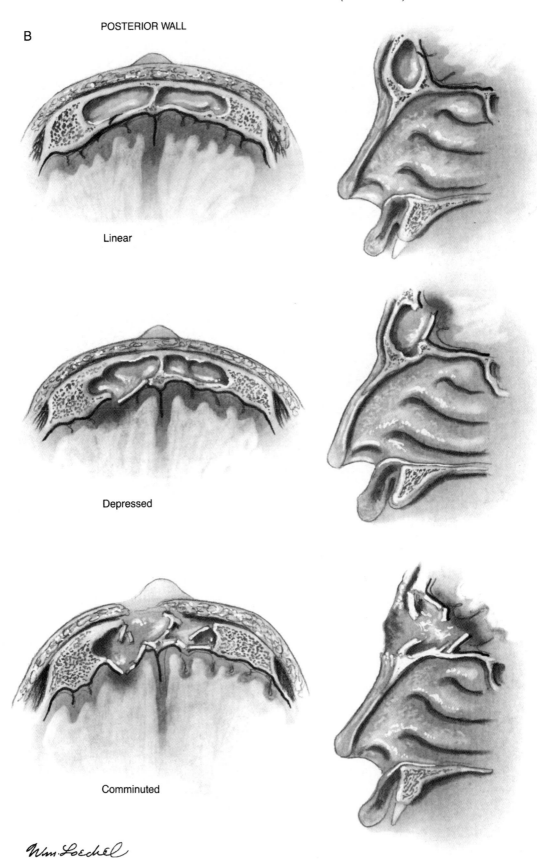

Linear

Depressed

Comminuted

Wm. Loechel

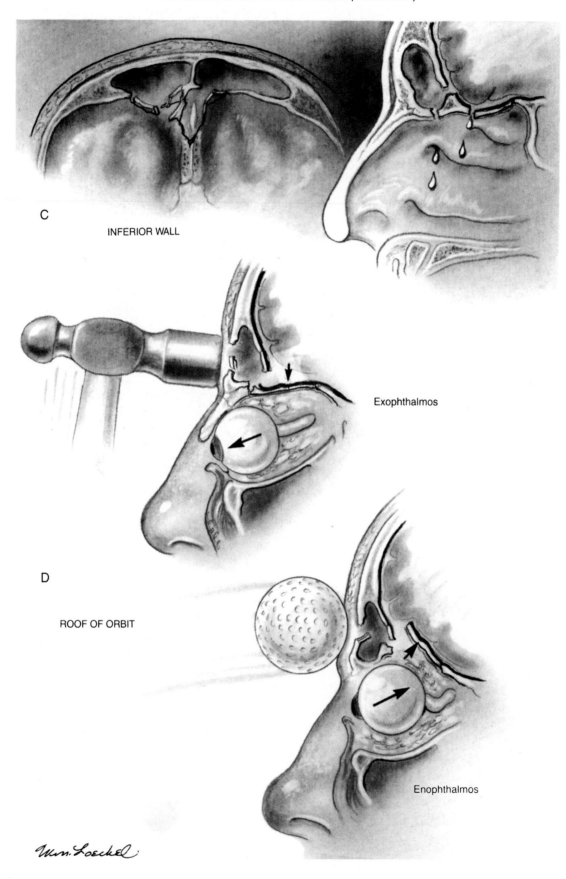

C

INFERIOR WALL

Exophthalmos

D

ROOF OF ORBIT

Enophthalmos

involve the cribriform and orbital plates and extend to the sphenoid bone. Dural tears, pneumocephalus, and cerebrospinal fluid leaks are common sequelae.

D One additional variation of frontal bone injury is the fracture that involves the eyebrow prominence and roof of the orbit. With such an injury, an eyebrow deformity, swelling, and ptosis of the upper eyelid can be expected. There can also be damage to levator, superior oblique, and superior rectus muscle function.

Fractures extending more posteriorly can present with a blow-out injury, and with such defects of the orbital plate, brain and dura can herniate into the orbit and cause a pulsating exophthalmos. If the fracture rotates upward into the anterior cranial fossa, elevation of the eye associated with an enophthalmos can occur. If the force of the fracture is transmitted farther posteriorly, the optic nerve and those vessels and nerves transmitted through the superior orbital fissure are at risk.

Anterior Wall Fractures of the Frontal Sinus

CHAPTER **75**

Repair of Anterior Wall Fracture of the Frontal Sinus With Plate Fixation
Alternative Technique Using Coronal Approach and Ex-Vivo Plating
Alternative Technique Using Titanium Mesh

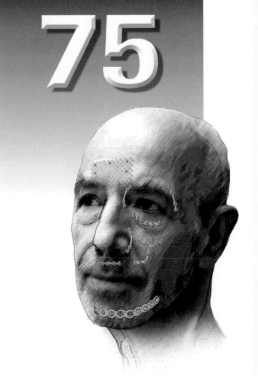

INDICATIONS

Fractures with minimal displacement that are confined to the anterior wall of the frontal sinus usually can be treated with conservative medical management. However, if the fracture causes a deformity, it should be reduced, and if the bones are unstable, they should be repaired with an appropriate method of fixation.

There is also an opportunity during the fracture repair to explore the sinus and directly evaluate the extent of the injury.

Several methods of fixation are available. For the simple fracture(s) in which one or several segments are depressed, one or several miniplates will be satisfactory. An open procedure is preferred although endoscopic techniques can be applied. When the fracture is associated with many displaced fragments (comminuted), a generous exposure is usually required. Multiple plates can be used, but it is probably more prudent to use a titanium mesh technique.

PROCEDURE

Lacerations of the forehead can often be used for exposure, but if none are present, incisions should be planned and marked out appropriately. The surgeon has the choice of an extended medial canthal incision (see Chapter 67), an "open sky" incision (see Chapter 70), a coronal incision as described in Chapter 76 or a "butterfly" subbrow approach. The site and length of the incision depend on the area of injury and the estimated exposure necessary for the repair.

A For most patients with low anterior wall fractures, the surgeon should mark a curvilinear incision along the frontal process of the maxilla upward to the medial part of the eyebrow. If necessary, the line of incision can then be extended laterally beneath the brow or medially across the nasofrontal angle to become continuous with a similar incision of the opposite side ("open sky").

B To help with hemostasis, the area of exploration is infiltrated with 1% lidocaine containing epinephrine. After 5 to 10 minutes, an incision is made through the skin and subcutaneous tissues. The angular vessels are identified and cauterized. The dissection then proceeds beneath the hair follicles, above the orbicularis oculi muscle, and across the prominence of the brow. The supraorbital and supratrochlear vessels and nerves are usually identified, and although they are kept deep and lateral to the dissection, neurovascular branches to the forehead skin may have to be sacrificed. The dissection then enters a plane between the galea and periosteum, and at this point, the surgeon has the option of directly exposing the fracture or continuing more superiorly until the dissection is above the area of damage. The periosteum then can be elevated retrograde to expose the fragments, but the surgeon should attempt to preserve as much as possible of the vascularized periosteal attachments. The mucoperiosteal lining that lies on the deeper portion of the fracture should also be kept intact.

The defect created by the fracture is cleaned with suction irrigation and the sinus is exposed with a focused light source. The surgeon should subsequently evaluate the possibility of the fracture extending to the posterior and/or inferior wall and resulting in cerebrospinal fluid leak. If such injury has occurred, other approaches should be considered (see Chapters 76 through 80).

C Fragments of frontal bone are elevated into position with skin hooks and small elevators. Thin plates are then bent to appropriate contour and adjusted so that at least two screws can be placed in solid bone adjacent to the fragment.

With the plate held against the fragments, holes confined to the outer cortex and diploë, are then made an appropriate-size drill. The screws should be just long enough to pass through the outer cortex and the diploë and engage the inner cortex. Because noncompression plates are usually used, the surgeon has the option of applying the screws first to the fragment and then to the adjoining bone. If there are many fragments, multiple plates will be needed to achieve a satisfactory fixation, but only the minimum number of plates necessary should be used to hold the bones in position.

For closure, the periosteum is advanced over the plates with 3-0 chromic sutures. The subcutaneous layer is closed with fine chromic sutures and the skin with running or interrupted 5-0 nylon sutures. Incisions are covered with antibiotic ointment. A light compression dressing of fluffs and a stretch gauze or small suction drain is applied. Prophylactic antibiotics are administered for 5 to 7 days. The dressings should be changed in 24 hours and the wound inspected at that time. Another dressing should be applied for at least 72 hours. Sutures are removed in 5 to 7 days.

PITFALLS

1. An accurate diagnosis, substantiated by imaging studies, is important if the direct approach to the frontal bone fracture is to be used. If the fracture extends to the posterior or inferior walls, other methods should be employed (see Chapters 76 through 80).

2. The surgeon should ensure that the wound is clean by washing the wound thoroughly with saline and mechanically removing any obvious particles or foreign material. This will help avoid postoperative infection.

3. If lacerations are present and sufficiently long, they can often be used for exposure and repair. Lacerations can also be extended in crease or furrow lines. However, if extension of the laceration would cross a crease or furrow line, then one of the subbrow approaches should be considered.

4. Use only that part of the incision that is necessary to expose and repair the injury. If the fracture is confined to a small area, the incision should be just long enough to explore and reduce the fracture and apply the smallest plate.

5. The dissection should avoid injury to the hairs of the eyebrow, the orbicularis oculi, and the levator aponeurosis and muscle. Generally the dissection is beneath the hair follicles and above the

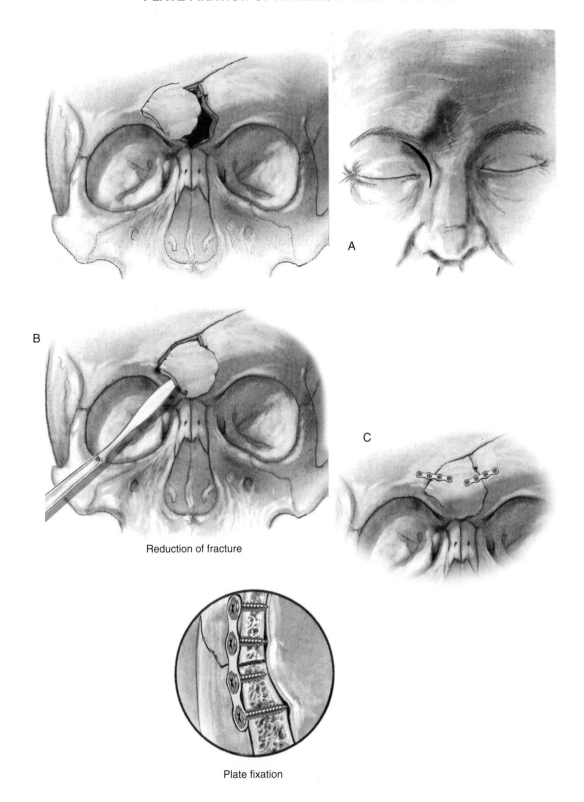

A

B

Reduction of fracture

C

Plate fixation

orbicularis oculi. The periosteum of the frontal bone can be exposed above the prominence of the brow.

6. Expose only enough bone to apply a plate. The more periosteum that is attached, the more rapidly the bone will heal and the less chance there is of avascular necrosis. For these same reasons, the mucoperiosteal lining should be retained during the reduction and fixation process.

7. The surgeon should be particularly aware of cerebrospinal fluid leaks and extension of the fracture to the nasofrontal duct. Occasionally Gelfoam can be placed against the dura and an appropriate repair effected. If not, the surgeon should close the wound and use an alternate approach, such as obliteration of the sinus with abdominal fat (see Chapter 76). Injury to the nasofrontal duct may be treated with obliteration or reconstruction of the nasofrontal duct with a tube or one of the flap techniques (see Chapter 80).

8. Thin, malleable miniplates should be applied to the thicker areas of bone. The plate should be bent to fit closely to the forehead so that it is not palpated or seen following fixation. If this becomes a problem later, the plate may have to be removed.

9. Postoperatively there is a tendency for swelling of the forehead and brow region. These effects can be minimized by a light compression dressing of fluffs or stretch gauze. The dressing should be applied over the forehead and, to achieve proper pressure, extended over the ear region. Dressings should be removed and replaced at 24 and 72 hours, at which times the wounds are inspected for adequacy of healing.

COMPLICATIONS

1. Lacerations of the forehead are often associated with soft tissue damage and embedded foreign material. These conditions predispose to subsequent infection. To avoid this problem, wounds should be debrided and prophylactic antibiotics administered for 5 to 7 days. If an infection develops, the physician should obtain cultures and check for appropriateness of antibiotics. The area may require further debridement and drainage. Unsightly scars that develop later can be corrected with appropriate scar revision surgery.

2. Fractures extending to the posterior wall of the frontal sinus can cause dural or intracranial damage. Fractures directed inferiorly can cause obstruction to the nasofrontal duct, stasis, and sinusitis. These conditions must be recognized and treated appropriately if the surgeon is to avoid and minimize the adverse sequelae (see Chapters 76 through 80).

3. The subbrow approach unfortunately can damage branches of the supraorbital nerves and vessels that enter the forehead tissues. Loss of sensation is variable, and although return of function can be expected, the patient should be warned about the possibility of anesthesia or paresthesia of the region.

4. Depression of the frontal bone in the early postoperative period can be treated by another reduction and fixation. Later, when the bone has healed, the defect can be repaired with bone cement or onlay grafts of autogenous rib or outer cortical plate from nearby parietal bone (see Chapter 82).

5. The rigid plate may be palpable or visible beneath the skin. If this occurs, the plate should be removed.

ALTERNATIVE TECHNIQUE USING CORONAL APPROACH AND EX-VIVO PLATING

Comminuted fractures of the anterior frontal bone require an approach that provides adequate exposure and opportunities for different methods of fixation. This additional exposure can be obtained through an "open sky" described in Chapter 70 or through a subbrow incision, but the preferred approach is through a coronal flap also described in Chapter 43.

a After preparation of the surgical field, a narrow area is shaved behind the hairline; the incision is marked and infiltrated with 1% lidocaine with epinephrine. Starting at the pretragal area, a gentle curved incision is made above the forehead behind the hairline to the pretragal area of the opposite side. Hemostasis is achieved with Raney Clips or electrocautery. The dissection is carried out in a subgaleal plane above the periosteum. Care is taken to avoid injury to the seventh nerve. Bleeding from the superficial temporal artery is controlled with silk ligatures.

b–f An incision is made through the periostem just above the fracture and the periosteum is elevated off of the fragments. If the fragments are comminuted and cannot be stabilized for plating, they are removed one by one and held with clamps or fingers in anatomic position while plates are applied for fixation. This procedure is usually performed on the back table away from the surgical field and because the plates are applied outside the body it is called an "ex-vivo" technique. Once the affected frontal bone is reconstructed, the bone is placed back in position and secured with additional plates to the surrounding stable cortex. The periosteum is closed with 3-0 chromic sutures, a flat suction drain inserted and the flap returned and closed in layers.

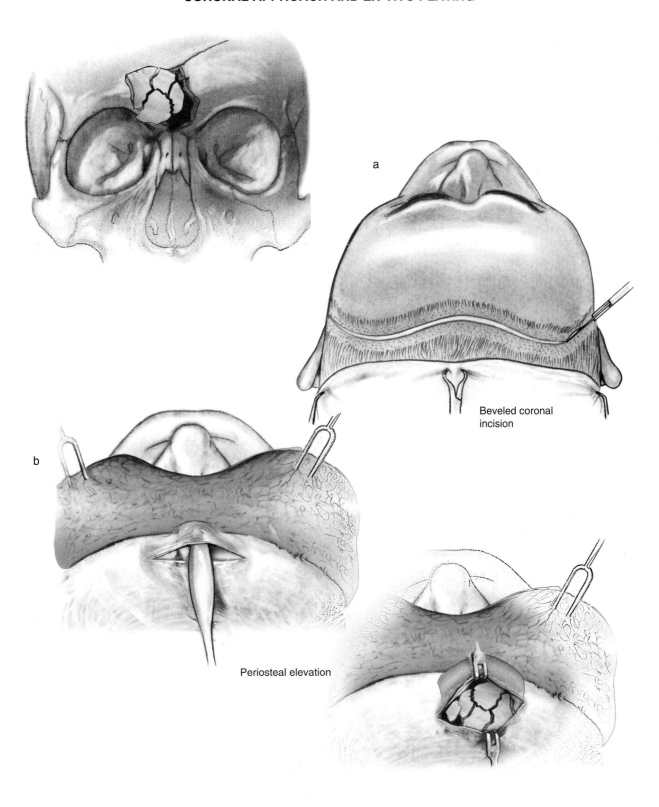

a

Beveled coronal
incision

b

Periosteal elevation

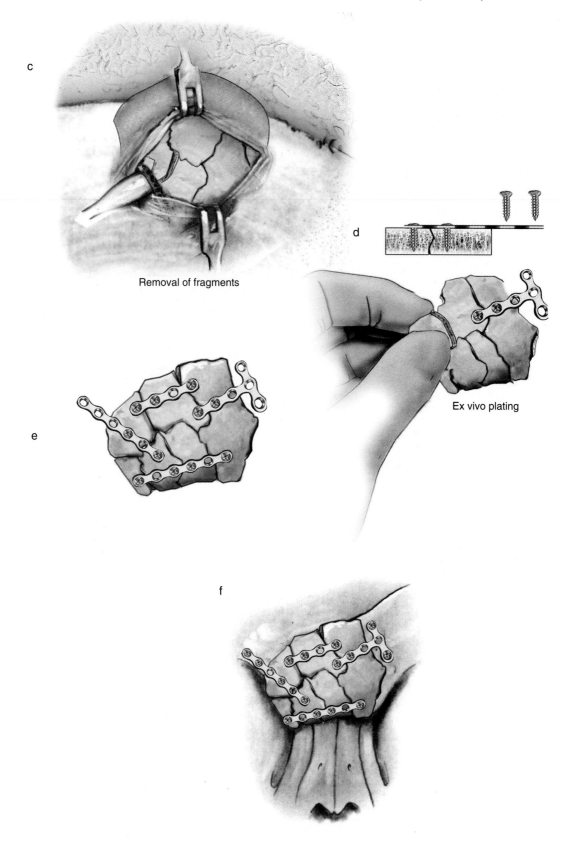

c

Removal of fragments

d

Ex vivo plating

e

f

ALTERNATIVE TECHNIQUE USING TITANIUM MESH

The application of titanium mesh is more efficient and just as effective as using multiple plates. The low profile of the mesh is also an advantage.

a'–c' After obtaining exposure of the fracture site using the coronal approach described earlier, a piece of titanium mesh is fitted over the area to be reconstructed, bent to the contour of the frontal bone and cut to size. Small single skin hooks are used to hold the bone fragments against the mesh, while 3 mm drill holes are made through the mesh perforations into the bone. The fragments of bone are then secured to the mesh and the mesh is secured to the adjacent stable bone. The periosteum is closed over the mesh, small flat suction drain inserted, and the coronal flap returned to be closed in layers.

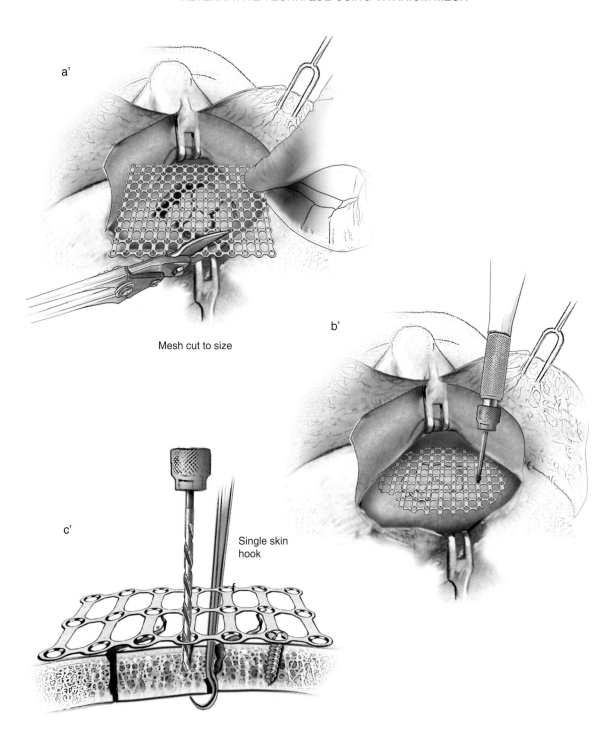

a'

Mesh cut to size

b'

c'

Single skin hook

Posterior Wall Fractures of the Frontal Sinus

CHAPTER

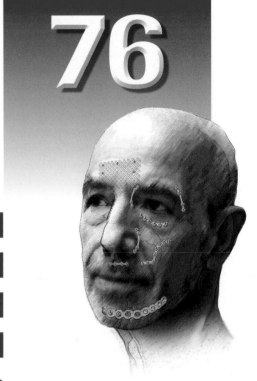

76

Repair of Posterior Wall Fracture of the Frontal Sinus With Coronal Osteoplastic Flap and Fat Obliteration

INDICATIONS

Posterior wall fractures of the frontal sinus are often associated with other fractures of the craniofacial skeleton. The diagnosis and extent of injury should be evaluated jointly with members of the neurosurgical department.

The isolated posterior wall fracture is rare, but if it is limited and nondisplaced, it can be managed conservatively. If the displacement is of a mild to moderate degree, then an external osteoplastic flap approach should be considered. For the more significant comminuted fractures that are associated with obvious dural tears, cerebrospinal fluid leaks, and pneumocephalus, a formal craniotomy may be required. When

the surgeon is not certain of the degree of damage, the procedure can start with an osteoplastic flap and, if necessary, be converted (with neurosurgery) into a more formal craniotomy.

The osteoplastic frontal flap provides excellent exposure of the posterior and inferior walls of the frontal sinus. Small dural tears can be repaired, and if the surgeon is to obliterate the sinus, the mucosa can be removed and the sinus filled with fat. It is also possible through this frontal flap approach to reduce fragments on the posterior wall and repair cerebrospinal fluid leaks directly with Gelfoam, fibrin glue, and/or fascial plugs. The osteoplastic flap has the advantages of being vascularized and healing rapidly, with an incision that can be readily concealed behind the hairline.

PROCEDURE

The osteoplastic flap is a variation of the coronal flap described in Chapter 43. The incision should parallel the coronal suture. It is marked behind the hairline in a gentle curve that is extended to a point several centimeters above the pretragal creases. The area for incision is prepared by limited shaving, antiseptic solutions, and application of drapes that keep the hair from the wound. Prior infiltration with 1% lidocaine containing 1:100,000 epinephrine will help with hemostasis.

A,B The knife blade should follow the direction of the hair follicles. The incision is made through the skin, subcutaneous tissues, and galea. Branches of the superficial temporal artery are ligated with fine silk sutures; other bleeding sites are controlled with pinpoint cauterization. The forehead flap is subsequently elevated in a plane between the galea and periosteum. Laterally the dissection is extended along the superficial temporalis fascia and inferiorly to the attachment of the fascia to the zygomatic arch, carefully avoiding injury to the seventh nerve. In the midline, the elevation proceeds to the eyebrows, exposing branches of the supertrochlear and supraorbital vessels that penetrate the bone flap.

C,D A template is used to make the periosteal cuts. This template is derived by cutting a replica of the frontal sinus from a "six-foot" Caldwell radiograph. The periosteum is incised at the border of the template and then elevated approximately 3 to 4 mm inferiorly. The exposed frontal bone is marked about 1 to 2 mm just beyond the edge of the periosteum. This will place the osteotomy 1 to 2 mm inside the original margin of the template. Using a medium-size oscillating saw, cuts are made obliquely so that the bevel of the cut is directed to the anterior portion of the inferior sinus. Attachments at the supraorbital ridges are released with osteotomes.

E,F A curved osteotome is then inserted beneath the bone flap at the level of the intersinus septum, and with the osteotome directed anteriorly, the anterior wall of the sinus is freed from the septum. The bone flap is then elevated, and if the procedure has been performed properly, fracture lines will develop on the superior wall of the orbit just beneath the supraorbital rim.

G,H Blood is carefully suctioned from the sinus. The mucosa is then elevated off all fragments using a Freer elevator and Takahashi rongeurs. A microscope is helpful in cleaning mucosa from the deep supraorbital crevices and cells. The posterior wall fragments are teased into position. Finally, the surface of the bone should be abraded with cutting burs and small dural tears covered with Gelfilm, fibrin glue, and/or fascia.

I The most popular material for obliteration of the sinus is abdominal fat. This fat is usually harvested separately in a sterile field through an oblique incision just beneath the belt line. The skin is undermined in all directions. The fat is grasped with a Babcock or Allis clamp and excised with a knife or scissors. Care is taken not to enter the underlying musculature. All bleeding should be controlled with cauterization. A small Penrose or suction drain should be applied to the wound and secured to the edges of the incision. The incision is closed in layers, using 3-0 chromic for the subcutaneous tissues and 5-0 nylon for the skin.

J,K Before inserting the fat into the sinus, the sinus is again inspected for cerebrospinal fluid leaks and mucosal remnants. The mucosa at the nasofrontal duct is turned down into the duct system. The fat is then placed into the sinus, filling all crevices and openings. The flap is replaced, and any fat that protrudes through the osteotomy is excised.

Using 3-0 chromic sutures, the periosteum of the bone flap is then tightly secured to the periosteum of the frontal bone. The forehead flap is repositioned and closed by application of 3-0 chromic sutures to the galea and 3-0 or 4-0 chromic sutures to the subcutaneous tissues. The skin is closed with a running 5-0 nylon suture. Flat suction drains are used if there is a question of blood accumulation. Alternatively, a light compression dressing of fluffs and stretch gauze is applied across the forehead and temples and around the ears. The dressing is inspected at 24 hours, replaced, and left on for another 72 hours. Such a dressing usually reduces postoperative swelling. Antibiotics are prescribed for 5 to 7 days, or longer in the case of a repair complicated by cerebrospinal fluid leakage.

PITFALLS

1. Many patients with posterior frontal wall fractures have intracranial damage. The surgeon should ensure that their medical status is stable and that there is reasonable certainty the procedure will not cause additional problems. Neurosurgical consultation is helpful.

2. Fracture of the anterior wall of the frontal sinus may compromise the development of the osteoplastic flap. In such cases, the surgeon can sometimes use the fracture line to create a smaller flap. After obliteration of the sinus, the anterior wall fracture can be repaired with a mesh or plating technique (see Chapter 75).

3. The initial frontal osteotomy should not enter the dura. An accurate template is mandatory, and the physician should make sure the Caldwell radiograph is taken at 6 ft. The size of the sinus can also be evaluated by companion imaging studies. The osteotomy

A

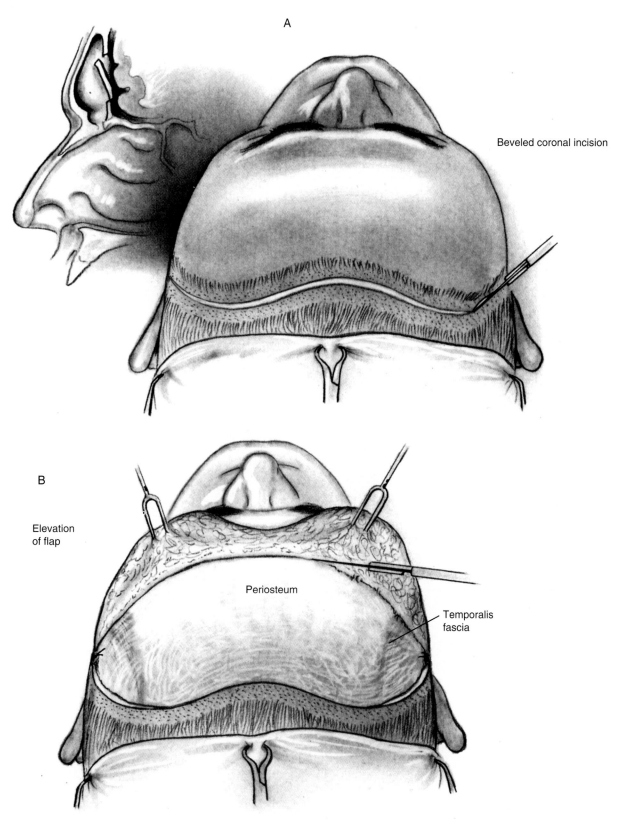

Beveled coronal incision

B

Elevation
of flap

Periosteum

Temporalis
fascia

Wm. Loechel

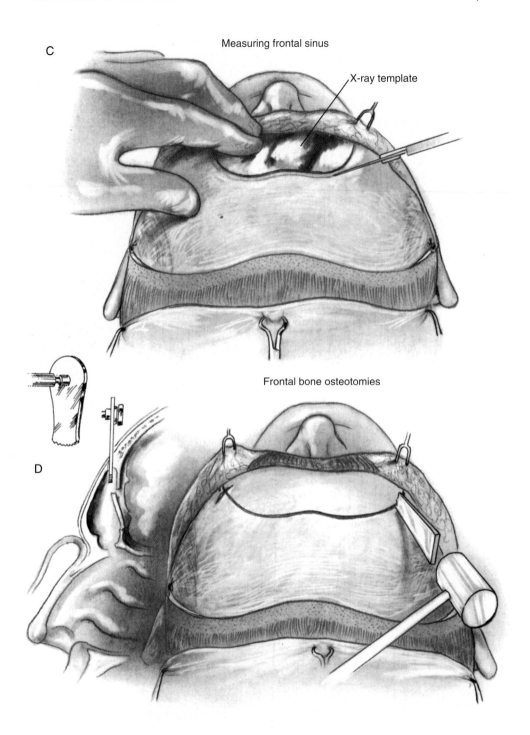

C Measuring frontal sinus

X-ray template

D Frontal bone osteotomies

Wm Loechel

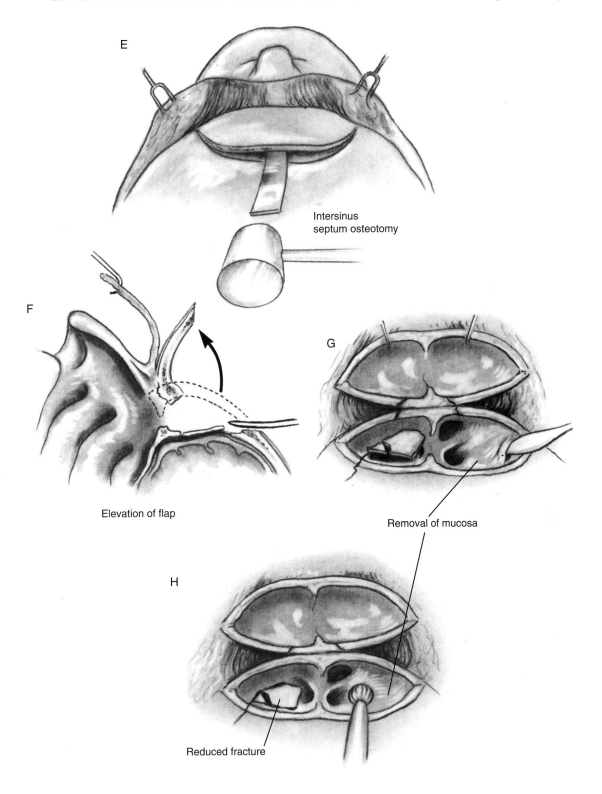

E

Intersinus
septum osteotomy

F

Elevation of flap

G

Removal of mucosa

H

Reduced fracture

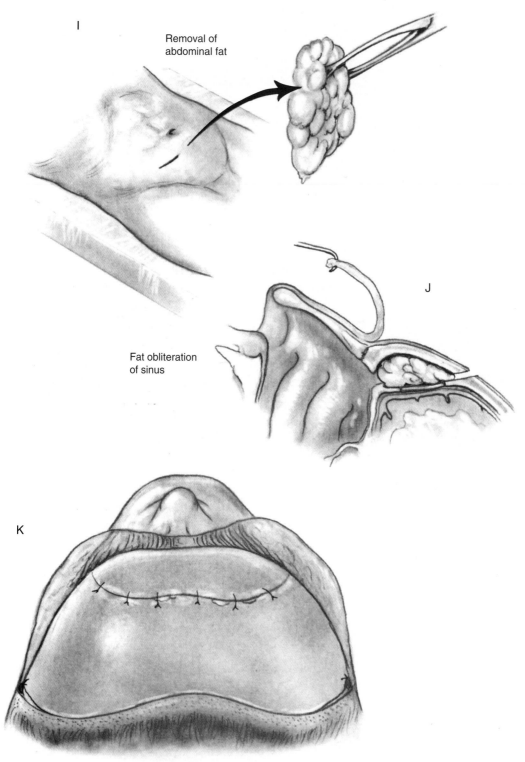

I

Removal of
abdominal fat

J

Fat obliteration
of sinus

K

Periosteal closure

should start 2 mm beneath the outline of the template and beveling the osteotomy while entering the sinus. Use of the oscillating saw also provides a margin of safety.

4. Make sure all mucosa is removed from the sinus. Failure to do so can later lead to mucoceles or mucopyoceles. Use of the microscope and removal of a layer of bone with the cutting burs ensures that the bone has been completely cleaned of mucous membrane. If multiple comminuted fragments make it impossible to remove all mucous membrane, the surgeon should consider a frontoethmoidectomy and reconstruction of the nasofrontal duct (see Chapter 80). The surgeon still has the option, if the frontal sinus does not clear, to later perform an osteoplastic flap and fat obliteration procedure.

5. Before obliterating the sinus with fat, the surgeon should ensure that the bones are in correct position and that dural tears have been repaired. If a significant cerebrospinal fluid leak is still present, it is more prudent to lift up the bone and suture the dura closed or have a neurosurgeon assist through a standard neurosurgical approach.

6. After replacing the bone flap, make sure that all fat is removed from the osteotomy site. Fat left between bone fragments will prevent fusion of the bone and cause instability and possibly a forehead deformity at a later time.

7. Periosteal coverage of the osteotomy will help in the healing process. This can be facilitated by making the osteotomy several millimeters from the edge of periosteum, and at the end of the procedure, the periosteum can be advanced over the bone defect.

8. Light compression dressings applied to the forehead region can be used to prevent edema. If dressings are not used, the patient can develop a supraorbital swelling that can persist for 4 to 6 months following surgery.

9. Make sure that the abdominal wound is dry and well drained. Infections are common but can be prevented by taking measures to avoid accumulation of blood and serous fluid.

10. CT scans should be obtained at prescribed intervals following surgery to ensure completeness and persistence in obliteration. The fat can be measured by MRI or computed tomographic (CT) absorption criteria. If the fat disappears and the patient is asymptomatic, no treatment is necessary. However, the patient must be watched cautiously for signs and symptoms of sinusitis and cerebrospinal fluid rhinorrhea. Follow-up appointments should be scheduled quarterly. If the fat persists in the sinus, periodic evaluations can be carried out on an annual or biannual basis.

COMPLICATIONS

1. Sinusitis is possible, especially if there has been tissue damage and contamination. Under such conditions, the surgeon should consider debridement of the wound and alternative methods of repair (see Chapter 80). If obliteration is performed, the surgeon must carefully apply atraumatic techniques, completely close all dead space, and administer intravenous antibiotics. If sinusitis develops, the infection should be cultured and treated with appropriate antibiotics. Chronic infection should be managed by reexploration, removal of diseased tissue, and reobliteration or reconstruction of the nasofrontal duct.

2. Loss of fat grafts can potentially lead to mucocele formation. Mucosa can grow from the nasofrontal duct into the sinus, and without adequate drainage, mucoceles or mucopyoceles will develop. This complication can be avoided by making sure that the fat is in contact with a well-vascularized bed and the grafts are handled in a relatively atraumatic fashion. If the fat should be absorbed, the sinus must be studied carefully by serial CT scans for the development of sinusitis and mucocele formation.

3. Deformity of the forehead can develop, especially if there is an associated fracture of the anterior table. This can be avoided by noting such fractures on CT scans prior to the initiation of the procedure and by using appropriate reduction and treatment methods. Forehead deformities, however, are also possible as a result of the osteotomy. Therefore the osteotomy should be made as thin as possible and beveled so that the bone flap will not slip. If the bone flap becomes depressed beneath the level of the frontal bone, miniplates should be applied directly to the outer cotex. Correction of a late deformity is discussed elsewhere (see Chapter 82).

4. Cerebrospinal fluid leaks are usually controlled by direct closure of the dura and/or fat obliteration. If the patient continues to have a cerebrospinal fluid leak or evidence of pneumocephalus, it is possible that other fractures are present or the obliteration is not satisfactory. Imaging studies should be obtained to determine the cause of the problem. If the condition does not improve with conservative management, additional repair procedures should be considered.

5. Anesthesia and hypoesthesia of the forehead are common following the osteoplastic flap. Some patients experience a return of function; others do not. Loss of forehead movement also can occur from damage to the frontal branch of the facial nerve. Such injury can be avoided by gentle retraction of tissues and keeping the planes of dissection close or deep to the temporalis fascia (see Chapter 43).

CHAPTER 77

Cranialization Technique for Posterior Wall Fractures of the Frontal Sinus

INDICATIONS

Posterior wall injuries can occasionally be isolated to the posterior wall and skull base, but they more often appear as through-and-through fractures with contamination and comminution of bone. In this latter type of injury, the viability of the soft tissues and bone may be questionable, and following debridement, there can be a significant defect. Under such conditions, a reasonable option is to fill the sinus with a vascularized obliteration.

Several techniques are available. The surgeon can remove the anterior and posterior walls of the frontal sinus and collapse the forehead tissues onto the anterior fossa. He or she can also reconstruct the anterior wall of the frontal sinus and fill the sinus with a transposed temporalis muscle galea flap (see Chapter 78) or, as an alternative, remove the posterior wall of the frontal sinus and obliterate or cranialize the sinus with the anterior displacement of brain. The collapse of the forehead (often called a *Reidel procedure*) causes a severe deformity that is difficult to correct at a later time. Filling of the defect with a temporalis muscle galea flap provides a limited amount of tissue and causes a depression of the temple region. It can also predispose to alopecia over the donor site. The cranialization procedure eliminates the sinus and allows for expansion of the injured brain. Meanwhile, it provides for protection of the frontal lobes and a normal appearance of the forehead. The disadvantage of the cranialization technique is that the anterior fossa will be located above the nasofrontal duct, and this relationship can predispose to contamination of the cranial cavity from the respiratory tract below.

PROCEDURE

Using general orotracheal anesthesia, the approach is identical to that carried out for the coronal incision and osteoplastic flap (see Chapter 76). Intravenous antibiotics are administered during and after the operative procedure.

A–C After exposure of the sinus, all depressed bone fragments from the posterior wall are removed. Necrotic brain tissues are debrided, and the dura is repaired with fine nonabsorbable sutures, fibrin glue, and/or fascial grafts. The remaining mucosa of the sinus is elevated and excised from the floor and anterior wall. The frontal intersinus septum is removed with burs and rongeurs. A layer of bone is excised from the walls of the sinus with cutting burs.

D If the anterior wall is fractured, fragments are stabilized with mesh or plates as described in Chapter 75. The nasofrontal duct mucosa is pushed into the duct, and the duct is then plugged with temporalis muscle or fascia. In patients with large frontal sinuses, abdominal fat grafts are placed anteriorly to help obliterate the cavity; this will reduce the degree of displacement necessary for the brain to fill the sinus. The frontal osteoplastic flap is returned to its normal position. The periosteum is closed with 3-0 chromic sutures. The superficial layers of soft tissue are approximated and treated with topical antibiotic dressings. Postoperatively the patient should receive intravenous antibiotics for 3 to 5 days and oral antibiotics for at least an additional 10 days. Flat suction drains are applied. Alternatively, a light pressure

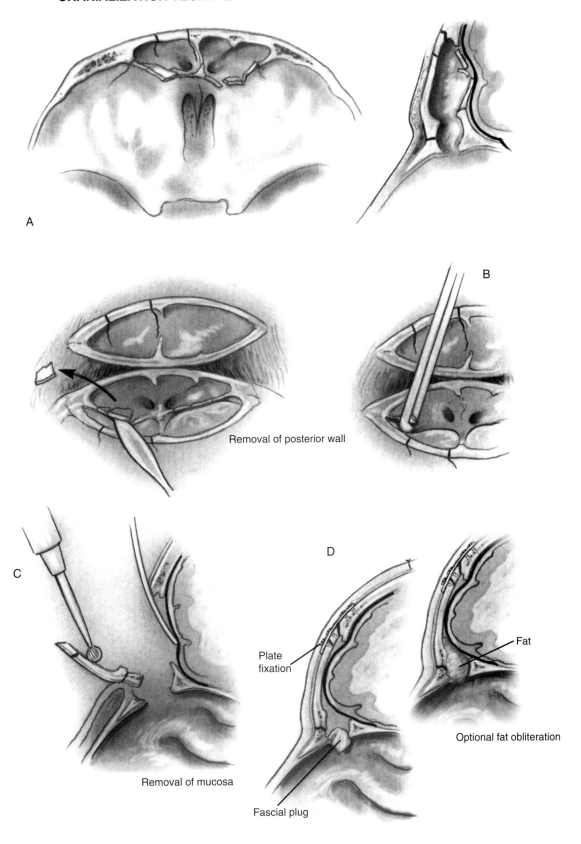

A

Removal of posterior wall

B

C

Removal of mucosa

D

Plate
fixation

Fascial plug

Fat

Optional fat obliteration

dressing is maintained for 5 to 7 days to control edema, but it should be checked and replaced during the first 24 hours and 2 to 3 days thereafter. Sutures are removed at 7 days. CT scans are obtained at several weeks and every few months until the physician is assured of a stable reconstruction.

PITFALLS

1. The anterior wall of the frontal sinus must be reconstructed to restore normal forehead contour and to protect the brain. Most fragments should be kept attached to the periosteum, especially because the overlying mucosa will be removed. Small, loose, contaminated fragments of bone can be treated with a povidone-iodine solution, followed by a wash in physiologic saline. They can be stabilized using appropriate methods of fixation. Plate fixation often provides the best stability, but the surgeon must avoid extension of the screws beyond the inner table and injury to the underlying dura.

2. Complete obliteration of the sinus and nasofrontal duct is very important if the surgeon is to avoid infection. Bony ledges that restrict anterior displacement of the frontal lobes should be excised, and all mucosa should be removed from the walls of the sinus. The opening of the nasofrontal duct should then be packed with fascia and fat added to ensure obliteration of the sinus cavity.

3. The patient must be treated with prophylactic antibiotics and watched carefully for intracranial complications. Intravenous antibiotics should be started early during the procedure and continued postoperatively. Because the patient has essentially had a craniotomy, he or she should be watched closely for 24 to 48 hours for any changes in sensorium that would indicate bleeding, infection, or other damage to the brain.

COMPLICATIONS

1. As with other frontal sinus procedures, the patient may later develop sinusitis and/or mucoceles. These complications can be avoided by removal of all mucosa, obliteration of the nasofrontal duct with fat or fascia, and complete obliteration of the sinus with brain tissue. If the sinus is large and the brain displacement only sufficient to obliterate a portion of the sinus, abdominal fat or, in the case of infection, vascularized periosteal or temporalis muscle galea flaps should be used to fill the defect (see Chapter 78).

Postoperative CT scans should be obtained to evaluate the completeness and permanence of the procedure. If infection or a mucocele develops, then reexploration, exenteration, and obliteration with fat and/or muscle should be contemplated. Acute infection should be treated with appropriate antibiotics.

2. Deformity of the forehead can be a problem, especially if the anterior wall of the frontal sinus has been comminuted. This complication can be minimized by keeping the fragments well vascularized with periosteum and achieving an accurate (and stable) fixation. Plate or mesh fixation is usually helpful in obtaining rigidity and protection of the anterior fossa.

3. Intracranial infections can occur, especially if the forehead tissues are severely damaged, the dura is torn and accompanied by a cerebrospinal fluid leak, and the wound is open or contaminated by foreign material. To prevent meningitis and/or brain abscess, foreign material must be removed and devitalized tissue debrided. The dura must be directly closed or patched with fascia. A complete obliteration and adequate antibiotic coverage will also help avoid these adverse sequelae.

CHAPTER 78

Repair of Posterior Wall Fractures of the Frontal Sinus With a Temporalis Muscle Galea Flap

INDICATIONS

Severe damage to the posterior wall of the frontal sinus associated with anterior wall injury, dural tears, and brain damage requires special techniques. As described earlier, the main objective is to separate the cranial cavity from the aerodigestive tract. Dural replacement and obliteration of dead space must be provided. The forehead tissues can be collapsed, the posterior wall of the sinus removed, and the brain allowed to expand forward (see Chapter 77), or the sinus can be filled with fat or flap tissue. Free grafts (i.e., fat or muscle) probably should be avoided in infected or grossly contaminated sinuses; these grafts require a well-vascularized bed, and if this is not available, the tissues will not survive. A flap with its own blood supply is thus preferred.

Flap coverage can be obtained from several sources. Adjacent musculocutaneous flaps can be used, but these rotations cause deformity and additional scars. Pericranial flaps developed from forehead periosteum are available, but these flaps are limited in length and thickness and require a passageway anteriorly through the frontal bone. The temporalis muscle galea flap appears to be an effective, easy, accessible alternative for soft tissue coverage over skull base defects in which a reliable separation of cranial and facial compartments is desirable.

The temporalis muscle galea flap has several unique advantages over other methods. This flap is well vascularized, receiving contributions from the superficial temporal artery, the middle temporal branch of the superficial artery, and the anterior and posterior deep temporal arteries. Its length can be increased by extending the flap to include the parietal (and occipital) pericranium and galea. It can be used to repair cranial defects either alone or in combination with skin, cartilage, or bone grafts. Disadvantages are that the flap dissection is tedious and there can be loss of hair, skin, and/or sensation in the parietal region overlying the area of surgery. Although one flap can usually cover more than one-half of the floor of the anterior cranial fossa, additional areas to be repaired require another flap from the opposite side.

PROCEDURE

A,B Surgery is performed under general anesthesia. The parietotemporal area is shaved, and the skin is prepared with a standard antiseptic solution and draped as a sterile field. The surgeon then marks out the incision lines for development of the temporalis galea flap. If a coronal incision is chosen as an approach to the frontal sinus injury, then a limb is extended posteriorly, at a right angle to the coronal incision, about 5 to 6 cm above the pinna. If a butterfly (subbrow) approach is chosen, then a hemicoronal incision and a posterior limb should be employed. The design of the flap should protect the superficial temporal artery.

C,D The osteoplastic frontal flap should be planned so that the periosteum can be attached to the bone fragments and the bone later repaired with mesh or miniplates (see Chapter 75). The sinus should be cleaned of blood and examined and the extent of damage noted. Fragments should be elevated from the posterior wall, and necrotic brain should be debrided. Dural tears should be repaired when possible with fine nonabsorbable sutures, fibrin glue, and/or fascial patch closure.

All mucosa should be removed from the sinus and an extra margin of ensurance obtained by excising a layer of bone with cutting burs. The intersinus septum should be removed. At the frontonasal duct, the mucosa should be stripped and inverted down into the duct.

E–G The temporalis muscle galea flap is prepared by cutting through the scalp markings into a subcutaneous plane. Skin flaps are then developed superiorly and inferiorly at a level that preserves the hair follicles but does not damage the underlying temporalis muscle, galea, or superficial temporal vessels. With the skin flaps retracted superiorly, inferiorly, and posteriorly, the galea is incised. Up to 10 × 20 cm of tissue, based on the temporalis muscle, can be prepared.

The flap incision should be carried through the galea to the surface of the pericranium. The flap is then elevated anteriorly in a plane between the galea and pericranium, and at the superior temporal line, the periosteum is elevated, allowing the temporalis muscle to be elevated from the temporal fossa. The temporalis fascia, temporalis muscle, and periosteum of the temporal fossa are then rotated toward the forehead. Additional relaxation is obtained by severing the temporalis muscle just lateral to the frontal process of the zygoma. The deep temporal artery and branches of the superficial temporal artery should be preserved.

The galea and temporalis muscle are subsequently rotated to obliterate the sinus and cover any dural defect. If necessary, the galea is sutured directly to the dura with nonabsorbable sutures. A nonconstricting passageway into the anterior fossa is obtained by removing portions of the frontal, greater swing of the sphenoid and the squamous portion of the temporal bone with bone cutting rongeurs. The opening should be large enough to accommodate the flap pedicle and provide for some swelling in the postoperative period.

H The fractures of the anterior wall are repaired with plates or titanium mesh. The frontal osteoplastic flap is replaced with interrupted heavy chromic sutures through the periosteum. The subcutaneous tissues are approximated with 4-0 chromic sutures and the skin with 5-0 nylon sutures. Penrose or suction drains should be at the inferiormost portion of the coronal incision. Prophylactic intravenous antibiotics are used both during the procedure and afterward for 5 days. The patient is then continued on oral antibiotics for 7 to 10 days. Sutures are removed at 7 days.

PITFALLS

1. The dissection of the temporalis muscle galea flap can potentially injure the hair of the parietal region. To prevent alopecia, the dissection should be carried just beneath the roots of the hair follicles.

2. Avoid injury to the superficial temporal artery. In making the incision, proceed cautiously through the skin. The superficial temporal artery usually lies in a subcutaneous plane very close to the skin.

3. Retain vascular attachments between the galea/pericranium and the temporalis fascia. The layers decussate near the edge of the temporal fossa at the superior temporal line, but if the surgeon performs a subperiosteal dissection into the fossa, damage can be minimized. The dissection should be limited to an area above the zygomatic arch, as a deeper dissection may injure the deep temporal artery.

4. Transfer of the flap into the anterior fossa requires a passageway through the frontal, sphenoid, and temporal bones. In designing this defect, the surgeon should allow for swelling of the muscle and fascial tissues.

5. Remove all mucosa of the frontal sinus and invert the mucosa near the area of the nasofrontal duct into the duct. The bone should be debrided completely with a cutting bur. The flap, combined with anterior displacement of the dura and brain, should completely obliterate the sinus.

COMPLICATIONS

1. Alopecia will develop if the hair follicles are damaged. This complication can usually be avoided by carefully dissecting between the hair follicles and the deeper subcutaneous tissues. Gentle handling of the skin flaps will preserve the blood supply to the area. A temporary alopecia is often seen near the incision lines. If alopecia persists, the surgeon can undermine and advance the tissues or, if the area of hair loss is large, employ a skin expander and sequentially advance the hair-bearing areas over the area of deficit.

2. A mass representing the muscle that is rotated into the anterior cranial fossa will appear in the temporal fossa. This projection of soft tissue will become less noticeable with time. If the deformity is bothersome and persists beyond 6 months, the base of the temporalis muscle flap can be incised and rotated back into its normal position. The distal portion of the flap should retain viability from its new attachment to the frontal sinus and anterior cranial fossa structures.

3. The flap reconstruction of the sinus is susceptible to all of the problems associated with obliteration of the sinus by other techniques. These complications are discussed in Chapters 76 and 77.

OBLITERATION WITH TEMPORALIS MUSCLE GALEA FLAP

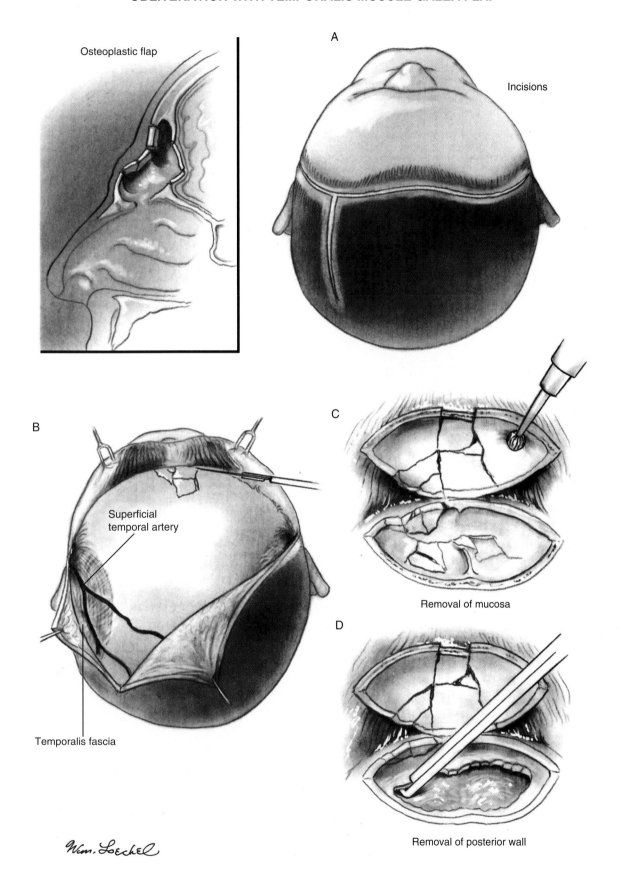

Osteoplastic flap

A

Incisions

B

Superficial
temporal artery

Temporalis fascia

C

Removal of mucosa

D

Removal of posterior wall

Wm. Loechel

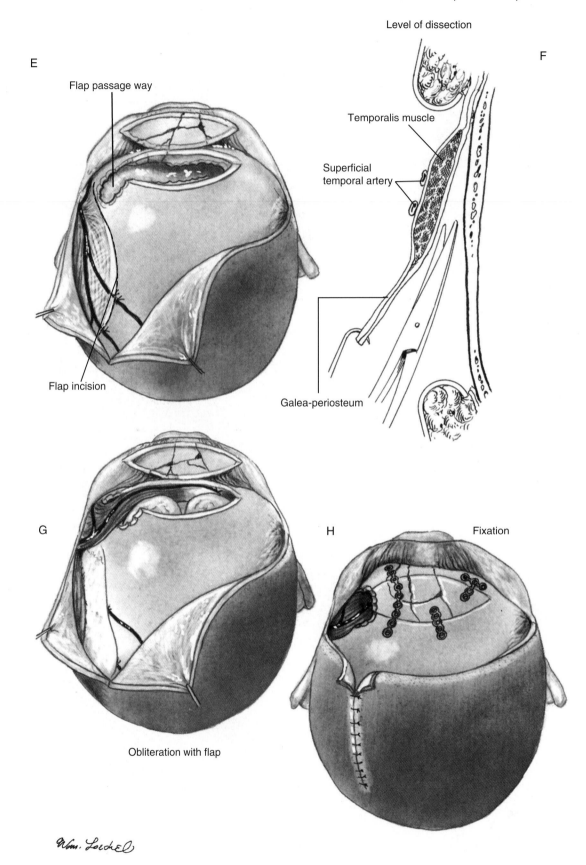

E

Flap passage way

Flap incision

Level of dissection

F

Temporalis muscle

Superficial temporal artery

Galea-periosteum

G

Obliteration with flap

H

Fixation

CHAPTER

79

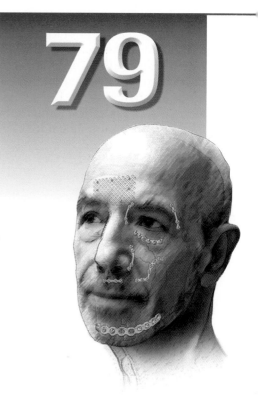

Fat Obliteration of Inferior Wall Fracture of the Frontal Sinus Using a Coronal Osteoplastic Flap
Alternative Technique of Subfrontal Approach

In Consultation With Mark Hornyak, MD

INDICATIONS

Inferior wall fractures can potentially interfere with the function of the nasofrontal duct. Obstruction of the duct can subsequently cause failure to aerate the sinus, stasis of secretions, and sinusitis. The infection can spread by way of Breschet's veins to the cranial cavity and through fracture lines to the orbit and adjoining structures. Thus with inferior wall fractures, obliteration of the sinus and reconstruction of the nasofrontal duct are important considerations.

The procedure of choice is dictated by the conditions associated with the injury. In nondisplaced, limited fractures, the surgeon can easily explore the sinus from below, enlarge the duct orifice, and either stent the duct with a chest tube or reconstruct it with a flap derived from the lining of adjacent nasal mucous membranes (see Chapter 80). When there is also damage to the anterior and/or posterior wall, the coronal osteoplastic flap is better suited for evaluating and correcting the pathologic abnormality; the mucosa can then be removed and the sinus obliterated with fat. Alternatively the frontal sinus can be explored through a subfrontal approach, which is also useful for exploration of the anterior skull base.

PROCEDURE

A–D The technique of a coronal incision and an osteoplastic flap is described elsewhere (see Chapter 76). As in other frontal fractures, it is important to ensure that the fragments are exposed and there is complete removal of the sinus mucosa. This often requires a microscopic dissection and removal of a layer of bone with cutting burs. The mucosa of the nasofrontal duct should be inverted and the duct plugged with fat or additional fascia. The sinus is then obliterated with fat and the flap returned to a normal position. Postoperative care is similar to that used in other obliteration procedures.

PITFALLS

1. Fractures of the inferior wall rarely occur alone. For this reason, the surgeon must be prepared to repair concurrent injuries of the anterior and/or posterior wall and also fractures that extend to the cribriform and orbital plates.

2. Care must be taken in manipulation or removal of bone fragments. Bone along the floor of the frontal sinus is thin and firmly attached to the dura. Thus when removing the bone, the surgeon must be careful not to tear or penetrate the underlying dura. If the dura is torn, it should be repaired with Gelfoam, fibrin glue and/or fascial plugs.

3. If the surgeon chooses to obliterate the sinus, all mucosa should be removed. The bone should be cleaned of mucosa with a microscope, and additional layers of bone should be removed with a cutting bur. If it is not possible to do this, then a reconstruction of the nasofrontal duct should be considered (see Chapter 80).

4. Some anatomic variations preclude removal of all mucosa. Occasionally, the mucosa lies deep within supraorbital crevices that extend beyond the orbit. The boundaries of the mucosa are not easily determined, and in such cases, obliteration should then cover only the anterior cells. The deep extensions of the sinus usually drain through a posterior group of cells that should subsequently function in a normal fashion.

COMPLICATIONS

1. Acute sinusitis is an important complication, as infection can spread into the meninges and orbit. The surgeon should avoid obliteration of a contaminated open wound with fat, although vascularized muscle/periosteal flaps can be considered. Antibiotic prophylaxis is mandatory. The patient should be followed during the postoperative period for infection and treated accordingly.

2. Chronic sinusitis, characterized by mucoceles and mucopyoceles, can develop at any time following the procedure. For these reasons, patients with inferior wall injuries should be followed with CT scans for infection and/or loss of fat and cyst formation. If the patient develops these complications, medical therapy should be initiated. Failure to control the disease process should prompt appropriate surgical procedures.

3. Cerebrospinal fluid leaks can continue or develop in the postoperative period. Most leaks will stop within 2 weeks, but if the leak persists, its exact anatomic location should be determined. Most leaks can be repaired from the osteoplastic frontal flap or frontoethmoid approaches or alternatively with transnasal endoscopy (see Chapters 84, 85, 90, and 91).

4. Loss of smell is commonly associated with the inferior wall injury. It is suspected that there is a disruption of the neural elements as they pass through the cribriform plate. The prognosis for recovery of smell is poor, and no known medical or surgical measures are available to treat this complication.

5. Deformity of the forehead can occur as a result of associated injury to the anterior plate of the frontal sinus and/or displacement of the osteoplastic flap. These complications are discussed in Chapter 82.

ALTERNATIVE TECHNIQUE OF SUBFRONTAL APPROACH

a–e Although the coronal incision with or without an osteoplastic flap is desirable for most frontal bone fractures, the subfrontal approach, popularized by Raveh and associates (1978), should also be considered. This procedure is designed to directly expose the area of injury especially when it involves inferior wall fractures of the frontal sinus and the anterior skull base. In most cases it is possible with this procedure to remove the lower portion of the frontal bone, parts or all of the frontal bar and the nasal bones as block, exposing the anterior cranial floor. Removal of the ethmoid cells will expose the sphenoid bone and optic canals. Additional exposure is also possible by placing bur holes above the frontal sinus and, with superiorly placed osteotomies, remove the lower frontal complex.

For the subfrontal procedure, the area to be explored requires careful evaluation using MRI and coronal and axial CT scans. A multidisciplinary neurosurgical and facial trauma team is desirable to develop strategies for exploration and placement of osteotomies. Miniplates can be applied prior to the osteotomy

CORONAL OSTEOPLASTIC FLAP FOR POSTERIOR WALL FRACTURES

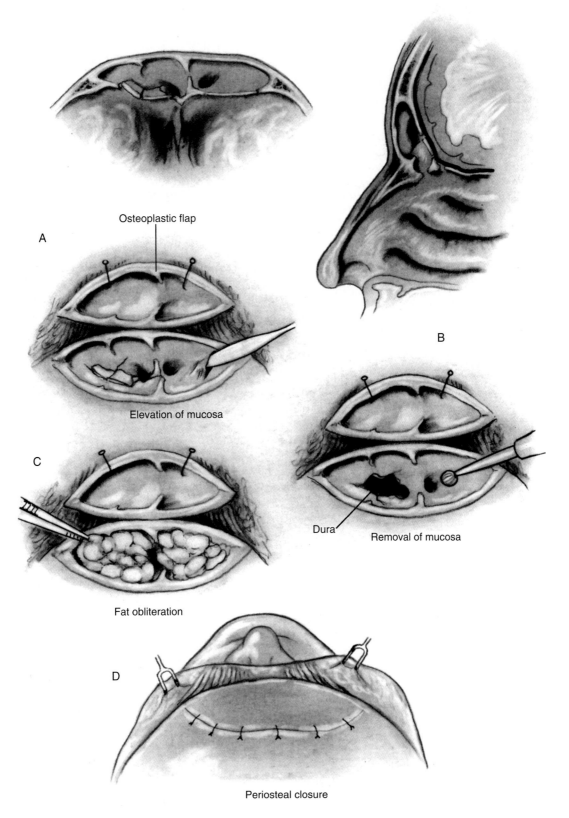

A

Osteoplastic flap

Elevation of mucosa

B

C

Dura

Removal of mucosa

Fat obliteration

D

Periosteal closure

Wm. Loechel

since these drill holes will give an exact guidance later for replacement of the bone.

The size and extent of the subfrontal bone block that will be removed is variable and will depend on those strategies developed during the planning of the case. A portion or most of the frontal bone is taken out, but to get additional exposure of the sphenoid bone, planum sphenoidale, and optic canals, the surgeon needs to perform an ethmoidectomy. The surgeon subsequently has the option of removing or reducing displaced bone fragments of the skull base, repairing dura or decompressing the optic nerve. The frontal sinus can then be managed by obliteration or reconstruction of the nasofrontal duct. Periosteal flaps can be used to reinforce the reconstruction.

At the completion of the repair(s), the frontal bone block is replaced in anatomic position and secured with miniplates. The coronal flap is returned and the tissues closed in layers.

Postoperatively, the patient is provided with intravenous antibiotics and observed for neurologic changes. Serial CT scans are used to evaluate progress.

Most complications are addressed in the earlier described procedures (see Chapters 71 through 75). The surgeon must, however, observe for meningitis, persistent CSF leaks, tension pneumocephalus, and subdural hematoma and be prepared to manage these untoward sequelae (see chapters 81 through 86).

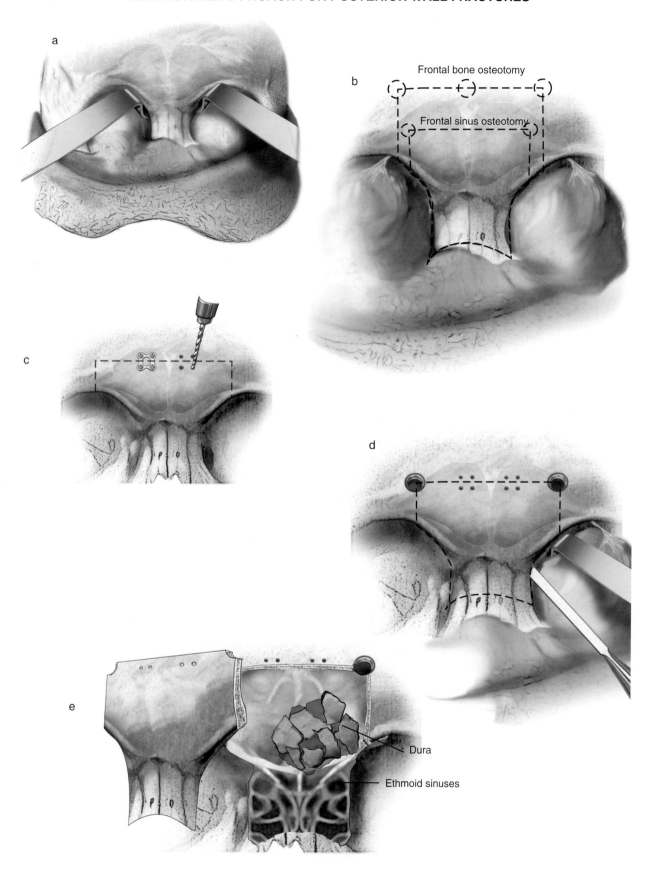

a

b

Frontal bone osteotomy

Frontal sinus osteotomy

c

d

e

Dura

Ethmoid sinuses

Treatment of Inferior Wall Fracture of the Frontal Sinus by Reconstruction of the Nasofrontal Duct
Alternative Technique Using Nasal Mucosal Flaps

INDICATIONS

Fractures of the frontal sinus that extend to the inferior wall threaten the integrity and function of the naso-frontal duct. This opening and passageway is essential for removal of secretions and aeration of the sinus. Failure of the duct system can cause stasis of secretions and sinusitis. There is also the possibility of developing a mucocele or mucopyocele. Infection can potentially spread through the transosseous veins to the cranial cavity and orbit.

If the inferior wall fracture appears to compromise the nasofrontal duct, the surgeon can obliterate the sinus with fat, brain, and/or muscle flaps, as described in Chapters 76 through 79, or proceed with reconstruction of the nasofrontal duct. When the frontal sinus injury is associated with contamination and infection threatens the free graft obliteration, duct repair should be considered. Also, if it is impossible to remove all of the mucosa, which can happen in severely comminuted injuries, then it is more prudent to avoid obliteration and fabricate a new duct. However, it should be recognized that duct patency following reconstruction may fail many years later, and for this reason, the surgeon should evaluate the sinus for clearing and aeration regularly during the postoperative period.

PROCEDURE

Reconstruction of the nasofrontal duct can be approached through the coronal osteoplastic frontal flap (Chapter 76), a Lynch frontoethmoid incision (Chapters 63 and 64), or with transnasal endoscopy. Exposure using the frontoethmoid approach is relatively fast; it also provides an opportunity to create an adjacent mucosal flap.

A Using general anesthesia, a curvilinear incision is mapped out one-half the distance from the medial caruncle to the dorsum of the nose. The area is then infiltrated with 1% lidocaine containing 1:100,000 epinephrine. Pledgets of 4% cocaine containing epinephrine (see Chapter 52) are applied to the nose to help in the control of bleeding.

B,C The incision is carried through the skin and subcutaneous tissues. The angular vessels are either cauterized or ligated. The periosteum overlying the nasal bones and the frontal process of the maxilla is incised and elevated with Joseph elevators to expose the nasal bones, nasofrontal suture line, and a portion of the anterior frontal bone. The trochlea is then detached, and the periosteum is elevated off the medial wall of the orbit. Bleeding from the anterior ethmoidal artery is controlled with gentle pressure, bipolar cautery, or a vascular clip. The posterior ethmoidal artery, a landmark for the location of the optic nerve, is kept intact.

The floor of the frontal bone is then opened by elevating the fragments or cutting through them with burs. The opening is enlarged to expose the floor region to at least the nasofrontal duct. Exenteration of the posterior ethmoidal cells ensures that the duct has been opened and enlarged appropriately. A complete external ethmoidectomy can be accomplished with curettage and Kerrison and Takahashi rongeurs.

D,E The nasal cavity is entered inferiorly. The anterior portion of the middle turbinate and portions of the frontal process of the maxilla and nasal bone should be removed to provide a passageway that will accommodate a No. 26 chest tube. At the same time the surgeon should avoid injury to the anterior and posterior lacrimal crest and lacrimal sac.

Oozing of blood should be treated with a 4% cocaine packing containing epinephrine or with bipolar cauterization. Once the passageway is adequate, a No. 26 chest tube can be inserted from the sinus opening into the nose. The tube is grasped with a clamp and pulled inferiorly so that the flange rests on the floor of the frontal sinus. A high flange should be avoided and excess flange removed with scissors. The other end of the tubing should be cut so that it projects just beyond the nares. The chest tube is then secured to the intermembranous septum with a 2-0 silk suture.

The periosteum over the osteotomy is closed with a 3-0 chromic suture. The subcutaneous tissues are approximated with 4-0 chromic sutures, and the skin is coapted with 6-0 nylon sutures. The nose should be kept clean with cotton-tipped applicators and 3% hydrogen peroxide. If blood clots form in the tubing, they should be removed with 3% hydrogen peroxide and suctioning. Antibiotics are prescribed for 10 to 14 days. Sutures are removed at 7 days and the tube at 4 to 6 weeks.

PITFALLS

1. Avoid placing the tube next to an area of dural injury. The tube should be contoured and positioned so that it stents and drains but does not come in contact with the exposed dura.

2. The opening from the sinus into the nose must be large and either stented or reconstructed with flaps if it is to provide a permanent airway. A No. 26 chest tube generally will keep the passageway open, and within 4 to 6 weeks, a reepithelialized fistula will have occurred. The surgeon has the option of developing nasal flaps, which can be rotated and immediately used to layer the edges of the opening with mucosa (see later).

3. Blood clots will form and must be removed from the tube. Failure to do so will cause swelling and periorbital pain. Blood clots can often be avoided by placing the flange of the tube at a low level within the sinus. Also, the surgeon should avoid through-and-through sutures that will cause debris to collect in the tube. Small clots can usually be removed with forceps and suction tips.

4. Keep the nares clean postoperatively with 3% hydrogen peroxide and cotton-tipped applicators. Crusts tend to develop around the suture, and if they are not removed, infection can occur.

5. The tube should be kept in position for at least 4 to 6 weeks. Usually the tube will be "caught" at the osteotomy site, but it should still be held firmly to the intermembranous septum or columella with a 2-0 silk suture.

6. Close the periosteum over the frontal process of the maxilla with a heavy chromic suture. This will return the trochlea to its normal position and reduce the incidence of postoperative diplopia.

COMPLICATIONS

1. Indwelling tubes can be associated with an infection, such as sinusitis, meningitis, and periorbital cellulitis. This complication can be avoided by strategic placement of the tube for drainage and by keeping the tube open and free from clots during the postoperative period. The surgeon should also avoid irrigations that tend to force bacteria into the adjoining tissues. Prophylactic antibiotics will help prevent infection, but if infection does develop, adequate drainage must be instituted and new cultures obtained to determine the appropriate specific treatment of the bacteria.

2. Cerebrospinal fluid leaks may be seen in the postoperative period, but most will stop within several days. Prophylactic antibiotics should be used. If the leakage persists for more than 2 weeks, exploration and repair should be considered (see Chapters 84, 85, 90, and 91).

3. Diplopia following frontoethmoidectomy should be transient, and vision should return to normal as the trochlea reattaches to the wall of the orbit. If diplopia persists, an ophthalmologic consultation is advised.

4. Although long-term results with tube reconstruction of the nasofrontal duct are excellent, there is also a possibility of developing obstruction of the duct, sinusitis, and sequelae such as mucocele and meningitis. These complications can be avoided by establishing an opening of more than adequate size and by providing epithelialization around the tube with a local mucosal flap. Failures can be attributed to extensive

NASOFRONTAL DUCT RECONSTRUCTION

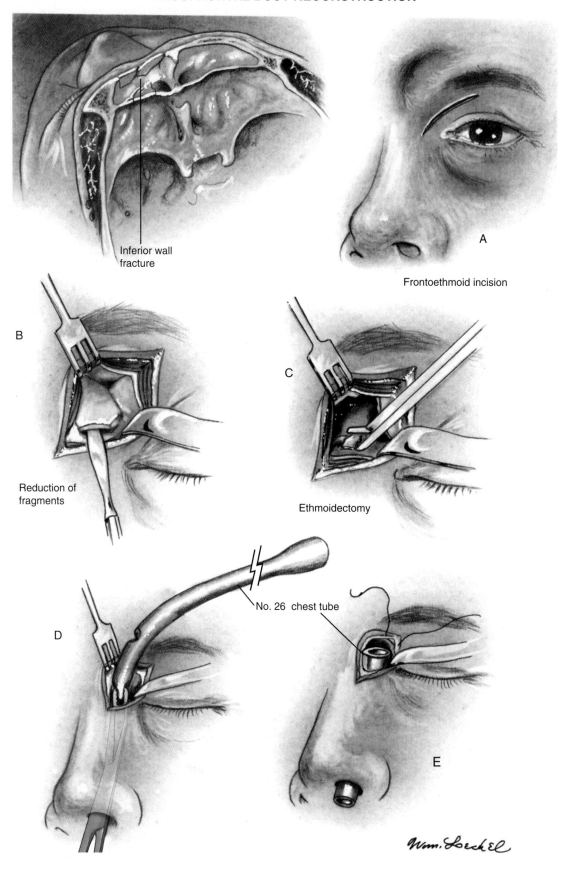

Inferior wall
fracture

A

Frontoethmoid incision

B

Reduction of
fragments

C

Ethmoidectomy

D

No. 26 chest tube

E

local damage or inflammatory conditions of the nose, such as rhinitis and polyps. If the sinuses fail to show signs of aeration, then the surgeon must consider obliteration with fat and/or local or regional flaps.

5. Hypertrophic scars, although rare, can develop in the frontoethmoid incision line. This problem can sometimes be prevented by making an irregular line of incision. If an unsightly scar develops, it can be treated with local injections of triamcinolone (40 mg/mL). If the scar is still unsatisfactory, then zigzag plasty or Z-plasty revision should be performed (see Chapters 13 and 73).

ALTERNATIVE TECHNIQUE USING NASAL MUCOSAL FLAPS

Although there are advantages to using a tube in the reconstruction of the nasofrontal duct, some disadvantages must also be considered. Placement of the tube may be difficult, and if the tube comes in contact with damaged dura and with cerebrospinal fluid leakage, there can be a problem with bacterial contamination and meningitis. Injury of the dura is also possible, and in such a situation, it is more prudent to reconstruct the duct with local flaps.

a–c The exposure is identical to that obtained for the tube reconstruction procedure. However, the surgeon must avoid injury to the nasal mucosa that lies beneath the nasal bones and anterior and inferior to the middle turbinate. Nasal endoscopy may be helpful in avoiding such injury. Working through the nose, parallel incisions about 2 cm apart are made along the upper nasal vault. These incisions are extended inferiorly to the level of the lower lateral cartilages. The tissues are then cut horizontally, and a flap based superiorly is elevated and rotated on itself into the frontal sinus. Closure of the periosteum and wound and postoperative care are identical to those used for the chest tube placement technique.

NASOFRONTAL DUCT RECONSTRUCTION *(Continued)*

ALTERNATIVE TECHNIQUE
USING NASAL MUCOSAL FLAP

a

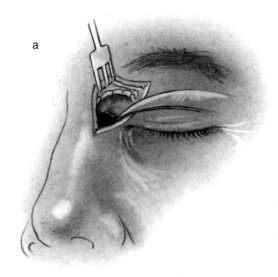

Frontoethmoid approach

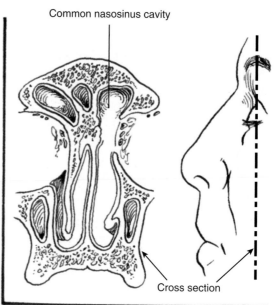

Common nasosinus cavity

Cross section

b

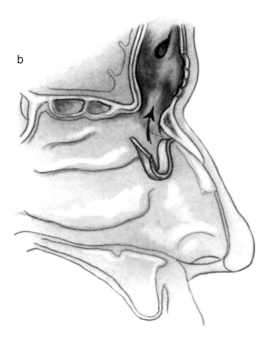

c

Development and rotation of flap

Superior Orbital Wall Fractures

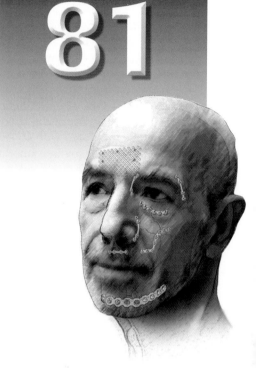

Repair of Superior Orbital Wall Fractures Using a Transorbital Approach
Alternative Technique Using Frontotemporal (Frontopterional) Craniotomy

In Consultation With Mark Hornyak, MD

INDICATIONS

Fractures of the orbital plate of the frontal bone can be isolated injuries or associated with fractures of the frontal sinus or zygoma that extend into the orbit. If the frontal sinus is small, the fracture will usually involve the orbital roof and floor of the anterior cranial fossa. If the frontal sinus is large, the fracture can cause damage to the inferior wall of the sinus and adversely affect the function of the nasofrontal duct.

Fracture of the superior orbital wall will often affect changes in orbital volume and displacement of the globe, clinically apparent as enophthalmos or exophthalmos. In fractures extending to the anterior fossa, there is usually a history of unconsciousness, and the patient may appear with pulsations of soft tissues within the orbit. Proptosis as a result of brain herniation can also be a problem. Fractures occurring more medially can present with cerebrospinal fluid (CSF) leaks. Levator and superior rectus injuries are also possible.

Superior orbital wall fractures that are confined to the rim and frontal sinus can often be explored and repaired by a direct transorbital subbrow, subfrontal or frontal osteoplastic flap approach (see Chapter 79). For more extensive areas of injury, the surgeon should consider a craniotomy. Frontotemporal (pterional) craniotomy provides an excellent exposure with which to repair other areas of the ipsilateral anterior cranial fossa including decompression of the ipsilateral superior orbital fissure and/or optic nerve (see Chapters 87 and 88). Bilateral exposure may require bifrontal craniotomy.

PROCEDURE

Under orotracheal anesthesia, the face is prepared and draped as a sterile field. The eyes should be exposed so that the surgeon can evaluate the relative position and mobility of the globes. Incisions can be designed either through the lateral eyebrow or as in a subbrow approach in which an incision is made about 3 cm in length beneath the medial part of the eyebrow. The incisions should then be infiltrated with 1% lidocaine containing 1:100,000 epinephrine for assistance in hemostasis.

A To avoid injury to the hair follicles, the skin should be incised either below or parallel to the orientation of the hair follicles. The incision is then carried through the orbicularis oculi. Angular vessels should either be ligated or cauterized. The periosteum is incised and elevated off the rim toward the orbit. Laterally the surgeon should elevate the lacrimal gland off the lacrimal fossa. Medially the trochlea is released from its attachment. Additional exposure is obtained by elevating the periosteum off the frontal bone. If possible, the branches of the supraorbital and supratrochlea nerves and arteries should be preserved.

B–D If the fracture does not involve the nasofrontal duct and displacement of the fracture is minimal without any evidence of CSF leak, then the rim of the orbit should be reduced and stabilized with miniplates or a contoured a piece of titanium mesh. If the superior orbital wall (roof) is fractured and/or displaced, this thin plate of bone can be reinforced with a piece of polypropylene mesh or with an extension of the titanium mesh.

The periosteum and subcutaneous tissues are closed with 4-0 chromic sutures. The skin is coapted with a 6-0 nylon suture. A light pressure dressing consisting of eye ointment, eye pads, stretch gauze, and fluffs is helpful in controlling postoperative edema. The wound should be evaluated at 24 and 72 hours. Prophylactic antibiotics are recommended for 5 days. Skin sutures are removed at 5 to 7 days.

PITFALLS

1. An accurate diagnosis is essential for application of proper treatment. If the fracture involves the nasofrontal duct, a coronal incision, osteoplastic flap,

and obliteration of sinus with fat or reconstruction of the duct are preferred (see Chapters 79 and 80). If the fracture involves the anterior fossa, the surgeon must consider combining the exploration and reduction of the frontal fracture with a craniotomy (see later).

2. Forces applied to the orbital rim can be transmitted posteriorly, resulting in compression of the optic nerve. For these reasons, vision must be evaluated preoperatively. During the reduction, the surgeon should be careful to elevate the orbital rim forward and avoid any posterior displacement of the fractures.

3. In patients with enophthalmos and/or exophthalmos, the surgeon has to consider a defect involving the anterior cranial fossa. The orbital plate can be displaced either upward or downward. In such situations, an osteoplastic flap or craniotomy (as described later) should be utilized for the repair.

4. Dystopia of the globe can be caused by downward or upward displacement of the superior orbital wall, alone or in combination with a floor injury. In planning reconstruction of the superior orbital wall, the surgeon should release those pressures that cause a downward displacement of the globe. Zygoma and inferior orbital rim fractures should be concurrently reduced and repaired to help in the support of the orbital tissues.

COMPLICATIONS

1. The initial fracture or the repair of the supraorbital rim can result in hypoesthesia or anesthesia of the forehead. When performing surgery, the surgeon should attempt to identify and avoid injury to the supraorbital nerve. In many patients function will return, whereas in others, there will be paresthesias and even permanent loss of sensation. Additional medical or surgical intervention has not proven to be effective.

2. If the orbital rim is not accurately reduced and stabilized, a brow deformity can occur. In the early postoperative period, open reduction, refracture, and repair are indicated. If healing of the bone has been completed, the surgeon must then consider removing projections with a cutting bur and filling in the defects with bone cement or cranial bone grafts (see Chapter 82).

3. Most swelling of the eyelid and weakness of levator function will improve with time. A subperiosteal dissection along the orbital rim should avoid injury to the neuromuscular units. If ptosis continues to be a problem, ophthalmologic consultation is advised.

4. Fractures extending to the nasofrontal duct and the anterior fossa can later be associated with sinusitis and/or CSF leaks. These complications are described in Chapter 76.

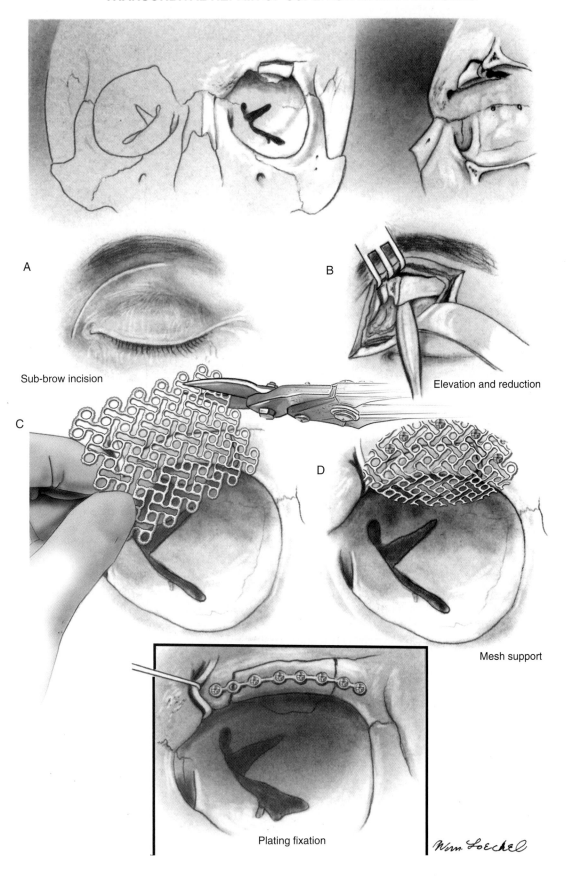

A

Sub-brow incision

B

Elevation and reduction

C

D

Mesh support

Plating fixation

Wm. Loechel

ALTERNATIVE TECHNIQUE USING FRONTOTEMPORAL (PTERIONAL) CRANIOTOMY

a,b Craniotomy for repair of the superior orbital wall (roof) is indicated when there is a suspicion of a large dural tear (i.e., CSF leak and/or pneumocephalus), displacement of the roof affecting position of the globe and when there are associated injuries requiring craniotomy. The procedure is carried out under general anesthesia with rigid skull fixation. For the frontotemporal craniotomy a unilateral coronal skin incision is designed 2 cm behind the hairline extending from just anterior to the tragus to the midline. A small area of hair is shaved, and the head is prepared and draped as a sterile field. The incision is beveled in the direction of the hair follicles and the temporalis fascia and muscle are divided with the skin incision. A plane is developed below the galea preserving the pericranium. The myocutaneous flap is elevated and held in position with fish hooks or self-retaining retractors. The pericranium is then elevated separately from the cranium as a vascularized, pedicled flap to be used in any repair at the completion of the procedure.

Bur holes are then placed to develop a bone flap. One bur hole is made at the pterion (or "keyhole") just behind the frontal process of the zygoma, a second in the temporal bone at the root of the zygoma, and a third just below the superior temporal line in the squamosal temporal bone. The dura is then dissected free from the inner table of the skull. A high-speed drill with a foot-plate tool is used to divide the bone. The frontotemporal bone flap is removed providing exposure to the anterior and middle fossa. Extradural bleeding is controlled with hemostatic products, bone wax, bipolar cautery, and dural tacking sutures.

c,d The dura is carefully elevated from the orbital roof medially toward the cribriform plate. Fragments of bone along the roof may be removed or elevated and replaced in anatomic position. No fixation is necessary. For large bony defects where the orbital bone cannot be replaced, the orbital roof can be reconstructed by fashioning a plate from malleable titanium mesh or other rigid substrate. It should be secured with screws or nonabsorbable suture to prevent herniation of cranial contents into the orbit or vice versa. The dura should be meticulously closed with 4-0 nonabsorbable sutures. If a defect is present, a piece of temporalis fascia, fascia lata, or commercially available dural substitute may be used for water-tight closure or to reinforce the area. For large defects, the previously harvested pericranial flap can be folded between the subfrontal dura and the orbital roof and then secured with suture to provide wide coverage with a viable tissue graft.

e The bone flap is replaced and secured to the adjacent cranium with titanium miniplates. The temporalis muscle and scalp are closed in layers, and a dressing is applied.

In performing this procedure transcranial exposure of the orbital roof requires elevation of the frontal lobe of the brain. Excessive brain retraction can lead to intracerebral hematoma and severe brain injury. Adequate exposure is achieved with brain relaxation and with bone removal. Surgery for fracture alone should not be performed acutely if the patient has any significant brain injury. Exradural removal of the sphenoid ridge can provide more exposure with less brain retraction.

Also if the frontal portion of the craniotomy is carried more medially, the frontal sinus may be opened. If the opening is small, it can be repaired by stripping the exposed mucosa and keeping it from the epidural space with a pedicled pericranial graft. Large openings may require cranialization and exenteration of the frontal sinus with closure of the nasofrontal duct as well as pericranial flap graft (see Chapters 76 through 79).

Most complications can be prevented. Epidural and subdural hematomas are usually prevented with meticulous hemostasis during the procedure. Intracerebral hematomas can be the result of excessive brain retraction and can be prevented with brain relaxation techniques and bone removal. Small hematomas are often been treated conservatively, while larger hematomas require craniotomy and evacuation.

Postoperative CSF leakage can usually be prevented by meticulous closure of the dura and proper handling of opened perinasal sinuses. However, if a leak occurs, initial treatment is bed rest with head elevated to 30°. Lumbar CSF drainage may be helpful but can also cause severe pneumocephalus as air rushes into the head replacing the CSF that is drained. If the site of CSF egress can be identified, a transnasal endoscopic procedure can be performed in an attempt to repair the leak extracranially (see Chapter 90). Often, a craniotomy is necessary to isolate and repair the dural defect and opening into the paranasal sinuses.

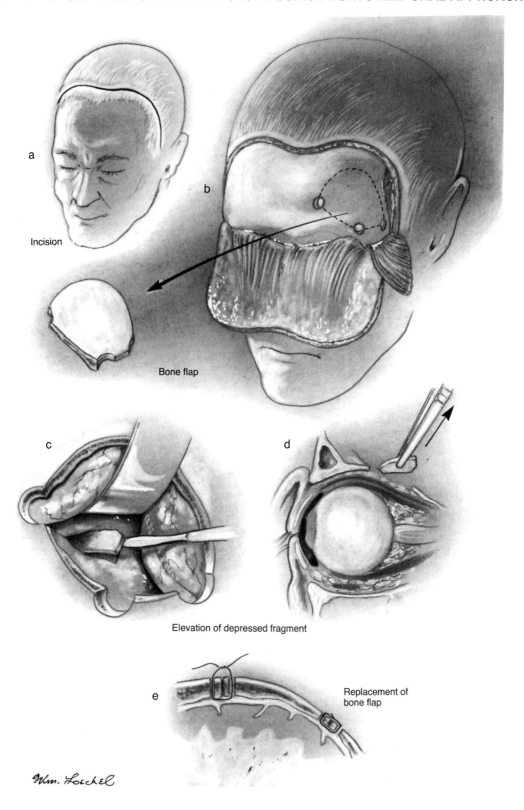

a

Incision

b

Bone flap

c

d

Elevation of depressed fragment

e

Replacement of
bone flap

Wm. Loechel

Forehead Deformity

Repair of Forehead Deformity With Bone Cement
Alternative Technique Using Bone Grafts

INDICATIONS

A posttraumatic deformity involving the fronto-orbital region can develop as a result of inadequate reduction and fixation and/or from absorption of bone. The defect is usually not noticeable early after the repair, but the affected patient will return months or years later complaining of a projection or depression of the frontal or brow region. For a small defect, we prefer recontouring of the forehead with bone cement. For larger defects that may extend into the sinus, we would prefer split cranial or rib grafts. The method for rib graft procurement is described in Chapter 38.

PROCEDURE

A Exposure of the fronto-orbital defect is usually obtained through a coronal forehead flap (see Chapters 43 and 75). The incision is about 2 cm behind the hairline, with a potential extension to the supra-auricular areas. The incision line should be shaved and the patient's head prepared and draped as a sterile field. The incision is carried into a subperiosteal plane. Hemostasis is achieved with electric cautery or hemostatic clips. Laterally the dissection is superficial to the temporalis fascia. The flap (with frontal bone periosteum) is then elevated forward and rotated over the face and is held in position with fish hooks or self-retaining retractors.

B–E The defect to be corrected is cleaned of soft tissues. Any projections beyond the desired contour are removed with a cutting bur. The bone cement powder and liquid are mixed according to directions. When the polymer has a pasty consistency, it is scooped onto a spatula or wooden tongue blade and molded into the defect. Hemostasis is very important or else blood will dilute the mixture and affect its ultimate consistency. Any irregularities of the implant can be corrected with a cutting bur. The wound is closed in layers. A flat suction drain is applied, and the patient is treated with prophylactic antibiotics for 5 to 7 days.

PITFALLS

1. In preparing for the reconstruction, the surgeon should ensure that the sinus is completely obliterated or functioning normally. The patient should be free of cerebrospinal fluid leaks or other defects of the anterior fossa. Care should also be taken during the preparation of the recipient site to avoid injury to the sinus and/or underlying dura.

2. To avoid problems with recurrent sinus infections, bone substitutes should be placed over viable bone and/or soft tissue. Be careful to prevent penetration of cement into the adjacent sinus or contact with contaminated tissues.

3. Although some bone cements will dry in a "wet bed," it is preferable to obtain a dry recipient area before applying the mixture. Under these conditions, the cement sets faster and dries with a more solid consistency.

COMPLICATIONS

1. Deformity can develop when the bone cement is too little or too excessive in amount, or when the underlying bone undergoes resorption. If a defect is noticed, additional application of cement can be considered. If there is an excess of implant, the surgeon can remove the projected areas with cutting burs. Revisional surgery, however, should be delayed until the grafted site area has stabilized, which may take months after the repair.

2. A bone cement implant affected by infection is unusual, but if this complication occurs, the material will have to be removed and the area treated with appropriate drainage. Intravenous antibiotics should be administered. Prophylactic antibiotics and aseptic techniques should help prevent this complication from occurring.

ALTERNATIVE TECHNIQUE USING BONE GRAFTS

This technique is preferred when there are large defects often in continuity with the sinus cavity. For most patients, a coronal incision and elevation of the forehead flap will provide optimal exposure. Nevertheless, for those patients with scars already present over the forehead region or for those who are balding, direct approaches should be considered.

a The coronal incision and method to expose the anterior plate of the frontal bone are described in Chapter 75. If the deformity involves the orbital rim, additional exposure can be obtained by extending the dissection along the zygomaticofrontal process and the frontal process of the maxillary bone. To provide for the harvest of the graft, the dissection should also be extended posteriorly over the parietal bone and upper portion of the temporal bone. The periosteum along the frontal bone should be incised just above the area of deformity, as this will later provide for a periosteal closure over the area of reconstruction.

b The deformity should be measured by cutting a 4 × 4 gauze sponge to the size of the defect and transposing this sponge to the donor site. The area to be harvested is then outlined with a marking solution.

The donor bone is obtained by forming an island of bone with cutting burs (see Chapters 59 and 62). A "trough" is developed by removing additional bone from around the donor site. The block of outer cortical bone is then removed with osteotomes or an oscillating saw. Bleeding is controlled by application of bone wax to the inner table of parietal cortex.

c,e Always harvest a larger graft than anticipated. Donor bone should then be carved in phases until the bone fills and fits the defect. If too much bone is removed in the shaping of the graft, additional small pieces can be harvested and inserted into the forehead gaps. The graft is subsequently placed over the defect to be repaired and contoured with burs so that it fits the defect. The recipient site can also be carved to help with the fit. The periosteum is then closed with heavy chromic (2-0 or 3-0) sutures; usually this closure will hold the graft in desirable position. Alternatively, one can use miniplates to secure the graft to adjacent bone or lag screws to secure the graft to underlying bone (see Chapter 24). The donor site can be repaired with bone cement as described earlier.

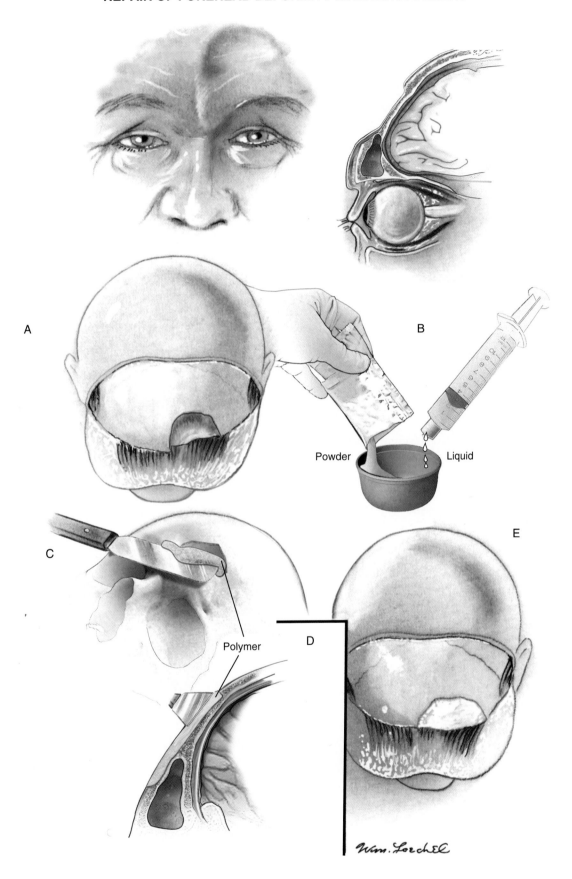

Powder

Liquid

A

B

C

D

E

Polymer

REPAIR OF FOREHEAD DEFORMITY WITH BONE GRAFT

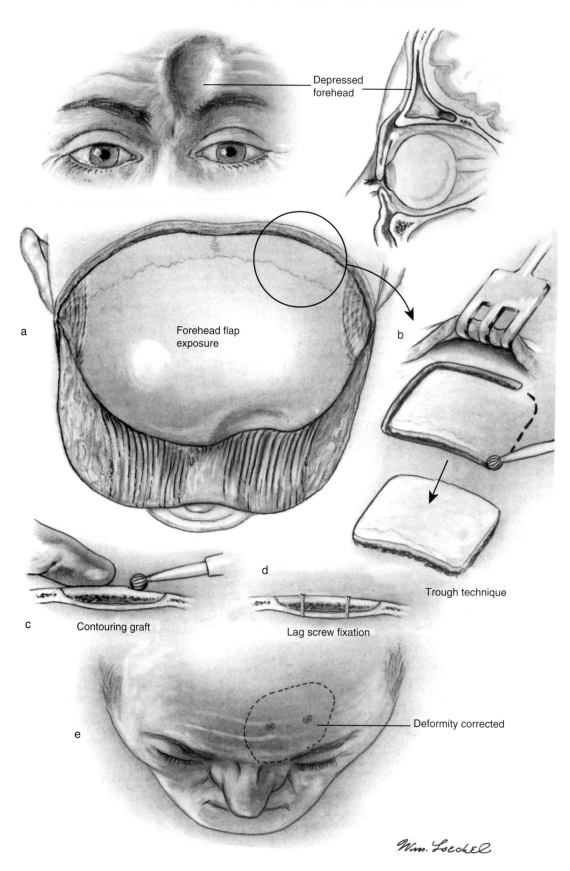

Depressed forehead

a Forehead flap exposure

b

Trough technique

c Contouring graft

d Lag screw fixation

e Deformity corrected

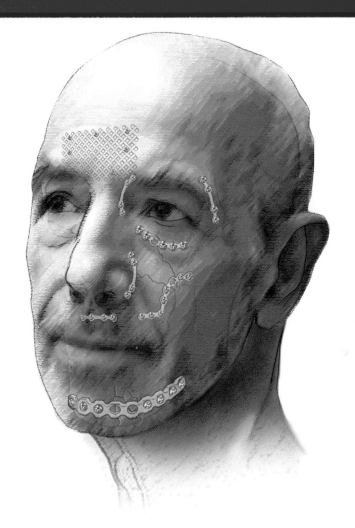

PART TEN

Sphenoid Fractures

Classification and Pathophysiology of Sphenoid Fractures

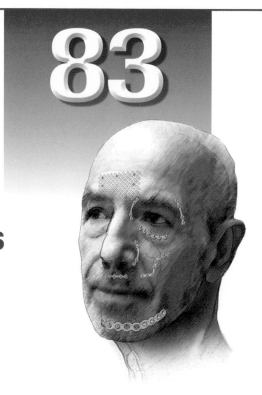

CHAPTER 83

General Considerations

The sphenoid bone appears to be protected by its central position within the craniofacial skeleton, but its multiple attachments to the cranium and face make it particularly vulnerable to fracture. Sphenoid injuries are commonly associated with maxillary, zygomatic, ethmoid, frontal, and temporal bone fractures, and thus the sphenoid injury often presents with a variety of additional deformities and neural and vascular deficits. Successful management depends on early diagnosis and appropriate medical and surgical regimens.

Sphenoid fractures often present with specific syndromes. Injury to the body of the sphenoid can cause a cerebrospinal fluid leak from the nose and/or damage to the optic nerve. Fractures involving the greater wing of the sphenoid and superior orbital fissure can result in injury to the recurrent branch of the lacrimal artery; the superior and inferior ophthalmic veins; the oculomotor (III), trochlea (IV), and abducens

(VI) nerves; and the lacrimal, frontal, and nasociliary branches and sympathetic fibers of the ophthalmic nerve (V^1). The multiple neuropathies generally affect pupillary and extraocular functions. Also, a greater wing fracture can extend to the foramen ovale and foramen spinosum and cause problems with the maxillary and mandibular nerves, the middle and accessory meningeal arteries, and the lesser petrosal nerve, resulting in problems with jaw strength and facial sensation. Pterygoid plate displacement can affect mastication, and if the hamulus is involved, the tensor veli palatini will fail to open and close the eustachian tube. This can lead to fluid and/or blood accumulation within the middle ear.

The location and extent of the sphenoid bone fracture are best evaluated by a combination of MRIs and CT scans. Clinical management depends specifically on the problem created by the injury. In most cases, expectant waiting with appropriate prophylactic antibiotic therapy is indicated. In others, there is a need for immediate, aggressive medical and/or surgical decompression of one or several nerves. Persistent cerebrospinal fluid leakage may require exploration and repair of a dural tear. Diplopia may require reduction of one of the orbital walls, prisms, and/or exercises with eye muscle surgery. Masticatory dysfunction may require a reduction of the pterygoid plates, but if a neural deficit is the cause, it is probably best treated with prosthetic and rehabilitative techniques.

SPHENOID FRACTURES

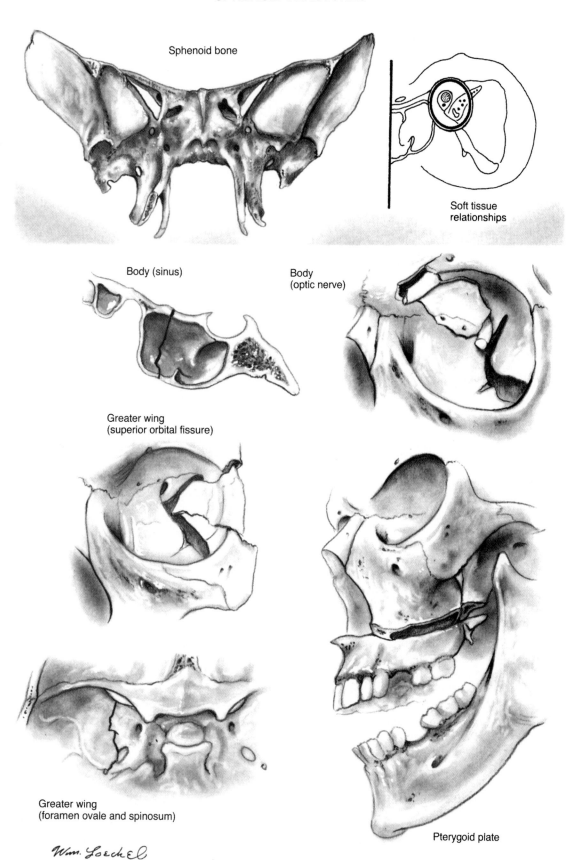

Sphenoid bone

Soft tissue relationships

Body (sinus)

Body (optic nerve)

Greater wing (superior orbital fissure)

Greater wing (foramen ovale and spinosum)

Pterygoid plate

Wm. Loechel

489

Cerebrospinal Fluid Leaks
Examination of Cerebrospinal Fluid Leak Using Intrathecal Fluorescein Dye and Endoscope
Alternative Technique Using Intranasal Pledgets

In Consultation With Adam Folbe, MD

INDICATIONS

A variety of sites within the skull base and a small amount of fluid leaking through these sites make it very difficult to diagnose a cerebrospinal fluid leak (CSF). Leaks can occur in the anterior fossa through the frontal sinus, cribiform plate or sphenoid sinus, or in the middle fossa through the middle ear and eustachian tube. In many patients, the surgeon cannot be certain that there is a leak, and the site of dural tear may not be evident. Some clues can be obtained from the history and physical examination of the patient and imaging studies, but it first must be determined that it is cerebrospinal fluid. Rhinorrhea should thus be collected and evaluated for biochemical markers found only in CSF. One of these markers, beta-2 transferrin, which is highly sensitive and accurate is expensive, and only a few laboratories in this country perform the test. The results usually take 3 to 7 days. Another protein found in CSF is beta-trace protein. Immunoelectrophoretic procedures to identify beta-trace protein are less expensive and more widely available than the testing for beta-2 protein. Although both tests are sensitive and specific for the presence of a CSF leak, the tests cannot help determine the site of the defect.

Imaging studies are particularly important for evaluating fractures and accumulation of fluid within the paranasal sinuses. High-resolution CT scans have been shown to accurately identify the site of CSF leak; however, a boney skull base defect does not necessarily mean that there is a dural defect. Recently, MR cisternography has become popular because it is a noninvasive method and is reasonably effective in localizing a CSF leak. Nevertheless, leaks can be difficult to identify and may require special intrathecal tests that rely on contrast and radioactive materials or colored dyes.

Many methods are available. A contrast material such as metrizamide is excellent for showing large leaks; the material will also accumulate within the adjacent sinuses or upper aerodigestive tract. Radioactive materials with a small molecular structure (e.g., sodium iodide I-123, ytterbium Yb-169 pentetate, and indium In-111) are useful in identifying very small leaks, but interpretation of data is often confounded by high background counts of contaminated blood and/or secretions. Iodinated I-131 serum albumin (RISA) is quite accurate in showing leaks but can be reactive and is not recommended (or approved by the Food and Drug Administration) for routine use. Some of the dyes that are visually detectable provide sensitive methods of evaluation, but these substances carry a risk of central nervous system reactions. Thus each test substance has its own risk-benefit relationship, and although this may vary among individual patients, the information should be shared with them.

Our preference is to first identify the presence of a leak using a high-resolution CT scan and beta-2 transferrin or beta-trace protein; if a leak is not demonstrated but is still suspected, an intrathecal fluorescein dye test is next considered.

PROCEDURE

Sedation should be light, as patient cooperation is important in performing the test. Special equipment such as a mechanical table or chair, headlight, nasal preparation tray, and lumbar puncture tray should be available.

For the patient in the sitting or recumbent position, the nose is sprayed with 4% lidocaine and 1/4% oxymetazoline hydrochloride (Neo-Synephrine). The nasal mucous membranes are then treated with 4% cocaine containing epinephrine, and the nose is blocked with 1% lidocaine containing 1:100,000 epinephrine. This nasal preparation is identical to that used in the preparation for rhinoplasty (see Chapter 54). The patient is then placed in a sitting or a lateral knees-up position for the lumbar puncture. The lumbar area is prepared with antiseptic solution, and the skin over the area of L4-5 is infiltrated with 2% lidocaine. A neurosurgeon or neurologist usually performs the puncture. With the index finger of the hand on the iliac crest, the thumb palpates the fourth lumbar interspace. A 22-gauge needle is then inserted between L4 and L5 and directed slightly upward. Proper penetration is assured by a free flow of spinal fluid. A 10-mL syringe is then filled with 0.3 to 0.5 mL of 5% fluorescein and attached to the spinal needle. The fluorescein is gradually diluted with the withdrawal of 9.5 mL of spinal fluid (barbotage technique). One or two milliliters of the diluted solution are then injected and the syringe is again filled with aspirated spinal fluid. This is repeated several times until the dilution does not change color within the syringe. The remainder of the fluid is then injected and the area covered with an adhesive dressing. The dye is injected over 10 minutes at a rate of approximately 1 mL/min.

A The patient is placed in a position to increase intracranial pressure and circulate the dye. Usually, the patient lays head down and performs a valsalva maneuver every 10 to 15 minutes. After approximately 30 minutes, a nasal endoscpe is used to look for the presence of fluorescein in the nasal cavity. The endoscopy includes a thorough exam including the inferior nasal cavity and nasopharynx, sphenoethmoidal recess, and the cribiform which is medial to the middle turbinate. If a leak present, the patient is taken to the operating room, for repair of the leak (see Chapters 90 and 91). If a leak is not observed, the patient is checked every 15 minutes for 1 hour. If suspicion remains high, but no dye is seen, the patient is taken to the operating room for a closer inspection and possible surgery.

PITFALLS

1. Fluorescein can cause reactions such as paresthesias, weakness, and seizures. The lumbar puncture can be associated with moderate to severe headaches for several days to several weeks. The patient should be informed of these potential sequelae but should also be told that the effects are usually temporary and there should be no permanent damage.

2. Patient cooperation is important for a valid test. The patient will be asked to move into specific positions and to hold still during the spinal puncture and during the insertion and removal of the pledgets.

3. The fluorescein should be diluted and injected very slowly, and no more than 0.3 to 0.5 mL should be used. The dilution should have a concentration of no more than 0.5 mL of fluorescein to 10 mL of spinal fluid, and even at that concentration, only a few milliliters should be injected. The solution within the syringe is again diluted and the process repeated until the color of the fluid is not changed by the aspirated spinal fluid.

4. The intrathecal mixing of fluorescein takes approximately 30 minutes. If a significant leak is suspected from the history, the surgeon should gradually approach the head-down position.

5. The patient should be observed after the test for adverse sequelae from the intrathecal substance. If the patient has a history of seizures, antiseizure medications should be utilized preoperatively and adequate levels of medication maintained during and after the test. If the patient develops signs or symptoms of inflammation, administration of steroids may be indicated.

COMPLICATIONS

1. Although the threat of impending meningitis necessitates early identification and control of the

INTRATHECAL DYE TEST

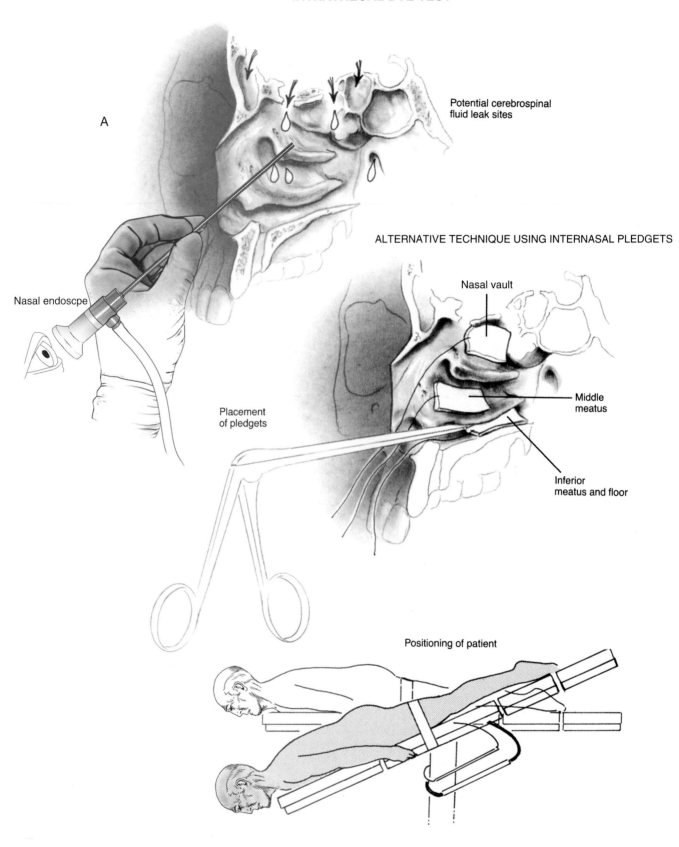

A

Potential cerebrospinal
fluid leak sites

Nasal endoscpe

Placement
of pledgets

ALTERNATIVE TECHNIQUE USING INTERNASAL PLEDGETS

Nasal vault

Middle
meatus

Inferior
meatus and floor

Positioning of patient

fistula, the test itself may cause meningitis. The mechanism is not well understood. Meningitis can occur from just the lumbar puncture, from a reversal of the flow through the fistula, and/or from contaminated fluorescein solutions. If evidence of meningitis develops, cultures should be obtained and the patient immediately treated with appropriate antibiotics.

   2. The lumbar puncture can be associated with headache. The complication is not predictable, and although the amount of aspirated spinal fluid is sometimes related to the degree and length of time that the headache persists, this will vary among subjects. The headache can be reduced by having the patient lie flat in the postoperative period. Analgesics should be administered and the patient kept well hydrated.

   3. Intrathecal fluorescein has been reported to cause transient reactions within the central nervous system (e.g., paresthesias, weakness of the extremities, and seizures). It appears that the complications probably can be minimized or avoided by using small amounts of dye, diluting the dye, and injecting it slowly. Patients who have a history of seizures should be maintained on antiseizure medications before and after the procedure. Adequate levels of the antiseizure drug should be maintained throughout the day. Steroids may be injected, if necessary, to control some of the inflammatory phases of the reaction.

ALTERNATIVE TECHNIQUE USING INTRANASAL PLEDGETS

The localization of fluorescein can also be carried out by the application of intranasal pledgets and Wood's light examination. For this procedure, ½ × ½ inch square cottonoid pads moistened with saline are placed on both sides of the nose. The first set is placed superiorly in the nasal vault near the superior meatus. They should be close to the cribiform plate and superior and anterior wall of the sphenoid sinus. Another set is placed in the middle meatus and a third along the floor of the nose near the eustachian tube. The attached strings are left hanging from the nose. The fluoroscein is injected intrathecally as described earlier and the pledgets inspected after the valsalva maneuvers. Pledgets are replaced ever 10 to 15 minutes. An operating room table is useful in the procedure since the patient may be tilted up and down mixing the dye with spinal fluid while increasing pressure in the down position. The pledget technique is also useful in evaluating leakage using clear radioactive materials that cannot be visualized with an endoscope. The radioactivity of the pledgets is then measured using scintigraphic techniques.

CHAPTER 85

Transnasal Repair of a Sphenoid Bone Cerebrospinal Fluid Leak Using Endoscopic Technique

In Consultation With Adam Folbe, MD

INDICATIONS

Fractures through the body of the sphenoid can be associated with dural tears, pneumocephalus, and cerebrospinal fluid leakage. Early recognition of this problem is important if the sequela of meningitis is to be avoided. The injury should be delineated by imaging studies, and special intrathecal tests should be used to demonstrate the site and degree of the leak. The pathophysiologic and diagnostic considerations are discussed in Chapters 83 and 84.

In general, the patient is treated first with reduction and fixation of the facial fractures; antibiotics are administered to prevent meningitis. Most cerebrospinal fluid leaks cease within 1 to 2 weeks, but if the leakage persists, a surgical repair must be considered.

In the past, three popular approaches for repair of a sphenoid bone cerebrospinal fluid leak were (1) transseptal, (2) transethmoidal or frontoethmoid (see Chapter 90), and (3) frontal craniotomy (see Chapter 91). The transantral-ethmoidal approach is also possible but provides little, if any, advantage over the others and can lead to greater instability when there are facial fractures. Currently, the most widely used approach is a transnasal transsphenoidal approach. The approach is described in detail below. As discussed in Chapter 84, there are many ways to indentify the site of the CSF leak.

Along with high-resolution CT, the use of intraoperative CT navigation has made the approach seemingly safer and more accessible. However, the CT navigation is a tool and should not replace the surgeon's experience and knowledge of the complex anatomy.

PROCEDURE

A,B For the sphenoidotomy, the nose is prepared as for a standard endoscopic sinus surgery. After general anesthesia has been obtained, pledgets (0.5 × 3 cm), which have been soaked in topical decongestants, are placed in two places: high in the nasal vault along the nasal septum medial to the middle turbinate and low along the nasal septum and floor of nasal cavity. Next, approximately 3 to 4 mL of 1% lidocaine with 1:100,000 epinepherine is injected into the tail of the middle turbinate for further vasoconstriction. If the middle turbinate obscures exposure of the sphenoid, the inferior third of the middle turbinate is resected.

C The sphenoid ostium is located just medial to the superior turbinate. However, trauma may distort the anatomy. The safest place to enter the sphenoid sinus is medially and inferiorly. Using an endoscope, a wide view of the posterior wall of the nasal cavity

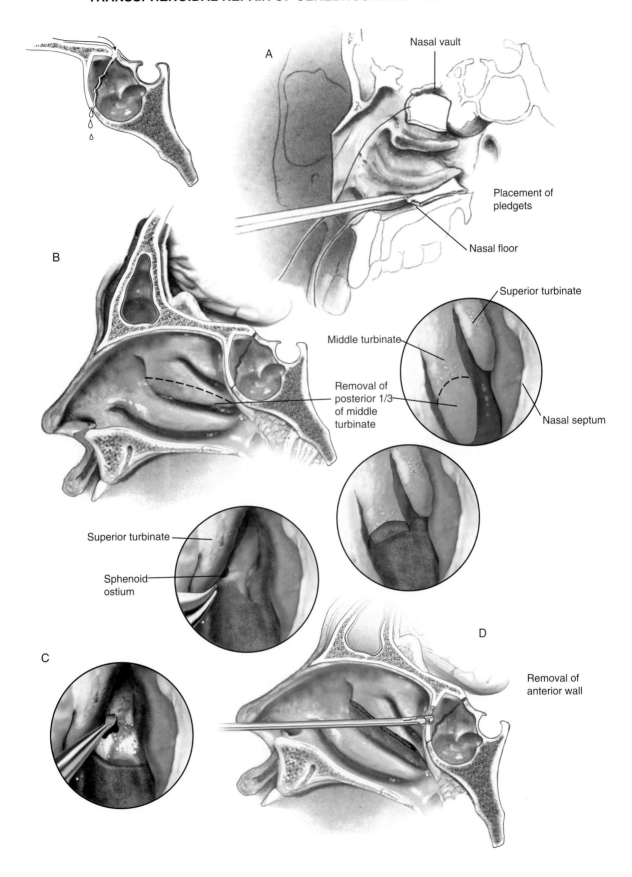

A

Nasal vault

Placement of pledgets

Nasal floor

B

Superior turbinate

Middle turbinate

Removal of posterior 1/3 of middle turbinate

Nasal septum

Superior turbinate

Sphenoid ostium

C

D

Removal of anterior wall

is displayed. A Cottle elevator is then marched up the posterior wall just lateral to the nasal septum. Without much pressure, the Cottle gently enters the sphenoid sinus and the posterior wall is carefully palpated. Useful measurements for the sphenoid sinus are 7 cm to the anterior wall and 9 cm to the posterior wall.

D,E The ostium is enlarged inferiorly and medially using the microdebridder, Hajek, and Takashi rongeurs. Next, placing the endoscope into the sinus, the surgeon can confirm the large superior and lateral extent of the sinus. Also, at this point, the surgeon can identify the optic-carotid recess and verify if the nerve and/or artery are dehiscent. After these structures are confirmed, the ostium is enlarged superiorly and laterally. During this step, the surgeon may expose and ligate the sphenopalatine artery. Simple suction cautery is adequate for hemostasis.

F If a three or four hand approach is needed, the above procedure is performed on the opposite side. Then, the posterior 1.5 to 2 cm of the septum is removed, as well as the sphenoid rostrum. Next, all of the mucosa is removed from the sphenoid sinus, especially the lateral recess of the sinus. Failure to remove the mucosa may prevent the graft from scarring into place, and it may lead to possible mucocele formation in the future.

G The cerebrospinal fluid leak should then be identified. To patch the defect, our preference is a sheet of acellular dermis, approximately 0.5 to 2 mm in thickness. After reconstitution in normal saline, the sheet is cut to approximately twice the size of the defect. Then, the piece is placed into the defect, so that a portion is intracranial, and the oversized edges are placed against the exposed bone. Layers of moist gel foam are placed against the graft filling the sinus. A 10 cm merocel is placed in the nose to support the graft and left in place for 5 to 7 days.

Postoperatively the patient is placed in the head-up position and told to avoid any straining, sneezing, coughing, or blowing of the nose. The patient is given a stool softener and placed on antibiotics for approximately 2 weeks. After removal of the nasal packing the nose is treated with saline mists at least three times daily.

PITFALLS

1. Exposure of the sphenoid sinus endoscopically requires knowledge of the anatomy of the nose and paranasal sinuses and experience with an endoscope.

2. The sphenoid sinus lies in the midline, on a line drawn 30° from the floor of the nose. The rostrum is an important landmark. The position of the midline septum of the sphenoid, however, is quite variable, and the anatomy of the septum should be evaluated on computed tomographic (CT) scans. Once in the sphenoid sinus, the surgeon should recognize the optic nerve ridge and projection of the carotid artery.

3. Postoperative mechanical debridement should be avoided for the first 3 to 4 weeks, as this may disrupt the graft. Patients, however, are started on nasal saline irrigations 2 weeks after the procedure.

COMPLICATIONS

1. Failure to stop the leakage can result in meningitis and/or pneumocephalus. All patients should be followed closely after the procedure, and if meningitis is suspected, a CT scan should be used to reevaluate the defect and intracranial tear. A lumbar puncture should be performed to analyze the spinal fluid and obtain cultures for appropriate antibiotic therapy.

2. Recurrent or persistent cerebrospinal fluid leakage requires reevaluation and repair. However, the surgeon should make sure that the leak is from the same place as before and there are no other leaks compounding the clinical picture. Imaging studies and intrathecal tests should be considered. A repair from below is still desirable, as the intracranial exposure carries more risk for morbidity and complication. The sphenoidotomy can be repeated, or alternatively, the surgeon can consider the frontoethmoidectomy or transantral ethmoidectomy approaches.

3. Injury to the optic nerve and/or carotid artery can be avoided by an appreciation of the anatomic relationships. Exposure provided by magnification and lighting from the endoscope is important, and such an approach should delineate the anatomy of the walls. The mucosa should always be stripped under direct visualization, as this will help avoid injury to any of the adjacent structures.

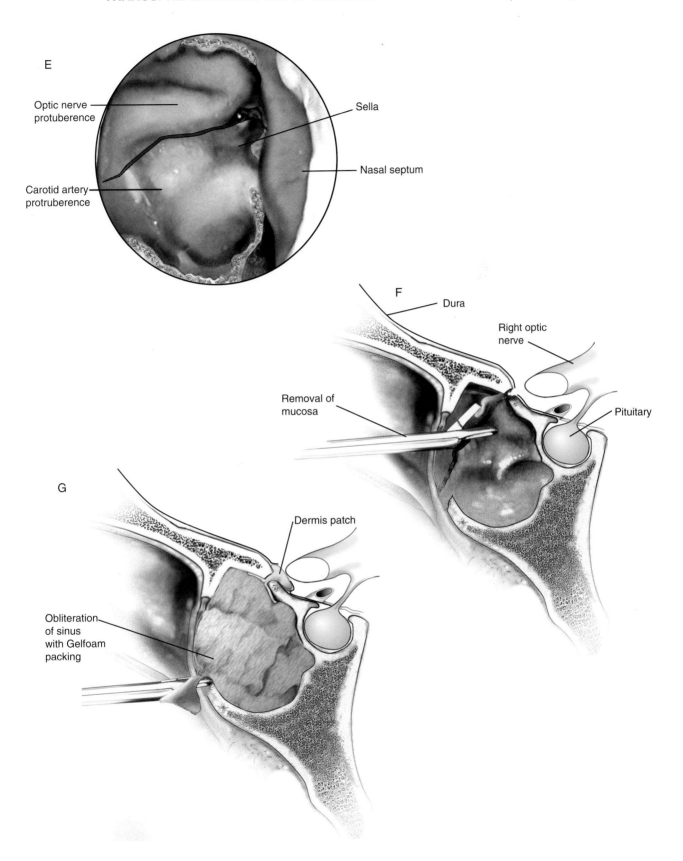

E

Optic nerve
protuberence

Carotid artery
protruberence

Sella

Nasal septum

F

Dura

Right optic
nerve

Removal of
mucosa

Pituitary

G

Dermis patch

Obliteration
of sinus
with Gelfoam
packing

Optic Nerve Injuries

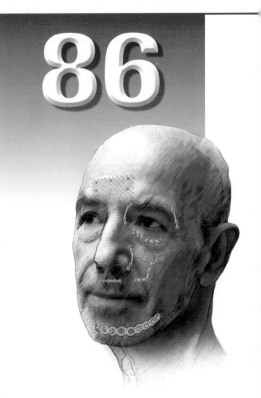

CHAPTER

86

Decompression of the Optic Nerve Using a Transethmoidal Approach
Alternative Transnasal Endoscopic Technique of Decompression

In Consultation With Adam Folbe, MD

INDICATIONS

Sudden or progressive loss of vision in the absence of globe injury often indicates optic nerve damage. The patient may demonstrate a Marcus Gunn pupil (afferent pupillary defect), but the physician should not expect optic nerve pallor or atrophy for several weeks. Evoked visual potentials are often markedly diminished or absent. The clinical picture may be complicated by other ocular injuries, and the impact these injuries have on vision must be determined.

A variety of mechanisms have been used to describe optic nerve damage. The optic nerve may be mechanically impacted by displacement of adjacent bone fragments, or it may be contused or compressed by blood clots or swelling within the optic canal. There is also a possibility that the nerve has been lacerated and severed from its attachments.

From a treatment standpoint, it is important to evaluate whether the nerve is severed or compressed, but this is often difficult to determine by clinical and/ or radiographic methods. A history of immediate loss of vision suggests a laceration or cutting, whereas a history of gradual loss is more consistent with a compression phenomenon. Major displacements of sphenoid bone fragments on imaging studies may imply an impaction or tearing of the nerve. All of this information is helpful, but because the surgeon cannot be certain of the pathologic condition, medical and/or surgical trials of therapy are indicated.

Our usual approach is to evaluate the history, physical examination, and radiographic information (sinus radiographs, axial and coronal computed tomographic (CT) scans and MRI scans). Ophthalmologic consultation is obtained. Most patients are started on megadose steroids (i.e., 100 mg dexamethasone followed by 50 mg every 6 hours for three doses). If the patient responds, the steroids are tapered. If the patient does not respond or there is a relapse after a gradual improvement, then the steroids are stopped (or tapered), and a surgical decompression is considered.

The transethmoidal approach is preferred when the injury to the sphenoid also involves the medial and inferior walls of the orbit. The exposure is indicated when there is a need to repair other facial fractures. The intracranial approach is best employed when there are associated cranial bone injuries and, in particular, dural tears, frontal bone fractures, and injury to the orbital plate (see Chapter 87). The transnasal endoscopic approach (see later) can be used when the anatomy is retained and under elective conditions.

PROCEDURE

The patient is placed in a supine position, and anesthesia is provided by way of an orotracheal tube. The nasal mucous membranes are treated with 4% cocaine containing epinephrine (see Chapter 54), and the medial canthal area is injected with 1% lidocaine containing 1:100,000 epinephrine. The head is extended, and the patient is placed in Trendelenburg position. The head and neck are then prepared with antiseptic solutions and draped as a sterile field.

A With the surgeon sitting at the head of the table, a curvilinear incision is made one half the distance between the inner caruncle of the eye and the dorsum of the nose. The incision is carried through the subcutaneous tissues; the angular vessels are ligated, and bleeding is stopped with cautery. The incision can also be extended to the shadow area beneath the brow.

B,C The periosteum is elevated off the nasal bones and the frontal process of the maxilla. The lamina papyracea and lacrimal bones are exposed, and the lacrimal sac is retracted laterally. The trochlea is released from its attachment. The periosteum is elevated off the medial wall of the orbit with a Freer elevator. The

anterior ethmoidal artery is clipped or avulsed, and bleeding is controlled by gentle pressure. Posteriorly the dissection should expose, but not injure, the posterior ethmoidal artery.

D,E A frontoethmoidectomy is then performed by removing portions of the floor of the frontal sinus, the nasal bone, and the frontal process of the maxilla. The frontal sinus is opened by a small drill hole and enlarged with Kerrison rongeurs. The inferiorly located ethmoid cells are then removed with Takahashi rongeurs. The curved posterior wall of the frontal bone should be visualized and followed inferiorly and posteriorly along the base of the skull. The undersurface of the cribriform plate is exposed.

F–H The operating microscope with a 300-mm lens is used for the remainder of the procedure. Self-retaining retractors are helpful in holding the soft tissues of the orbit from the sinus cavity. We prefer to open the sphenoid sinus with Hajek rongeurs, which in turn exposes the intersinus septum and those landmarks that identify the optic nerve and carotid artery. The transverse bulge superiorly shows the course of the optic nerve; a wider bulge laterally and posteriorly represents the carotid artery canal.

With the optic nerve bulge identified within the sphenoid sinus and the posterior ethmoidal artery visualized within the orbit, the posterior ethmoidal artery is clipped or treated with a bipolar cautery. The bone along the posteromedial wall of the orbit is then removed, exposing more of the sphenoid sinus. The periorbita is elevated 1 or 2 mm at a time, and immediately posterior to the posterior ethmoidal artery, the surgeon will see the optic nerve sheath entering the optic canal. The entrance to the canal (ring) is quite thick, and diamond burs on a long drill handle should be used to open this area. The more posteriorly and medially directed portion of the canal is thinned with burs and extracted with small elevators. Approximately one half to three fourths of the canal is opened. Any displaced bone spicules are removed.

Bleeding should be minimal, and nasal packing should not be needed. The periosteum is closed with 3-0 chromic sutures, and the trochlea should be returned to its anatomic position. The subcutaneous tissues and skin are closed in layers.

The patient should be treated with prophylactic antibiotics and the eye checked periodically for visual function and for changes in pressure on the globe. The patient can be discharged in 24 to 48 hours.

PITFALLS

1. The optic nerve decompression procedure requires exquisite attention to detail. The patient must be

TRANSETHMOIDAL DECOMPRESSION OF THE OPTIC NERVE

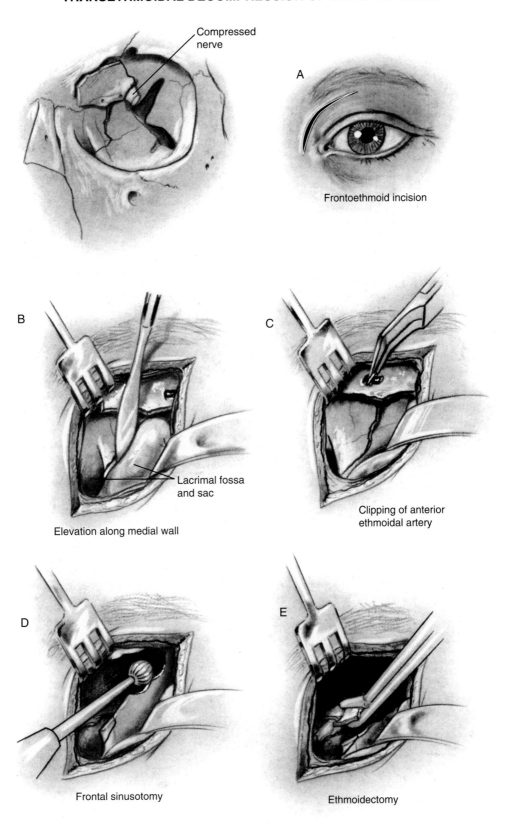

Compressed nerve

A

Frontoethmoid incision

B

Lacrimal fossa and sac

Elevation along medial wall

C

Clipping of anterior ethmoidal artery

D

Frontal sinusotomy

E

Ethmoidectomy

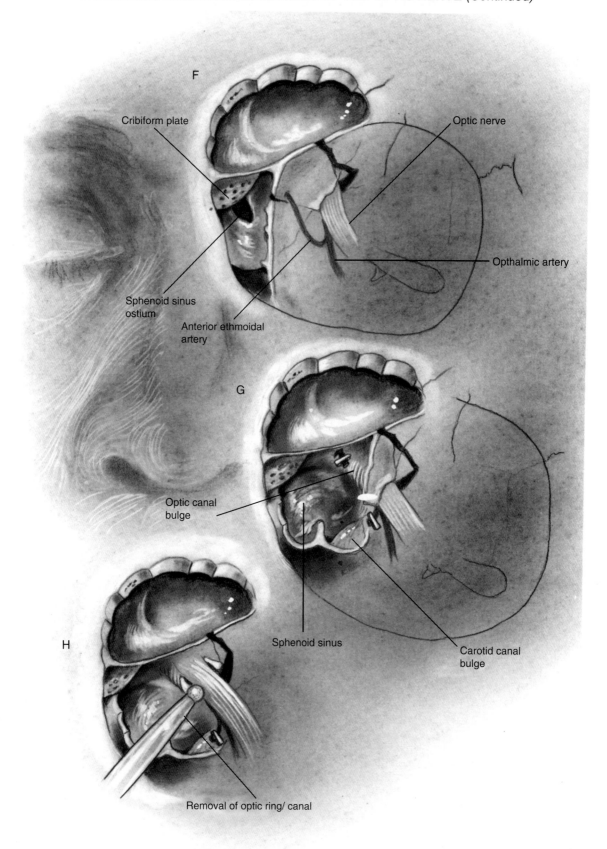

F

Cribiform plate

Optic nerve

Opthalmic artery

Sphenoid sinus ostium

Anterior ethmoidal artery

G

Optic canal bulge

Sphenoid sinus

Carotid canal bulge

H

Removal of optic ring/ canal

in an appropriate position; therefore a motorized table and mechanical chair should be available for rapid, frequent, and exact changes in position of the patient and/or surgeon during the procedure. Overhead lighting should be supplemented by a bright, adjustable headlight. Self-retaining retractors; long, thin suctions; and microinstruments, such as those used in pituitary and/or ear surgery, are helpful. A long-handled, smooth-cutting drill is also important. As soon as the surgeon penetrates the sphenoid sinus and/or posterior ethmoidal cells, lighting and magnification through a microscope will help in the visualization and dissection.

2. There are two important methods of defining the location and extent of the optic nerve. Although distances measured from the orbital rim can be variable, the posterior ethmoidal artery and its relationship to the nerve are fairly constant, and in almost all cases, the nerve lies 3 to 10 mm directly posterior to the artery. The bulge on the superior wall of the sphenoid sinus is also a reliable landmark. Thus if the surgeon works below the posterior ethmoidal artery and toward this bulge, the optic nerve and ring should be readily discernable.

3. Avoid injury to the carotid artery. The carotid canal lies on the lateral wall of the sphenoid, below and posterior to the optic canal. Once this bulge is identified, the surgeon should keep the drill a distance from this area.

4. Although the optic nerve can be visualized by a pure transethmoidal/transphenoidal approach, the additional orientation obtained by removing all or part of the medial wall of the orbit is desirable. The posterior ethmoidal vessel is easily identified and can act as a "pointer" directly to the nerve. The procedure rarely requires removal of the lateral wall of the nose or entrance through the anterior wall of the maxilla; these additional exposures may cause more bleeding and morbidity.

5. Removal of the medial wall of the orbit will cause an enlargement of the orbit to some degree, and this will predispose the patient to a postoperative enophthalmos. The amount of wall removed often determines the degree of enophthalmos. Generally the resection should be as conservative as possible, yet still expose the important landmarks. If necessary, the surgeon can remove a portion of the wall and then replace it into the area of deficit following the procedure. It should also be noted that with practice, sections of the medial wall can be retained, and eventually only that section between the posterior ethmoidal vessel and optic nerve will have to be resected.

6. The question of whether to open the optic nerve sheath is controversial. Removal of one half to three fourths of the optic canal makes the nerve fairly mobile. This suggests that with an adequate decompression, an opening of the sheath is probably not necessary. Moreover, a cut through the sheath often causes a cerebrospinal fluid leak (CSF) which may persist or cause complications in the postoperative period.

7. Bleeding can be avoided by ligature of the vessels with vascular clips or by letting the vessels clot off with gentle pressure. If cautery is to be used, we prefer the bipolar cautery applied directly to the ends of the vessels. This avoids additional injury to the optic and other cranial nerves.

COMPLICATIONS

1. If the medial wall of the orbit is removed, enophthalmos will most likely occur. This complication can be avoided by limiting the resection of the wall, replacing the wall, or (in experienced hands) removing only a small portion of the wall in front of and behind the posterior ethmoidal artery. If enophthalmos develops and is a problem to the patient, the surgeon can later reconstruct the orbit with bone grafts (see Chapter 64).

2. Postoperative bleeding can cause accumulation of blood in the retro-orbital space. Significant amounts of bleeding can compromise and obstruct the ophthalmic vessels and thereby further threaten visual acuity. The problem is suspected when increasing proptosis and/or pain out of proportion to the procedure is observed, and if this occurs, the incision should be opened and the blood removed. Hemostasis should be obtained with a bipolar cautery.

3. Epistaxis can often be controlled by judicious use of nasal packing. Nasal tampons or 1/4-in gauze treated with bacitracin ointment, placed appropriately within the nose, are standard methods of control (see Chapter 52).

ALTERNATIVE TRANSNASAL ENDOSCOPIC TECHNIQUE OF DECOMPRESSION

The nasal mucus membranes are prepared with oxymetazoline pledgets as described in Chapter 85. The lateral wall of the nasal cavity is also injected with 1% lidocaine comtaing 1;100,000 epinephrine. The uncinate process is medialized and removed exposing the natural osteum of the maxillary sinus. To help with the exposure, the inferior third of the middle turbinate is removed and the ethmoid cells are exenterated to expose the medial wall of the orbit. The anterior wall of the sphenoid sinus is subsequently removed (see Chapter 85).

a With exposure of the lamina papyracea and identification of the anterior and posterior ethmoidal arteries, the lamina is removed inferior to these vessels in an anterior to posterior direction. A higher dissection would require coagulation of one or both arteries. The lamina will thicken as the dissection proceeds toward the apex of the orbit and a diamond bur is used to thin the bone near the optic ring. Once the bone is thinned, a Cottle elevator or curette can be used to remove the bone from the optic sheath.

b–e Working in the sphenoid sinus, the bulge of the optic canal is identified along the upper lateral wall of the sphenoid sinus superior to the carotid bulge. In some patients, the optic canal will be found in the posterior ethmoid or in an Onodi cell, which can be visualized on preoperative CT scan. This cell (area) must be opened to expose the canal at the apex of the orbit and medially to remove the intersinus part of the canal. The decompression continues from the orbital apex in the lateral part of the sphenoid sinus medially toward the optic chiasm. Care is taken not to go too far medially as a CSF leak can occur. Small leaks can be treated with Gelfoam whereas larger leaks require more aggressive techniques described in Chapter 85.

A tampon treated with antibiotic/steroid ointment should then be placed in the nose and removed in 48 to 72 hours. The patient should be treated with antibiotics and steroids continued. After removal of the tampon, the nose should be gently irrigated with normal saline and examined and cleaned postoperatively for clots and mucus plugs.

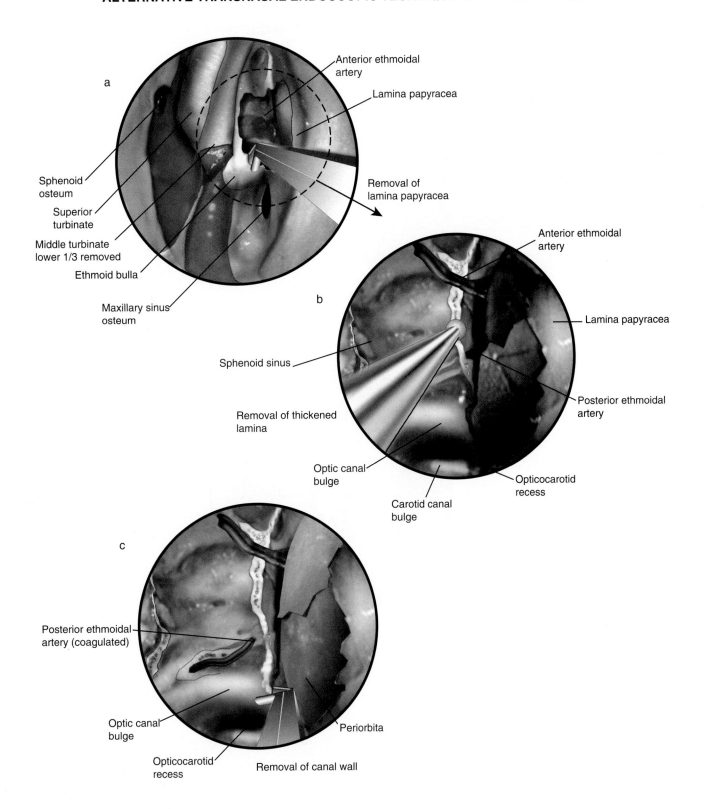

a

Anterior ethmoidal artery

Lamina papyracea

Removal of lamina papyracea

Sphenoid osteum

Superior turbinate

Middle turbinate lower 1/3 removed

Ethmoid bulla

Maxillary sinus osteum

b

Anterior ethmoidal artery

Lamina papyracea

Sphenoid sinus

Posterior ethmoidal artery

Removal of thickened lamina

Optic canal bulge

Opticocarotid recess

Carotid canal bulge

c

Posterior ethmoidal artery (coagulated)

Optic canal bulge

Periorbita

Opticocarotid recess

Removal of canal wall

ALTERNATIVE TRANSNASAL ENDOSCOPIC TECHNIQUE OF DECOMPRESSION

d

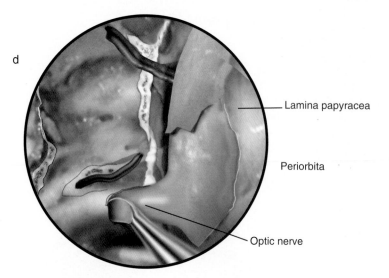

Lamina papyracea

Periorbita

Optic nerve

Cottle used to
remove optic
canal wall

e

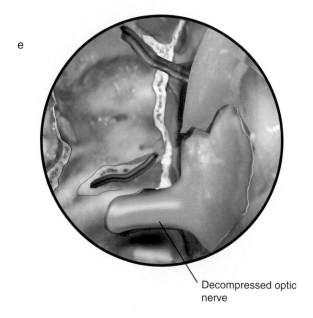

Decompressed optic
nerve

CHAPTER 87

Decompression of the Optic Nerve Using a Frontotemporal Craniotomy

In Consultation With Mark Hornyak, MD

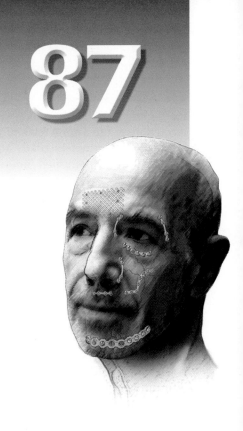

INDICATIONS

Sphenoid fractures associated with optic nerve injury present with loss of vision and can be treated either by a transethmoidal or subfrontal approach (see Chapters 79 and 86) or by a craniotomy. The rationale and indications for surgical decompression are discussed in Chapter 86. The transcranial techniques are useful when injury of the optic nerve is associated with fractures of the greater and lesser wings of the sphenoid. Frontotemporal (pterional) craniotomy is typically preferred. The approach is also indicated when there is damage to the dura, frontal sinus, orbital roof, or other structures that require craniotomy for repair. It also has an advantage over the frontoethmoid and/or subfrontal approach when important craniofacial landmarks along the base of the skull are lost or distorted by the injury, as they can be visualized along their intracranial course.

PROCEDURE

A,B The surgery is carried out under general anesthesia with rigid skull fixation. For the frontotemporal craniotomy, a unilateral coronal skin incision is designed 2 cm behind the hairline, extending from just anterior to the tragus to the midline. A small area of hair is shaved, and the head is prepared and draped as a sterile field. The incision is beveled in the direction of the hair follicles, and a subperiosteal plane is developed over the skull. An interfascial dissection is performed over the temporalis muscle to preserve the frontalis branch of the facial nerve. The scalp flap is elevated and held anteriorly with fish hooks or self-retaining retractors. The temporalis muscle is then freed anteriorly and reflected inferiorly, separate from the scalp flap.

Bur holes are then placed to develop a bone flap. One bur hole is at the pterion (or "keyhole") just behind the frontal process of the zygoma, a second in the temporal bone at the root of the zygoma, and a third just below the superior temporal line in the squamosal temporal bone. The dura is then dissected free from the inner table of the skull and a highspeed drill with a footplate tool is used to divide the bone as outlined. The frontotemporal bone flap is removed providing exposure to the anterior and middle fossa dura. Extradural bleeding is controlled with hemostatic products, bone wax, bipolar electrocautery, and dural tacking sutures.

C,D The dura is elevated from the floor of the frontal fossa and the middle fossa along the sphenoid ridge. The lateral sphenoid ridge (part of the greater wing) can be removed with bone rongeurs. The medial sphenoid ridge (part of lesser wing) is removed with the high-speed drill. Meticulous technique is necessary, typically using the operative microscope for magnification and illumination and a variety of sizes of both cutting and abrasive drill bits under constant irrigation. As the sphenoidal resection is carried medially, extradural retraction of the frontal and temporal lobes of the brain will be necessary; safe and adequate retraction requires brain relaxation. The sphenoid bone removal is continued medially and the superior orbital fissure will be identified inferiorly. Further medial bone removal is carried out toward the anterior clinoid process. Removal of the anterior clinoid process will expose the junction of the optic sheath with cranial base dura. When the extradural anatomy is obscure, it may be safer to open the anterior fossa dura to visualize the optic nerve and perform an intradural anterior clinoidectomy to decompress the optic nerve. The optic canal is then decompressed (either extra- or intradurally) by completely removing the anterior clinoid process and optic strut, and removing the posterior roof of the orbit.

Bleeding should be controlled, dural openings and tears should be carefully repaired, and openings into the paranasal sinuses closed with muscle, fat, or periosteum. The bone flap is held in place with titanium plates. For favorable cosmetic results, the temporosphenoidal cranial defect should be covered to prevent displacement of the temporalis muscle into the defect. The cranioplasty can be fashioned from malleable titanium mesh or any rigid substrate. The temporalis muscle should be carefully reapproximated, the scalp is closed in layers, and a dressing is applied.

PITFALLS

1. If the craniotomy for optic nerve decompression should be more than 1 cm from the midline, the sagittal sinus should not present a problem. If more exposure is necessary to repair the frontal fossa and a bifrontal bone flap is needed, then the sagittal sinus will be at risk. In such cases, we prefer to place a bur hole on each side of the sinus, 1.5 cm lateral to the midline and along the posterior edge of the planned bone flap. The sinus is dissected free from the inner surface of the flap, and the cut between these bur holes made last. If the sinus damaged, a large piece of Gelfoam placed over the sinus and covered with a cottonoid pledget will usually provide sufficient hemostasis.

2. If the bony dissection is confined to the orbital roof and the roof of the optic canal, the carotid artery should not present a problem. If a greater dissection is needed, this portion should be done intradurally with direct visualization of these critical neurovascular structures.

3. Cerebrospinal fluid leaks can be prevented by meticulous closure of the dura in all areas. Dural leaks into the orbit are ordinarily not a problem, but if the leak does extend over a paranasal sinus, cerebrospinal fluid rhinorrhea can occur. Thus an opening into the air-bearing sinuses should be carefully closed.

4. Protection of olfaction is provided by doing a unilateral craniotomy and by staying away from the cribriform plate and the olfactory fibers.

COMPLICATIONS

1. Dural tears may occur when the dura is dissected from the bone flap, when the craniotomy flap is cut, and when the dura is elevated from the floor of the frontal fossa. Careful dissection will decrease the possibility of a dural tear, but if one does occur, prudent management is to provide a watertight closure with fine nonabsorbable sutures.

2. Postoperative epidural or subdural hematomas result from inadequate control of bleeding. Careful use of the electrocautery and bone wax is mandatory. A hematoma presents clinically as a decrease in conscious state or a progressive neurologic deficit. The diagnosis should be confirmed by a nonenhanced CT scan. Immediate evacuation of the hematoma is the treatment of choice.

3. Cerebrospinal fluid leaks may be prevented by meticulous closure of dural tears and careful closure of openings into the sinuses. If a leak occurs, treatment consists of bed rest with the head elevated 30°. Occasionally lumbar puncture drainage may be helpful. If the leak does not stop, a craniotomy is necessary for repair of the dura. The use of prophylactic antibiotics to prevent meningitis is controversial.

FRONTOTEMPORAL DECOMPRESSION OF THE OPTIC NERVE

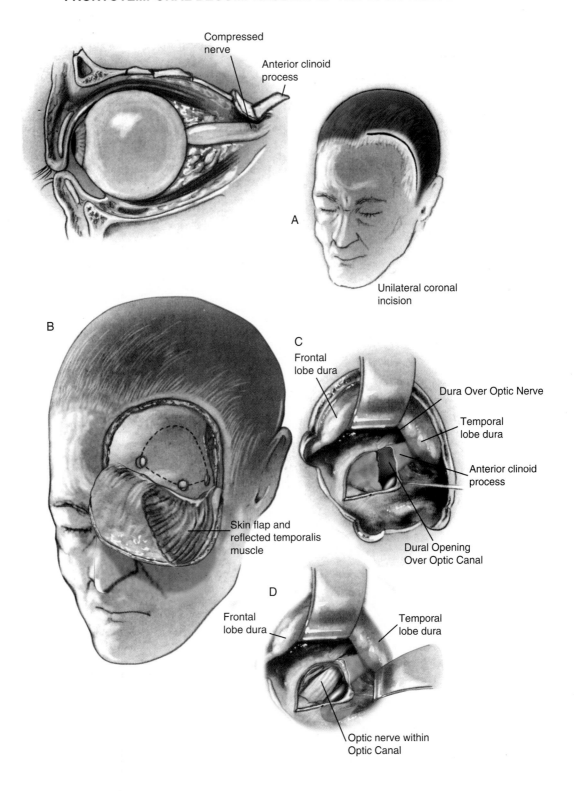

Compressed nerve

Anterior clinoid process

A

Unilateral coronal incision

B

Skin flap and reflected temporalis muscle

C

Frontal lobe dura

Dura Over Optic Nerve

Temporal lobe dura

Anterior clinoid process

Dural Opening Over Optic Canal

D

Frontal lobe dura

Temporal lobe dura

Optic nerve within Optic Canal

CHAPTER

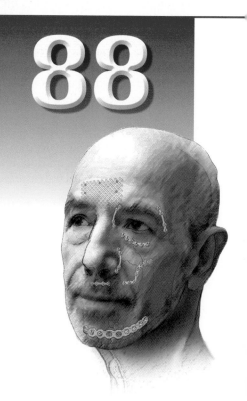

Decompression of the Superior Orbital Fissure Using a Frontotemporal Approach

In Consultation With Mark Hornyak, MD

INDICATIONS

Sphenoid fractures associated with frontozygomatic injuries can often involve the lateral superior orbital wall, causing injury to the superior orbital fissure. Such a fracture can affect cranial nerves III, IV, V_1, and/or VI and result in various degrees of ophthalmoplegia. Sometimes there is an associated optic nerve injury, ocular injury, or dural tear.

In those patients in whom the orbital injury is localized to the superior orbital fissure on high-resolution computed tomographic (CT) scan, and in whom vision is otherwise salvageable, a decompression procedure can be contemplated. The role of high-dose corticosteroids is controversial, but if desired, a trial of an 18- to 24-hour course of 100 mg dexamethasone followed by 50 mg every 6 hours for three doses can be given, and if there is no response, surgical decompression is performed. A frontotemporal (pterional) craniotomy is direct and also offers the opportunity to decompress the optic nerve and/or repair other associated cranial base fractures on the involved side (see also Chapter 87).

PROCEDURE

A The surgery is carried out under general anesthesia with rigid skull fixation. For the frontotemporal craniotomy, a unilateral coronal skin incision is designed 2 cm behind the hairline, extending from just anterior to the tragus to the midline. A small area of hair is shaved, and the head is prepared and draped as a sterile field. The incision is beveled in the direction of the hair follicles, and a subperiosteal plane is developed over the skull. An interfascial dissection is performed over the temporalis muscle to preserve the frontalis branch of the facial nerve. The scalp flap is elevated and held anteriorly with fish hooks or self-retaining retractors. The temporalis muscle is then freed anteriorly and reflected inferiorly, separate from the scalp flap.

B Bur holes are then placed to develop a bone flap. One bur hole is at the pterion (or "keyhole") just behind the frontal process of the zygoma, a second in the temporal bone at the root of the zygoma, and a third just below the superior temporal line in the squamosal temporal bone. The dura is then dissected free from the inner table of the skull using a high-speed drill and a foot-plate tool to divide the bone as outlined. The frontotemporal bone flap is removed providing exposure to the anterior and middle fossa dura. Extradural bleeding is controlled with hemostatic products, bone wax, bipolar electrocautery, and dural tacking sutures. A zygomatic osteotomy is usually not necessary, but when greater exposure of the middle fossa floor is needed, it can be performed with the frontotemporal craniotomy.

C The dura is elevated from the floor of the frontal fossa and the middle fossa along the sphenoid ridge exposing the superior orbital fissure.

D Loose fragments from the lateral orbital wall are carefully reduced or removed, and the area lateral to the superior orbital fissure is opened with Kerrison rongeurs.

The bone flap is replaced and held in place with titanium plates. A cranioplasty is performed if needed to reconstruct the squamosal temporal bone that is removed. The temporalis muscle is lifted back into its anatomical position and the zygomatic arch secured with titanium plates. The temporalis muscle is reapproximated, the scalp is closed in layers, and a dressing is applied.

PITFALLS

1. Because the procedure has the risk of a craniotomy, it should be performed only when the patient is stable and eye functions can be expected to return to normal.

2. Zygomatic osteotomy provides good exposure to the inferior portion of the middle fossa when necessary. If more exposure is needed superiorly, the lateral orbital rim can be osteotomized and repaired after decompression. This direct approach also provides an opportunity to explore both sides of the orbital wall.

3. The frontalis branch of the facial nerve is located anterior to the incision and should be protected with a subfascial dissection of the temporalis muscle.

4. Avoid extensive dissection of the temporalis muscle. The superficial blood supply will be interrupted with the facial flap, and the deep blood supply beneath the muscle flap should be protected.

5. The cranial nerves passing through the superior orbital fissure first pass through the cavernous sinus. If the cavernous sinus is involved in the injury, or is opened during the decompression, bleeding can be difficult to control and blood loss can be high. Preparation is important by cross-matching units of blood for possible transfusion. Having hemostatic products available (we prefer powdered gelatin with topical thrombin) and elevating the head can be instrumental in quickly controlling cavernous sinus bleeding.

6. Rarely, the base of the squamosal temporal bone is aerated with mastoid-like air cells. When these are encountered, they provide an egress for CSF and can leak to otorrhea and rhinorrhea Most leaks can be blocked simply with bone wax. Wax should be applied liberally and rechecked prior to closure.

7. The greater superficial petrosal nerve runs along the floor of the middle fossa and can be injured during elevation of the temporal lobe dura. Avoid unnecessary dissection to preserve nerve integrity. If dissection is needed, care should be taken to avoid traction on the geniculate ganglion of the facial nerve, which can lead to severe facial weakness.

COMPLICATIONS

1. Dural tears may occur when the craniotomy is cut and the dura is elevated from the floor of the middle fossa. Careful dissection will decrease the possibility of a dural tear. If a tear occurs, the tear can be closed with sutures or covered with a temporalis muscle flap. The patient should subsequently be confined to bed with the head elevated 30 degrees. If a leak develops, lumbar puncture drainage may be helpful. If the leak does not stop, a craniotomy may be necessary for repair of the dura. Prophylactic antibiotics to prevent meningitis may be administered.

2. Postoperative epidural or subdural hematomas result from inadequate control of bleeding. Careful use of the electrocautery and bone wax is mandatory. A hematoma usually presents as a decrease in consciousness or a progressive neurologic deficit. The diagnosis can be confirmed with a nonenhanced CT scan. Immediate evacuation of the blood is the treatment of choice.

3. Injury to the superior orbital fissure may result in ophthalmic nerve dysfunction and an anesthetic eye. Furthermore, injury to the greater superficial petrosal nerve will cause loss of lacrimation. Either complication increases the risk of exposure injury to the cornea. Patients with any dysfunction of these nerves need to be educated in eye care, prescribed artificial tear and lubricants, and followed carefully to avoid permanent corneal injury.

DECOMPRESSION OF SUPERIOR ORBITAL FISSURE

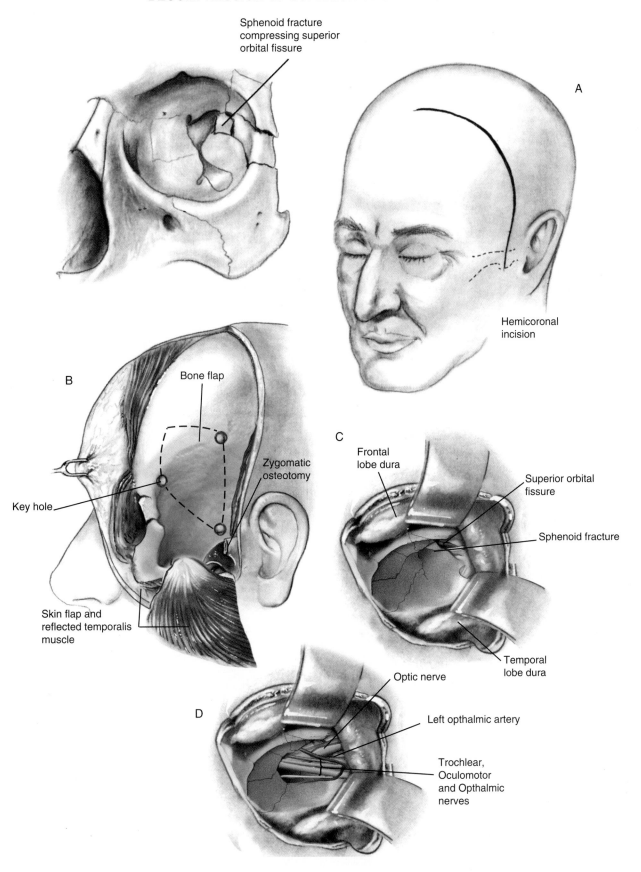

Sphenoid fracture compressing superior orbital fissure

A

Hemicoronal incision

B

Bone flap

Zygomatic osteotomy

Key hole

Skin flap and reflected temporalis muscle

C

Frontal lobe dura

Superior orbital fissure

Sphenoid fracture

Temporal lobe dura

D

Optic nerve

Left opthalmic artery

Trochlear, Oculomotor and Opthalmic nerves

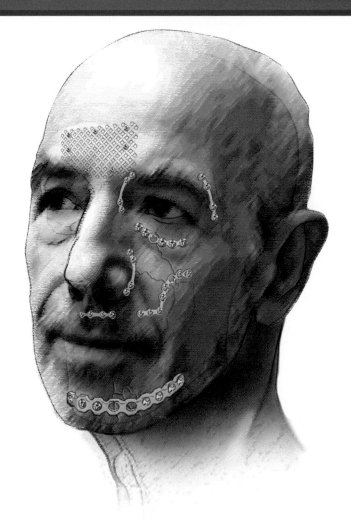

PART ELEVEN

Ethmoid Fractures

Classification and Pathophysiology of Ethmoid Fractures

CHAPTER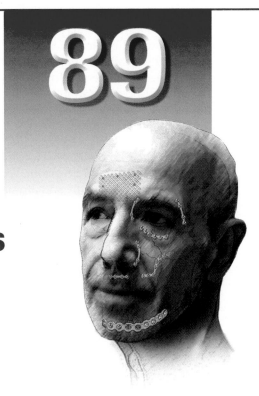

89

General Considerations

The tent-like ethmoid bone can be fractured at its central support (the nasal septum), its lateral support (the lamina papyracea), or its roof (the cribriform plate). Damage involving the cribriform plate is often associated with anosmia, cerebrospinal fluid leak, pneumocephalus, and loss of consciousness. The cerebrospinal fluid leak can also result in untoward sequelae such as meningitis or brain abscess, requiring immediate treatment. The care of septal, naso-orbital, cribriform plate and lamina papyracea injuries is discussed in Chapters 52 through 54, 67 through 69, 79, 84, and 85.

As for the cerebrospinal fluid leak, several pathophysiologic processes can take place. If the dura is torn, pressure differences will force the fluid into the upper respiratory-digestive tract. If the dura is partially torn, constant intracranial arterial and respiratory pressures can slowly separate the dural fibers and cause a delayed presentation of the leak. A hematoma may form over the area of injury, and as it dissolves, the fluid becomes noted.

Many dural tears heal spontaneously without sequelae. The main problem with a cerebrospinal fluid leak is that there is no way to predict which leak will stop and which will be associated with intracranial infection. Thus for most patients, it is important to localize the site and nature of the injury and, if the leak does not stop, to prepare for surgical exploration and repair. The leak of the cribriform plate must be distinguished from other leaks in the frontal sinus, the sphenoid sinus, the roof of the orbit, and temporal bone.

A–D The history and physical examination are helpful. Gushing clear fluid from the nose associated with a change in head position suggests a fluid collection in one or several of the paranasal sinuses. Anosmia is often associated with leaks through the cribriform plate. Visual problems suggest injury to the tuberculum sella, sphenoid sinus, or posterior ethmoidal sinus. Loss of cochlear, vestibular, or facial nerve function indicates a temporal bone injury. Paresthesia or anesthesia of the face and forehead suggests damage to one or several branches of the trigeminal nerve.

On physical examination of the nose, the surgeon should shrink the mucous membranes with 1/4% oxymetazoline hydrochloride (Neo-Synephrine) and observe for a clear fluid discharge. Leakage superiorly from the vault area and/or from the superior meatus is indicative of a cribriform plate, ethmoid, or sphenoid injury. Leakage from the middle meatus is often associated with a flow of fluid from the frontal sinus by way of the nasofrontal duct. Fluid coming from behind the inferior turbinate may indicate a eustachian tube transit from a dural tear of the temporal bone. In most patients, the cerebrospinal fluid flow can be increased by placing the patient in the head-down position; a stream or drops of fluid may be observed at the tip of the nose. In some patients, fluid may be seen behind the tympanic membrane.

With small leaks, cerebrospinal fluid may be difficult to collect and analyze. However, if the fluid can be collected, it should be evaluated in the laboratory and compared chemically and physically to the known properties of spinal fluid. Glucose-sensitive sticks are not usually diagnostic, as glucose can vary in cerebrospinal fluid and in lacrimal and nasal secretions. A handkerchief test in which the surgeon observes different rings can be suggestive; mucus generally will cause rings, and in contrast to a cloth soaked with spinal fluid, the handkerchief will stiffen with drying. A specimen that contains beta 2 transferrin is usually diagnostic of cerebral spinal fluid.

The site and size of the defect must be obtained by special imaging and/or dye studies (see Chapter 84). Coronal and horizontal computed tomographic (CT) scans and MRIs are useful in demonstrating sites of injury. The studies may also show the accumulation of fluid in adjoining sinuses. Metrizamide in combination with a CT scan is very helpful in defining the larger leaks. Sodium iodide I-123, ytterbium Yb-169 pentetate, In-111, and technetium Tc-99m tests are sensitive, but because of high background counts, interpretation can be difficult. Fluorescein dye is also a useful method, but the surgeon must be aware of a potential reaction to the intrathecally placed substance.

Patients with cerebrospinal fluid leaks should have an early reduction of any associated facial fractures, and most of the time the leak will stop in 2 to 3 weeks. Although there is controversy regarding the use of prophylactic antibiotics, we prescribe them at least during the early observation period. If the cerebrospinal fluid leak persists beyond several weeks, we assume that it will not stop, and for these leaks, site localization and surgical repair must be considered.

SITES AND SIGNS OF CEREBROSPINAL

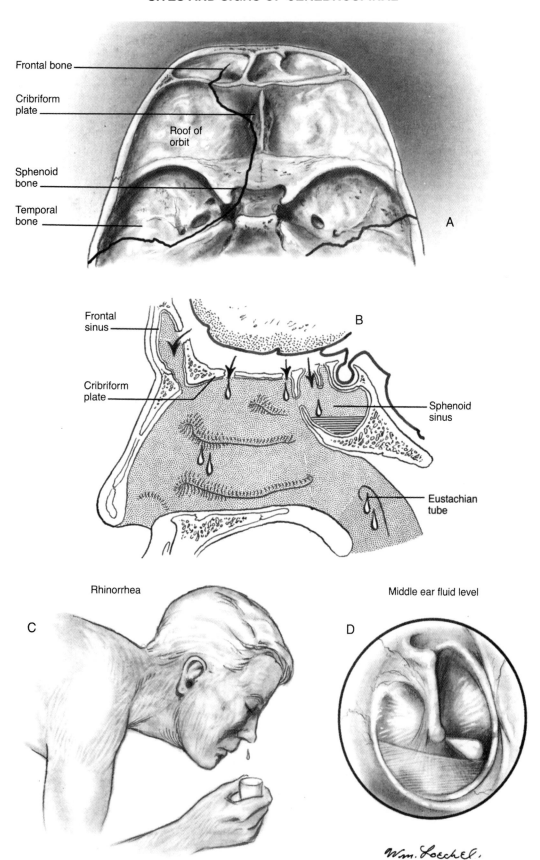

Frontal bone

Cribriform plate

Roof of orbit

Sphenoid bone

Temporal bone

A

Frontal sinus

Cribriform plate

Sphenoid sinus

Eustachian tube

B

Rhinorrhea

C

Middle ear fluid level

D

Wm. Loechel.

Management of Ethmoid Fractures

CHAPTER

90

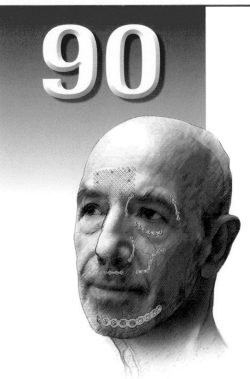

Repair of a Cribriform Plate Cerebrospinal Fluid Leak Using a Transnasal Endoscopic Technique
Alternative Technique Using Frontoethmoidal Approach

In Consultation With Adam Folbe, MD

INDICATIONS

Cerebrospinal fluid leakage following trauma can occur in many sites along the skull base but is commonly found associated with dural tears along the cribriform plate. Early management requires reduction of facial fractures and antibiotic coverage. If the leakage persists, the patient should be treated additionally with bed rest and elevation of the head of the bed. Some surgeons suggest a lumbar drain. For a leakage that continues for more than several weeks, the site of leakage should be determined and a repair carried out by either an intracranial or extracranial approach.

Brain herniation evident on a computed tomographic (CT) scan and associated with a leak is also an indication for exploration and repair. Diagnostic tests for cerebrospinal fluid leaks are described in Chapters 84 and 89. The same intrathecal fluorescein that is often used in the diagnostic test can also be useful for intraoperative identification of the site of the leak.

For uncomplicated cerebrospinal fluid leaks, we prefer a transnasal endoscopic technique and elective use of a CT navigation system. The navigation system however should not be a substitute for knowledge of anterior skull base anatomy.

Endoscopic surgery is often easier to perform than the external frontoethmoiodectomy and is associated with less morbidity and a high success rate. The frontoethmoidectomy is useful when there are other midfacial injuries that require further reduction and fixation (see later). A craniotomy described in Chapter 91 is reserved for those patients with herniation of brain tissues and displaced fragments of the skull base in which an open reduction is required. Also, the intracranial approach must be considered when extracranial procedures fail to repair the leak.

PROCEDURE

With the patient under general anesthesia and in a supine position, the patient's head is slightly extended. A navigation system (if available) is calibrated. The head is then prepared and draped for a sterile (clean) field.

The nasal cavity is then treated with pledgets soaked in ¼% oxymetazoline hydrochloride or 4% cocaine containing epinephrine placed on the lateral wall of the nose. A solution of 1% lidocaine containing 1:100,000 epinephrine is also injected near the tail of the middle turbinate for vasoconstriction of branches of the sphenopalatine artery.

Repair of a leak in the cribriform plate and/or fovea ethmoidalis is best treated with visualization of the medial orbital wall and the attachment of the middle turbinate. The first part of the procedure is to perform a standard endoscopic maxillary antrostomy and anterior ethmoidectomy with exposure of the medial floor of the orbit. If the defect is more posterior, then the basal lamella should be removed and posterior ethmoidectomy completed. To facilitate exposure of the cribrifom plate, the middle turbinate should be removed, but care must be taken not to create a larger defect in the thin lateral lamella.

A–D To perform the maxillary antrostomy, the uncinate process is fractured medially and inferiorly and removed with a back-biter or microdebrider. Once the natural osteum is exposed, the antrostomy is enlarged with cutting instruments to show the maxillary sinus and the inferior/medial part of the orbital wall.

E–G With the middle turbinate pushed medially, the ethmoid bulla is removed and the basal lamella is identified. The lamella is then removed and the posterior ethmoid cells visualized and excised to expose the skull base.

H To obtain optimal exposure, the middle turbinate is removed and the superior turbinate either excised or pushed laterally. The sphenoid sinus osteum is then seen, and if a leak is suspected in the sphenoid sinus, the anterior wall of the sinus is removed. This maneuver will allow excellent exposure of most of the anterior skull base.

It is important to have visualization of the entire defect. The technique of fluoroscein dye placed intrathecally is helpful in identifying the exact site. Once the defect is visualized, the mucosa is removed from the edges. A saline soaked cotton pledget is placed along the defect to stop any bleeding and palpate edges.

I As in Chapter 85, acellular dermis is used to plug the defect. A piece is cut to size and hydrated according to directions. The dermis is then placed into the defect so that a portion is through the defect and the oversized edges are placed against the exposed bone. Gelfoam is then layered over the graft. As an option, one can plug the leak with a piece of temporalis fascia and/or rotate adjacent mucosal flaps over the graft. A 10-cm tampon made of merocel is placed in the nose to support the graft and left in place for 5 to 7 days.

Postoperatively the patient is placed in the head-up position and told to avoid any straining, sneezing or blowing of the nose. The patient is given a stool softener and placed on antibiotics for 2 weeks. After removal of the nasal tampon, the nose is treated with saline mists at least three times daily.

PITFALLS

1. Exposure is an important component of the operation. The patient's head must be positioned to access the skull base and the surgeon should prepare for removal of the middle turbinate, visualization of the medial wall of the orbit and a "clean" ethmoidectomy. Ear and sphenoid instruments are helpful in placing the graft and if necessary, rotating mucosal flaps.

2. If the surgeon finds that the leakage is coming from the sphenoid sinus, the anterior wall of the sphenoid sinus should be removed to show the defect. Once the leakage is identified, treatment is very similar to that following the sphenoidal approach (see Chapter 85).

3. Although the surgeon may know preoperatively that the leak is at the cribriform plate, it may be difficult to find the leak at the time of surgery. Fluorescein dye injected into the spinal fluid, as described in Chapter 84, should be helpful in distinguishing the cerebrospinal fluid leakage from other fluids.

4. The closure of the defect is important. The intracranial placement of acellular dermis or fascia acts as a plug and a mucosal flap can provide additional protection and coverage to the defect.

REPAIR OF CEREBROSPINAL LEAK USING TRANSNASAL ENDOSCOPIC TECHNIQUE

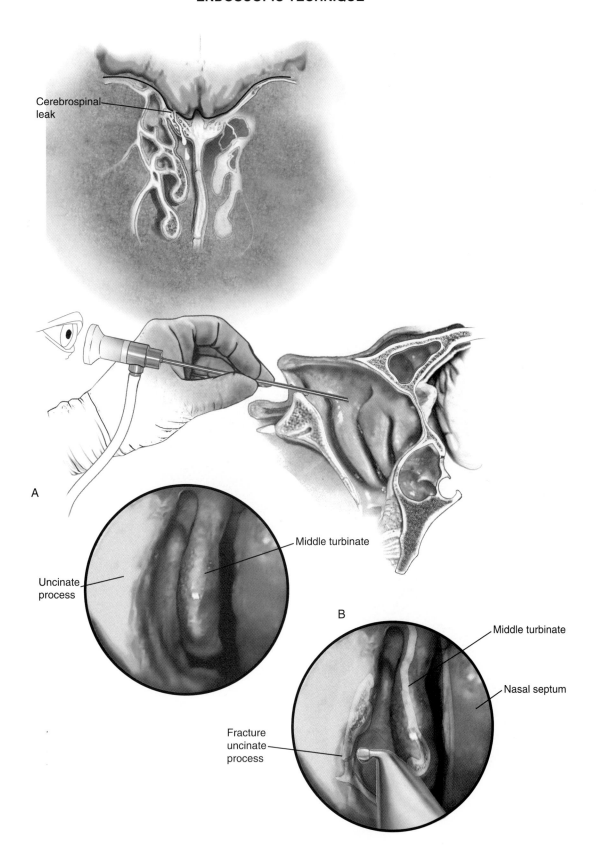

Cerebrospinal leak

A

Uncinate process

Middle turbinate

B

Middle turbinate

Nasal septum

Fracture uncinate process

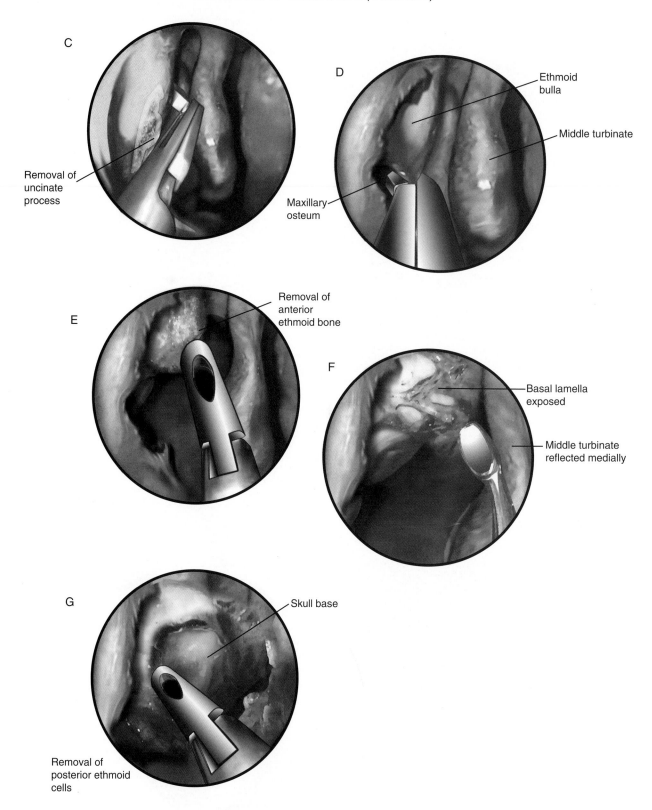

C — Removal of uncinate process

D — Ethmoid bulla; Middle turbinate; Maxillary osteum

E — Removal of anterior ethmoid bone

F — Basal lamella exposed; Middle turbinate reflected medially

G — Skull base; Removal of posterior ethmoid cells

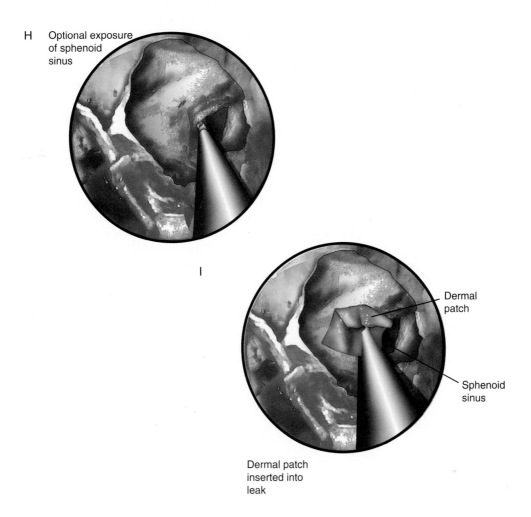

H   Optional exposure
of sphenoid
sinus

I

Dermal
patch

Sphenoid
sinus

Dermal patch
inserted into
leak

5. Do not allow the patient to participate in any activities that will increase the cerebrospinal fluid pressure. During the postoperative period, the patient's head should be elevated, and the patient should be given instructions to avoid sneezing, blowing the nose, and straining.

COMPLICATIONS

1. Failure to close the leakage may result in meningitis and/or pneumocephalus. For this reason, the patient must be maintained on antibiotics and vital signs followed closely for several days. Any change in clinical status should be evaluated by CT scan, and if meningitis is suspected, a lumbar puncture should be performed. Additional spinal fluid should be obtained for cell counts and for cultures to determine appropriate antibiotic treatment.

2. Recurrence or persistence of the cerebrospinal fluid leak requires additional attempts at closure. In general, a failed extracranial procedure indicates a need for a subsequent intracranial approach. However, the surgeon should make sure that the leak is still in the same place as originally suspected and that there are no additional sites. More testing with intrathecal substances may be necessary.

3. It is important to carefully remove mucosa from the area around the leak. If this mucosa gets trapped by the flap, it can cause an intracranial or extracranial mucocele.

ALTERNATIVE TECHNIQUE USING FRONTOETHMOIDECTOMY APPROACH

With the patient in the supine position under general anesthesia, a curvilinear incision is marked one-half the distance between the caruncle and dorsum of the nose. The nose is prepared with both a topical and local anesthetic (i.e., treatment of the mucus membranes with 4% cocaine containing epinephrine, along with a block consisting of 1% lidocaine containing 1:100,000 epinephrine) (see Chapter 52). The medial canthal incision is also infiltrated with the anesthetic solution. The face is washed with an antiseptic solution and isolated with towels as in a sterile field.

a–c A microscope using a 300-mm lens is then brought into position. The surgeon can sit at the head of the table or stand to the side. The standard external frontoethmoidectomy is performed as described in

Chapters 80. The opening into the ethmoid and frontal region is enlarged with rongeurs and cutting burs so that there is adequate exposure of the posterior wall of the frontal sinus. The curvature of the frontal sinus plate is then followed inferiorly toward the cribriform plate. Additional ethmoid cells are removed, as well as portions of the lamina papyracea. The superior and middle turbinate are examined and, if necessary, removed to provide sufficient exposure. Tissues adjacent to the cribriform plate should be salvaged and used later for flap closure. Bleeding is controlled by packing with 1/2-in gauze soaked in the 4% cocaine solution. Larger vessels such as the anterior ethmoidal artery are cauterized with a bipolar cautery.

d,e Using magnification, the cribriform plate is cleaned free of mucosal attachments. As the plate is exposed, the surgeon should inspect carefully for evidence of cerebrospinal fluid leakage. If the presence or site of leakage is uncertain, it is possible to dye the spinal fluid with fluorescein, as described in Chapter 84.

The cribriform plate should be completely exposed by removing all adjacent cells and mucosa with Takahashi rongeurs and cleaning the area with a diamond bur. The hole over the leakage should be devoid of mucosa and opened slightly to expose the dural tear. We then place a small piece of acellular dermis or temporalis fascia through the hole with either a duckbill elevator or an alligator forceps. The fluid pressure from within the cranium keeps the implant in position and closes the defect. As an option, another piece of fascia or dermis is then placed, using similar ear instruments, on the undersurface of the cribriform plate. Additional coverage can also be obtained by rotation (and/or advancement) of a flap of adjacent mucosa or turbinate. If these tissues are not available, then Gelfoam is packed over the defect. A merocel tampon or layers of 1/2-in gauze treated with bacitracin ointment are used to hold the tissues in position.

The periosteum over the frontoethmoidectomy is closed with 3-0 chromic sutures. The subcutaneous tissues are closed with 4-0 chromic and the skin with 5-0 nylon sutures. The patient is kept with his or her head elevated for 5 days. When the packing is removed, the nose is treated with saline mists. The patient is maintained on antibiotics for approximately 2 weeks and during this time is told to refrain from lifting, sneezing, straining, or blowing the nose. A stool softener is provided. Follow-up examination should be performed weekly during the first month and then monthly for at least 6 months.

ALTERNATIVE TECHNIQUE USING FRONTOETHMOIDAL APPROACH

a   Incision

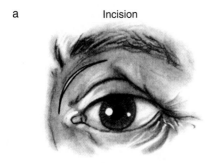

b

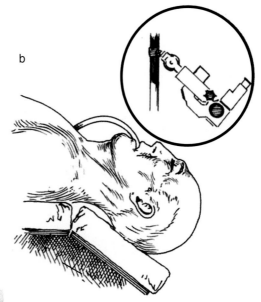

Frontoethmoidectomy

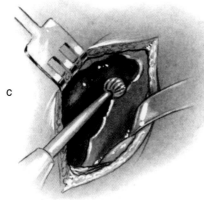

c

Exposure of leak

d

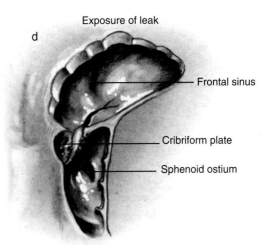

Frontal sinus

Cribriform plate

Sphenoid ostium

Placement of
tissue plug

Dura

e

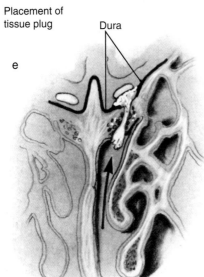

Wm. Loechel

527

Repair of a Cribriform Plate Cerebrospinal Fluid Leak Using a Frontotemporal Approach

In Consultation With Mark Hornyak, MD

INDICATIONS

Cerebrospinal fluid (CSF) leaks require repair if they persist following craniofacial trauma. One of the most common sites of CSF rhinorrhea is the cribriform plate. Fractures through the cribriform are often associated with anosmia and can typically be identified on high-resolution CT scans (see Chapter 90). Indications for the transnasal endoscopic, frontoethmoid, and subfrontal approaches are discussed in Chapters 79, 85, and 90. The cranial approach is indicated when the endoscopic, subfrontal, and/or frontoethmoid approaches fail or when there is significant injury to the skull base resulting in dural tears, displaced fragments, and compression of cranial nerves. The frontotemporal (pterional) craniotomy is an excellent method to expose unilateral damage to the floor of the anterior fossa. A bicorporal craniotomy may be necessary if fractures are bilateral, involve the frontal sinus, or cannot be fully delineated on preoperative imaging.

PROCEDURE

A,B The frontotemporal approach is identical to that used for the repair of the roof of the orbit (see Chapter 81). The incision and bone flap are carried more medially in order to provide better access to the cribriform. A pedicle pericranial flap graft should be raised, as it is almost always needed to repair the anterior cranial base.

Using the operative microscope, the dura is carefully elevated off the frontal bone and orbital roof toward the cribriform plate. If the elevation causes more tearing of the dura, the dura can be opened, and the cribriform defect exposed from the intradural side. Raising the dura from the cribriform will invariably create a dural opening. This defect, along with any traumatic lacerations should be repaired primarily. Ideally the dura should have a watertight closure with fine nonabsorbable sutures. If this is not possible, or to reinforce a repair, other techniques can be employed. From the intradural side, an inlay graft of muscle, facia, pericranium, or other dural substitute is placed under the frontal lobe covering the defect. Intracranial fluid pressure will usually press the graft against the dura allowing healing to occur. Extradurally, similar grafting materials can be used as an onlay, or a vascularized, pedicled pericranial flap can be folded under the dura and sutured in place, covering the bony cribriform defect with viable tissue.

Significant bony defects should also be repaired with suitable tissue plugs. Large defects may require the use of titanium mesh or split cranial bone, which can be obtained from the bone flap.

The bone flap is replaced and fixated with titanium plates. The temporalis muscle is reapproximated, the scalp is closed in layers, and a dressing is applied.

A

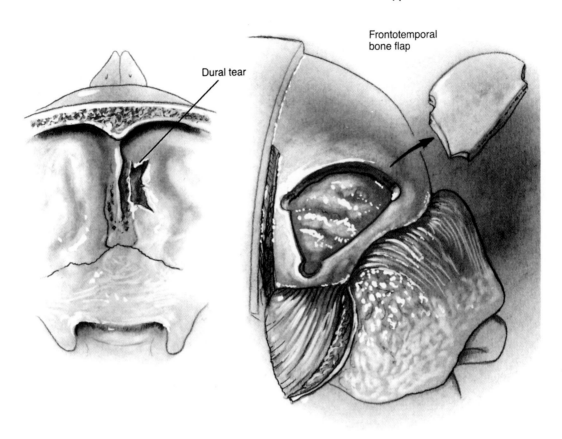

Dural tear

Frontotemporal bone flap

B

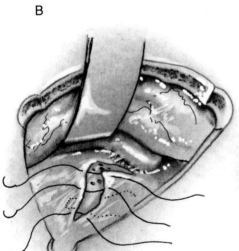

Repair of dura

OPTIONAL METHOD
USING TISSUE PLUG

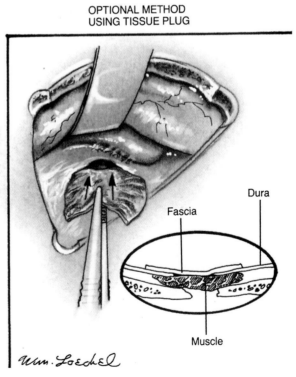

Fascia

Dura

Muscle

PITFALLS

1. As with any of the approaches, the site of leakage should be determined preoperatively. The leak may be difficult to identify at the time of surgery, and preoperative studies that provide the exact location of the leak are extremely helpful.

2. Tears over the cribriform plate pose special problems. Sometimes these tears are small and difficult to see but may be the cause of the leak. On the other hand, the cribriform area may be normal and may only appear pathologically abnormal as the surgeon elevates and separates the olfactory filaments. Any obvious tears must be repaired with suture or grafts.

3. Tears or fractures that extend to the posterior ethmoid, sphenoid, and sella area are difficult to repair. Tissue patches should be applied, but if the leak persists postoperatively, the surgeon must consider a transnasal endoscopic, subfrontal or frontoethmoidal exposures, and a packing from the undersurface of the cranium (see Chapters 79, 85, and 90).

COMPLICATIONS

1. Occasionally the surgeon fails to eradicate the CSF leak, or the leak recurs following surgery. The surgeon may repair the area suspected to be the source of the leak, but the leak may actually be coming from a different area. This is why an accurate preoperative evaluation is necessary for a successful repair.

Sometimes the closure is not sufficiently watertight, or the patch does not hold. In such cases, a short period of bed rest, elevation of the head, and lumbar drainage may be indicated. The patient should avoid nose-blowing. Antibiotic coverage is optional. If the leak continues after these conservative measures, the surgeon should repeat localization studies. The location of the leak often requires a new operative approach.

2. Infection can present clinically as meningitis in the postoperative period. This often signifies a continuation of the leak, and identification and localization studies should be carried out. If a leak is present, it should be treated with standard medical or surgical methods. The bacteria associated with meningitis should be cultured by obtaining CSF from a lumbar puncture and the patient subsequently treated with antibiotics appropriate for the organism.

PART TWELVE

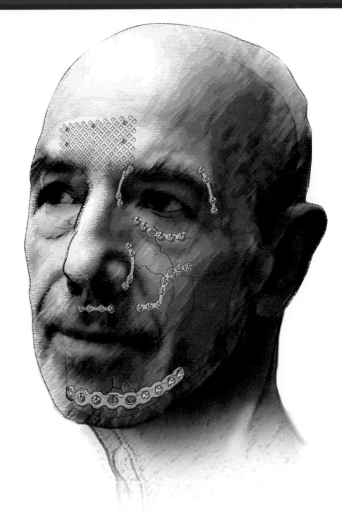

Temporal Bone Fractures

Classification and Pathophysiology of Temporal Bone Fractures

CHAPTER 92

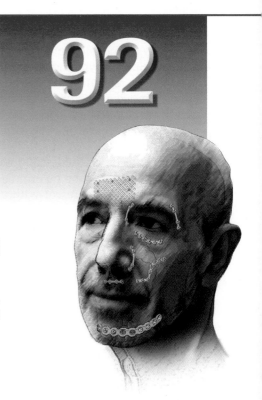

General Considerations

In Consultation With Michigan Ear Institute (Michael J. LaRouere, MD, Dennis I. Bojrab, MD, Ilke Naumann, MD, and Robert Hong, MD, PhD)

Temporal bone fractures occur infrequently with skull injuries, but they are important to identify and classify for appropriate treatment. These fractures are more common in young men and occasionally occur bilaterally. Causes of temporal bone fractures with decreasing frequency are motor vehicle accidents, falls, assaults, and weapons. Whereas most trauma is a blunt type, gunshots are usually associated with penetrating wounds.

The temporal bone is believed to be the hardest bone in the human body, and since a significant amount of force is required to cause a fracture, concomitant injuries are common and should be suspected. Upon arrival in the emergency department, routine protocols should be followed, including methods to secure the airway and stabilize the cervical spine (see Chapters 3 through 7). Two major emergent complications can occur in association with a temporal bone fracture: bleeding and brain injury, resulting in increased intracranial pressure or herniation. Profuse bleeding from

ear canal may indicate carotid artery or jugular bulb/ sigmoid sinus injury. Packing the ear canal followed by an angiogram with possible neurovascular intervention may be necessary. Brain herniation may be a sign of increased intracranial pressure. Management of intracranial injuries such as subdural or epidural hematoma, brain contusions, and pneumocephalus takes precedence over temporal bone related injuries.

Once the patient is stabilized, a complete history and neurotologic exam is performed. Information is obtained from the patient or witnesses regarding onset of facial weakness, hearing loss, tinnitus, vertigo and rhinorrhea (cerebral spinal fluid leak) in relation to the trauma.

The exam should evaluate the patient for Battle's sign (hematoma over the mastoid) or Raccoon eyes (periorbital hematoma as a sign of a base of skull fracture). The ear canal should be cleared of blood and debris allowing visualization of the ear canal and tympanic membrane. Hemotympanum, step off fractures in the ear canal, and tympanic membrane perforation should be noted. Tuning forks can be helpful to determine types of hearing loss, but formal audiometry should be performed when possible. Conductive hearing loss should eventually be distinguished from sensorineural hearing loss and be evaluated for corrective causes such as fluid or blood in the middle ear, perforation of the tympanic membrane, or oscicular chain disruption. Nystagmus may indicate an otic capsule injury.

With regard to facial nerve function, it is important to distinguish between paresis (some movement) and paralysis (no movement). Holding the examiners hand tightly over the forehead and instructing the patient to raise the eye brows will allow differentiation of movement from the contralateral side. The facial nerve should be carefully examined prior to the injection of any topical anesthetics and before suturing facial lacerations.

Cerebral spinal fluid (CSF) leaks from the ear and/or nose need to be determined. Temporal bone fractures commonly present with otorrhea especially if the otic capsule is violated. The diagnosis is made clinically with clear fluid dripping from the ear canal, through a laceration, or from one side of the nose. The Halo sign, also called ring sign, will appear on the patient's pillow as CSF separates from blood. Additional laboratory testing of beta-2 transferrin can confirm a suspected leak (see Chapter 84). CSF leaks not responding to conservative measures will require surgical intervention (see Chapter 93).

Radiographic examination is essential to confirm the diagnosis. Although a head CT in the Emergency Department can be helpful for determining intracranial injury, high-resolution CT (HRCT) without contrast specifically for the temporal bone is the test of choice to evaluate for fracture. HRCT demonstrates excellent bony anatomy and can show damage to cochlea, vestibule, fallopian canal, carotid canal, jugular bulb, and tegmen. MR imaging has low specificity and sensitivity in evaluating temporal bone fractures, but it is superior for demonstrating intracranial pathology such as subdural or epidural hematomas and cerebral contusions.

In patients with suspected carotid artery injury, a CT angiogram should be performed urgently (see Chapters 3 and 11). A standard arteriogram remains the gold standard in diagnosing thrombosis, dissections, or pseudo-aneurisms and can directly lead to treatment with embolization or stenting.

A–C Several classification systems have been described to predict complications and long-term outcomes resulting from temporal bone fractures. Most commonly longitudinal, transverse, and mixed fractures have been described. Longitudinal fractures paralleling the long axis of the petrous pyramid are seen most of the time and result from a temporoparietal impact. Facial nerve injury is not common in these patients. In contrast, transverse fractures which are perpendicular to the axis of the petrous pyramid, and related to a fronto-occipital impact more commonly cause facial nerve injury. A newer classification based on CT scans emphasizes otic capsule sparing versus otic capsule violating fractures. Otic capsule violating fractures are more likely to lead to acute vertigo and long-term sequelae of sensorineural hearing loss and facial nerve injury. A third classification relates to petrous versus nonpetrous fractures. The onset of complications (sensorineural hearing loss, facial paralysis, vertigo) is more common in the petrous group. Of the three classification systems, the otic capsule violating/nonviolating classification appears to have the most clinical value.

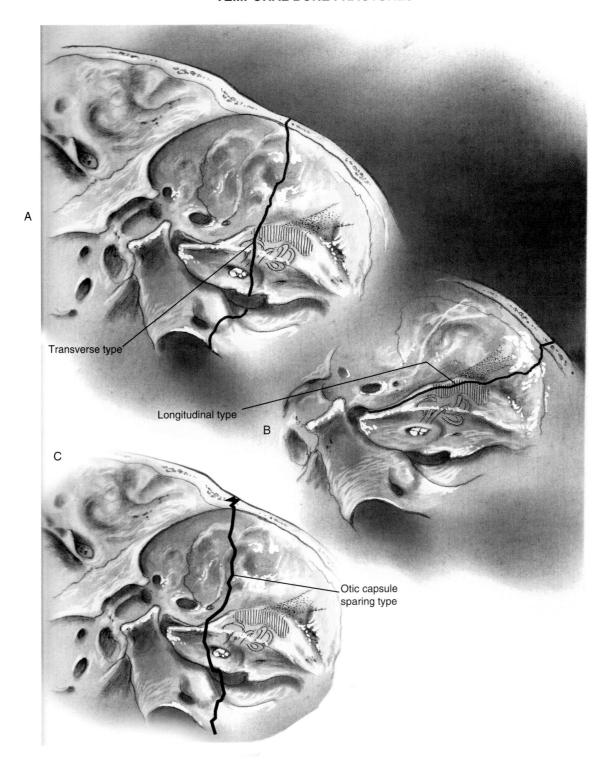

A

Transverse type

Longitudinal type

B

C

Otic capsule
sparing type

Management Strategies of Temporal Bone Fractures

CHAPTER

93

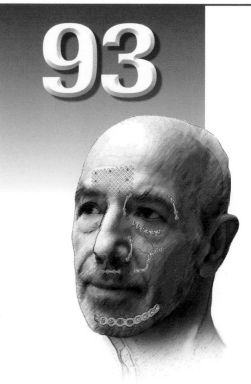

Decompression and Repair of Facial Nerve
Alternative Technique for Repair of Cerebral Spinal Leak of Middle Fossa

In Consultation With Michigan Ear Institute (Michael J LaRouere, MD, Dennis I Bojrab, MD, Ilka Naumann, MD, and Robert Hong, MD, PhD)

INDICATIONS

The time of onset of facial nerve dysfunction and the physical examination are essential for determining prognosis and treatment of facial nerve injuries resulting from temporal bone fractures. Facial nerve injuries are classified as either immediate or delayed. An immediate paralysis is more likely caused by a nerve transection, or severe compression of the nerve by bone fragments, whereas delayed paralysis or pareses is more likely caused by edema, hematoma, inflammation, or mild bony compression. Weakness that occurs during the first few hours after trauma is usually considered an immediate type.

The degree of paralysis is an important predictor of ultimate facial function and the need for surgical intervention. If there is any facial motion (House Brackmann 1-V), the likelihood of a good return of facial function is high. If there is complete paralysis (House Brackmann VI), the overall prognosis for the return of function is poor. Patients with complete paralysis require electrical nerve testing and potentially surgical intervention.

In order to determine the location and additional information on degree of injury, the patient should undergo radiographic and electrodiagnostic tests. High-resolution CT (HRCT), studies using fine cuts 1 mm or less, are important for imaging temporal bone fractures and suspected site(s) of facial nerve injury. MRI with gadolinium complements CT and is useful for intracranial pathology. MRI can reveal temporal lobe contusions that can complicate anticipated surgical intervention in trauma patients with facial nerve injuries.

Our preferred electrodiagnostic test is electroneuronography (ENoG), which is considered an accurate test for qualitative and objective measurement of neural degeneration. A maximal transcutaneous stimulus is applied near the stylomastoid foramen, and the muscle response is then measured using bipolar electrodes placed near the nasolabial groove. The peak-to-peak amplitude wave is then measured and compared to the contralateral side. A reduction of >90% amplitude correlates with a poor prognosis for spontaneous recovery. ENoG should only be used when there is a complete paralysis (House Brackmann VI) as an incomplete paresis predicts a good functional outcome. ENoG should not be performed prior to 72 hours after the trauma, which is the time required for Wallerian degeneration to take place.

Currently, our practice is to obtain ENoG testing on all patients (both immediate and delayed) who have a complete facial paralysis. If ENoG shows >90% degeneration, then the EMG tracing is examined for voluntary muscle action potentials. If action potentials are present, there still is the possibility of good functional return. If action potentials are absent, facial nerve decompression is recommended. If patients have <90% degeneration present or show >90% degeneration but have voluntary muscle action potentials, nerve decompression is usually not advocated until >90% degeneration and absent action potentials are noted. Testing is usually carried out periodically over the first 2 weeks following trauma.

More difficult decisions involve patients who are seen 2 weeks or later following temporal bone trauma. If patients have a complete paralysis, EMG testing is done. If there is no activity or fibrillation potentials are noted, facial nerve decompression is still indicated. We have had good results with decompression and/or repair of the facial up to 1 year post injury with good results.

PROCEDURE

A–E The authors preferred approach for exploring, decompressing, and repairing facial nerve injuries caused by temporal bone fractures is a combined middle cranial fossa and transmastoid approach. This allows exposure of the course of the nerve and excellent access to the perigeniculate are where injury is most likely to occur.

After appropriate head placement, stabilization, and sterile preparation, a postauricular incision is extended into the temporal area. Soft tissue is reflected anteriorly to the level of the ear canal. A simple mastoidectomy is performed and the facial nerve is decompressed with diamond burrs from the stylomastoid foramen to the second genu. Bone is removed from the posterior-lateral aspect of the nerve near the stylomastoid foramen. Bone removal is continued in a more anterior-lateral direction to the second genu, thus avoiding damage to the labyrinth. The facial recess is drilled out with diamond burrs preserving the chorda tympani nerve and the annulus. The tympanic segment of the facial nerve is then uncovered and decompressed.

If the incus and the malleus head are removed for additional exposure an ossicular chain reconstruction will need to be performed. The facial recess exposure obtained during the decompression also provides an excellent opportunity to repair any ossicular chain disruption (see Chapter 94).

a–e For the middle cranial fossa exposure the operating team is repositioned, the head is stabilized and a skin flap developed posteriorly while a temporalis muscle flap is reflected anteriorly. A bony window centered two-thirds above and anterior to the external auditory canal is removed with diamond burrs. Care is taken to avoid damage to the dura; the bone is stored in an antibiotic solution. The dura is then elevated medially and held in place with a House-Urban retractor. The arcuate eminence and facial hiatus are identified. The arcuate eminence is generally 1 cm posterior and 0.5 cm medial to the facial hiatus. The superior semicircular canal is then thinned with diamond burrs to obtain a blue-line effect. Bone is then removed from over the geniculate ganglion and the labyrinthine portion of the facial nerve. The internal auditory canal may or may not be opened depending on the extent of the trauma.

Hematomas are evacuated and bony spicules are removed. The nerve sheath is opened (neurolysis) to allow for decompression along the entire aspect of the nerve. Transected nerve ends are freshened, approximated, and sutured with 8-0 Nylon through the epineurium. Tensionless re-approximation is desired and this can usually be achieved by mobilizing and elevating the nerve from the Fallopian canal. However if there is a 1 cm or greater gap, cable grafts are usually necessary. The great auricular nerve or sural nerves are excellent grafts. If sutures cannot be applied the nerve and/or grafts can be approximated with fibrin.

The brain retractor is removed and the dura relaxed. The craniotomy flap is plated in position and the adjoining soft tissue flaps replaced and closed in layers. The mastoid exposure is also closed in layers and a mastoid/craniotomy dressing applied. Prophylactic antibiotics are usually provided for 5 days.

DECOMPRESSION OF FACIAL NERVE

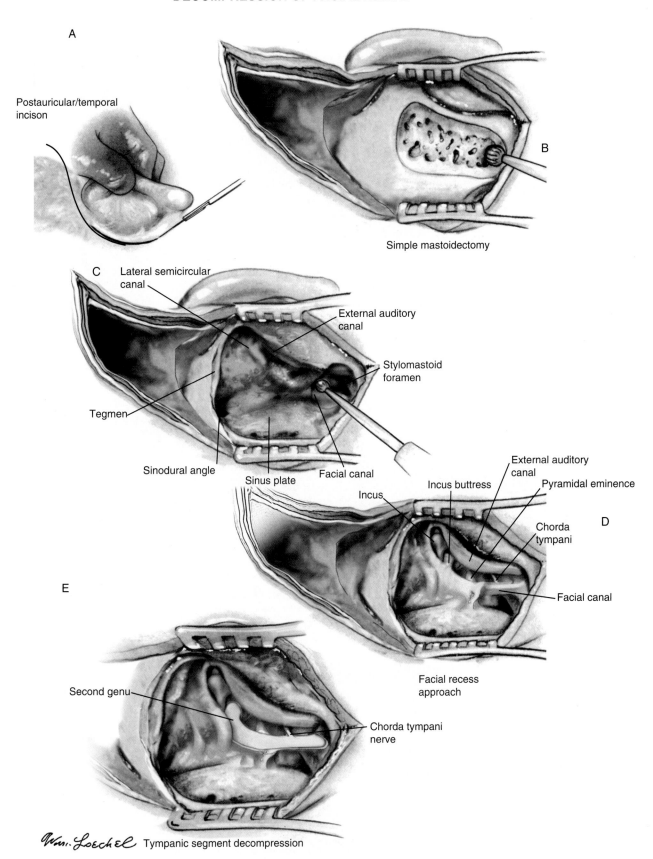

A

Postauricular/temporal incison

B

Simple mastoidectomy

C

Lateral semicircular canal

External auditory canal

Stylomastoid foramen

Tegmen

Sinodural angle

Sinus plate

Facial canal

D

Incus

Incus buttress

External auditory canal

Pyramidal eminence

Chorda tympani

Facial canal

Facial recess approach

E

Second genu

Chorda tympani nerve

Wm. Loechel Tympanic segment decompression

MIDDLE FOSSA APPROACH

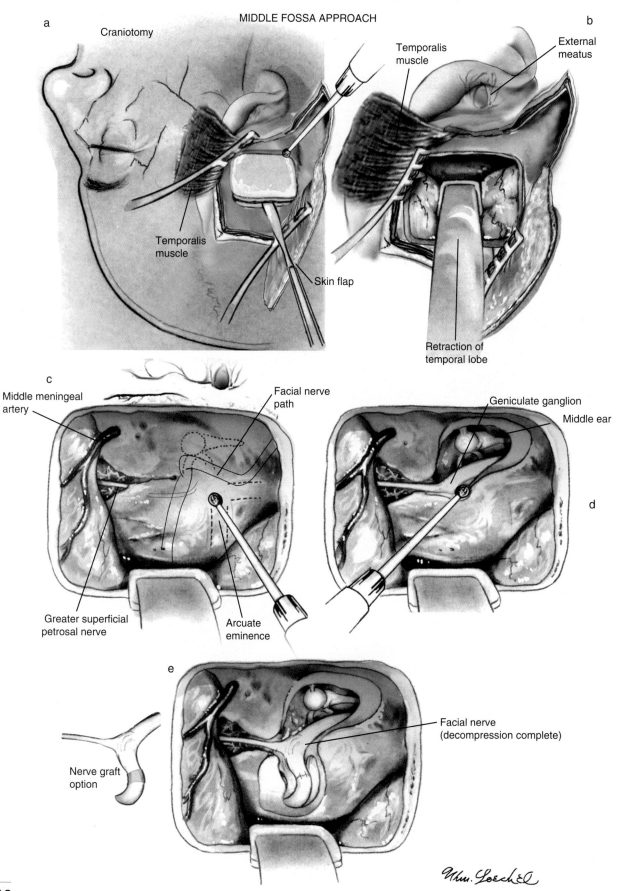

a

Craniotomy

Temporalis
muscle

Skin flap

b

Temporalis
muscle

External
meatus

Retraction of
temporal lobe

c

Middle meningeal
artery

Facial nerve
path

Greater superficial
petrosal nerve

Arcuate
eminence

Geniculate ganglion

Middle ear

d

e

Nerve graft
option

Facial nerve
(decompression complete)

PITFALLS

1. If the patient has no hearing in the traumatized ear; a translabyrinthine approach can be used, exposing the facial nerve along its entire course throughout the temporal bone. If the patient has neurological complications precluding an intracranial approach then a transmastoid approach with removal of the incus and the head of the malleus, along with an extended facial recess approach can be employed.

2. There is general consensus supporting conservative treatment in patients with an incomplete paralysis or unstable patients. Oral or intravenous steroids in doses up to 1 mg/kg for 10 to 21 days are used. In cases of delayed paralysis antivirals have been used but their efficacy remains controversial.

3. The overall status of the patient is of utmost importance. Prior to any surgical intervention, intracranial injuries should be excluded by clinical examination and MRI scans (temporal lobe contusions and hematomas). As soon as the patient is stable, surgical decompression (if indicated) should be performed. Typically the earlier the intervention, the better the outcome, although late decompression many months after the injury can still be beneficial.

4. During the procedure, even if peripheral electrical testing is abnormal or absent, facial nerve monitoring should be used. The facial nerve may often stimulate without clinical evidence of motion. The use of stimulating dissectors is also helpful, even weeks or months after trauma in locating the nerve intratemporally, isolating the location of the conduction block and predicting outcome of nerve surgery.

5. A facial nerve that has been transected between the brain stem and internal auditory canal is difficult to isolate proximal and distal to the injury, making repair of this injury problematic.

6. Attention should also be given to eye protection. Early gold weight implantation is recommended as recovery will take months to occur. The authors' recommendation is to perform the gold weight implantation at the time of decompression.

7. If patients do not achieve good facial movement after 9 to 12 months, other procedures can be offered. These include 12-7 nerve grafts, temporalis muscle transposition (see Chapters 14 and 15) or static procedures such as rhytidectomy or fascial slings.

COMPLICATIONS

1. As in all craniotomies, the patient needs to be followed closely for bleeding and/or infection. Neurological status should be checked periodically and any changes investigated with appropriate imaging studies. Drainage procedures should be contemplated for subdural/epidural hematomas and meningitis should be treated with culture-specific antibiotics.

2. Permanent and complete loss of facial nerve function can still occur following surgery. In many patients, there is recovery with some degree of weakness and synkinesis. The nerve will repair itself at a rate of about 1 mm per day, and the more intact the axon cylinders are, the better the prognosis. As to the decompression, the surgeon should remove all areas of obstruction while ensuring a sufficient blood supply for the reparative processes. Special suturing/grafting techniques must be used for those cases characterized by disruptive or avulsive neural injury. Residual paralysis, depending upon degree, can be treated with dynamic and/or static reconstructive procedures in conjunction with gold weight protection of the eye.

3. Ossicular chain damage is a possibility as a result of the original injury. Disruptions and/or tympanic membrane tears should be recognized and treated at the time of the facial nerve repair. (see Chapter 94).

4. Cerebral spinal fluid leaks can occur and usually are managed conservatively with bed rest and/or lumbar drain. A persistent leak may require exploration and repair as discussed below.

ALTERNATIVE TECHNIQUE FOR REPAIR OF CEREBRAL SPINAL LEAK OF MIDDLE FOSSA

a'–c' The initial treatment of a cerebral spinal fluid leak is observation as most leaks seal spontaneously. Bed rest, keeping the head elevated to 45 degrees at all times, stool softener, and avoiding coughing and nose blowing will increase the success of spontaneous closure. Surgical management is needed for leaks of more than 10 days as the risk of meningitis increases significantly after 7 to 10 days. In the authors practice oral or intravenous antibiotics are not routinely used but patients with lacerations in the ear canal should be placed routinely on antibiotic containing ear drops.

Since the majority of leaks occur in the tegmen it is sometimes possible to accomplish a repair using a mastoidectomy approach with fascia plugging. However, when this approach fails or there is need to explore other areas of the temporal bone, the middle fossa exposure described above is preferred. Using this technique, the dura is elevated, and the dural laceration is repaired with artificial dura and fibrin glue or its equivalent. Defects in the temporal bone are repaired with fascia/hydroxyappetite/fascia seal. If the patient has a profound hearing loss or the leak does not seal with conventional surgery, then packing the middle ear with fascia and a fat graft in the mastoid will prevent further leakage through the Eustachian tube. A lumbar drain can be used as an adjunctive measure if surgical repair is tenuous or fails.

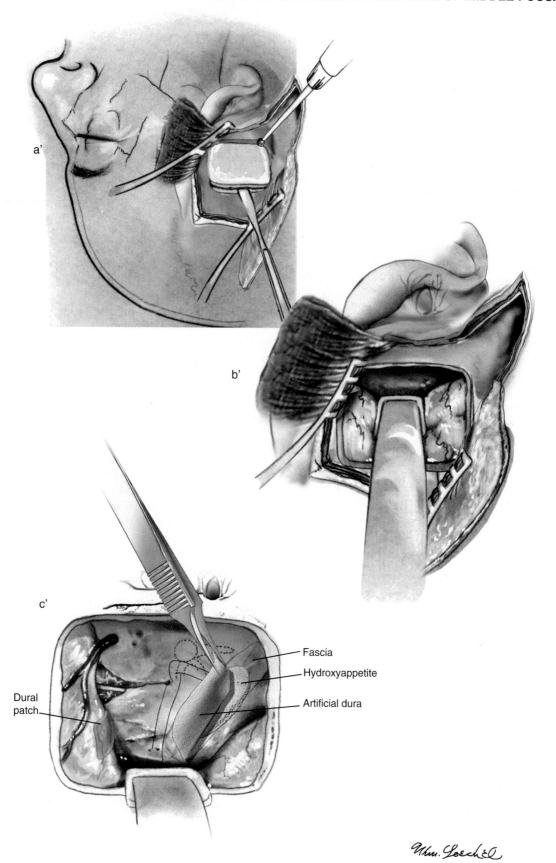

a'

b'

c'

Dural
patch

Fascia

Hydroxyappetite

Artificial dura

Repair of Tympanic Membrane Perforation
Alternative Technique for Repair of Ossicular Chain Disruption

In Consultation With Michigan Ear Institute (Dennis I. Bojrab, MD, Michael J. LaRouere, MD, Robert Hong, MD, PhD, and Ilke Naumann, MD)

INDICATIONS

Hearing loss following temporal bone trauma often depends on the location and severity of injury. Conductive hearing loss is more frequent than sensorineural loss, but many patients present with a mixed type after injury. In the past, longitudinal fractures of the temporal bone were thought to miss the otic capsule and cause mostly a conductive loss, while transverse fractures were thought to usually involve the otic capsule and cause sensorineural loss. However, these designations have not proven to be useful, and with new imaging techniques (CT and MRI), it can be determined that fractures of the otic capsule and/or petrous pyramid better correlate with sensorineural loss, while those through the middle ear associate more with conductive loss.

The type of loss is important in determining prognosis and treatment options. Posttraumatic conductive hearing loss may occur secondary to blood (hemotympanum) or fluid (either middle ear effusion or cerebrospinal fluid [CSF]) behind the tympanic membrane, rupture of the tympanic membrane, or disruption of the ossicular chain (incudostapedial joint dislocation or incus dislocation). Other less common findings include fracture of the stapes superstructure and malleus and, at later time, posttraumatic cholesteatoma and ossicular fixation secondary to osteoneogenesis, tympanosclerosis, or fibrosis. Most fluid/blood within the middle ear space will clear with conservative management, whereas the tympanic membrane perforation and damage to the ossicular chain usually require reconstructive techniques.

Sensorineural hearing loss with the exception of perilymph fistula is usually not responsive to medical or surgical therapy. Steroids can be given, but their efficacy is controversial. Some senorineural losses will improve regardless of treatment. Conductive loss, on the other hand, will often respond to appropriate medical and/or surgical intervention.

The history and examination of the patient with temporal bone trauma is necessary for an accurate diagnosis, but this requires the cooperation of witnesses and the participation of the patient. Unfortunately, patients with head trauma are often sedated, intubated, or comatose, making it difficult to obtain a complete history and physical examination. A preliminary examination should at least include otoscopy to assess for fractures within the external auditory canal, hemotympanum, middle ear effusion, and tympanic membrane perforation. The patient should also be evaluated for dizziness and nystgmus. A high-resolution CT scan without contrast should be used to evaluate for opacification (fluid) in the middle ear space or a fracture involving the otic capsule. Tuning fork tests can give some preliminary information, but the patient should undergo (when awake and cooperative) a complete audiometric workup including pure tone, speech discrimination, and tympanometry. An auditory brainstem response (ABR) for comatose patients with a high suspicion for hearing loss may be useful.

Early management will depend upon the diagnosis. Conductive hearing loss in patients will often resolve spontaneously if due to blood/fluid behind the tympanic membrane. It is even possible for patients with tympanic membrane perforation and/or ossicular chain disruption to repair the defect(s). Thus, a period of watchful waiting, anywhere from 6 weeks to 3 months, with a repeat audiogram is recommended before undertaking further surgery.

If persistent fluid is found on otoscopy behind an intact tympanic membrane after several months, the diagnosis of a CSF leak should be considered. A salty taste in a patient's mouth or clear rhinorrhea should increase suspicion of this condition. The temporal bone CT scan should be carefully reviewed for fractures of the skull base that may lead to a CSF leak, and a MRI should be obtained in cases with sizable tegmen defects to rule out brain herniation through the defect before any repair is contemplated.

If a tympanic membrane perforation has not healed after 3 months, surgery, typically in the form of an underlay tympanoplasty (described below), is performed. The surgeon should be prepared to evaluate and reconstruct the ossicular chain and remove a middle ear cholesteatoma should this have developed.

The early management of the patient with posttraumatic sensorineural hearing loss is somewhat controversial. Oral steroids or intratympanic steroid injections can be used, but their efficacy is either weak or not available. Suspected early perilymph fistula is treated with bed rest, stool softeners and avoidance of nose blowing and straining.

If a unilateral profound sensorineural loss persists after several months, the patient should be evaluated for hearing rehabilitation using a contralateral routing of signals (CROS) hearing aid or a BAHA (bone-anchored assistive hearing device). In patients with bilateral severe-profound loss, hearing aids should be tried, but when loss is severe and not responding to amplification, cochlear implantation can be recommended. In patients with persistent fluctuating sensorineural loss, a perilymph fistula should be confirmed by a positive fistula test and should be considered for a tympanomastoidectomy with a plugging of the leak. Occasionally these patients are confused with those having a posttraumatic endolymphatic hydrops, and

in that situation, Electrocorticography (ECoG) should be used to distinguish the pathology. Patients with endolymphatic hydrops are usually treated conservatively with diet, diuretics, and antivertiginous drugs before considering surgery (i.e., endolymphatic sac decompression).

PROCEDURE

A–H The procedure may be performed under local or general anesthesia. A solution of 1% lidocaine with 1:100,000 epinephrine is injected postauricularly and in all four quadrants of the external auditory canal. The ear is prepped and draped in a sterile fashion.

For small posterior perforations of the tympanic membrane, a transcanal approach with underlay tympanoplasty may be performed. A piece of temporalis fascia is harvested, pressed, dried, and set aside for later use in grafting. The edges of the tympanic membrane perforation are freshened using a right-angled hook. A tympanomeatal flap is raised about 5 mm lateral to the annulus, extending from 6 o'clock to 12 o'clock along the posterior external auditory canal skin. The middle ear space is entered, deep to the annulus, with care taken to preserve the chorda tympani. The ossicles are palpated to assess for mobility. The fascia graft is placed under the annulus and medial to the tympanic membrane perforation, and bolstered with gelfoam (soaked in Ciprodex) in the middle ear space. The tympanomeatal flap is laid back down in anatomic position. Additional pieces of gelfoam are placed lateral to the tympanic membrane-graft complex in the ear canal, followed by bacitracin ointment and a cotton ball.

For larger perforations or anterior perforations, a postauricular approach with over-under tympanoplasty is preferred. The edges of the tympanic membrane perforation are freshened. A postauricular incision is made about 5 mm behind the postauricular sulcus. Temporalis fascia is harvested, pressed, dried, and set aside for grafting. The plane of the loose areolar tissue overlying the temporalis fascia is extended inferiorly to the mastoid tip. A "T" incision is made down to the bone, with the horizontal portion of the "T" extending posteriorly from the zygomatic root along the linea temporalis, and the vertical portion located just posterior to the external auditory canal, extending from the linea temporalis to the mastoid tip. A vascular strip based on the posterior external auditory canal skin is raised postauricularly, extending from the tympanomastoid to the tympanosquamous suture lines. A tympanomeatal flap is raised and the middle ear space entered. The tympanic membrane is dissected off of the malleus. The ossicles are palpated to assess mobility. The fascia graft is placed under the annulus

REPAIR OF TYMPANIC MEMBRANE PERFORATION

Otoscopic view of perforation

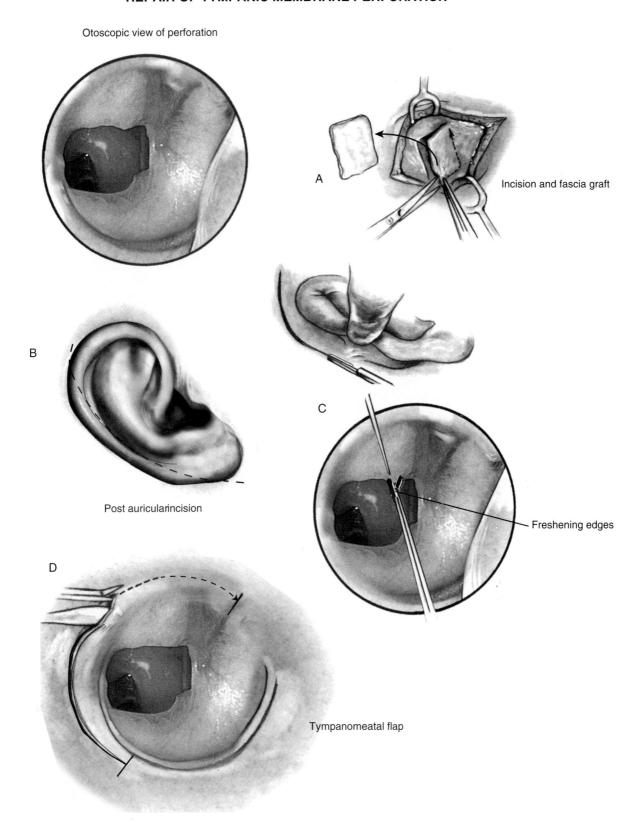

Incision and fascia graft

A

B

Post auricularincision

C

Freshening edges

D

Tympanomeatal flap

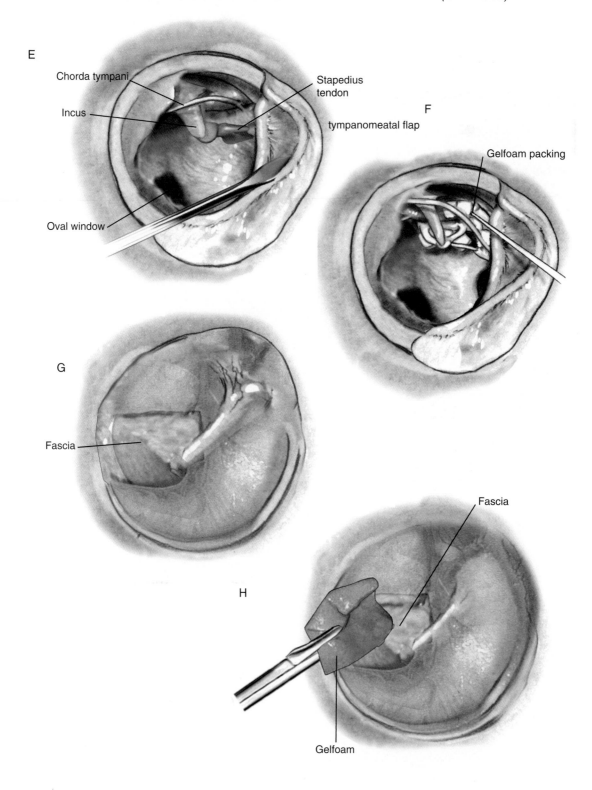

E

Chorda tympani

Incus

Stapedius tendon

tympanomeatal flap

F

Gelfoam packing

Oval window

G

Fascia

Fascia

H

Gelfoam

Wm. Loechel

and over the malleus, medial to the tympanic membrane perforation. When the malleus is severely retracted or there is severe middle ear mucosal disease, a piece of silastic sheeting is placed over the promontory to help create a middle ear space. Gelfoam is placed in the middle ear to bolster the graft medially. The tympanomeatal flap and vascular strip are placed back in anatomic position, with additional gelfoam placed lateral to the tympanic membrane-graft complex. The postauricular incision is closed. Bacitracin ointment is placed in the ear canal followed by a mastoid dressing.

PITFALLS

1. Conductive hearing loss following trauma will usually improve with time as the blood/fluid leaves the middle ear space and the tympanic membrane heals a perforation. It is even possible for the ossicular chain to repair defects with fibrosis and new bone formation. It is therefore prudent to wait and see before undertaking a surgical procedure.

2. Conductive hearing loss that fails to respond to conservative management can be associated with several defects. The surgeon in preparing for a tympanic membrane perforation must be aware of the possibility of ossicular chain disruption malleus fixation and/or cholesteatoma and be prepared to use procedures applicable to these problems.

3. Most perforations with large conductive hearing losses are better treated with middle ear exploration combined with over/under technique. Other, usually smaller, perforations can be managed by packing the middle ear with Gelfoam and placing a small piece of fascia underneath the perforation. Isolated perforations in the absence of temporal bone injury can often be managed with microscopic examination, elevation of inwardly displaced flaps and scaffolding with a paper patch treated with antibiotic solution.

4. The fascia should fit beyond the defect of the drumhead. The fascia is easier to manipulate if it is thinned and dried. Properly prepared fascia will provide for a thinner drumhead and improved acoustic properties.

5. The fascia should be in contact with the vascular supply from the external auditory canal. The blood supply around the perforation may be limited and a better vascular supply may be found on the walls of the canal. A vascular strip (flap) provides for improved vascularity.

6. The fascia graft should be tightly "sandwiched" by the gelfoam below and external to the graft. Failure to do so may lead to retraction and foreshortening of the drumhead. Tight packing will help prevent this from occurring.

COMPLICATIONS

1. Infection can cause the dissolution of the graft and potentially a toxic/sensorineural hearing loss and meningitis. For the most part, infection can be prevented by sterile atraumatic techniques. The middle and external ear should be packed with antibiotic-soaked dressings, and prophylactic antibiotics should be used for 2 days. If the patient develops signs of infection, the packing should be removed, cultures obtained, and the ear treated with appropriate antibiotic drops.

2. As with any ear surgery, hearing may be worse following this procedure. Conductive hearing loss may persist or return as a complication of failure to heal or fibrosis. Sensorineural hearing loss, tinnitus facial weakness, and dizziness may also occur. Patients should be made aware of these possibilities prior to the start of surgery.

3. A new perforation is always a possibility. If the eustachian tube fails to function properly, the middle ear will develop fluid and cause undue pressure on the new tympanic membrane. This can cause a graft failure. If the surgeon suspects that this has occurred, the patient must be checked out for rhinosinusitis, obstruction in and around the eustachian tube (i.e., adenoids), and obstruction caused by deflection of the septum. These conditions must be treated prior to embarking on another repair procedure. The patient can also be given the option of living with the perforation and/or using a hearing aid.

ALTERNATIVE TECHNIQUE FOR REPAIR OF OSSICULAR CHAIN DISRUPTION

a–e Middle ear exploration may be performed using either local or general anesthesia. Either a transcanal or postauricular approach as described above may be used for access to the middle ear space. Intraoperative palpation and visualization of the ossicular chain after entry into the middle ear space is important to determine ossicular chain disruption and/or fixation. If either an incudostapedial and/or incudomalleolar joint dislocation is found, reconstruction may be performed using either an incus interposition homograft or prosthetic implant. With the incus interposition, the incus is shaped by the surgeon and repositioned to fit snugly between the capitulum of the stapes and the malleus/tympanic membrane Alternatively, a prosthesis can be used and the authors prefer a Grace Alto Bojrab Titanium + Hydroxyapatite PORP (Grace Medical, Memphis, TN). With this prosthesis, the titanium shaft of the prosthesis is seated over the capitulum of the stapes, the hydoxyapatite head is placed directly under the tympanic membrane, and the titanium hook extension is locked under the malleus for additional stability. If a stapes superstructure fracture is observed, reconstruction is performed with a Grace Alto Bojrab TORP and a footplate shoe. For the rare malleus fracture, reconstruction may be performed with a Grace Alto Bojrab PORP; if the malleus is severely fractured and unstable, the titanium hook extension can be removed and a cartilage cap can be placed over the prosthesis for additional stability. These prostheses have the advantage of being light and have provided excellent long-term hearing results. After the ossicular chain is reconstructed, the tympanomeatal flap and vascular strip are laid back in anatomic position, and closure proceeds as previously described in the section on technique of tympanoplasty.

REPAIR OF OSSICULAR CHAIN DISRUPTION

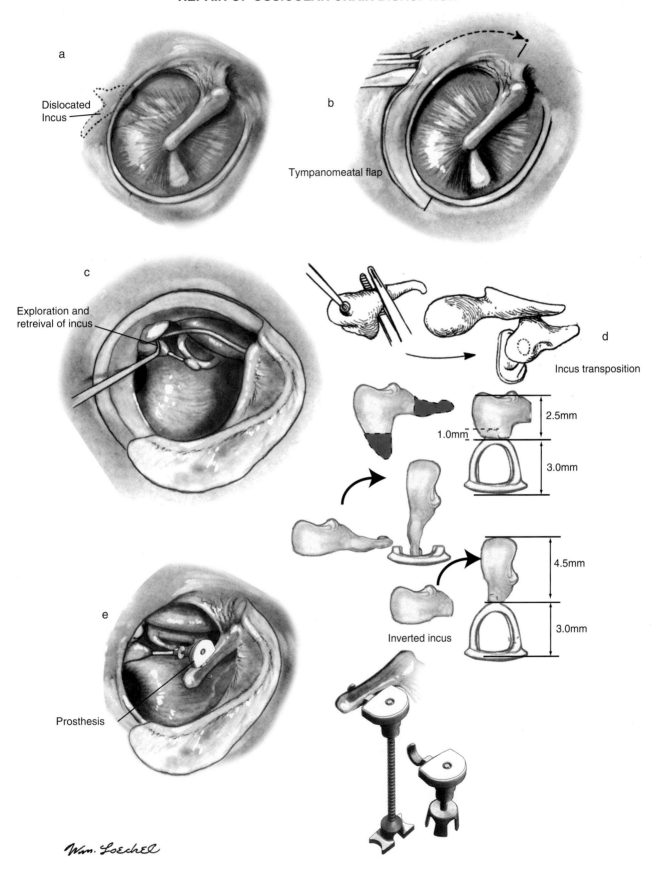

a

Dislocated Incus

b

Tympanomeatal flap

c

Exploration and retreival of incus

d

Incus transposition

2.5mm

1.0mm

3.0mm

Inverted incus

4.5mm

3.0mm

e

Prosthesis

Wm. Loechel

Treatment of Canalithiasis With a Plugging of the Posterior Semicircular Canal
Alternative Technique of Transmastoid Labyrinthectomy

In Consultation With Michigan Ear Institute (Dennis I. Bojrab, MD, Michael J. LaRouere, MD, Robert Hong, MD, PhD, and Ilka Naumann, MD)

INDICATIONS

Dizziness following temporal bone trauma can be the result of different pathologies, and to provide appropriate treatment, it is important to understand why this symptom is occurring. It is thus critical to determine whether the dizziness arises from the peripheral or central nervous system and whether the dizziness is of vestibular or nonvestibular origin.

Vestibular dizziness can be the result of damage to the membranous labyrinth, blood supply to the inner ear or nerves leading from the inner ear to the brain. When both vestibular and cochlear symptoms occur in the absence of temporal bone fracture, the broad terminology (labyrinthine) otitic concussion is used to characterize the injury.

Another common cause of peripheral vestibular dizziness is posttraumatic benign paroxysmal positional vertigo or canalithiasis. For this to occur,

shearing forces cause release of the otoconia or ultimately degeneration of the otoconia with subsequent release into the semicircular canals. This results in episodic vertigo triggered by change of the head position, which causes shifting of the otoconia within the semicircular canals. Perilymphatic fistula or delayed posttraumatic endolymphatic hydrops are also causes of dizziness of peripheral origin but are often associated with fluctuating sensorineural hearing loss.

Brain concussion or what is called closed head injury syndrome is usually the main central cause of central posttraumatic dizziness. A brain concussion is frequently associated with a nonspecific dizziness (as opposed to true vertigo) with symptoms of headache, fatigue, and difficulty in concentration. The visual system also may be affected by brain injury and can cause problems with balance and dizziness.

Nonvestibular dizziness can also occur following temporal bone injury and is common in patients with hypotension or vascular insufficiency. Other causes are neck trauma, over medication, or side effects of drugs.

For an accurate diagnosis, a full history should be obtained, paying particular attention to the difference between dizziness (unsteadiness, light headedness) often implicated with a central etiology versus vertigo that is more consistent with peripheral etiology. True vertigo is also found with nausea and vomiting, symptoms that usually improve quickly within days. Patients with concussion type injury often describe positional vertigo as less severe in nature and more persistent over time. Posttraumatic benign paroxysmal positional vertigo will be described as episodic vertigo lasting seconds, often triggered by certain head positions. Posttraumatic sensorineural hearing loss in conjunction with vertigo will be more consistent with perilymph fistula, delayed endolymphatic hydrops, or labyrinth concussion.

The physical examination should include a complete neurologic examination, otoscopy, an evaluation of hearing with tuning forks, and an assessment of nystagmus with Frenzel glasses. In addition, the examiner should evaluate the facial nerve, intraocular motion, visual acuity, bedside calorics, a fistula test, a Dix-Hallpike test, and a Romberg test. Cerebellar testing is part of the neurologic evaluation. Electronystagmography, or even better, videonystagmography are important in accessing function of the superior vestibular nerve. Vestibular evoked myogenic potentials (VEMPS) are important to assess function of the inferior vestibular nerve. Dynamic posturography may be considered to evaluate the patient's overall balance function. The diagnosis of delayed endolymphatic hydrops should be considered with electrocochleography (ECoG).

Since most patients will get better with time, they can be managed conservatively using antiemetics, vestibular suppressants (i.e., valium, and intravenous fluids). For those patients who do not respond to conservative management, the diagnosis should be reevaluated for surgical intervention. Important considerations are labyrinthine fistula, persistent labyrinthine dysfunction of unknown idiopathic etiology and benign paroxysmal vertigo.

Benign paroxysmal positional vertigo should be initially managed with the Epley maneuver. This canalith repositioning procedure is successful in many patients and should be followed by instruction to sleep in the upright position and a neck brace to stabilize the head at least for 48 hours. In patients who have remission Brandt-Darhoff exercises can be used. In patients who repeatedly fail the Epley maneuver a posterior canal plugging procedure should be considered.

PROCEDURE

A–D This procedure is performed under general anesthesia through an intact canal wall mastoidectomy, described for facial nerve decompression in Chapter 93. The semicircular canals are exposed. The posterior semicircular canal near its ampulla is "blue-lined" by thinning the canal bone to eggshell thickness. The canal is opened for about 3 mm and fascia and then bone pate' placed to occlude the canal. The success of this procedure depends on stopping endolymph flow in this canal. The mastoidectomy incision is closed in layers and a mastoid dressing applied for 2 days.

PITFALLS

1. Canalithiasis can affect any semicircular canal but seems to respond best surgically when it only involves the posterior canal. Positioning tests should be performed prior to surgery to rule out superior and lateral canal involvement.

2. Prior to surgery the patient should be treated with Brandt-Darhoff exercises and particle repositioning maneuvers. Also since symptoms will frequently clear over time, the surgeon should delay surgery until there are no other options.

3. The patient should be informed that there will likely be dizziness for a while following the procedure and will do better with postoperative vestibular exercises. Although sensorineural hearing loss is rare, the patients should be informed of this possibility.

COMPLICATIONS

1. Persistent dizziness may occur especially if there are other causes of dizziness. An accurate diagnosis is important to obtain optimal results.

2. Sensorineural hearing loss is rare but can occur from the surgical procedure.

3. Incomplete occlusion of the canal can cause recurrence of benign paroxysmal positional vertigo and, in such cases, repeat surgery may be necessary.

ALTERNATIVE TECHNIQUE OF TRANSMASTOID LABYRINTHECTOMY

a–e This procedure is performed for persistent incapacitating dizziness of peripheral labyrinthine origin associated usually with sensorineural hearing loss. Our preferred labyrinthectomy technique is under general anesthesia through a mastoidectomy. An intact canal wall mastoidectomy is performed with high speed drilling and suction irrigation. The lateral

PLUGGING OF POSTERIOR SEMICIRCULAR CANAL

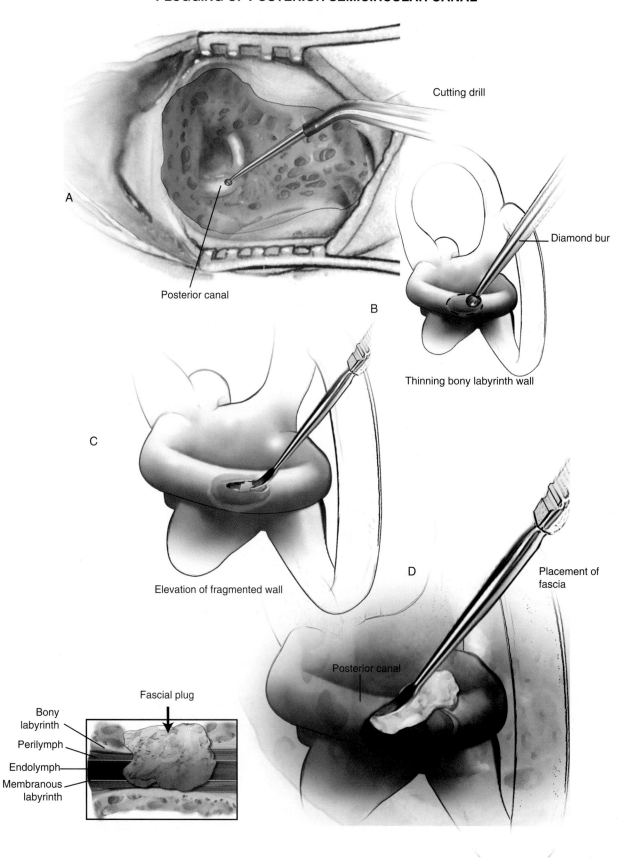

Cutting drill

Posterior canal

Diamond bur

Thinning bony labyrinth wall

B

C

Elevation of fragmented wall

D

Placement of fascia

Posterior canal

Fascial plug

Bony labyrinth

Perilymph

Endolymph

Membranous labyrinth

A

semicircular canal is then "blue-lined" and opened. The canal is followed to the posterior semicircular canal, which is then opened to the common crus. The common crus is followed to the superior semicircular canal which is open to the ampulla. Ultimately all of the canals are open to their ampullated ends and then into the vestibule. The neuroepithelium of the canals (cupulae of posterior, superior, and lateral canals) is removed. The saccule and utricle are excised from the vestibule. Postoperatively there will be some dizziness or vertigo, but this will improve with time and vestibular rehabilitation. Hearing loss is inevitable with this procedure.

ALTERNATIVE TECHNIQUE OF TRANSMASTOID LABYRINTHECTOMY

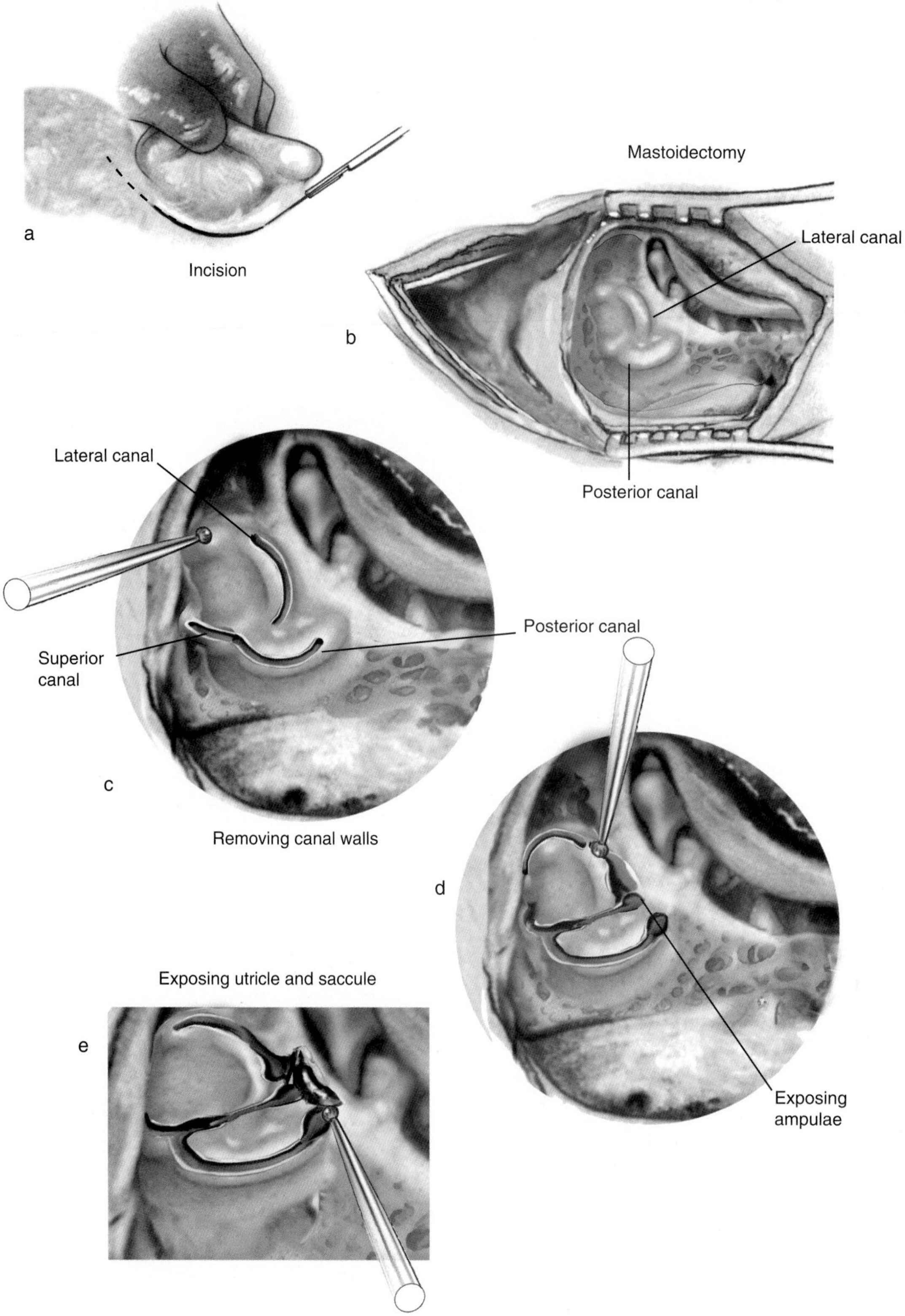

a

Incision

Mastoidectomy

Lateral canal

b

Posterior canal

Lateral canal

Superior canal

Posterior canal

c

Removing canal walls

d

Exposing ampulae

Exposing utricle and saccule

e

Wm. Loechel

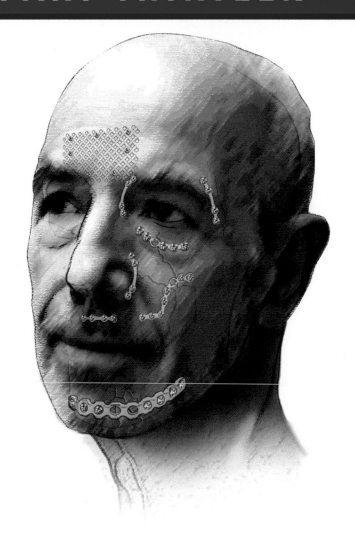

PART THIRTEEN

Laryngeal Injuries

Classification and Pathophysiology of Laryngeal Injuries

CHAPTER **96**

General Considerations

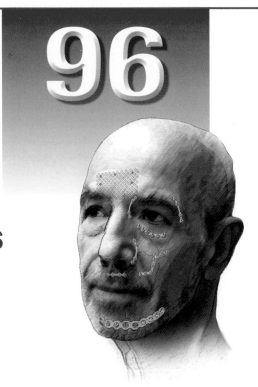

A The larynx, by virtue of its anterior position in the neck, is susceptible to both blunt and penetrating trauma. The risk is even greater when the neck is hyperextended, as the mandible and sternum no longer provide a natural protection in this position. Moreover, the larynx can be easily crushed against the rigid cervical spine.

From an anatomic standpoint, the larynx can better tolerate a lateral blow. The vertically oriented muscular and ligamentous slings provide some freedom of mobility and, consequently, protection from laterally directed forces. Laryngeal calcification and rigidity, which are related to age, can also be factors. Additional pathophysiologic considerations include (1) the soft tissue contents and shape of the neck that define a protective cushion and (2) the lamina angle that describes the projection of the larynx and point of potential impact.

Although laryngeal injury can occur alone, it is often associated with other types of trauma. The cervical spine can be damaged and must be evaluated early

when a laryngeal fracture is suspected. Displacement of the larynx can also be associated with a laryngotracheal separation, pharyngoesophageal tears, and damage to the recurrent laryngeal nerve. Penetrating injuries of the neck can tear the laryngeal skeleton and, additionally, cause damage to a variety of nerves and vessels that pass through the cervical region.

Laryngeal injuries are usually classified according to site of soft tissue and skeletal damage. Supraglottic, glottic, subglottic, and laryngotracheal patterns are described, but more commonly, a variety of combinations can occur. The diagnosis is usually made on the basis of a careful examination and imaging studies. Laryngoscopy is used to confirm pathologic findings. The classification that follows is useful in defining and understanding the injury and planning for specific treatment protocols.

B **SOFT TISSUE.** Soft tissue injury commonly develops from blunt trauma and manifests as edema and/or hematoma involving the aryepiglottic folds, arytenoids, and false and true vocal cords. In addition, superficial lacerations of the laryngeal mucosa can occur.

C SUPRAGLOTTIC. Supraglottic injuries are fractures of the hyoid bone and thyroid cartilage that are usually oriented in a caudal-cephalic direction. The injury is generally associated with a depression or widening of the thyroid notch and loss of the thyroid prominence. If there is a disruption of the thyrohyoid membrane and/or thyroepiglottic ligament, the epiglottis and soft tissues of the anterior larynx can be displaced posteriorly. Tears of the false cords, aryepiglottic folds, pharyngeal walls, and ventricles are common. The injury pattern is often complicated by avulsion-dislocation of the arytenoid cartilages.

D TRANSGLOTTIC. Transglottic injuries are injuries of the vocal cord region and are usually divided into anterior and posterior types. The anterior glottic damage is characterized by midline vertical fractures of the thyroid cartilage with lacerations that extend into the true cords, false cords, and aryepiglottic folds. The larynx is foreshortened in the anteroposterior diameter, and vocal cord mobility is affected. If the lateral walls of the larynx are involved, there can be posterior displacement of the thyroid ala into the piriform sinus, with ipsilateral avulsion-dislocation of the arytenoid.

Fractures isolated to the posterior larynx present with disruptions of the interarytenoid and thyroarytenoid muscles. They are often associated with dislocation and exposure of the arytenoid cartilages. Compression-induced cricoarytenoid damage to the recurrent laryngeal nerves can occur.

E SUBGLOTTIC. Isolated injuries to the subglottic larynx are unusual and are often seen in combination with thyroid cartilage injuries or the laryngotracheal separation pattern. Typically, anterior cricoid arch fractures occur in the midline or paramedian position and result in loss of the cricoid prominence. Displacement of cartilage fragments and submucosal edema often compromises the subglottic lumen. Both cricothyroid and cricotracheal membrane tears may be seen. One or both cricoarytenoid joints can be affected.

F LARYNGOTRACHEAL. Laryngotracheal injuries develop from excessive shearing forces with the neck in a hyperextended position (i.e., a "clothesline" injury). The cricotracheal separation often involves damage to the strap muscles, the recurrent laryngeal nerves, and even the anterior esophageal wall. Characteristically the trachea retracts substernally, whereas the larynx migrates upward for a distance of approximately 6 to 10 cm.

Most laryngeal injuries are managed conservatively, but if there are significant mucosal lacerations and tears and/or displacement of cartilage, open reduction and fixation must be considered. The objectives of surgery are to restore respiration and/or phonatory function. The degree of injury and prognosis should direct the individual evaluation and treatment protocol.

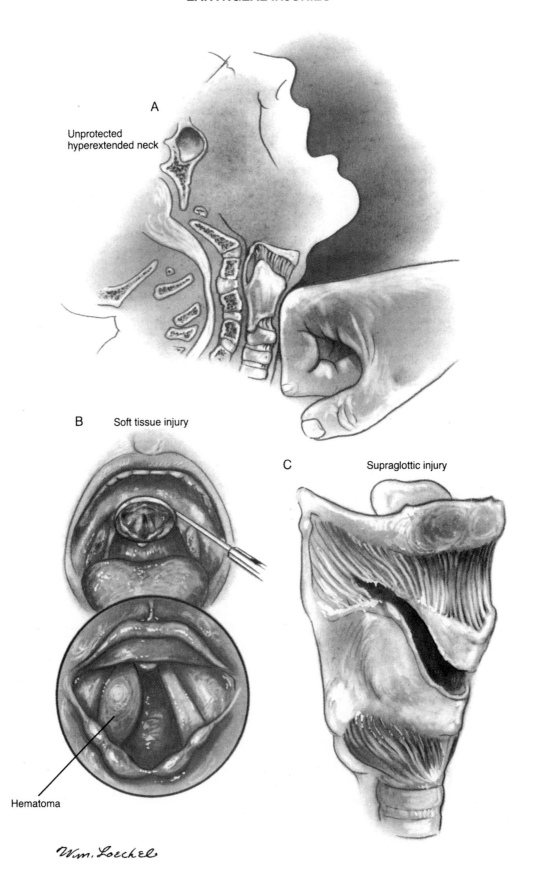

A

Unprotected
hyperextended neck

B   Soft tissue injury

C   Supraglottic injury

Hematoma

Wm. Loechel

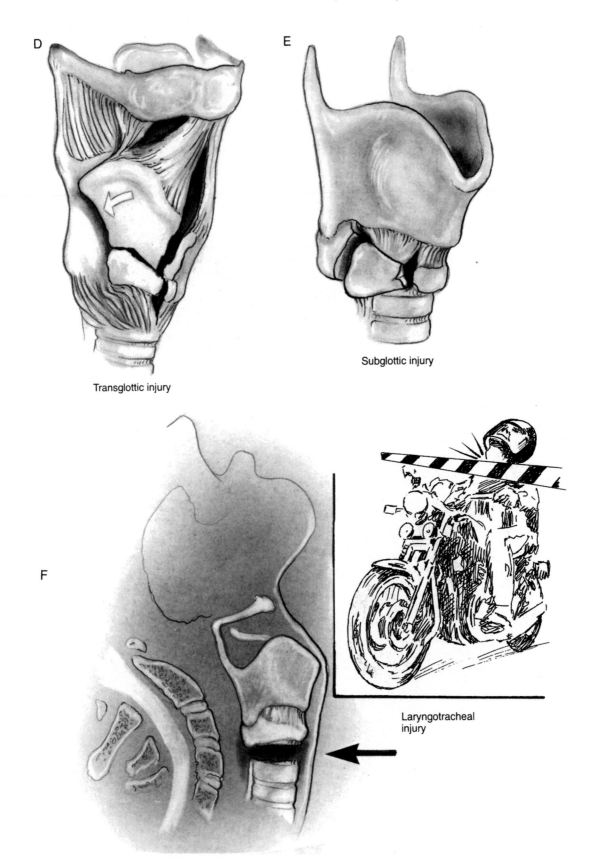

D

Transglottic injury

E

Subglottic injury

F

Laryngotracheal injury

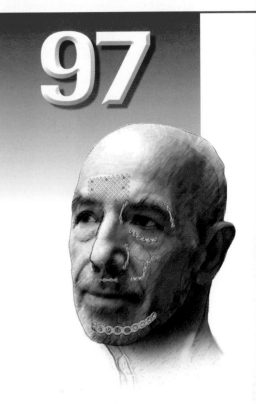

CHAPTER

97

Open Reduction and Repair of Endolaryngeal Injury by Thyrotomy

In Consultation With Terry Shibuya, MD

INDICATIONS

Proper evaluation and treatment of an endolaryngeal injury is essential for restoring the injured patient to optimal speaking and swallowing function. Additionally, it is important to reduce the possibility of laryngeal or tracheal stenosis by addressing the injury within 24 to 48 hours. Treament of the injury should start by securing the airway, and this is usually achieved by performing a tracheostomy under local anesthesia (see Chapter 7). Following the tracheostomy, the examination (direct laryngoscopy/esophagoscopy/bronchoscopy) is performed to assess the extent of the injury.

The goal of surgery is to restore the larynx to a preinjury anatomical state as best as possible. This means reducing fractured cartilage and bone into proper anatomical relationships and providing an epithelium-lined internal covering to reduce subsequent scarring. An open reduction and repair is indicated in the following cases: (1) the airway is obstructed necessitating tracheotomy, (2) extensive and subcutaneous emphysema due to open injury, (3) fractured and dislocated cartilaginous structures, and (4) lacerated or disrupted laryngeal mucosa. The traditional approach used for repair is through a midline thyrotomy. This provides easy access and optimal exposure to the internal larynx. Via this approach, injuries can be directly evaluated and repaired using a variety of reconstructive techniques.

PROCEDURE

A,B Control of the airway is usually obtained with a local tracheostomy. Oral intubation is typically avoided to prevent potential injury to the damaged endolaryngeal structures and to avoid the risk of inducing further airway obstruction in an already damage upper airway. Once the airway has been secured, a 5- to 7-cm transverse skin incision is marked out in a natural crease line at the midthyroid cartilage level. Subcutaneous infiltration with 1% lidocaine containing 1:100,000 epinephrine is performed to enhance hemostasis. The incision is carried through skin, subcutaneous tissue, the superficial cervical fascia, and the platysmal layer. Superior and inferior subplatysmal flaps are then elevated to the level of the hyoid superiorly and to the level of the first tracheal ring inferiorly. Self-retaining retractors or fish hooks are then placed to retract the flaps superiorly and inferiorly and to assist with the exposure.

C–E The dissection proceeds through the strap muscle to access the perichondrium of the thyroid and cricoid cartilages. This is performed by splitting the strap muscles in the midline and following the midline raphe to the thyroid cartilage. Army-navy tractors and self-retaining retractor are used to assist exposing the thyroid cartilage. Hemostasis is maintained to provide optimal visualization of the surgical field. Once the thyroid cartilage is exposed, a marking pen is used to outline the midline thyrotomy incision. If a fracture of the thyroid cartilage already exists in the median or paramedian plane, it can be used alternatively for the endolaryngeal exposure. Typically the thyrotomy is performed with an oscillating saw. Care is taken to prevent premature laryngeal penetration. The midline thyrotomy can be extended superiorly through the thyrohyoid membrane or inferiorly through the cricothyroid membranes for accessing injuries in these regions. After the thyrotomy is performed, wide double skin hooks are used to retract the thyroid ala laterally. This provides sufficient exposure for the surgeon to incise the inner perichondrial layer. Usually the incision begins at the inferior boarder of the thyroid cartilage, through the cricothyroid membrane, and then extends superiorly through the anterior commissure to the superior border of the thyroid cartilage. If further exposure is required to repair the injury, the anterior commissure can be extended along the inferolateral border of the epiglottis (depending on the side of injury) and further extended along the aryepiglottic fold. This will enhance exposure and preserves epiglottic mucosa.

F The laryngeal injury should be assessed and a plan developed for the repair. A key principle for repair is preserving mucosa, covering exposed cartilage, and delicate handling of the soft tissue. Mucosal tissues are primarily repaired with 4-0 chromic suture.

The arytenoids should be inspected. Since the vocal processes insert on the arytenoids, anatomical positioning is very important. If an arytenoid is subluxated, it should be repositioned on to the cricoid facet in proper anatomical position. If the injury involves the cricoid, the vocal process should be secured in the paramedian position to provide an adequate airway and voice. For these reconstructions to be successful, the contralateral vocal cord must be mobile and function normally. Only in the setting of a severe injury should submucosal resection of the injured arytenoid and mucoscal closure be considered.

Advancement flaps can be performed to close small areas of mucosal loss. For larger defects, epiglottic flaps may be considered (see Chapter 101). Mucosal defects that are too large for coverage by a local mucosal flap may require free mucosal or split-thickness grafts applied with an internal stent (see Chapter 98). Severe injures may require regional or free tissue transfers, similar to reconstruction after a cancer ablative surgery. It is important to remember that debridement of tissue should always be conservative, and rarely should a cartilaginous fragment be removed.

Fractures of the hyoid bone, thyroid, and cricoid should be replaced in anatomic position and stabilized with heavy chromic, polyglactin, or wire sutures. Titanium and resorbable plates/screws may be used. Internal stents, T tubes, or keels may be necessary (see Chapters 98 through 100).

G The thyrotomy is closed by approximating the outer perichondrium with interrupted 3-0 chromic sutures, but if more stability is needed, the cartilage can be approximated with 2-0 nylon suture or stainless steel wire applied in a figure of eight fashion. If the cartilage is sufficiently calcified, one can use titanium or resorbable plates and screws. The strap muscles are approximated with 3-0 chromic suture and a two-layered skin closure is accomplished with 3-0 vicryl and 5-0 nylon sutures. Typically a suction drain is placed into the wound in the deeper layers reducing the chance of hematoma and/or subcutaneous emphysema. A nasogastric feeding tube is placed intraoperatively into the stomach. Prophylactic antibiotics are given for 7 to 10 days. The patient is not given anything orally until 7 days, allowing the mucosa to heal.

PITFALLS

1. Surgery should ideally be performed within 24 hours of injury. The tissues of the larynx have a poor blood supply and are prone to infection and necrosis. The sooner the repair is performed, the less chance there is of contamination and stricturing.

2. Failure to precisely divide the junction of the vocal cords in the midline can lead to transection of a portion of the anterior membranous vocal cord and a foreshortening and alteration in vibratory characteristics. Excessive mucosal disruption can predispose to anterior glottic webbing.

3. Usually suturing of the perichondrium over the thyroid lamina is sufficient for closure of the thyrotomy.

REPAIR OF LARYNGEAL INJURY USING THYROTOMY APPROACH

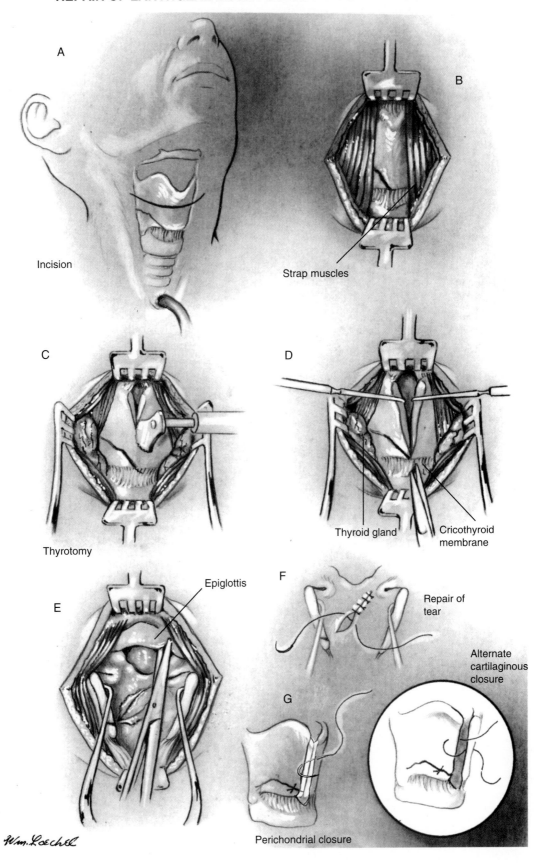

A

Incision

B

Strap muscles

C

Thyrotomy

D

Thyroid gland

Cricothyroid membrane

E

Epiglottis

F

Repair of tear

Alternate cartilaginous closure

G

Perichondrial closure

Wm. Loechel

Overtightening the sutures applied to the thyroid ala can pull through the cartilage or lead to overriding of the cartilaginous anterior segments which can also cause vocal cord asymmetries. Plating with titanium or resorbable plates can reduce the chance of cartilage segment migration.

4. Failure to approximate the mucosal edges, improper mucosal handling, or inadequate assessment of the need for mucosal free grafting can lead to cartilage exposure with subsequent chondritis and laryngeal stenosis. Use of a stent with a mucosal graft is discussed in Chapter 98.

5. Recognition of comminuted cartilaginous fragments and collapse of the airway is important. If such a condition develops, the surgeon must consider an internal keel or stent fixation technique (see Chapters 98 through 100).

6. Injuries to the cricoid require extension of the incision to include the cricoid area. These techniques are described in Chapter 102.

COMPLICATIONS

1. Stenosis of the airway is possible despite laryngeal repair. This complication may be reduced by meticulous handling of the soft tissues and precise reduction and fixation techniques. If this stenosis develops, further surgical repair and correction may be necessary.

2. Granulation tissue formation following the thyrotomy and repair may be prevented by making sure all exposed mucosal surfaces are covered. Free mucosal grafts or skin grafts may be added along with a stent to reduce this possible development. If the granulations become excessive, this can be removed endoscopically with either microlaryngeal instruments or laser. Broad-spectrum antibiotics should also be used as well to prevent infection.

3. Vocal cord paralysis and fixation are potential complications that can affect the voice and/or respiration. The physician must distinguish between the two by careful examination of laryngeal-vocal cord movements and by palpation of the arytenoid (and/or vocal cord) under anesthesia. Videostroboscopy and/or electrodiagnostics may also help in diagnosis. In the case of a unilateral vocal cord paralysis, the surgeon should wait at least 6 to 9 months for a return of function. If vocal cord function does not return, then a vocal cord can be placed in the paramedian position by either injection or open neck medialization (see Chapter 103). For bilateral vocal cord paralysis, there are several options which may be discussed with the patient including tracheotomy or partial cordectomy (Kashima procedure).

Internal Fixation of a Laryngeal Injury With a Montgomery Silicone Stent

Alternative Technique Using a Soft Stent

In Consultation With Terry Shibuya, MD

INDICATIONS

The internal laryngeal soft stent usually provides skeletal support when there is extensive comminution of laryngeal fractures or when the fracture is unstable despite open reduction and internal fixation. The stent may be used to stabilize skin or mucosal free grafts applied to denuded areas of the larynx and used to prevent mucosal web formation. Ideally the stent should be stable enough to provide internal support and help permit restoration of epithelial bridging of the injured mucosa. The stent should move with the larynx during respiration and deglutition and should also be well tolerated by the patient. It should be easy to place and easy to remove once healing has been completed.

A wide variety of conforming alloplastic laryngeal stents has been described. The prefabricated Montgomery silicone stent is primarily used to provide relatively rigid support to unstable laryngeal fractures with or without mucosal or split-thickness grafts. A surgeon-devised soft stent (see later) may also be used to stabilize a fracture of the larynx and support mucosal or skin grafts. Each type is for a different purpose. A Montgomery T tube works well for injuries of the trachea and cricoid (see Chapter 99). For individuals

with an uncomplicated midline glottic injury, avulsion of the true or false cords (or both), and the potential for anterior web formation, a Teflon keel is desirable (see Chapter 100).

PROCEDURE

A The hard silicone stent is used for individuals who require primarily stabilization of a reduced laryngeal skeleton. Such stents are available in a variety of sizes to fit almost any larynx in a patient of any age, male or female. The stent can be covered with a mucosal or split-thickness skin graft around the stent and secured with absorbable sutures.

B–D Using a thyrotomy approach, described in Chapter 97, the larynx is exposed for placement of the stent. The stent should be transfixed within the larynx by passing an 18-gauge spinal needle through the skin, platysma, thyrohyoid muscle, and thyroid lamina at a level superior to the glottis and anterior to the arytenoids. The needle is then passed through the upper aspect of the stent and out through the contralateral thyroid lamina, strap muscles, and soft tissue of the opposite side. Two No. O polypropylene sutures are subsequently passed through the cannula (needle), the cannula is withdrawn, and the ends of the suture are secured with Silastic buttons. A similar maneuver is performed through the lower aspect of the stent. The second set of sutures is also held into position with button fixation. The surgeon can also secure the buttons to the laryngeal skeleton; this will fix the stent to the mobile cartilages, but it will also require additional surgery for removal. The wounds are closed in layers. As an alternative to using O polypropylene suture to secure the stent in place, one can use 26-gauge wire.

PITFALLS

1. Avoid overtightening the sutures that hold the stent in position. This can result in pressure necrosis of the surrounding mucoperichondrium and free graft. Under such conditions, infection can occur, causing loss of soft tissues and chondritis of the laryngeal skeleton.

2. Avoid overtightening of sutures on the skin which can lead to ischemic changes and permanent skin markings. If the sutures/wires holding the stent become loose or break, then the stent can migrate and cause respiratory obstruction. To avoid these problems the wires should be checked weekly and the position of the stent ensured by fiberoptic laryngoscopy examination. If a suture breaks, a new one should be affixed immediately.

3. The procedure to remove the stent should not be taken lightly. The pull suture within the stent can break, the stent can break, or the stent can be displaced inferiorly. Just in case the pull suture within the stent should break, the suture should be reinforced with a wire suture at the time of placement of the stent. For removal of the stent, an endoscope is used. The stent and pull suture should be grasped with a large forceps, the fixation sutures released and the stent removed from the larynx.

COMPLICATIONS

1. Granulation tissues often occur adjacent to the stent. This reaction is partially the result of stasis of secretions and contact of tissue with a foreign body. Antibiotic coverage is helpful. The stent should also be removed as soon as it has fulfilled its purpose. Residual granulations can be managed by endoscopic surgery or laser removal. Recurrence of granulations and/or collapse of the endolarynx may require reinsertion of another stent or keel.

2. Stenosis can also follow laryngeal injury and stent fixation. If it is recognized early, dilatation and/or reinsertion of the stent for a longer period may be successful. However, if the stenosis persists and affects respiration and/or phonatory functions, surgical removal of the stenosis and reconstruction with or without stents or keels may be indicated.

3. Skin ulceration and scars can develop from the buttons and wires used for stabilization. Such areas on the skin should be kept clean with application of 3% hydrogen peroxide followed by antibiotic ointment. Unsightly scars can later be revised by excision and reorientation of the scars in crease lines.

ALTERNATIVE TECHNIQUE USING A SOFT STENT

a A soft stent is made from a finger cot or a size eight or six surgical glove finger, depending on the size of the larynx. The "container" is stretched open with a nasal speculum while a surgical prep sponge is cut to appropriate size, rolled, and inserted into it with bayonet forceps. The stent should be checked to ensure that it is soft and conforming. A 2-0 silk suture is then secured around the open end of the stent to retain the sponge and is cut long to allow for uncomplicated endoscopic retrieval at a later date. Depending on need, a split-thickness skin (0.0014 in), dermal, or mucosal graft can be wrapped around the stent, trimmed, and secured with 4-0 chromic suture.

The procedure for inserting and securing the soft stent is the same as that described for the Montgomery hard stent. The stent is secured in the larynx and to the skin surface of the neck using the identical technique with O polypropylene sutures. One of the main dangers of using the soft stent is that the glove or finger cot can disintegrate over time or rupture. If this occurs, the surgical sponge can migrate into the distal airway, be swallowed or expectorated out. Removal of the soft stent should be under general anesthesia via a tracheostomy tube. Again the stent should be grasped with a forceps prior to the suture release to prevent inferior migration of the stent. Once the sutures are released, the stent can be removed safely.

REPAIR OF LARYNGEAL INJURY WITH STENTS

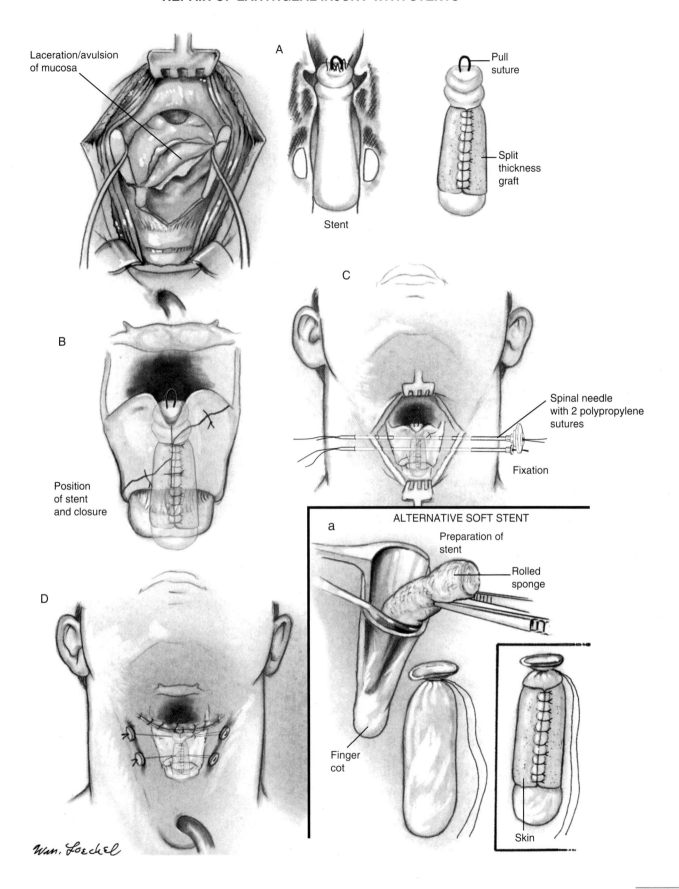

Laceration/avulsion of mucosa

A

Pull suture

Split thickness graft

Stent

B

Position of stent and closure

C

Spinal needle with 2 polypropylene sutures

Fixation

D

ALTERNATIVE SOFT STENT

a

Preparation of stent

Rolled sponge

Finger cot

Skin

Wm. Loechel

Internal Fixation of a Laryngeal Injury With a Montgomery T Tube

In Consultation With Terry Shibuya, MD

INDICATIONS

The silicone Montgomery tracheal T tube is best applied to the management of complex tracheal and subglottic injuries. Its primary role has been to serve as a lumen keeper and for stenting segmental subglottic resections and comminuted cricoid fractures. The T tube may also be used for tracheomalacia, with the expectation that long-term stenting will allow for the development of fibrocartilage formation, thus strengthening the tissue and reducing the collapse of the cartilaginous framework.

PROCEDURE

A The T tube is a flexible, hollow silicone tube in the shape of a "T" that comes in a variety of lengths and diameters (8 to 16 mm). Its superior and inferior vertical sections are of unequal length. The horizontal limb is of a smaller diameter. The tube's size can be adjusted by trimming any of the ends.

In sizing the T tube, the largest outer diameter stent that easily accommodates the airway should be selected. The superior and inferior limbs of the tube should be cut so that their ends overlie a normal laryngotracheal mucosa. When this technique is selected for subglottic stenting, the stent should be extended just slightly below the glottis. This allows the supraglottic and glottic valves to function and prevents aspiration.

B–E Insertion of the T tube requires a tracheostomy and endolaryngeal exposure. The tracheostomy is created below the site of injury. If a tracheostomy tract already exists, but it is small, it may require dilatation for T tube insertion. The tracheostomy opening can also be enlarged with surgical revision.

Topical anesthesia with sedation is preferred. The application of 4% topical lidocaine to the laryngeal mucosa will help control bronchospasm and laryngospasm. A number eight ventilating bronchoscope is passed, and the airway is secured. The tracheostomy tube is removed. Next, the T tube is grasped with a hemostat near the junction of the upper vertical and horizontal limbs so that the curve of the hemostat is in a position to direct the lower vertical limb inferiorly through the tracheostoma. With continued advancement of the hemostat, the superior limb of the stent will become intraluminal; this can be confirmed bronchoscopically. While holding the tube in position, a second, much smaller hemostat is applied to the horizontal limb. This will prevent dislodgement of the tube into the tracheobronchial tree. The first hemostat can then be released. Usually the tube will position itself in the airway, but if adjustments are necessary, an alligator forceps can be passed through the bronchoscope and the upper limb directed into the appropriate position.

Postoperatively the patient is placed on oral antibiotic for 5 to 7 days. To reduce the likelihood of crusting and obstruction, the horizontal limb of the T tube is corked as soon as possible. If crusts form, application of mucolytic agents may be helpful. In general, the T tube should remain in place for 6 to 12 months, with interval changes for cleaning made every 3 months until removal. This can be done under local anesthesia and sedation or under general anesthesia by simply tugging steadily on the horizontal limb and pulling anteriorly. At the time of decannulation, it is recommended that the T tube be replaced with a small tracheostomy tube (No. 4 cuffless) for at least 4 weeks to allow adequate time to reassess the airway for possible restenosis. Decannulation is then carried out after the patient has tolerated a trial of capping/occluding the tracheostomy tube overtime.

PITFALLS

1. Working through a small stoma makes T tube insertion and manipulation difficult, if not impossible. Employ proper dilatation techniques before attempting insertion.

2. A tube that is too small in diameter will not provide adequate internal stenting; a tube that is too large will be difficult to manipulate into position and is likely to result in significant mucosal trauma and possible displacement of skeletal segments.

3. A long upper limb can interfere with epiglottic and vocal cord closure, resulting in aspiration. If the cut end sits too close to the vocal cords, it may result in mucosal irritation and ulceration, with the potential for granulation tissues and laryngeal stenosis.

4. Do not use the T tube technique with free mucosal or skin grafts. The manipulations required for insertion predispose the graft to shearing and displacement. An open procedure using a silicone stent or a soft sponge stent is recommended for subglottic injuries of this type (see Chapter 98).

5. A close cooperative and communicative effort between the surgeon and the anesthesiologist is essential during the procedure to ensure safe and controlled airway management.

6. The horizontal limbs of the T tube should extend 3 to 4 cm beyond the surface of the skin. Short limbs can predispose to retrodisplacement of the tube during vigorous coughing. Newer tubes with external ring cuffs help overcome this problem.

COMPLICATIONS

1. Displacement of mucosal and cartilaginous segments may occur during insertion. For this reason, direct visualization by bronchoscopy and careful guidance of the upper limb with laryngeal instrumentation will aid in a smooth and precise manipulation.

2. Aspiration can occur. Under such conditions, the patient should be fed a clear liquid diet. An efficient cough can be facilitated by occluding the horizontal limb of the tube. Usually the patient learns to compensate, and as aspiration is diminished or disappears, the patient can progress to a regular diet.

3. Restenosis may occur following T tube removal and can be managed early with dilatation. Failure to keep the airway open may necessitate a more formal reconstructive procedure (see Chapter 109).

4. The T tube can become displaced with coughing and choking. If the tube enters a bronchus and/or kinks, the patient can develop respiratory difficulty. If this occurs, the surgeon can open the tracheostomy with a nasal speculum, grasp the edge of the tube, and extract the tube. For tubes that are displaced even farther down the trachea, the surgeon will have to completely excise the tracheostomy site and gain control of the airway just beneath the area of tracheostomy.

5. Secretions can thicken, harden, and become obstructive. Management includes interval changes, administration of mucolytic agents, and appropriate suction techniques. For firmly adherent crusts, bronchoscopic removal may be necessary. Patient use of humidified air or oxygen will help reduce this problem.

INTERNAL FIXATION WITH MONTGOMERY T TUBE

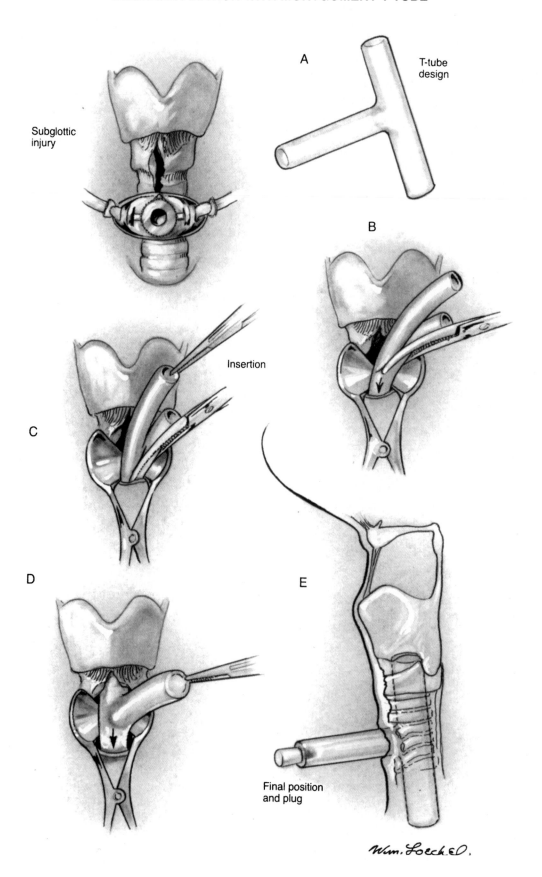

Subglottic injury

A

T-tube design

B

C

Insertion

D

E

Final position and plug

Wm. Loechel.

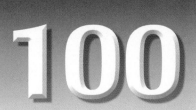

Internal Fixation of a Laryngeal Injury With a Teflon Keel

In Consultation With Terry Shibuya, MD

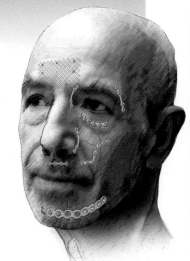

INDICATIONS

The alloplastic keel is best applied in cases of blunt laryngeal trauma in which the thyroid cartilage injury has resulted in lacerations or mucosal disruptions of the anterior commissure and/or both vocal cords. By interposing a thin conforming keel, there will be a reduced chance of anterior web formation. A properly positioned keel should permit intelligible speech when the tracheostomy is plugged and should not interfere with swallowing function.

PROCEDURE

The application of a keel is preceded by a prophylactic tracheostomy (see Chapter 7) and placement of a tracheotomy or anode tube. The keel is then aligned according to the size of the endolarynx. The length of the keel should correspond to a height from the superior aspect of the thyroid cartilage to the top of the cricoid cartilage. The depth of the keel should be approximately the distance from the anterior commissure to the vocal process of the arytenoid. Ready-made keels are available; additionally, the keel can also be fabricated from a standard septal splint that is trimmed according to the previously taken length and width measurements.

A–D The keel is placed by performing an open thyrotomy (see Chapter 97). The true and false vocal cords should be secured to the edge of the thyroid cartilage. The keel is then brought into position and held with a No. 0 polypropylene suture. The placement of the suture is such that the external flanged surface of the keel lies on the thyroid cartilage, and the superior leading edge lies between the vocal cords. The suture is subsequently passed through one flange of the keel, the thyroid cartilage, and the opposite flange of the keel. The needle is returned in a similar fashion to create a figure-of-eight configuration. The needle is then cut off from the suture, and the ends are tied over the thyroid prominence. A similar procedure is performed over the lower part of the thyroid laminae. The thyroid cartilages are then approximated with heavy chromic sutures, and the platysma and skin are closed in layers. Placement of a subplatysmal suction drain or Penrose (1/2 in) for 1 to 2 days is desirable. Prophylactic antibiotics are given during keel retention, which is usually 2 to 3 weeks. The keel is removed after surgically exposing the thyroid cartilage and cutting the sutures that hold the keel in position.

PITFALLS

1. The keel should be used only when injury involves the anterior commissure. For patients who also have damage to the arytenoids or vocal cords, the surgeon should consider a stent with or without a graft (see Chapter 98).

2. After securing the retention sutures, it is imperative to check for proper seating of the upper and lower

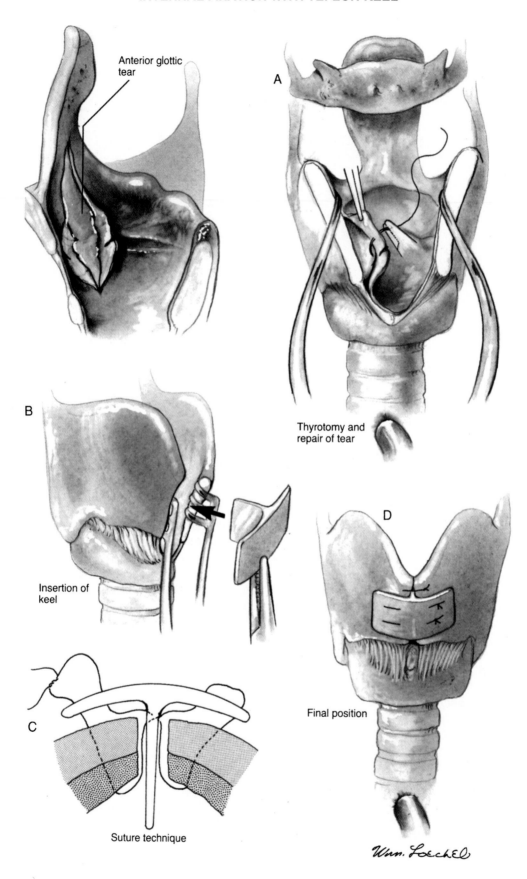

Anterior glottic tear

A

Thyrotomy and repair of tear

B

Insertion of keel

C

Suture technique

D

Final position

Wm. Loechel

ends of the keel. The leading keel angle should fit into the anterior commissure, and excessive tension should be avoided as the sutures are tied down.

3. Make sure that the vocal cords are secured to the thyroid cartilage at the same level. Vocal cord apposition following removal of the keel is the primary determinant of voice quality.

COMPLICATIONS

1. Granulation tissue formation may occur at the upper and lower ends of the keel and may develop, in part, from movement of the keel against opposing mucosa. If not corrected, this inflammatory process can also lead to web formation. Fixing the keel to the laryngeal skeleton and then removing the sutures later using an open technique will reduce the possibility of such sequelae.

2. The keel, if improperly placed, can cause exposure of thyroid cartilage and subsequent chondritis. This complication can be avoided by making sure the keel fits the opening (i.e., not too large or too small). Tight fixation should also prevent movement and further irritation of the tissues.

3. Aspiration may be a problem in some patients who are treated with a keel that is too large. One or several factors can contribute to the complication. The device itself can interfere with epiglottic closure and approximation of the true and false cords. An open tracheostomy will reduce subglottic pressures and afford little, if any, protection against entry of food or drink into the upper airway. Temporarily plugging the tracheostomy tube during eating or drinking may be helpful. If aspiration continues, the surgeon should consider either a redesign of the keel or an alternative technique.

Supraglottic Injury

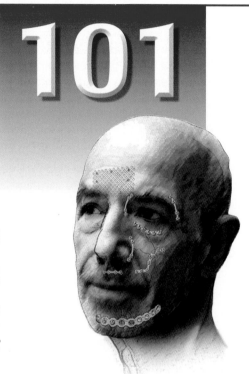

CHAPTER **101**

Treatment of Supraglottic Injury With Supraglottic Laryngectomy
Alternative Techniques of Anterior Pharyngotomy With Partial Supraglottic Resection and Epiglottic Base Resection

In Consultation With Terry Shibuya, MD

INDICATIONS

Surgical repair for a supraglottic injury due to an avulsion and/or laceration requires an understanding of the extent of injury and an assessment of vocal cord mobility. The epiglottis is important for the supraglottic valve mechanism that protects the larynx from aspiration. With its absence, the valve must be compensated with a more posterior excursion of the tongue, a more anterior displacement of the larynx, and complete closure by the true and false vocal cords. Attempts should be made to preserve the epiglottis, but when this is not possible, complete or partial resection may be necessary.

If there is an extensive comminution of the thyroid ala in which repair of the cartilage is not feasible, a conventional supraglottic laryngectomy is an option. If the thyroid cartilage fracture is limited to its superior half and vocal cord mobility (and glottic competence) can be established, the supraglottic injury can be managed by an interfragmentary repair and a partial supraglottic resection. If true vocal cord mobility is impaired and the epiglottis is dislocated, it is probably advisable to resect the inferior portion (petiole) and reattach the epiglottic base to the superior margin of the thyroid cartilage.

TECHNIQUE

Anesthesia is provided by a tracheostomy that is secured below the area of injury (see Chapter 7). This provides airway security and allows for better visualization of the injured supraglottic larynx. Additionally, a nasogastric tube is also inserted for feeding postoperatively as the patient is kept NPO for the next 7 to 10 days while wound healing occurs.

A–C A transverse skin incision is made in a skin crease at the midthyroid cartilage level. Subplatysmal flaps are elevated both superiorly and inferiorly to expose the hyoid bone and cricoid cartilage. For a pure supraglottic injury, the strap muscles are carefully mobilized from the thyroid ala and underlying cricoid. Sharp division of these muscles at a level just above the thyroid cartilage is carried out, followed by incising the thyroid cartilage perichondrium at its superior border. A subperichondrial flap is developed inferiorly with a Freer elevator, and the thyroid cartilage is exposed to visualize all fracture lines. Depending on the level of these fracture lines, transverse cartilage cuts are outlined between the superior thyroid notch and the attachment of the vocal cords, which occurs just below the midthyroid level. Vertical cuts are then made at least 1 cm medial to the superior horns to intersect with the transverse cuts on the thyroid cartilage. This should protect the internal laryngeal nerves and superior laryngeal arteries that penetrate the thyrohyoid membrane.

D–H The suprahyoid muscle attachments are next released with a dissection close and superior to the hyoid. The superior and inferior horns are cut from the body. The hyoid is grasped with an Allis clamp and excised. The hypopharynx is then entered by sharp dissection through the base of the vallecula (or piriform sinus), and the tip of the epiglottis is secured with an Allis clamp. An incision is carried out across the vallecula. The thyrohyoid membrane cuts are then completed, and with appropriate counter rotation, endolaryngeal cuts are made through the aryepiglottic folds, just above the arytenoids and the false vocal cords toward the thyroid angle. By sectioning intervening tissues, the supraglottic larynx is mobilized and extracted. This technique is similar to the procedure related to cancer ablative surgery.

Mucosal tears within the larynx should be carefully approximated with 4-0 chromic sutures. If primary repair cannot be implemented because of devitalized or avulsed segments of mucosa, the surgeon can use grafts with stents or, preferably, local flaps from the interarytenoid or piriform sinus region (see Chapter 98). Fractures of the remaining thyroid laminae should be identified and then reduced and fixed with titanium or resorbable miniplates, 28- or 30-gauge stainless steel wires or nylon suture (see Chapters 97 through 100).

I Two additional procedures can be used to minimize aspiration: laryngeal suspension and cricopharyngeal myotomy. Laryngeal suspension can be carried out by drop sutures from the mandibular symphysis adjusted to elevate the larynx 2 cm and thereby distribute the tension load. The net effect is anterosuperior rotation of the larynx, with protection from aspiration afforded by the overlying base of the tongue. Cricopharyngeal myotomy is carried out sharply with the No. 15 scalpel blade against a finger inserted on the mucosal surface of the cricopharyngeus muscle.

J,K Closure of the larynx is completed by approximating the thyroid cartilage perichondrium with the base of the tongue superiorly and the remnants of the thyrohyoid membrane laterally with interrupted 2-0 chromic sutures. A second layer of closure is accomplished by approximating the strap muscles loosely in the midline and to the tongue with interrupted 3-0 chromic sutures. A suction drain or 1/2-in Penrose drain is inserted, and the platysma and skin are closed with interrupted 3-0 chromic and 5-0 nylon sutures. Prophylactic antibiotics are given for 10 days and the patient is kept NPO while the wound heals.

PITFALLS

1. As in resection for neoplastic disease, supraglottic laryngectomy may be contraindicated in those elderly or debilitated persons or those with chronic lung disease who would otherwise not tolerate aspiration.

2. Care must be taken during the lateral part of the resection to preserve the superior laryngeal nerves. Sensory denervation can lead to aspiration problems.

3. Avoid tension on mucosal closures. If such a condition develops, it is more prudent to use local flaps or tissue advancements.

COMPLICATIONS

1. Supraglottic laryngectomy effectively removes the supraglottic valve mechanism during swallowing and predisposes to aspiration. This complication is more prone to occur in patients who have inadequate

LARYNGEAL INJURY TREATED WITH SUPRAGLOTTIC LARYNGECTOMY

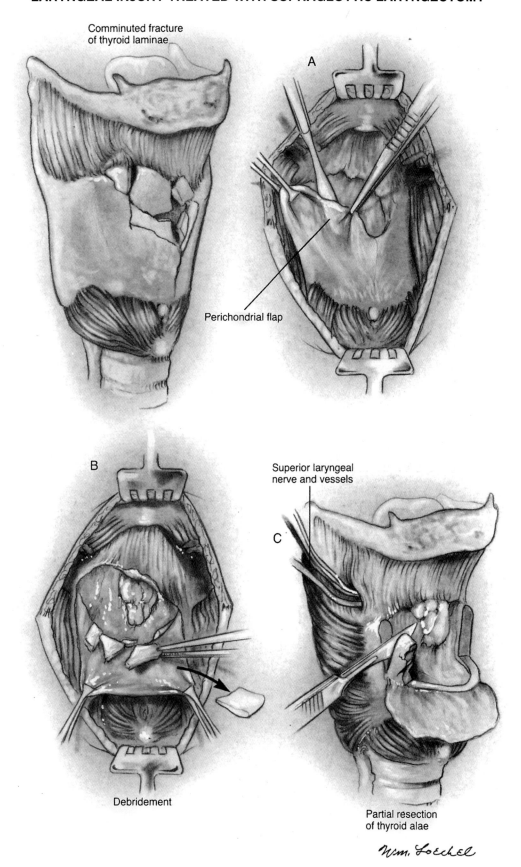

Comminuted fracture
of thyroid laminae

A

Perichondrial flap

B

Debridement

Superior laryngeal
nerve and vessels

C

Partial resection
of thyroid alae

Wm. Loechel

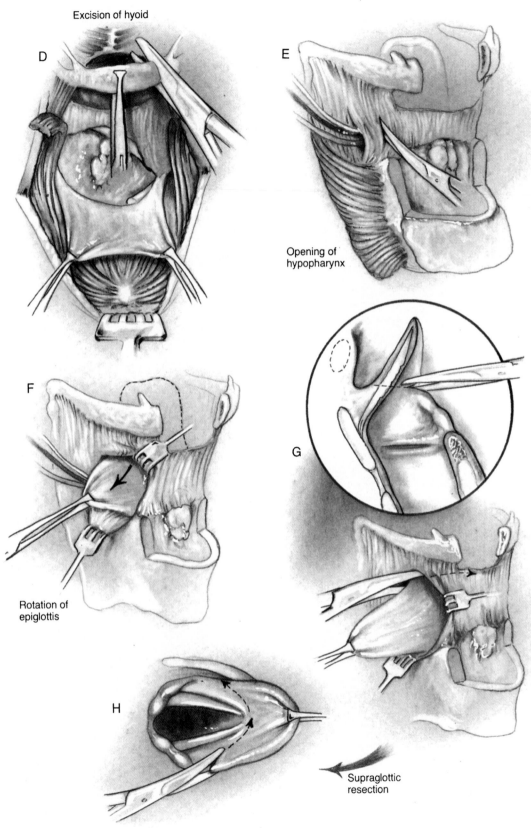

Excision of hyoid

D

E

Opening of
hypopharynx

F

G

Rotation of
epiglottis

H

Supraglottic
resection

Wm. Loechel

vocal cord mobility and poor lung function; in such patients, the procedure should be avoided. Aspiration can also be minimized by suspension techniques and cricopharyngeal myotomy. If it should occur in spite of these precautions, the surgeon must consider training the patient in supraglottic swallowing and appropriate modifications in diet.

2. Some degree of respiratory obstruction may be noted following supraglottic resection. Usually this is the result of swelling of the arytenoids and false cords, and in such cases, improvement will occur with time. Excessive folds or granulations can be removed microsurgically or with a laser technique.

ALTERNATIVE TECHNIQUE OF ANTERIOR PHARYNGOTOMY WITH PARTIAL SUPRAGLOTTIC RESECTION

A modified supraglottic resection for limited injuries to the supraglottic larynx can be carried out using suprahyoid, transhyoid, or infrahyoid approaches. The goal of this surgery is the conservative removal of devitalized segments while preserving epiglottic and vocal cord functions.

a,b The skin incision is placed in a transverse skin crease line near the upper border of the thyroid cartilage. Superior and inferior subplatysmal flaps are developed, and the strap muscles are separated away from the laryngeal complex. The insertions of the sternohyoid and a portion of the thyrohyoid muscles are sharply divided at the inferior border of the hyoid bone and reflected inferolaterally. An inferiorly based flap of thyrohyoid membrane incorporating perichondrium covering the thyroid laminae is developed to a level sufficient to expose the fracture lines of the superior part of the thyroid. Comminuted or unstable segments are resected; fractured but stable segments can be reinforced by microplate fixation.

An anterior pharyngotomy is then made by transversely incising the thyrohyoid membrane near its midportion, being careful to visualize and protect the neurovascular pedicle entering laterally. The surgeon then resects the area of irreversible injury (i.e., epiglottis, aryepiglottic folds, or false cords).

c In preparation for closure and laryngeal suspension, 28-gauge stainless steel wires or 0 polyprolene sutures are passed around the hyoid in front of the thyrohyoid membrane flap and through the anterior edge of the remaining thyroid ala. If the hyoid is fractured and unstable, the segments are removed, and suspension is employed from the mandibular symphysis. Closure of the pharynx is then carried out by approximating the base of the tongue to the inferior thyrohyoid membrane flap. If possible, the superior flap should be imbricated and closed with 2-0 chromic sutures over the lower flap. The tension on the suspension wires is adjusted and the wires are tied to provide for laryngeal elevation and a decrease in tension on the suture line. The strap muscles are reattached and approximated in the midline with 3-0 chromic sutures. A two-layered closure with drainage completes the procedure.

ALTERNATIVE TECHNIQUE OF EPIGLOTTIC BASE RESECTION

The approach to the epiglottic base is initiated in a manner similar to that described for thyrotomy (see Chapter 97). Essentially the surgeon resects the base and closes the defect with advancement of the remaining epiglottis. This technique is useful in repairing a defect or stenosis of the anterior glottic area (see Chapter 105).

a′–d′ A midline laryngofissure or a paramedian fracture line can provide appropriate access. Following careful separation of the thyroid ala and after endolaryngeal assessment and mucosal repair, a conservative resection of the preepiglottic space fat adjacent to the epiglottic base is performed. A transverse mucosal incision is then made at the level of intended cartilage resection, and a submucoperichondrial plane is developed superiorly about 5 mm onto the anterior surface of the epiglottis. Epiglottic mucosal flaps are developed on the anterior cartilaginous surface and then on the posterior surface just above the level of the original mucosal incision. The epiglottic base is resected while protecting the mucosal flaps with malleable retractors. A 2-0 chromic suture is next passed between the thyroid ala and the remaining epiglottic base from anterior to posterior and then back again to the contralateral ala in a horizontal mattress fashion. The epiglottis is tacked with additional sutures to the thyroid cartilage. The remainder of the closure and postoperative care are as described for thyrotomy (see Chapter 97).

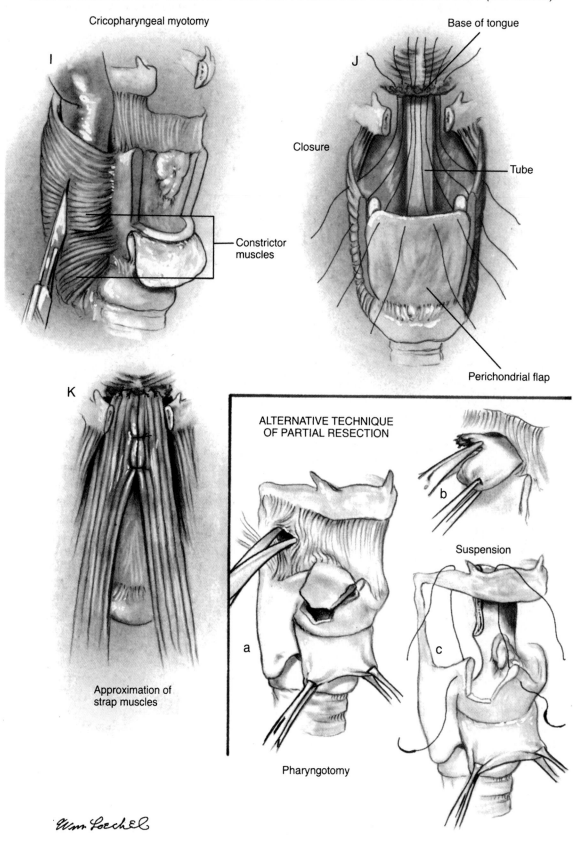

Cricopharyngeal myotomy

I

Constrictor muscles

Base of tongue

J

Closure

Tube

Perichondrial flap

K

Approximation of
strap muscles

ALTERNATIVE TECHNIQUE
OF PARTIAL RESECTION

b

Suspension

a

c

Pharyngotomy

Wm Loechel

ALTERNATIVE TECHNIQUE OF EPIGLOTTIC BASE RESECTION

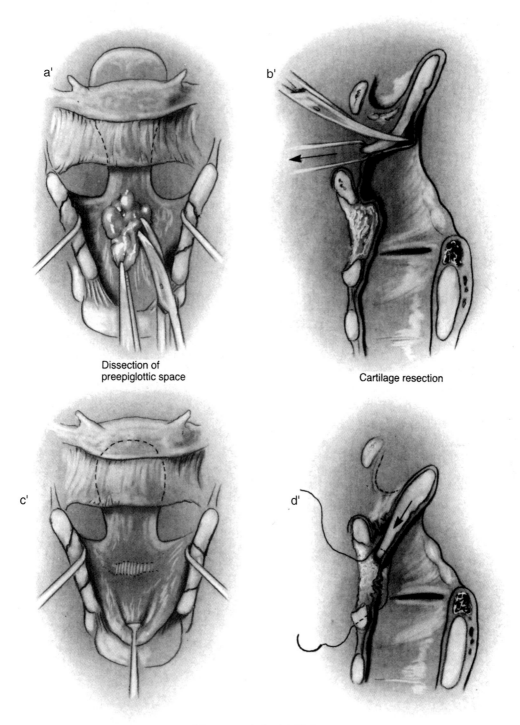

a'

Dissection of
preepiglottic space

b'

Cartilage resection

c'

d'

Advancement of epiglottic base

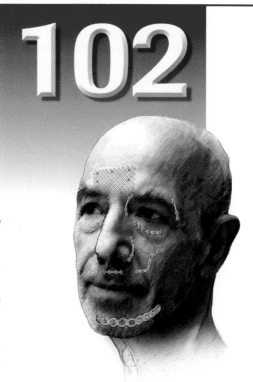

CHAPTER

102

Open Repair of
Subglottic Injury
Alternative Technique of
Hyoid Interposition Graft

In Consultation With Terry Shibuya, MD

INDICATIONS

Acute subglottic injuries are often an emergency characterized by early obstruction and respiratory distress. In such situations, control of the airway takes priority. Any cervical spine injury and the degree and extent of subglottic damage are evaluated by appropriate imaging studies and endoscopy. Only after the airway has been secured and the cervical spine cleared from injury should the subglottic injury may be addressed.

A variety of injuries may occur, including an isolated cricoid fracture, a comminuted cricoid arch, and/or laryngotracheal disruption. In general, limited cricoid arch fractures are managed by open reduction and fixation. A comminuted cricoid can be stabilized with microplates or may require a composite hyoid arch transposition with a thyrotracheal anastomosis. Extensive damage may require the use of a T tube or

laryngeal stent (see Chapter 98). Laryngotracheal disruption is usually managed with a direct cricotracheal repair.

PROCEDURE

A Following a tracheostomy placement (see Chapter 7), a transverse collar neck incision is outlined over the lower half of the thyroid cartilage. Superior and inferior subplatysmal flaps are developed to provide exposure of the thyroid and cricoid cartilages, as well as the first and second tracheal rings. An effort should be made to maintain soft tissue between the newly created tracheostomy site and the area of cricoid repair.

B–D The investing and pretracheal fascia are incised in the midline; the thyroid isthmus is divided, and the thyroid lobes are retracted laterally to expose the cartilaginous laryngeal structures. An initial endoscopy performed at the beginning of the case will help determine whether it will be necessary to perform a thyrotomy to access the larynx (e.g., for denuded mucosa requiring free grafting or grossly displaced fracture segments). If mucosal continuity has been maintained and there are minor displacements of the fracture segments, then reduction can be performed using the tip of the rigid bronchoscope or by manually reducing the exposed cartilage fragment into proper positioning. From this exposure, titanium miniplates or resorbable plates and screws can hold the cartilage fragments in proper position. Alternatively suture (0 polyprolene) or wires (30 or 32 gauge) can be used. Ideally, the screws, sutures, or wires do not penetrate the laryngeal/tracheal mucosa but only are placed deep enough for fixation.

If the larynx must be entered, the surgeon should extend the incision from the fracture line into the cricotracheal/cricothyroid membranes. Additional cuts through the thyroid cartilage in the midline will provide the necessary exposure for free grafting, mucosal repair (4-0 chromic suture), reduction of cartilage segments, and soft stent placement (see Chapters 97 and 98). Fractures of the thyroid laminae are usually stabilized extralumenally with titanium or resorbable miniplates (or alternatively with 30- to 32-gauge wire/0 polyprolene suture). Comminution of fractures and instability of the cricoid area can be treated by attaching the fragments to a titanium or resorbable plate shaped in the contour of the cricoid ring. Alternatively a hyoid graft may be placed and fixed in position and or T tube placement may be performed (see Chapter 99). Cricopharyngeal separation should be repaired by suturing the first ring of the trachea to the cricoid with strategic placements of 3-0 chromic sutures.

The cricothyroid membrane is repaired with 3-0 or 4-0 chromic sutures. A small drain is placed and the overlying soft tissues are approximated with additional 4-0 chromic sutures. The skin is closed with a 5-0 nylon suture, and prophylactic antibiotics are employed for 7 to 10 days. A nasogastric tube is placed and the patient is kept NPO for 7 to 10 days while the wound is healing.

PITFALLS

1. Failure to recognize associated injuries such as arytenoid dislocation, esophageal rupture, or cervical spine trauma can lead to complications of glottic incompetence, fistula, or neurologic injury. For this reason, the patient must be carefully evaluated with a detailed history, physical examination (including laryngoscopy), sequential endoscopy, and computed tomographic (CT) scans in the horizontal plane.

2. The integrity of the cricoid arch is essential for respiration. For these reasons, debridement should be minimized and reconstruction limited to simple techniques that will not disrupt the blood supply of the tissues. The larynx should not be entered for exploration unless there is a strong indication of failure in reduction and/or repair of intralaryngeal injury.

3. Make sure that the dissection of tissues is limited to the central portion of the cricoid, as the recurrent nerve can be injured laterally. This should be avoided.

4. An internal stent can be employed any time stability of the framework is in question. The T tube (see Chapter 99) is a very popular technique and is often indicated. Failure to stent can lead to a retrodisplacement of fracture segments and stenosis.

COMPLICATIONS

1. Subglottic stenosis is probably the most common significant complication following cricoid injury. Appropriate reduction of the fragments and fixation should help avoid this occurrence. Early stenosis can be treated with dilatation and steroid injections. Persistent stenosis may require resection of the involved segment and either an interposition graft or a fresh cricotracheal anastomosis.

2. Vocal cord paralysis and/or fixation are possible with cricoid injury. An accurate diagnosis should distinguish between the various conditions. If paralysis is present and vocal cord function does not return, then a vocal cord medialization procedure or vocal cord injection may be indicated (see Chapter 103). For bilateral paralysis, a partial cordectomy, arytenoidectomy, neuromuscular pedicle procedure, and tracheotomy are possible options (see Chapter 104).

ALTERNATIVE TECHNIQUE OF HYOID INTERPOSITION GRAFT

The hyoid bone is well suited for functioning as interpositional grafting. Its gentle curve and thickness are ideal for an anterior cricoid arch deficiency and its close proximity make it simple source for access. In using the hyoid autograft, we prefer to raise it based on a vascularized muscle pedicle composed of sternohyoid muscle with or without attached omohyoid (depending on the length of graft needed). In contrast to a free graft technique, the vascularized graft should provide optimal conditions for healing, thus lessening the chances of resorption and fibrous tissue replacement.

a–d In preparation for the graft, all devitalized cartilage fragments should be removed, preserving as much inner perichondrium as possible. Endolaryngeal

REPAIR OF CRICOID INJURY

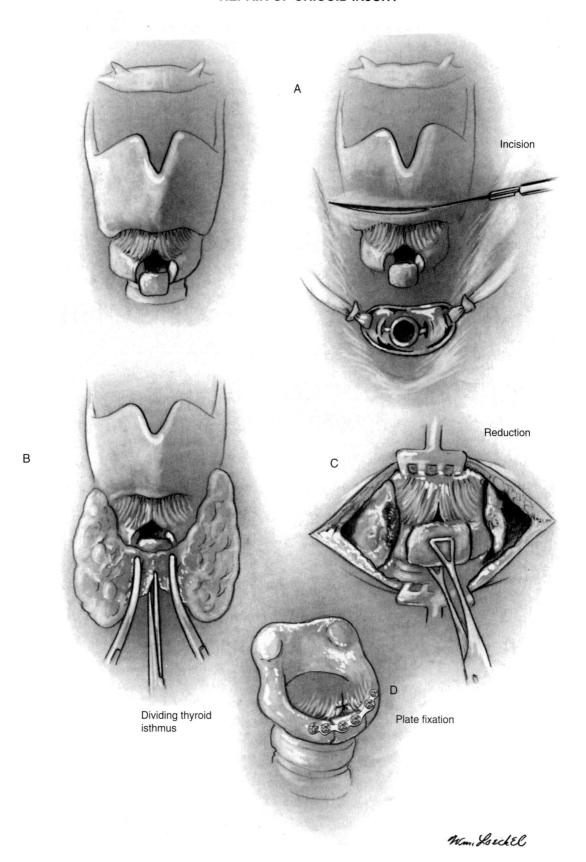

A

Incision

B

C

Reduction

Dividing thyroid
isthmus

D

Plate fixation

Wm. Loechel

mucosal tears are meticulously repaired with 4-0 chromic sutures, and the larger, more viable, cartilaginous segments are retained and stabilized with either wire (30- or 32-gauge stainless steel) or suture (0 polyprolene). Next the length of the cricoid defect is measured with a ruler, keeping the defect's anterior convexity in mind. This length is then mapped out over the body of the hyoid, but if necessary, it can extend beyond the lesser cornus laterally. The suprahyoid muscular attachments overlying the donor segment are released. Working from below, posterolaterally to anteromedially, the layers of fascia that invest the sternohyoid (and omohyoid) muscle are preserved and followed to the level of the hyoid. Care must be exercised to avoid injury to the superior laryngeal neurovascular bundle. Next, using sharp bone cutters, hyoid osteotomies are performed to the desired length. The underlying thyrohyoid muscle is next divided sharply, and its attachments to the overlying strap muscles are released. The compound hyoid bone-muscle pedicle graft is then rotated into the cricoid defect.

If the graft is oriented vertically, at titanium or resorbable miniplate is placed extralumenally to secure it to the thyroid cartilage above and the first tracheal ring below. Alternatively wire (30- or 32-gauge stainless steel wire) or suture (0 polyprolen) may be used. If the graft is to be oriented horizontally, it is secured to the ends of the remaining cricoid cartilage using a similar fixation technique. Additional graft stability can be obtained by approximating the medial borders of the sternohyoid muscles to each other with absorbable sutures. A standard two-layer closure with drainage is employed, and prophylactic antibiotics are given for 7 to 10 days. Again a nasogastic feeding tube is place and the patient is kept NPO for 7 to 10 days as well.

ALTERNATIVE TECHNIQUE OF HYOID GRAFT

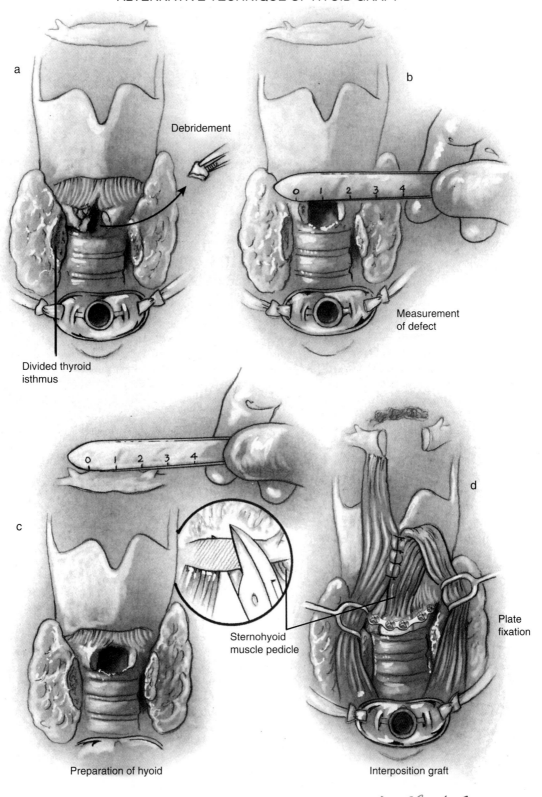

a

Debridement

Divided thyroid
isthmus

b

Measurement
of defect

c

Preparation of hyoid

Sternohyoid
muscle pedicle

d

Plate
fixation

Interposition graft

587

Vocal Cord Paralysis

CHAPTER

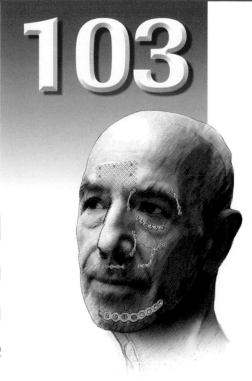

103

Treatment of Unilateral Vocal Cord Paralysis With Injection Medialization
Alternative Technique of Implant Medialization Thyroplasty

In Consultation With Adam Folbe, MD

INDICATIONS

Recurrent laryngeal nerve injury is often a consequence of laryngeal trauma, especially when there has been a laryngotracheal separation or cricoarytenoid compression. Paralysis limited to one side causes a weak voice and, in some patients, aspiration of food or drink. In bilateral paralysis, the voice remains strong, but the adducted vocal cords may compromise the airway and often cause obstruction.

Unilateral vocal cord paralysis is sometimes difficult to evaluate and distinguish from posterior glottic scarring. Moreover, the diagnosis of vocal cord paralysis can be confounded by associated injuries to the superior laryngeal nerve and swelling, laceration, and hematoma in and around the glottic chink.

The patient with cervical trauma should be evaluated for adequacy of the airway, and if there is obstruction (present or impending), he or she should be treated with cricothyrotomy or tracheostomy (see Chapters 6 and 7). The cervical spine should also be checked for injury. The vocal cords can then be inspected by flexible laryngoscopy or mirror examination, carefully recording the appearance and function of the cords. At a later time, the surgeon will want to palpate the mobility of the arytenoid joint by way of endoscopy and assay the thyroarytenoid muscle electrically with electromyography. Videotaping and voice recordings are desirable. Computed tomographic (CT) scans should be used to elucidate the anatomic integrity of the glottic area.

Isolated unilateral vocal cord paralysis should not cause any urgent problems, but the patient may complain of a weak voice, hoarseness, and occasionally, aspiration of fluids. Speech therapy may help, but vocal cord function that does not return within 6 to 9 months suggests a poor prognosis, and the surgeon should consider a surgical method of rehabilitation. Injection is an easy-to-perform and popular technique. Alternatively, an implant thyroplasty procedure can be considered.

PROCEDURE

Ideally the injection medialization procedure is performed in an office setting with topical/local anesthesia. However, based on the patient's anatomy, motivation, and cooperation, the procedure may have to be performed in an operating room with general anesthesia. Regardless of the method, the injection is placed lateral to the vocal fold, and anterior to the vocal process.

Awake Office Based Procedure

For preparation of the endoscopy and injection, Oxymetazaline and 4% lidocaine are sprayed into the nasal cavity. The oral cavity and pharynx is sprayed with the lidocaine solution. Subsequently, 3 mL of 4% lidocaine are injected transtracheally into the airway to anesthetize the subglottic area and vocal folds. A flexible laryngoscope is introduced into the airway through the nose to visualize the vocal cords. A monitor attached to the scope is set up to face the surgeon.

A–C A hydroxyl apatite gel (Radiess) is injected transtracheally using a 21-gauge needle. The needle is placed through the cricothyroid membrane and directed superiorly and laterally into position. Next, the material is slowly injected, and the fold is evaluated throughout the procedure to observe the degree of medialization. Overmedialization is key, because approximately 20% may resorb.

Operating Room Procedure Under General Anesthesia

The smallest endotracheal tube or jet ventilation is used. The patient is then placed in the supine position, and a laryngoscope is introduced into the larynx. The larynx is reevaluated and the laryngoscope fixed to a holder. A microscope with a 400-mm objective lens is then focused onto the vocal cord area.

a–c The aim of the vocal cord injection is to move the paralyzed vocal cord to the midline. The injection should thus be placed lateral to the thyroarytenoid muscle and anterior to the vocal process of the arytenoid. A syringe with a long laryngeal needle is loaded with the injectable. A spatula is used to lateralize the false vocal cord, exposing the ventricle. The needle of the syringe is then inserted and directed just lateral to the true vocal cord and anterior to the vocal process. The needle depth should be approximately 2 to 3 mm beneath the mucosa. As mentioned previously, the amount of injection should cause approximately 20% overcorrection to account fro the reabsorption of the material. Any material injected onto the surface of the vocal cord should be removed by suction to avoid aspiration. Postoperatively the patient is checked for respiratory difficulty. If the patient has any problem with breathing, steroids should be administered and the patient placed under close observation. If there are no complications, voice use can be restored as soon as the effects of anesthesia have disappeared.

PITFALLS

1. The diagnosis of vocal cord paralysis is important. The physician must be certain that the problem is a true recurrent laryngeal nerve paralysis, free of arthritis or stenosis. A normally functioning superior laryngeal nerve is preferred. Any question of fixation or stenosis should be resolved with electromyographic studies.

2. With regard to timing of treatment, the surgeon must wait at least 6 to 9 months for return of vocal cord function. If the patient is severely incapacitated by voice weakness and/or aspiration, it is possible to inject a temporary material such as fat, Gelfoam, or collagen (Cymetra), which will provide short-term effects. If, after 9 months, there is no return of function, a more permanent injection using hydroxyl apatite or a definitive medialization procedure can be considered.

3. Neurorrhaphy of the recurrent laryngeal nerve is controversial. If there is evidence of transection of the recurrent nerve, it is probably prudent to explore the recurrent laryngeal nerve and affect a microscopic repair. However, it should be noted that results are variable, and the injection medializaiton still may be needed at a later time.

4. Injection is ideal for the small to moderate deficiency. However, if the defect is large (e.g., following atrophy or removal of the vocal cord), the injection often is not sufficient. Under such conditions, the surgeon should consider an operative implant for thyroplasty technique (see later).

5. Underinjection or injecting until the vocal cord moves to the midline may result in immediate

TREATMENT OF UNILATERAL VOCAL CORD PARALYSIS
WITH INJECTION MEDIALIZATION

AWAKE OFFICE BASED PROCEDURE

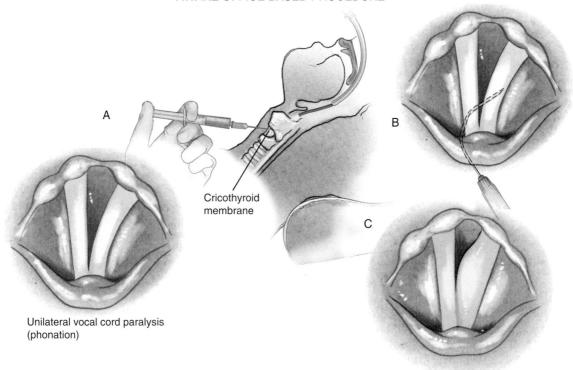

A

Cricothyroid
membrane

B

C

Unilateral vocal cord paralysis
(phonation)

OPERATING ROOM PROCEDURE UNDER GENERAL ANESTHESIA

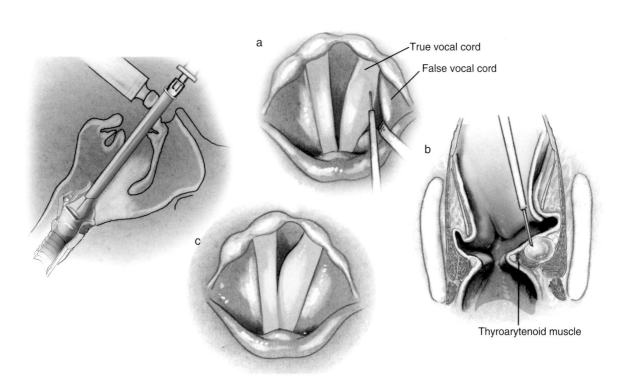

a

True vocal cord

False vocal cord

b

c

Thyroarytenoid muscle

improvement of voice. However, after 1 to 2 weeks, the voice may become weak because of reabsorption of implant material. For this reason, the surgeon should plan for a slight overinjection.

6. Avoid injection that is superficial or into the laminal propria; this can result in impaired mucosal wave. Also avoid injection of material into the airway as this can lead to aspiration.

ALTERNATIVE TECHNIQUE OF IMPLANT MEDIALIZATION THYROPLASTY

Adduction paralysis, complicated by loss of vocal cord tissues or an opening that is too large and not corrected by injection, should prompt the consideration of a permanent implant. The main advantage of the implant technique is the inert material is less apt to undergo reaction or displacement. Although one can use silastic, hydroxyapatite, or other alloplastic materials, we prefer to use 4-mm wide strips of polytetra-fluoroethylene (Gore Tex) cut from a cardiovascular patch graft.

The nasal passageway, oropharynx, hypopharynx, and larynx are anesthetized as described earlier. Next, under mild sedation, the patient is placed in a supine position. A flexible laryngoscope is placed and held in position to clearly visualize both vocal folds. Throughout the procedure, the patient should be able to phonate so that the surgeon can evaluate the position of the vocal folds.

a' Our technique of thyrotomy is performed through a horizontal curvilinear incision that is marked at the midportion of the thyroid cartilage. The tissues are infiltrated with 1% lidocaine containing 1:100,000 epinephrine. The incision is carried through the superficial layers and into a subplatysmal plane that is developed superiorly and inferiorly. The thyrohyoid muscles are retracted laterally to expose the prominence of the thyroid cartilage.

b'–d' The perichondrium of the thyroid cartilage is incised in the midline and then horizontally across the lamina of the affected side. The perichondrium is then raised with a Freer elevator. Using a 4-mm diamond burr, a small window is drilled through the thyroid cartilage. Careful attention is made to not violate the internal perichondrium. The window is placed approximately 3 to 5 mm superior to the inferior border of the thyroid cartilage and 10 mm posterior to the midline.

e' With the patient phonating, the Gore Tex strip is carefully positioned. Simultaneously, the surgeon watches the medialization of the vocal fold from a monitor connected to the laryngoscope. Once the desired amount of Gore Tex has been placed, the perichondrium is closed with 3-0 chromic sutures, and the thyroid lamina is approximated with 2-0 chromic sutures. A small Penrose drain is usually retained for 24 hours. If the displacement of the vocal cord is less than optimal, the Gore Tex should be adjusted and the evaluation repeated. The patient should be given prophylactic antibiotics for about 5 days.

TREATMENT OF UNILATERAL VOCAL CORD PARALYSIS *(Continued)*

ALTERNATIVE TECHNIQUE OF IMPLANT MEDIALIZATION THYROPLASTY

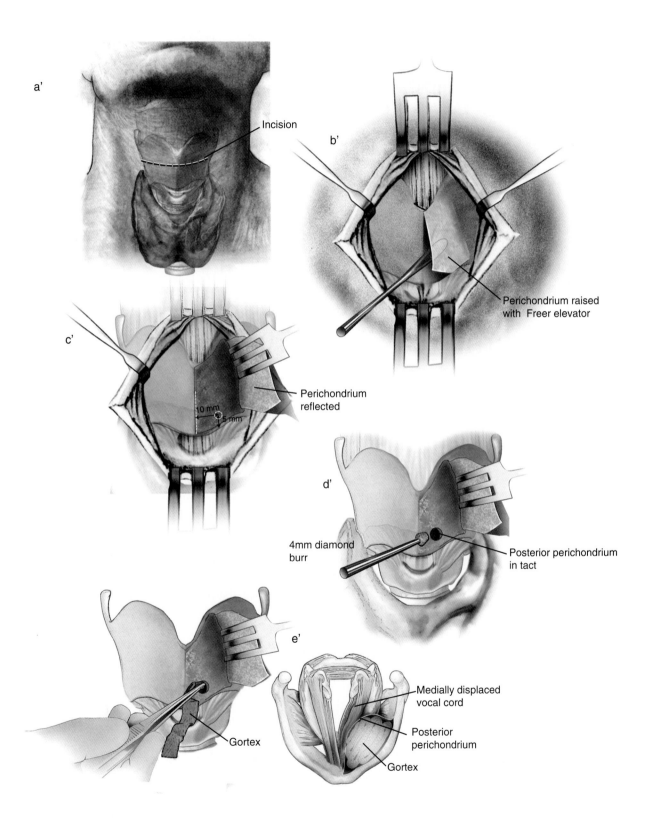

a'

Incision

b'

Perichondrium raised
with Freer elevator

c'

10 mm

5 mm

Perichondrium
reflected

d'

4mm diamond
burr

Posterior perichondrium
in tact

e'

Gortex

Medially displaced
vocal cord

Posterior
perichondrium

Gortex

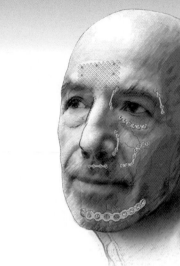

Treatment of Bilateral Vocal Cord Paralysis With Arytenoidectomy by Way of Thyrotomy
Alternative Techniques of Endoscopic Arytenoidectomy and Neuromuscular Pedicle Reinnervation

INDICATIONS

The presumed mechanism of bilateral vocal cord paralysis following trauma is a crush injury or an associated laryngotracheal separation. In most patients, there is a mild dyspnea with a strong voice; in others, there can be a moderate to severe respiratory obstruction. In this latter group, intubation and/or tracheostomy must be employed.

Although it is not predictable, many patients recover vocal cord function. The patient's prognosis can usually be established at about 6 to 9 months following injury, and it is at this time that plans can be made for static or dynamic lateralization of the vocal cord. The condition must be distinguished from fixation, and for this evaluation, the surgeon should perform endoscopic mobility studies. Electromyography, videotaping, and voice recordings are desirable.

Bilateral vocal cord paralysis is treated with an arytenoidectomy or a neuromuscular reinnervation procedure. Arytenoidectomy can be performed either through a thyrotomy or through a laryngoscope using microscopic or laser techniques. The thyrotomy provides

excellent exposure but can be complicated by postoperative hematoma and/or infection. The endoscopic method is easier to carry out but can be compromised by incomplete removal of the arytenoid and subsequently, an incomplete lateralization of the vocal cord.

The neuromuscular pedicle reinnervation method is more controversial than the arytenoidectomy. It has the advantage of being a dynamic method of rehabilitation, but the results are variable and less reliable. Nevertheless, if the procedure fails, there is still an opportunity to perform an arytenoidectomy. The neuromuscular pedicle reinnervation procedure will not work if there is any arytenoid ankylosis or interarytenoid fibrosis, and in patients with these conditions, the surgeon has a better chance of success with an arytenoidectomy.

PROCEDURE

The thyrotomy is usually performed under general anesthesia by way of a tracheostomy. The neck is prepared and draped as a sterile field. A transverse incision is marked across the thyroid and then infiltrated with 1% lidocaine containing 1:100,000 epinephrine for control of hemostasis.

A The incision should be extended through the platysma and a plane developed superiorly and inferiorly to expose the strap muscles. The sternohyoid and sternothyroid muscles are identified and retracted laterally. The thyroid cartilage perichondrium is incised in the midline, and a small opening is made in the cricothyroid membrane. The thyroid cartilage is then split with an oscillating saw, and from the subglottic space, the mucosa is incised in a cephalic direction between the vocal cords. Above the vocal cords, the incision can be directed to the side of the petiole. The thyroid laminae are retracted laterally with self-retaining retractors to expose the posterior wall of the larynx.

B,C The affected arytenoid is identified, and a vertical-to-oblique incision (1.5 cm) is made over the cartilage. The vocal process is exposed and freed from the thyroarytenoid muscle with small scissors. The vocal process is then grasped and pulled forward. The perichondrial tissues and the extrinsic arytenoid musculature are separated from the cartilage. Finally, the joint is cleaved and the arytenoid extracted from the wound. The mucosa is closed with two 4-0 chromic sutures.

D,E Lateralization of the vocal cord can be improved by suturing the vocal cord laterally to the thyroid lamina. For this procedure, the sternohyoid and sternothyroid muscles are retracted laterally from the thyroid laminae, and with a large curved needle, a 3-0 nonabsorbable suture is passed through the lamina and through the upper mucosal surface of the vocal cord. The needle should be directed several millimeters anterior to the arytenoid wound. The needle is then withdrawn and returned through the same mucosal hole to run submucosally around the vocal cord and then back out through the thyroid lamina. The suture is tied laterally to the thyroid lamina, and the position of the vocal cord is checked with a laryngoscope and adjusted accordingly.

The thyroid cartilage and perichondrium are approximated with 2-0 chromic sutures. The wound is then closed in layers, using 4-0 chromic and 5-0 nylon sutures, respectively, through the platysma and skin. A small Penrose drain should be used for 1 to 2 days. Prophylactic antibiotics are prescribed for 5 days. The tracheostomy can be removed when postoperative swelling is no longer a problem and the patient tolerates the plugging of the tube for at least 24 to 48 hours.

PITFALLS

1. Bilateral vocal cord paralysis must not be confused with fixation. The patient must be evaluated for arytenoid mobility and the absence of interarytenoid or subglottic stenosis. Electromyographic recordings may be a valuable adjunct in confirming the diagnosis.

2. Make sure that the arytenoid is completely removed and the vocal cord is adequately lateralized. Sometimes the arytenoid can be removed, and the vocal cord still remains near or across the midline. The degree of lateralization should be confirmed endoscopically before termination of the procedure.

3. A drain is important, as the wound is often contaminated, and there is a possibility of saliva leaking through the mucosa into the subcutaneous tissues. The drain can usually be removed in 24 to 48 hours.

4. The tracheostomy is helpful in establishing an airway and reducing subglottic pressures. The tube should be retained until healing is complete and the surgeon is assured that coughing or sudden increases in intrathoracic pressures will not disrupt the soft tissue closure. The timing of extubation is governed by plugging and exercise tolerance.

COMPLICATIONS

1. Infection and/or fistula formation are rare but can occur. To prevent these sequelae, prophylactic antibiotics should be prescribed and a drain employed for 1 to 2 days. The tracheostomy should be retained until healing is complete. If an infection develops in the postoperative period, the soft tissues of the neck should be opened and packed with antibiotic-treated gauze. Cultures should be obtained to determine the appropriate antibiotic treatment of specific pathogens.

2. Incomplete lateralization is probably one of the most common complications and can usually be avoided by complete removal of the arytenoid and the suture lateralization technique. However, if the vocal cord slips back into its original position, the surgeon can remove a portion of the cord with a partial cordectomy through microscopic or laser surgery.

3. Although rare, too much lateralization of the vocal cord can cause aspiration. For most patients, this will improve with time. If it continues, the physician should consider the injection medialization technique (see Chapter 103).

ALTERNATIVE TECHNIQUE USING ENDOSCOPIC ARYTENOIDECTOMY

The arytenoid can also be removed endoscopically by way of laser or surgical resection. The procedure requires expertise and special instrumentation. Exposure can be limited by a small mouth and elements of trismus, and bleeding can be difficult to control. Because of these problems, the arytenoid may

ARYTENOIDECTOMY FOR BILATERAL VOCAL CORD PARALYSIS

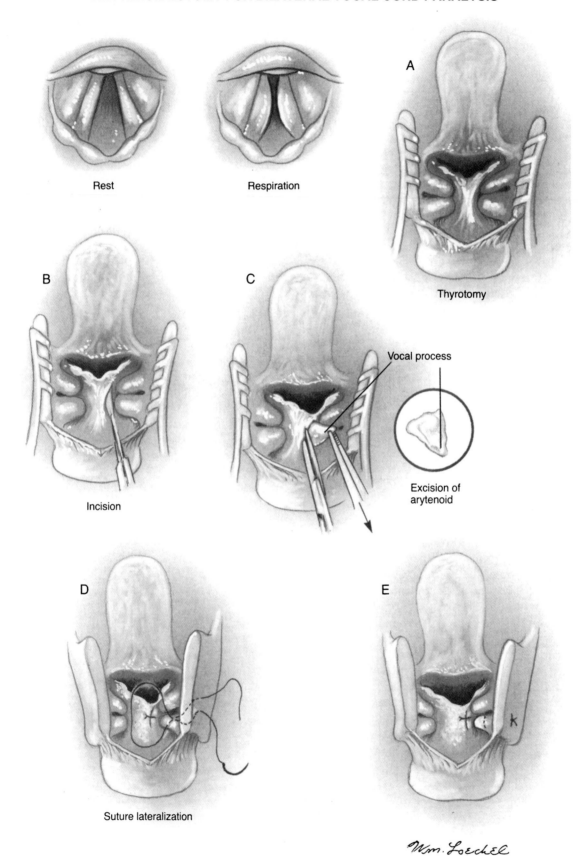

Rest

Respiration

A

Thyrotomy

B

Incision

C

Vocal process

Excision of arytenoid

D

Suture lateralization

E

Wm. Loechel

be only partially removed, and it may be difficult to achieve accurate positioning of the affected cord.

a,b Usually a tracheostomy is performed preliminarily to control anesthesia and prevent respiratory obstruction in the postoperative period. An operating laryngoscope is introduced to expose the glottic chink. An incision is made over the arytenoid, and the arytenoid is grasped with a laryngeal forceps. The cartilage is dissected free from the surrounding tissues. Bleeding can be controlled with an electric cautery, which will also cause more than usual tissue damage and will help develop more scarring and retraction of the vocal cord in the postoperative period. The mucosa is allowed to fall back into its normal position. Transcutaneous wire sutures can be used to lateralize the vocal cords, but because the amount of lateralization from the cauterization cannot be predicted, the lateralization procedure should be used sparingly. The laser method of removal requires special precautions and instrumentation. For this technique, a suitable laser surgery text should be consulted.

ALTERNATIVE TECHNIQUE USING NEUROMUSCULAR PEDICLE REINNERVATION

The lateralization procedure using a neuromuscular pedicle reinnervation requires a careful evaluation of vocal cord mobility. The procedure is contraindicated when there is arytenoid fixation. Results are variable, and the mechanism is still unclear. Although reinnervation may appear to be present, there is some evidence that the airway is actually tethered by the extralaryngeal muscle, and it is this contraction that opens the airway.

a' Tracheostomy is the preferred anesthesia route. The neck is prepared and draped as a sterile field. An incision is made at the midthyroid cartilage level and extended horizontally into a crease on the left side to later expose the left omohyoid muscle.

b' After infiltration with 1% lidocaine containing 1:100,000 epinephrine, the skin is incised through the platysma musculature. The omohyoid is identified at the anterior border of the sternocleidomastoid muscle. Using a blunt dissection, the sternocleidomastoid muscle is retracted posteriorly, exposing the jugular vein and fascia surrounding the vessel. Within this fascia, strands of ansa cervicalis will be found, and a nerve stimulator should be employed to help with this identification. The nerve and some fascia are then freed on a pedicle and kept attached to the omohyoid muscle. Using a microscope with a 250-mm objective lens, a 5- × 5-mm piece of omohyoid innervated by the nerve is excised and allowed to retract into the wound with the nerve pedicle.

c',d' The larynx is then rotated to the opposite side, and using the posterior edge of the lamina as a guide, the thyropharyngeal muscles are incised. A Senn retractor is used to rotate the lamina further, exposing the cricoarytenoid musculature. The arytenoid is palpated beneath the soft tissues. An incision is then made perpendicular to the long axis of the posterior cricoarytenoid muscle. Using the microscope, the omohyoid muscle pedicle is inserted into the defect and held with several 6-0 silk sutures. Tension should be avoided. The thyropharyngeal muscle is reattached to the lamina with chromic sutures (3-0) and the wound treated with a small Penrose drain. The platysma is closed with 4-0 chromic sutures and the skin with 5-0 nylon sutures.

Postoperatively a light dressing is applied. The dressing is removed in 24 to 48 hours. The patient is maintained on prophylactic antibiotics for 5 days. At about 1 or 2 weeks, attempts should be made to plug the tracheostomy tube. Extubation and exercise tolerance dictate the success of the procedure.

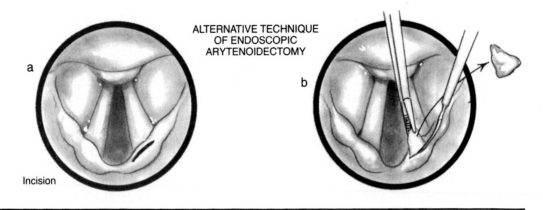

ALTERNATIVE TECHNIQUE
OF ENDOSCOPIC
ARYTENOIDECTOMY

a

Incision

b

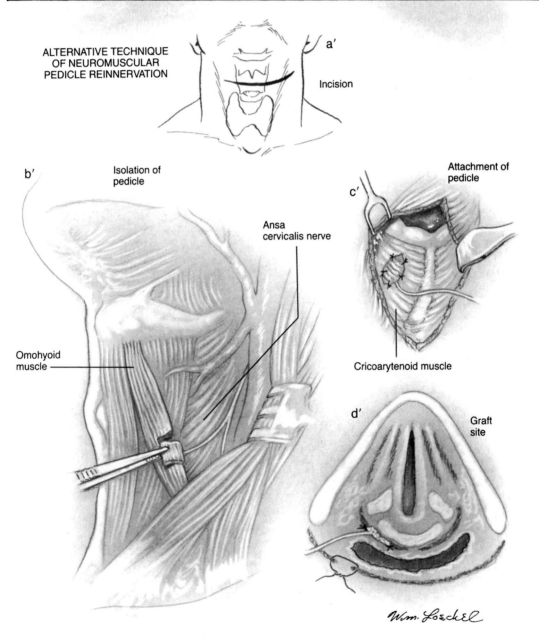

ALTERNATIVE TECHNIQUE
OF NEUROMUSCULAR
PEDICLE REINNERVATION

a'

Incision

b'

Isolation of
pedicle

Ansa
cervicalis nerve

Omohyoid
muscle

Attachment of
pedicle

c'

Cricoarytenoid muscle

d'

Graft
site

Wm. Loechel

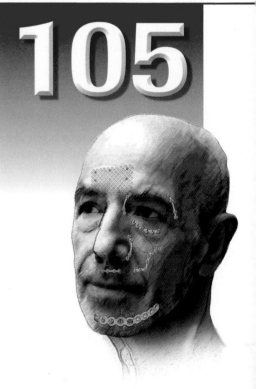

CHAPTER

105

Treatment of Anterior Glottic Stenosis With Advancement of Mucosa, Skin Grafts, and Epiglottic and Interposition Grafts

In Consultation With James Coticchia, MD

INDICATIONS

Depending on the site and degree of injury to the larynx, there can be a variety of soft tissue contractions and stenoses. Supraglottic stenosis is usually caused by a retrodisplacement of the epiglottis and is often associated with injury to the hyoid and upper portions of the thyroid cartilage. An anterior midthyroid cartilage injury will cause shortening of the larynx as thyroid cartilage and soft tissues fill the anterior commissure. Injury to the arytenoid can cause scarring and limitation of vocal cord motion. Below the vocal cords, cricoid or tracheal injury will present with narrowing and/or web formation.

In general, patients with stenosis at any level of the larynx complain of a weak voice, hoarseness, and reduced exercise tolerance. Severely injured patients have respiratory distress and have been previously treated with intubation and/or tracheostomy.

Management of stenosis in the anterior and supraglottic region requires thoughtful design and implementation. A variety of procedures are available, but most focus on resection of the scar and prevention of new scar formation. The majority of the defects can be closed by advancement or rotation of mucosal flaps. More severe injuries in which the airway has been compromised will need interpositional grafts. Posterior glottic and subglottic stenosis, which can complicate the glottic injury, are discussed elsewhere (see Chapters106 through 108).

PROCEDURE

Most approaches to laryngeal scarring will be through a standard thyrotomy (see Chapter 97). A tracheostomy is employed to provide general anesthesia and to control the airway during the postoperative period. A headlight or, even better, a microscope with its own lighting is valuable in performing the procedure.

A,B For the patient with limited supraglottic and anterior glottic stenosis, the thyroid laminae should be separated with self-retaining retractors. The larynx is entered, and small areas of scar tissue are removed. The surgeon has the option of applying a keel, as described in Chapter 100, or undermining and advancing the mucosal tissues with a primary closure using 4-0 or 5-0 chromic sutures. If the area of defect is large and cannot be covered with such flaps, a full-thickness skin graft is harvested from the supraclavicular fossa and carefully sutured with 5-0 or 6-0 chromic sutures to the edge of the normal mucosa. The surgeon can consider a soft or firm stent for holding the graft (see Chapter 98).

C In patients with more extensive damage, the epiglottis can be used to provide the mucosal covering. Through the same thyrotomy exposure, incisions are carried laterally along the superior edge of the thyroid laminae, separating the thyrohyoid membrane from the laminae. The preepiglottic space is entered and a dissection carried out through the vallecula and laterally along the hyoepiglottic fold. The petiole of the epiglottis is then pulled inferiorly, and the soft tissues are used to close the defect created by resection of the scar tissues. If the anterior portion of the thyroid lamina is deficient, the flap is sutured directly to the edge of the thyroid lamina with 3-0 absorbable sutures. If the defect mostly involves the mucosal and soft tissues, portions of the petiole can be resected and the flap advanced into the anterior glottic space. Several sutures can be placed through the soft tissues to secure the flap into position. The more superior edges of the flap are attached also to the thyroid lamina (see Chapter 101). In either case, the result should be a lining of the larynx with the laryngeal surface of the epiglottis.

D If the thyroid laminae are severely damaged, hyoid interposition graft must be considered. The thyrotomy again provides a reasonable approach. The area of scarred tissue (and damaged cartilage) is resected. The hyoid bone is palpated and skeletonized in the midline. The suprahyoid muscles are released with a sharp scissors by cutting very close to the surface of the cartilage. The posterior and medial borders of the sternohyoid and omohyoid muscles are freed up, carefully avoiding injury to the deeper superior laryngeal nerve. The hyoid is cut medially and laterally with a bone-cutting instrument. The deeper thyrohyoid muscle is separated from the hyoid bone. The hyoid and muscle pedicle are then rotated and tested in the laryngeal defect. If there is a denuded surface internally, it should be treated with splints and covered with mucosa or skin grafts. The cartilage graft can then be stabilized with permanent sutures (30-gauge stainless steel wires); the muscle pedicle is attached with 3-0 chromic sutures to the strap muscles of the opposite side. A Penrose drain is used; the platysma and skin are closed in layers.

Patients having anterior glottic reconstructive procedures should be treated with prophylactic antibiotics for 5 to 7 days. If stents are used to stabilize the laryngeal skeleton, they should be removed in 3 to 4 weeks. If they are used only to hold a skin and mucosa graft, they should be removed in 7 to 10 days. Such an approach will minimize the development of granulation tissues. Healing should be evaluated by direct and indirect laryngoscopy. The tracheostomy should be plugged on a trial basis, and when the airway is adequate and there is no aspiration, it can be removed.

PITFALLS

1. If possible, the surgeon should retain viable healthy tissues and try not to use stents or keels. Unfortunately the mucosa may be difficult to undermine and advance over the defect, and when the defect is >0.5 to 1 cm, a graft/stent technique will have to be applied.

2. The epiglottic mucosa provides a reasonably healthy flap that can be manipulated into a variety of defects of the anterior larynx. On the other hand, the anterior displacement of the epiglottis will affect the valve closure, and some aspiration can be expected to occur. This complication is usually transient and should disappear with time as the "supraglottic swallow" is learned. Intermittent plugging of the tracheostomy tube may be helpful.

3. The interposition hyoid graft should be secured to the thyroid laminae in such a way that it does not project or have the potential to become dislodged posteriorly into the larynx. Intralaryngeal stents will offer some security, but the grafts should still be stabilized with nylon or fine wire sutures to the thyroid laminae.

4. Avoid transposing too much tissue into the anterior larynx with the epiglottic and transposition techniques. If this should occur, the vocal cords may remain separated, the voice may be weak, and aspiration may occur. Therefore, it is prudent to place just enough tissue to compensate for the soft tissue defect.

GLOTTIC REPAIR USING FLAPS AND GRAFTS

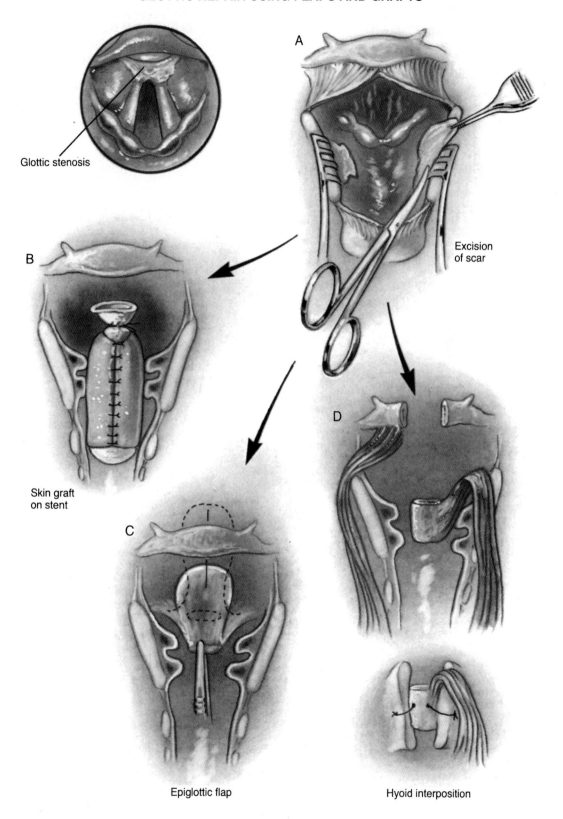

Glottic stenosis

A

Excision of scar

B

Skin graft on stent

C

Epiglottic flap

D

Hyoid interposition

5. Following any manipulation of the airway, repeat endoscopy or keel removal, patients should receive IV Decadron and a Medrol Dosepak on discharge.

COMPLICATIONS

1. Infection can destroy the local tissues, flaps, and/or grafts and cause recurrent scarring. To protect against this occurrence, the wound should be drained for 24 to 48 hours. Prophylactic antibiotics should be used for 5 to 7 days. Internal stents and keels should be used sparingly and removed as soon as possible. Patients with keel placement should receive broad spectrum lactamase stable antibiotics until the keel is removed. All patients should have aggressive antireflux management with a proton pump inhibitor and H_2 blocker at night.

2. Stenosis associated with voice change and respiratory problems can occur. Early recognition of the developing scar tissues should prompt the use of intralesional steroids and dilatation. Endolaryngeal surgery (with or without use of a laser) may be helpful. If a reoperation is necessary, the surgeon will have to consider a wider resection and use of skin/mucosal graft techniques.

3. Aspiration will sometimes occur when the glottic chink has been made too wide. This occurs primarily with epiglottic flaps and interpositional hyoid grafts. The complication can be avoided by placing just enough tissue to fill the defect. If the cords are only slightly lateralized, it might be possible to endoscopically remove some of the intervening tissues or even inject the cord to a more medial position (see Chapter 103).

106

Treatment of Posterior Glottic Stenosis With Interarytenoidopexy and Excision of Subglottic Webs

In Consultation With James Coticchia, MD

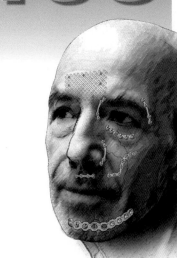

INDICATIONS

Vocal cord paralysis and fixation must be distinguished from each other if the surgeon is to select and apply the appropriate form of treatment. On indirect examination of the vocal cords, the paralyzed vocal cord will be associated with a "still arytenoid," and if seen sometime later, there will be atrophy and thinning of the vocal cord. If the patient with arytenoid fixation phonates, the corniculate process and the aryepiglottic fold will tend to move. The vocal cords will retain their anatomic appearance. Scarring may be observed in the interarytenoid space or in the posterior subglottic region. On direct laryngoscopy, the paralyzed vocal cords will separate on gentle pressure, and the arytenoid can be easily moved to a lateral position with a spatula. When the patient has a fixed cord, the vocal cord will be stiff and the arytenoid difficult to move in any direction. On electromyography, the fixed cord will be characterized by normal action potentials, whereas with paralysis, there will be fibrillation and polyphasic potentials.

The treatments of the two conditions are quite different. Bilateral vocal cord paralysis is often treated with a lateralizing procedure (see Chapter 104), whereas bilateral fixation requires removal of scar tissues between and below the arytenoid and either a flap or skin or mucosal graft coverage. Additionally, the patient may need a cordectomy with or without arytenoidectomy. Unilateral paralysis is generally treated with an injection or implant (see Chapter 103), whereas the unilateral fixed cord requires removal of scar tissue and resurfacing of the mucosa. If this latter procedure fails, the surgeon will also have to consider an implant technique.

PROCEDURE

A tracheostomy is performed to assist in anesthesia and provide a safe airway in the postoperative period. The neck is prepared and draped as a sterile field. A microscope is sometimes helpful in carrying out this reconstruction.

A After infiltration with 1% lidocaine containing 1:100,000 epinephrine, a horizontal incision is made at the level of the inferior aspect of the thyroid cartilage through the platysma to expose the thyroid cartilage, the cricothyroid membrane, and the cricoid. As described in Chapter 97, a vertical anterior splitting incision is made through the cricothyroid membrane and thyroid laminae. The mucosa is then cut in the midline. The thyroid laminae are separated with a self-retaining retractor, the pathologic condition is evaluated, and a procedure is designed to deal with the condition.

For the patient with interarytenoid scarring, the scar is outlined with marking solution. The scar is subsequently excised, and if the underlying interarytenoid muscle is involved, it is conservatively removed with the scar. Bleeding is controlled with an electric cautery.

B–D If the defect is large and involves the surface of the arytenoids, a free graft of skin or mucous membrane should be considered. The graft can be retained by temporary placement of an intralaryngeal soft stent (see Chapter 98). For a more limited injury, the defect can be closed by designing a sliding flap based on the postcricoid mucosa and/or by advancement of local tissues. The mucosa is approximated with 5-0 chromic sutures.

In patients in whom the stenosis is caused by a subglottic web, the scar should be completely resected. The mucous membranes should be undermined, mobilized off the posterior tracheal wall, and advanced superiorly to close over the defect. The mucosa should be approximated with 5-0 or 6-0 chromic sutures. Larger subglottic areas of scarring are discussed in Chapters 107 and 108.

Following repair of the larynx and/or subglottic area, the thyroid laminae are approximated with 2-0 chromic sutures. The perichondrium and platysma are closed with 3-0 chromic sutures and the skin with 5-0 nylon sutures. A subplatysmal 1/4-in Penrose drain is usually retained for 24 to 48 hours.

Postoperatively the patient is treated with prophylactic antibiotics. A light dressing is applied. The laryngeal stent should be evaluated and removed at approximately 7 to 10 days.

PITFALLS

1. An accurate diagnosis and understanding of the pathologic condition are essential for planning of the reconstructive procedure. Elective direct laryngoscopy/bronchoscopy is essential to evaluate the degree of stenosis and inflammation at the glottis airway. Patients with active airway inflammation should be treated with antibiotics, proton pump inhibitors, and a Medrol Dosepak. When stenosis is present, but there is normal recurrent nerve function, the surgeon should use methods that resect the scar or muscle and apply a mucosal reconstruction. Arytenoidectomy should be avoided, because if the arytenoid is resected with intact recurrent nerve function, the adductors may be unopposed and the glottic chink will tend to remain closed. This condition may later require a cordectomy to maintain an open airway. If the patient has a vocal cord paralysis associated with stenosis and there is an airway problem postoperatively, the surgeon will have to consider an arytenoidectomy and then decide whether to resect the vocal cord.

2. Mucosal flaps have a limited blood supply and must be handled with the utmost caution. The flaps should be designed with a broad base. Simple advancement flaps work best, and pedicle rotation flaps have less chance of survival. Closure should be meticulously performed with fine chromic sutures.

3. Avoid stents or splints. Small grafts can often be successful with just suture fixation. Splints tend to rub and cause pressure necrosis; they should only be used when the defects and grafts are large and there is a need to stabilize the larynx (i.e., with fractures of the larynx).

COMPLICATIONS

1. Failure of the technique will result in restenosis, a weak voice, and possibly respiratory difficulty. If such a complication appears to develop, it is probably prudent to perform laryngoscopy, dilate the area of stenosis, and inject the area with triamcinolone. If these attempts to prevent scarring are not successful, the surgeon will have to consider endoscopic and possibly open surgical approaches to effect a satisfactory result.

2. Infection can be avoided by prophylactic antibiotics and drainage of the subplatysmal space. If the patient develops an infection, the neck should be debrided and the wound packed with antibiotic-treated gauze. Cultures should be obtained and appropriate antibiotics administered.

3. To avoid adverse side effects of laryngopharyngeal reflux on wound healing, patients should be started on proton pump inhibitors at the time of initial endoscopy. Patients should be maintained on reflux treatment during the postoperative period to facilitate mucosal wound healing. Signs and symptoms of upper respiratory infection, particularly with cough, should be treated with broad spectrum oral antibiotics.

INTERARYTENOIDOPEXY FOR GLOTTIC STENOSIS

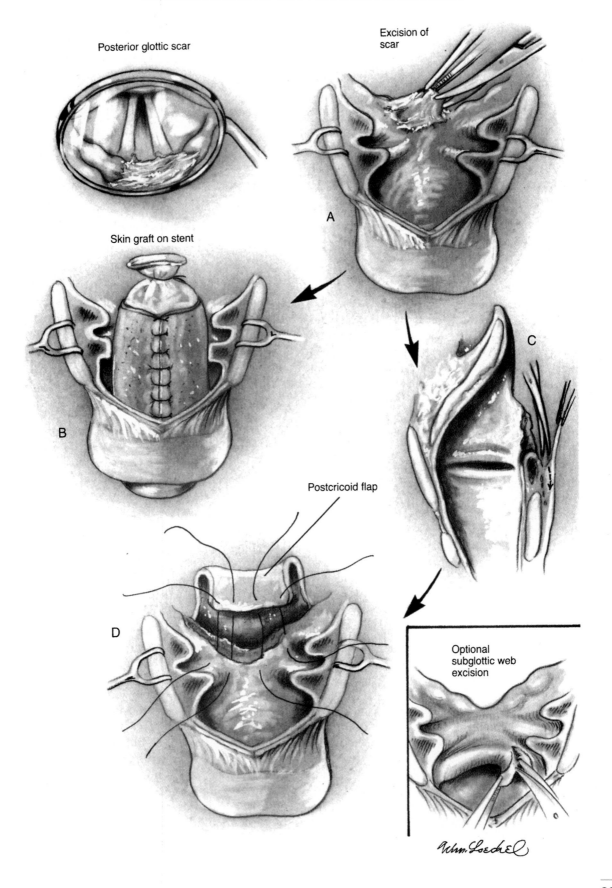

Posterior glottic scar

Excision of scar

Skin graft on stent

A

B

C

Postcricoid flap

D

Optional subglottic web excision

Treatment of Subglottic Stenosis With Endoscopic Laser or Surgical Excision and Dilatation

In Consultation With James Coticchia, MD

INDICATIONS

Stenosis of the subglottic region can result from external blunt trauma, intubation, and/or tracheotomy. Children, because of their narrow subglottic area, are prone to this type of injury; congenital stenosis itself may be an etiologic factor. Tube irritation, pressure necrosis, and infection are also important pathophysiologic considerations.

Early subglottic stenosis can usually be treated with endoscopic forceps or laser resection or by dilatation and intralesional injections of steroids. Failure of treatment may prompt the use of a stent, usually a T tube. If the T tube is not effective in relieving obstruction, the surgeon may have to proceed with external approaches, interpositional grafts, and/or other reconstructive techniques (see Chapters 108 and 109).

PROCEDURE

A low tracheostomy is performed preliminarily to gain control of the airway and provide for anesthesia during the treatment of the stenosis (see Chapter 7). Ideally the tracheostomy should be several centimeters below the area of stenosis so that secretions do not accumulate and predispose to infection. The low tracheostomy also protects the operative site from repeated trauma caused by suctioning and/or manipulation of the tube.

An operating laryngoscope, suitable for the patient's age and mouth opening, is inserted orally and into the larynx. The tip of the scope is then used to spread the vocal cords, and the subglottic area is evaluated. Bronchoscopy may also be applied to help determine the site and extent of injury. Microscopic control and stabilization with a laryngoscope holder are desirable.

A,B Using fine suction tips and a laryngeal forceps, granulation tissues are excised. Alternatively, the surgeon can ablate the involved area with a carbon dioxide laser and, with a microspot technique, preserve a flap for closure. In patients with scar formation, a flap can be developed with microsurgical instruments. Bleeding is controlled with pledgets of 4% cocaine solution. Electrocauterization can be used but only if bleeding cannot be controlled with cocaine and pressure. Following removal of the tissue, bronchoscopes are passed, and the size of the largest bronchoscope that effectively dilates the area is recorded. The subglottic region is then injected through the cricothyroid membrane with a 21-gauge needle containing 40 mg/mL of triamcinolone. The adequacy of the injection is checked with the laryngoscope or bronchoscope.

After the endoscopy, the patient should be maintained on a tracheal cleansing regimen. The tracheostomy should not be plugged until the surgeon is assured of an adequate airway. Prophylactic antibiotics are desirable. Reevaluation of the stenosis should be performed in about 2 weeks. The procedure can then be repeated, but if the subglottic region becomes progressively stenotic, the surgeon should consider a long-term lumen keeper or resection (see Chapters 108 and 109).

PITFALLS

1. Bronchoscopy is initially performed to evaluate the subglottic airway. Patients with >90% stenosis or thick long segments of stenosis are not good candidates for endoscopic procedures and are better served by open technique described in Chapters 108 and 109.

2. Treatment of subglottic stenosis should be based on the site and degree of injury and the maturity of scar formation. Soft scar and granulation tissues can usually be removed with endoscopic laser or surgery. Mature scarred areas may require a more aggressive approach (see Chapters 108 and 109).

3. The surgeon must ensure that the procedures are progressively enlarging the airway. This can be quantitated by bronchoscopic measurements and, if the surgeon chooses, by noting the size of the dilatator and/or bronchoscope that is used to pass through the area.

4. Failure to obtain progressive enlargement should prompt other techniques. The use of a T tube and/or resection must be considered (see Chapters 99, 108, and 109).

COMPLICATIONS

1. Restenosis is the most common complication. This can be avoided by making sure the tracheostomy is several centimeters below the area of endoscopic surgery, and the patient is covered prophylactically with broad-spectrum antibiotics. As the role of laryngopharyngeal reflux has been demonstrated to impair wound healing and lead to recurrent stenosis, preoperative and postoperative proton pump inhibitors are strongly advised. Also a Medrol Dosepak in the postoperative period may be of benefit in maintaining patency of the subglottic space. Reevaluation of the stenosis should take place at about 10 to 14 days, with the option of then excising more tissue and/or injecting the scar with steroid solution. Failure of these techniques should prompt laser methods or application of T-tube and/or resection procedures.

2. Bleeding can develop during and after the procedure. Intraoperative bleeding can be controlled with 4% cocaine pledgets and pressure, but if necessary, the surgeon can apply a laryngeal electrocautery. Blood can be kept from the lungs by keeping the tube cuff inflated and by surveillance and suctioning of the subglottic region. Postoperative bleeding should be treated by inflation of the cuff. If, after several hours, bleeding is still evident, the trachea should be reinspected with an endoscope, at which time hemostatic agents and cautery can be applied.

3. Complications regarding the T-tube procedure are described in Chapter 99.

ENDOSCOPIC EXCISION OF SUBGLOTTIC STENOSIS

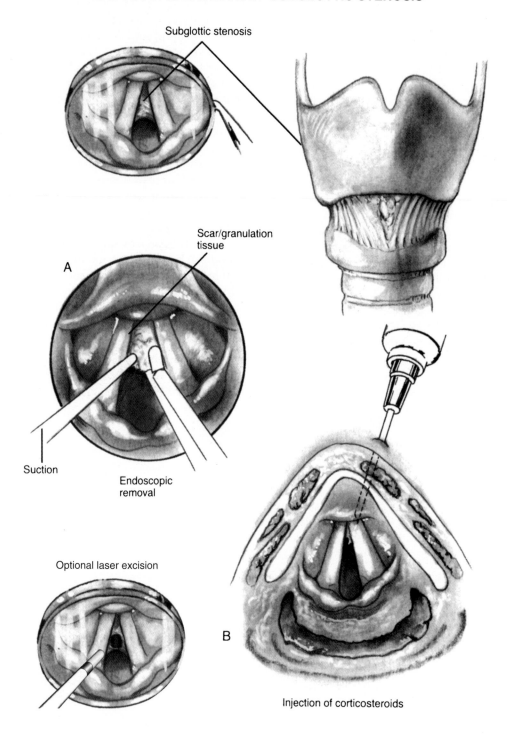

Subglottic stenosis

A

Scar/granulation tissue

Suction

Endoscopic removal

Optional laser excision

B

Injection of corticosteroids

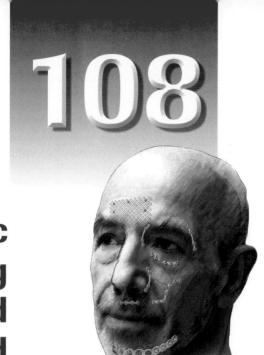

Treatment of Subglottic Stenosis Using Interposition Grafts and Tracheal–Cricothyroid Anastomosis

In Consultation With James Coticchia, MD

INDICATIONS

If excision of subglottic granulations and scar tissues and dilatation, with or without stenting, are unsuccessful, the next step should be a layngotracheal reconstruction (LTR) using a cartilage-splitting procedure with graft enlargement of the airway or resection of the stenosis and advancement of the trachea to the cricoid remnant and thyroid laminae. The interposition graft technique is best considered for conditions of limited damage. If the injury is extensive, involving most of the circumferential ring of cricoid or the first few rings of trachea, then resection followed by direct anastomosis is the best option. Indwelling stents have been described, and although they are important for distant bronchial problems, their efficacy in the trachea has yet to be demonstrated. Fixation of the vocal cords and/ or recurrent laryngeal nerve injury can complicate the preoperative analysis and affect therapeutic options.

PROCEDURE

Prior to starting the procedure, the tracheotomy tube is removed and replaced with a reinforced endotracheal tube in the midline. Patients without a tracheotomy should undergo a local tracheotomy at the beginning of the procedure. Since these patients already have a

significant degree of subglottic stenosis, any manipulation of the airway without a tracheotomy tube in place is not recommended.

A,B After securing the airway, attention is directed at obtaining auricular cartilage as the autologous augmentation graft. The cartilage is harvested medial to the anthelix. A 21-gauge needle with methylene blue is used to determine the anthelix, which is the lateral border of the cartilage graft. An incision is then performed over the posterior aspect of the conchal bowl and a combination of a 15 blade knife and Freer elevator is used to carefully elevate the posterior perichondrium and soft tissue. The cartilage of the choncal bowl can be safely harvested as long as the anthelix is maintained and the lateral border is preserved. The incision is closed with 4-0 Vicryl and 5-0 fast absorbing gut, a rubber band is secured inferiorly and a mastoid dressing is applied.

C,D A horizontal incision approximately 10 cm in length encompassing the tracheotomy is designed and carried down to the subplatysmal plane. Flaps are then elevated to above the superior aspect of the thyroid cartilage and approximately 2 cm distal to the tracheotomy site.

The tracheotomy stoma is carefully dissected to the anterior tracheal mucosa and discarded. All soft tissue in the midline is removed from the superior aspect of the tracheotomy site to above the superior aspect of the thyroid cartilage.

E A rigid bronchoscope with a video camera is carefully advanced to just above the stenotic segment. An assistant then passes a right angle clamp through the tracheotomy site until it is visualized from above with a bronchoscope. If the clamp is not visualized a flexible suction catheter may be passed from either above or below to help identify the lumen. Another option is to use a 16-gauge needle to help identify the lumen in cases of severe stenosis.

Once the clamp is visualized on the video monitor the clamp is spread in the airway. The trachea, cricoids, and thyroid cartilage are incised in the midline with a 12-gauge knife until the stenotic segment is divided. Care should be taken to preserve the anterior commissure. Once the anterior cricoid cartilage is divided, stay sutures are placed and retracted laterally.

F The next step is division of the posterior cricoid lamina. This is an important step as it allows the cricoid ring to be divided in two spots. To perform the posterior cricoid split the patient is placed in steep Trendelenburg, and with the use of a dual head oppositional microscope the posterior cricoid lamina is identified and palpated with a small hemostat. The posterior cricoid split is performed with a fresh 15 blade to the level of the posterior cricoid perichondrium. The posterior cricoid perichondrium is then divided with blunt dissection using a small hemostat. The blunt dissection and microscope prevent injury to the esophagus.

G A finger is then inserted to verify complete division of all posterior cricoids fibers. A Cotton Lorenz stent is then inserted into the airway to verify fit. As a general rule a 12-mm stent fits well into the adult airway. The stent is carefully advanced superiorly until it is just superior to the true vocal cords. This position is verified endoscopically. An estimate is then made of the position where the Jackson tracheotomy tube will enter the stent taking into account the curvature of the tracheotomy tube and the amount of soft tissue anterior to the tracheotomy tube. This position on the stent is marked and drilled out with an approximately 5- to 8-mm bit. The distal portion of the stent is then incised in the midline to allow removal of the Jackson tracheotomy tube. The Jackson tracheotomy tube is then placed inside the stent and any stent distal to the tracheotomy tube is trimmed.

Subsequently, the plane of anesthesia is lightened to the point that the patient is asleep but breathing spontaneously. Through-and-through holes are then drilled into the stent to provide anchor points for the tracheotomy tube to the stent; a 22-gauge wire is used

to secure the metal tracheotomy tube to the stent and then wires are then clamped.

The stent is inserted from below up, and the endotracheal tube is removed and the stent is then advanced inferiorly. A large clamp is useful to facilitate this maneuver. Once the stent is in position, the metal tracheotomy tube is carefully placed into the stent and then secured with the 22-gauge wires. To facilitate anesthesia a small endotracheal tube with a cuff can be placed through the metal tracheotomy tube. The cartilage graft is then secured to the widened anterior defect with 3-0 vicryl sutures. The incision is closed in layers and a through-and-through 1/2 in Penrose is secured with safety pins.

The patient is then transferred to the ICU with appropriate signs to prevent any attempts at manipulation of the metal tracheotomy tube. The Penrose drains are removed postoperative day five, and the patient is discharged with broad spectrum oral antibiotic proton pump inhibitors and an H_2 blocker.

Approximately 6 weeks after surgery the patient is returned to the operating room. After induction of general anesthesia a direct laryngoscopy is performed to evaluate wound healing and stent position. If conditions are optimal a Dedo laryngoscope is suspended and a microscope is used to visualize the stent. A long clamp is then inserted into the stent and clasped firmly. The assistant then cuts the wires and withdraws the wires and metal tracheotomy tube. The cotton Lorenz stent is removed from above and a Shiley tracheotomy tube is placed through the tracheostomy site. The patient is placed on high dose steroids and the tracheotomy tube is capped for 24 hours. If the patient does well, the capped tracheotomy tube is removed and the patient is observed for 48 hours.

H For those patients in whom there is an obvious destruction of most of the cartilage of the cricoid and trachea, a resection should be carried out. The approach is identical to that used in the hyoid interposition procedure described earlier.

Using a bronchoscope to isolate the inferior and superior extent of stenosis, the surgeon should make an incision at the lower level of the involved trauma. The trachea is then transected through the cartilage and the mucosa of the posterior wall. The superior resection is usually directed just above the anterior portion of the cricoid ring and through the cricothyroid membrane. The cut is made diagonally through the ring to preserve the posterior lamina. The intervening tissues are removed, carefully avoiding injury to the recurrent nerves.

I For closure of the defect, the trachea is mobilized upward and the larynx dropped downward. The inferior relaxation is accomplished by a sharp and

TREATMENT OF SUBGLOTTIC STENOSIS USING INTERPOSITION GRAFTS

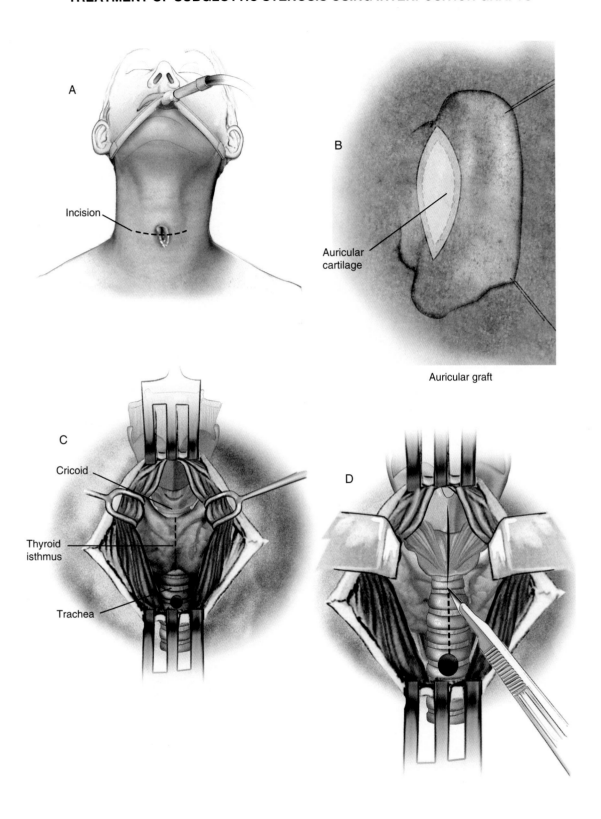

A

Incision

B

Auricular
cartilage

Auricular graft

C

Cricoid

Thyroid
isthmus

Trachea

D

TREATMENT OF SUBGLOTTIC STENOSIS USING INTERPOSITION GRAFTS

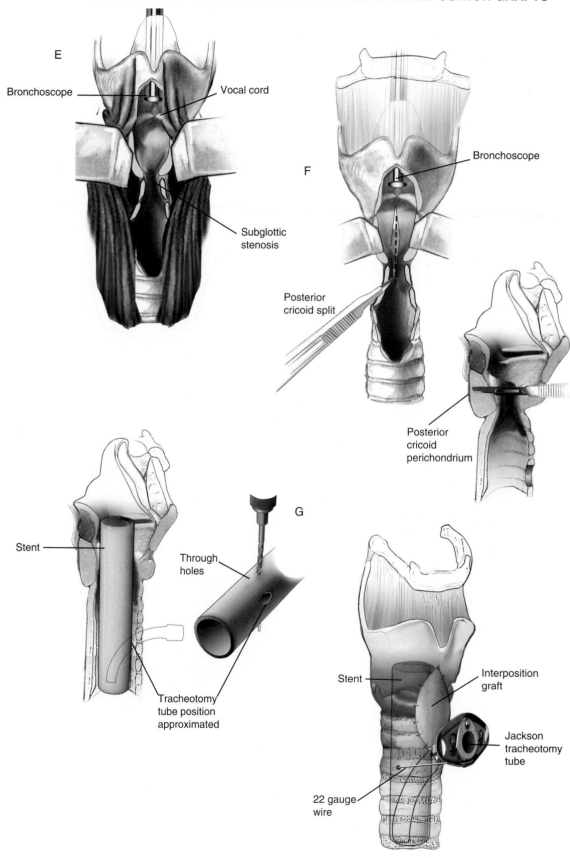

E

Bronchoscope

Vocal cord

Subglottic stenosis

F

Bronchoscope

Posterior cricoid split

Posterior cricoid perichondrium

Stent

Through holes

G

Tracheotomy tube position approximated

Stent

Interposition graft

Jackson tracheotomy tube

22 gauge wire

blunt dissection just deep to the pretracheal fascia. The larynx is released by incising the suprahyoid musculature free from the hyoid bone. The digastric and stylohyoid attachments are usually retained, whereas the body is cut free from the lesser and greater cornua.

J After mobilization of the inferior and superior portion of the airway, the trachea is sutured to the posterior cricoid lamina and the thyroid cartilage. The first sutures are placed posteriorly and the knots directed to the extraluminal surface. The sutures are then placed anteriorly to close the trachea to the thyroid lamina. The wound is irrigated with saline, and a 1/2-in Penrose drain is placed subplastymally. The wound is then closed in layers, with 4-0 chromic sutures through the platysma and 5-0 nylon sutures through the skin. The anode tube is replaced with a tracheostomy tube, and a light compression dressing is applied.

Postoperatively the patient is kept in the flexed position, which is facilitated with tapes running from the head to the chest. Antibiotics are used for 7 to 10 days. The drain is removed in 2 to 4 days and the nasogastric tube in about 10 days.

PITFALLS

1. Patients prior to laryngotracheal reconstruction should undergo direct laryngoscopy/bronchoscopy with biopsy. Particular attention should be directed at level and degree of subglottic stenosis and any supraglottic changes associated with laryngotracheal reflux and inflammation of the airway mucosa. Procedures should be delayed if there is any evidence of active inflammation of the airway. Patients should also be started on reflux medications at the time of endoscopy.

2. Patients with a history of gastroesophageal reflux or airway changes consistent with reflux should undergo a Barium swallow to rule out anatomical issues such as an undiagnosed hiatal hernia. If significant concerns remain, it may also be helpful to obtain a 24-hour pH probe.

3. Patients with significant comorbidities, that is diabetes or significant chronic bronchopulmonary disease are not good candidates for laryngotracheal reconstruction. In addition, patients who are noncompliant and unwilling to follow up postoperatively are at high risk of airway problems following decannulation and may be better served with a stable airway provided by the tracheostomy tube. Patients with other comorbidities should undergo rigorous medical evaluation prior to scheduling the laryngotracheal reconstruction.

4. Relaxation procedures will usually compensate for about 2 to 3 cm of tracheal deficit. If more resection is necessary, the surgeon must consider relaxation either by incising opposite sides of the tracheal rings (annular ligaments) or by releasing the hilum and pulmonary ligaments. For large resections, a thoracic surgeon should be consulted.

COMPLICATIONS

1. The most common complication postoperatively is stenosis of the subglottic region. This problem usually occurs within the first week or two following decanulation. Maintenance of a patient airway following LTR is best achieved by aggressive antireflux proton pump inhibitors twice daily and H2 blockers every evening. In addition, patients are discharged on a Medrol Dosepak and prophylactic oral antibiotics. If patients develop stridor or other airway symptoms they should be admitted and placed on high dose IV steroids and IV antibiotics. This may decrease the need for further surgical intervention of the airway.

2. Another complication that may be encountered is development of a tracheoesophageal fistula. In our experience this problem is best avoided by bluntly separating the posterior perichondrium of the cricoid cartilage. Should a tracheoesophageal fistula develop an exploration is indicated, carefully identifying the party wall and reinforcing this area with local myofascial flaps and placement of a Dobhoff tube for feeding. The Dobhoff is left in place for 2 weeks at which point a barium swallow is obtained to verify closure of the fistula.

3. Hematoma of the cartilage donor site is commonly encountered in the initial postoperative period. This problem can usually be treated by needle aspiration followed by a tight mastoid dressing.

4. Recurrent laryngeal nerve paralysis can adversely affect the results. Knowledge of the anatomy of the recurrent nerve should prevent most injury, and particular care should be taken during retraction of the thyroid gland. The resection of the stenosis should be carried out in a subperichondrial plane. If the patient shows signs of nerve paralysis postoperatively, the surgeon should then wait 6 to 9 months, and if there is no return of function, one of the techniques described in Chapters 103 and 104 should be applied.

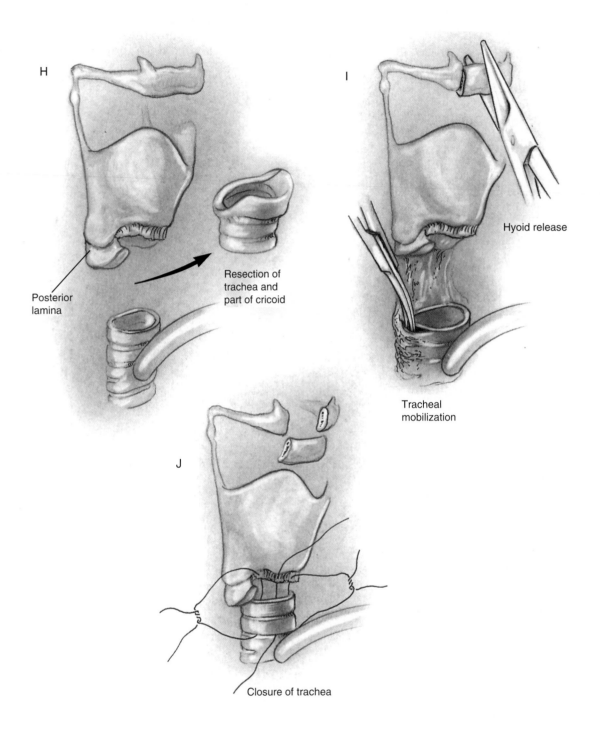

H

Posterior
lamina

Resection of
trachea and
part of cricoid

I

Hyoid release

Tracheal
mobilization

J

Closure of trachea

CHAPTER

109

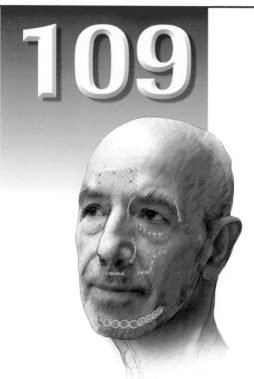

Treatment of Tracheal Stenosis With Segmental Resection and Anastomosis
Alternative Techniques of T-Tube Reconstruction and Wedge Resection

In Consultation With James Coticchia, MD

INDICATIONS

Tracheal stenosis is characterized by a narrowing of the trachea below the subglottic region and above the carina. Usually this is caused by intubation and/or tracheostomy, but occasionally it is the result of blunt or penetrating trauma. Pressure, necrosis at the tube tip, and scarring at the tracheostomy site are commonly implicated factors. Once the diagnosis is made, it is important to establish an airway below the area of

obstruction and then, with endoscopy, CT Scans, and basic swallowing and pulmonary function tests, determine the extent of injury and the degree of incapacitation. During initial bronchoscopy, evidence of infection or any granulation tissue should be addressed prior to definitive resection.

In general, resection of the trachea is indicated in acute trauma when there has been extensive damage and in cases of chronic stenosis in which there has been a collapse or buckling of at least 3 to 5 cm of the trachea. If the stenosis is caused by granulation tissues and early soft scar, excision and dilatation and even long-term stents (T tubes) can be used. If the lesion involves the anterior wall or less than two to three rings, the surgeon can use a wedge resection with or without an interpositional graft (see Chapter 108). The segmental resection is contraindicated in patients who are severely debilitated, who require permanent tracheostomy, and in whom there is laryngeal incompetence.

PROCEDURE

A Anesthesia is administered through an anode tube placed through a prior tracheostomy. The neck is extended by placing a blanket roll under the shoulders. The neck and chest are prepared and draped as a sterile field.

B The incision is designed to remove the old tracheostomy wound. A collar incision is thus created, and a vertical incision is also drawn down to the jugular notch. The area is infiltrated with 1% lidocaine containing 1:100,000 epinephrine to assist in hemostasis.

C The dissection is carried through the platysma layer, and a superior flap is elevated to the level of the thyroid cartilage. Two inferolateral flaps are developed in a similar plane to expose the strap muscles. The sternohyoid and sternothyroid muscles are retracted laterally and the tracheostomy separated from the adjacent scar tissues. Pretracheal fascia is incised and the trachea exposed inferiorly. If the thyroid gland is obscuring vision, it should be divided and ligated to expose the upper trachea and cricoid.

D At this point, the anesthesiologist should introduce a nasotracheal tube. Under visual guidance, the anode tube is removed and the endotracheal tube passed through the stenosis. Vertical incisions through the area of stenosis will help pass the tube.

Having achieved control of the airway below the stenosis, vertical incisions are then used to assess the extent of stenosis in the area to be resected. Tracheal rings are usually removed by way of subperiosteal dissection from the adjacent scar tissues. The mucosa on the posterior wall is dissected free from the tracheoesophageal space.

E Closure is initiated by relaxation techniques. The inferior release is accomplished by a sharp and blunt dissection beneath the pretracheal fascia. This can be facilitated by a finger dissection below the clavicle and sternum. Above, the body of the hyoid is separated from the lesser and greater cornua and freed from the suprahyoid musculature as described in Chapter 108.

F,G The trachea is closed with extralumenally placed 3-0 polyglactin sutures. The sutures are first positioned posteriorly and left loose. The anterior sutures are then placed, and the sutures are tied sequentially from posterior to anterior. Additional relaxation can be obtained by removing the shoulder roll and flexing the head. The strap muscles are subsequently closed in the midline, and a medium-sized suction drain is placed between the strap muscles and platysma. The platysma is closed with 3-0 chromic sutures and the skin with 5-0 nylon sutures.

To reduce inflammation and postoperative granulation tissue patients should be given broad spectrum oral antibiotics and proton pump inhibitors. The endotracheal tube should be retained until the patient is alert and breathing without difficulty. Postoperative bucking and coughing should be avoided. A bandage should be placed from the head to the chest to hold the head in a position of flexion for 2 to 3 weeks. If a significant amount of mobilization is needed a suture should be secured from the mentum to the sternum to keep the neck flexed and to reduce tension on the anastomosis.

PITFALLS

1. The area of stenosis dictates the degree of resection. Because small lesions can be handled with limited excision and larger lesions require resection and anastomosis, the size of the lesion should be assessed with a bronchoscope before the resection is performed. The technique is described in Chapter 108.

2. Resections larger than 5.0 cm require additional relaxation techniques. For such procedures, annular ligaments between the trachea can be incised on alternate sides, and if more length is needed, the resection should be performed by relaxation of the right hilum and pulmonary ligaments.

3. Airway management is challenging. The surgeon has the option during the procedure to place an anode at the lower portion of stenosis or intubate directly by way of an oral endotracheal tube. The method of choice will be dictated by the pathologic condition. In general, the endotracheal tube is used during the anastomosis and removed soon after surgery. However, if there is concern (i.e., too much tension or poor anastomosis), a temporary tracheostomy tube can be placed below the area of resection.

4. The objectives of the procedure are to remove mucosa, cartilage, and scar tissue and bring the trachea together; recurrent nerve injury should be avoided. This can be accomplished by dissecting close to the cartilage and the mucosal surface.

5. For stenosis that does not require resection, other techniques can be employed. Portions of the

TREATMENT OF TRACHEAL STENOSIS WITH SEGMENTAL RESECTION

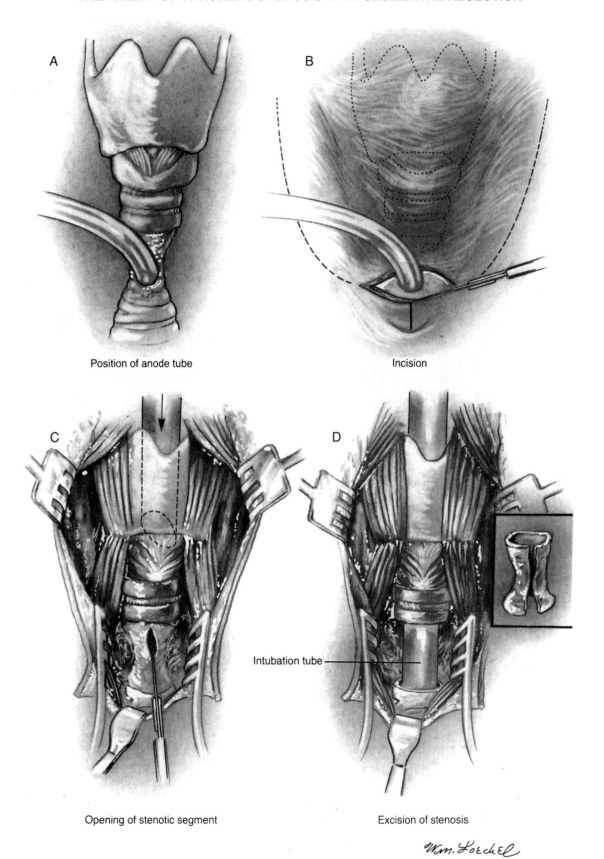

A

Position of anode tube

B

Incision

C

Opening of stenotic segment

D

Intubation tube

Excision of stenosis

Wm. Loechel

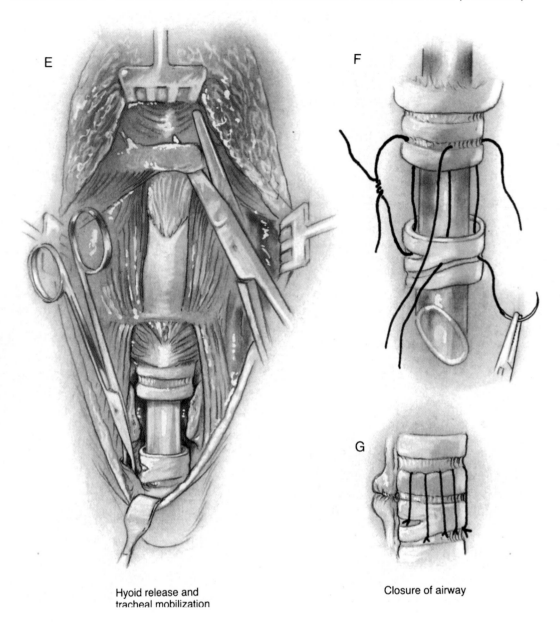

E

Hyoid release and
tracheal mobilization

F

G

Closure of airway

anterior tracheal wall can be removed with or without T tubes. Interpositional grafts can also be employed (see Chapter 108).

6. For high lesions involving the subglottic space, part of the cricoid can be resected with the trachea. This reconstruction is described in Chapter 108.

7. Tension is relieved at the suture line by any of a number of techniques: (1) upward mobilization of the trachea, (2) relaxation of the larynx, (3) neck flexion, and (4) annular ligament incisions on opposite sides of the trachea. If these are not sufficient, an intrathoracic procedure will have to be carried out to release the traction at the pulmonary hila.

8. Postoperative care is important. The patient should be in an intensive care unit, and bucking and coughing should be avoided. When the patient is stabilized, the endotracheal tube can be removed and the patient's head and neck kept in a flexed position until the wounds have healed.

COMPLICATIONS

1. One of the causes of recurrent stenosis is wound infection. Thus the chances for infection should be minimized by use of prophylactic antibiotics and drainage of the subplatysmal space. If infection develops, the wound should be opened and treated with debridement and packed with gauze. Pathogen-specific antibiotics should be employed. Limited scarring can be treated with endoscopic techniques. For recurrent significant stenosis, the surgeon should consider T-tube placement and/or permanent tracheostomy.

2. Separation at the suture line is rare, but if it occurs, the patient will develop granulation tissue and possibly respiratory distress. The tension should be relieved by one or several relaxation methods described above. Granulation tissues can be treated conservatively with endoscopic surgery or laser techniques.

3. Recurrent laryngeal nerve injury can develop and cause problems with laryngeal competence. After splitting the thyroid isthmus and thyroid laminae, the surgeon should remember the course of the nerve and its entry into the cricoarytenoid region. Injury should also be avoided by using a subperichondrial dissection and trying to remove only scarred cartilage and mucosa. If one or both nerves become impaired, one of the specialized techniques described in Chapters 103 or 104 can be employed.

4. Esophageal injury with tracheoesophageal fistula is possible, especially if the "party wall" is injured during the resection of the trachea. To avoid this problem, the dissection should be limited to the mucosa only. The nasogastric tube within the esophagus should give a clue as to the location and depth of the esophageal mucosa. However, if a fistula develops, repair with a muscle interposition must be considered.

5. Airway problems as a result of this procedure can also occur. The surgeon should thus be certain that the patient is breathing quietly and without distress on removal of the endotracheal tube. If there is any respiratory difficulty, the surgeon should inspect the airway to evaluate competency of the larynx (i.e., for recurrent laryngeal nerve injury). A formal endoscopy is necessary if a tracheal separation is suspected. In the presence of such a condition, endotracheal intubation or a new tracheostomy, or both, is indicated.

ALTERNATIVE TECHNIQUE OF T-TUBE RECONSTRUCTION

When the tracheal stenosis is soft and characterized more by malacia than by stenosis, a **T** tube should be considered. This procedure is also indicated when excision and dilatation (with or without stents) has failed and when there are lacerations and "weaknesses" of the tracheal walls from acute tracheal trauma.

a–d The procedure is usually carried out using endoscopic methods and exposure through the tracheostomy site. An endotracheal or tracheostomy tube is used for control of the airway. If the stenosis is at or above the tracheostomy site, the trachea should be explored by way of a horizontal incision. Strap muscles are separated from the midline, and the thyroid isthmus is divided. Bleeding is controlled by silk ligatures and/or cauterization. The area of stenosis is exposed, the pretracheal fascia is elevated, and the trachea is incised over the affected area. After excision of the stenosis and/or granulation tissues, the defect can be left open anteriorly or optionally reconstructed with a small cartilage graft. The **T** tube, used as a stent, is placed through the tracheostomy so that the upper limb is just above the area of resection (see Chapter 99). The soft tissues (i.e., strap muscles) are then approximated in the midline over the defect. A Penrose drain is inserted and the platysma and skin closed in layers.

Usually the **T** tube is left in place for several months. Radiographs should be obtained and a hairline radiolucency noted around the tube before it is removed. Crusting can be a problem and must be controlled with humidification and suctioning. If the **T** tube becomes plugged, it should be removed and temporarily replaced with a tracheostomy tube. **T**-tube complications are discussed in Chapter 99.

ALTERNATIVE TECHNIQUE OF WEDGE RESECTION

Stenosis characterized by exuberant soft tissues probably can be corrected by one of the endoscopic techniques with or without stenting. However, if the stenosis is limited to a small area of the trachea or an anterior area of the tracheal wall, a partial wedge resection can be considered. If the patient has any form of incompetency of the larynx, the procedure is probably contraindicated.

a',b' For the wedge resection, the tracheostomy tube is converted to an anode tube, and the tracheostomy opening is elliptically excised as part of the collar incision. The skin flaps are elevated in a subplatysmal plane, and the strap muscles are retracted from the midline. The tracheostomy site is dissected free from surrounding tissues. The level and length of stenosis should be confirmed by endoscopic methods. A transoral endotracheal tube is inserted beyond the area of stenosis, and the anode tube is removed. The anterior wall of the trachea is resected. The defect is closed with a cartilage-to-cartilage ring anastomosis using 3-0 chromic or polyglactin sutures.

TREATMENT OF TRACHEAL STENOSIS

ALTERNATIVE TECHNIQUE OF T-TUBE INSERTION

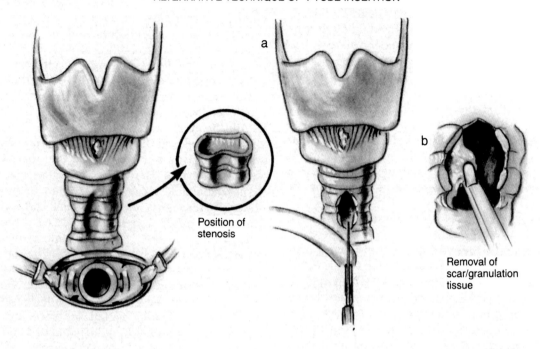

a

Position of
stenosis

b

Removal of
scar/granulation
tissue

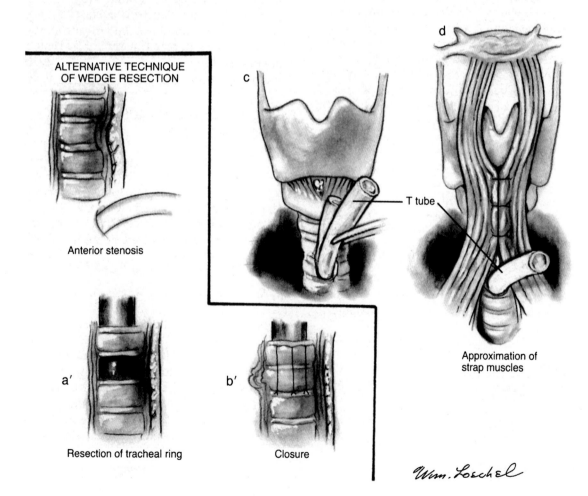

ALTERNATIVE TECHNIQUE
OF WEDGE RESECTION

Anterior stenosis

c

d

T tube

a′

Resection of tracheal ring

b′

Closure

Approximation of
strap muscles

Wm. Loschel

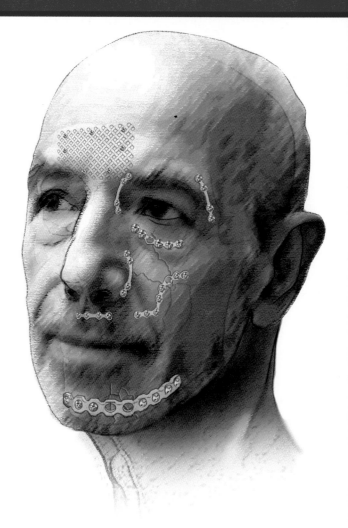

PART FOURTEEN

Children's Injuries

Pathophysiology of Children's Injuries

CHAPTER 110

General Considerations

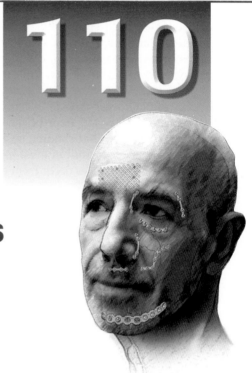

Children are different from adults, and because of these differences, the evaluation of craniofacial injuries and strategies for management require special consideration.

Children's anatomy dictates to a great extent the site and degree of injury. An important factor is the external force that can be put on the child's craniofacial skeleton. Since force is determined by mass and acceleration, the smaller the child, the lesser the impact and injury. The small stature of a child however becomes a disadvantage when confronted and attacked by an aggressive animal.

A–C The skeletal proportions also play an important role in defining the most likely site of injury. In early childhood, most of the craniofacial skeleton is made up of cranium and therefore the injury is most likely to occur to the cranial cavity and skull base rather than the facial bones. Sinuses are poorly developed, and this provides relative strength and stability to the buttresses and beams of the face. Maxillary fractures are thus rare in the small child. The nose has relatively a larger amount of cartilage compared to bone

resulting in flexibility and resistance to fracture. The developing mandible has a mixture of deciduous and permanent teeth providing little room for the thin cortex, thus predisposing this bone to easier fracture. Over time, the mandible will thicken (ridges) as a result of stress and develop areas resistant to fracture. In general, the bones of the child are fairly elastic and tend to develop a greenstick fracture rather than fragment and move out of place from an external force.

D,E From a physiologic standpoint, the craniofacial skeleton of the child develops from a coordination of growth centers and a functional matrix "in which the soft tissue envelope becomes filled with appropriate structures." Growth centers are found in the condyle of the mandible and in the septal/ethmoid areas, and injury to these areas can cause jaw deformity, malocclusion, and hypoplasia in the midface. Additional injury from surgery must be avoided. Development of teeth within the mandible must be considered, and to prevent injury, the surgeon must use arch bars, Ivy loops, or mini (micro) plates to the inferior border of the mandible. Care must be taken not to extract the deciduous teeth, and monocortical screws should just penetrate the cortex to avoid injury to the deeper structures. Since growth can be restricted by titanium plates, resorbable materials are now popular.

The behavior of children and parents also affects the possibility of injury. Parental supervision will frequently prevent the child from accident. Nevertheless, children cannot be monitored all the time and their inquisitiveness and fearlessness can lead to untoward sequela. Children are thus prone to falls, bicycle accidents, and injury from sports and fights. As an unrestrained passenger in a car they are also subject to severe craniofacial injury. Children are also prone to provoke animals into causing bites and around the house, the child can bite on electrical cords causing damage to the lip and floor of the mouth. It should also be recognized that children sustain frontal blows to the midface as a result of most injuries, whereas in the adults, most injuries occur from the side as a result of altercations.

The incidence of fracture will depend upon the age of the child with more occurring as the child matures. In general the child accounts for 5% of all craniofacial injury. Nasal fractures are the most common and outweigh mandible fractures 2-1. Maxillary, frontoethmoid, and zygomatic fractures are relatively rare.

In evaluating the child for degree and extent of injury, it should be noted the child has a relatively small airway and it does not take much displacement of soft tissues, that is tongue, larynx, etc. to cause respiratory difficulty. Surgeons should be prepared to insert a nasal trumpet, oral airway, or intubation tube. A tracheostomy or cricothyroidomy in some situations must be considered (Chapters 6 and 7).

A child has a relatively small blood volume and does not tolerate blood losses that could be managed in adults. It thus becomes prudent to establish early an intravenous line in which blood and blood substitution products can be administered. For optimal evaluation, cooperation of the child is desirable. Calm reassurance may be sufficient but in some cases judicious use of sedation may be necessary. In addition to a history and physical examination, it will be necessary to obtain appropriate imaging studies-CT scans and MRIs. Consultation with a neurosurgeon and/or ophthalmologist may be necessary.

FRACTURES IN CHILDREN

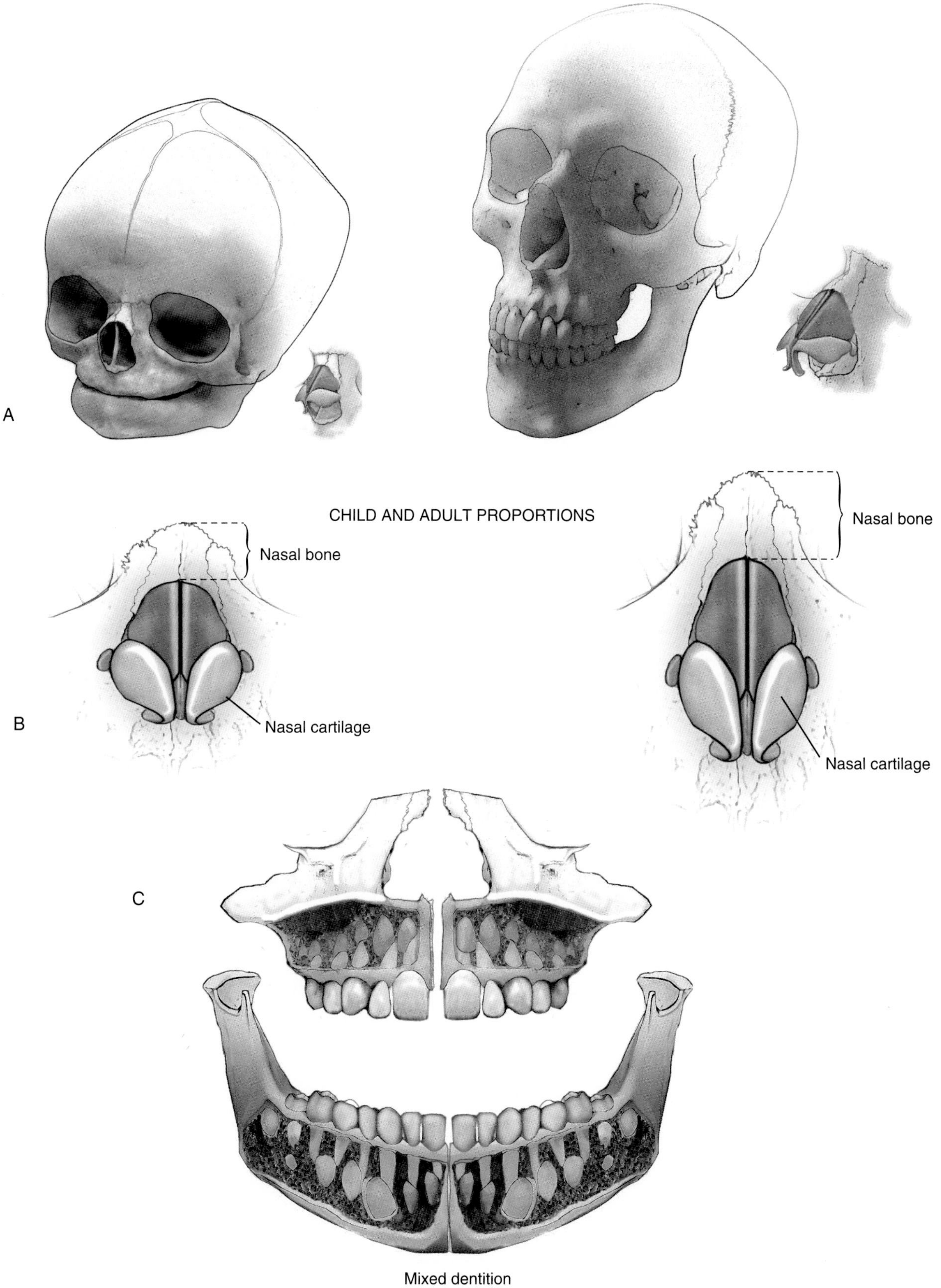

A

CHILD AND ADULT PROPORTIONS

Nasal bone

Nasal bone

Nasal cartilage

Nasal cartilage

B

C

Mixed dentition

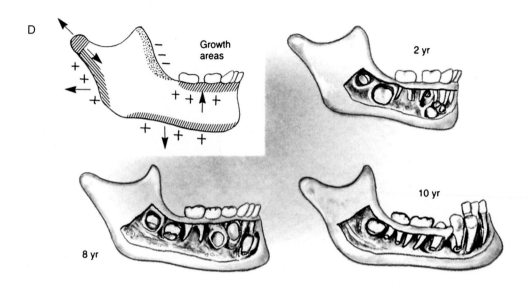

D

Growth areas

2 yr

8 yr

10 yr

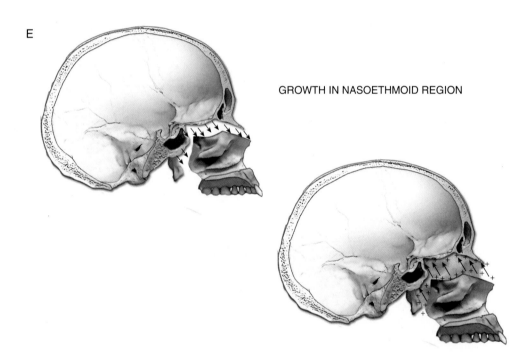

E

GROWTH IN NASOETHMOID REGION

General Techniques for Treating Facial Fractures in Children

CHAPTER

111

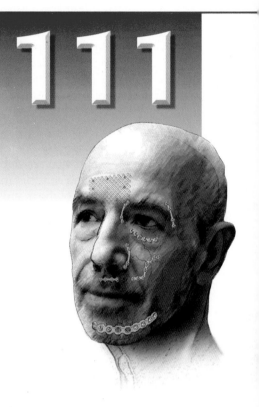

Open and Closed Repair of Facial Fractures in Children
Alternative Technique of Resorbable Plates

INDICATIONS

The mainstay of treating children's injury is conservative management. Management strategies rely on growth center activity, the development of a functional matrix, and rapid healing to correct and obtain structural and functional recovery. Fractures that are displaced and are not reduced easily will require intervention and, in most cases, some degree of stabilization to prevent displacement and encourage healing. In contrast to adults, periods of immobilization in children are short (2 to 4 weeks) and exercise becomes important in the rehabilitation process.

PROCEDURE

Mandibular Fractures

A Fractures of the symphysis, body, and angle of the mandible are usually treated conservatively with soft diet and analgesics assuming that the fracture is not displaced and/or mobile on mastication. For all others, the surgeon must consider some degree of intervention. This can take the form of intermaxillary fixation and/or open reduction and fixation with small plates and monocortical screws. Resorbable plating materials are desirable.

Surgical management depends upon the age of the child and degree of development of deciduous and permanent teeth. The following guidelines are suggested:

TIME	MANAGEMENT
0–2 years	During this period, teeth are unerupted and deciduous/permanent tooth buds are found within the body of the mandible. In such cases, a lingual splint should be applied with circummandibular wires. A lingual splint (Chapter 29) can be a device made of acrylic material applied to the alveolar ridge or a manufactured splint made from an impression of the jaws. Alternatively a resorbable miniplate or microplate can be placed below the tooth buds with monocortical screws applied to avoid injury to the deep tissues.
2–4 years	During this period, deciduous teeth erupt and permanent teeth are in the process of developing. Stable deciduous teeth can be placed in intermaxillary fixation with Ivy loops or arch bars or a mini (micro) plate can be placed along the lower border of the jaw. Monocortical screws are recommended. As an alternative, resorbable plates can be applied to avoid restriction of mandibular growth.
5–8 years	During this time, roots of deciduous teeth are being reabsorbed and these teeth are being shed from the jaw. There still are unerupted permanent teeth. Intermaxillary fixation can be applied to molars that are stable in their socket, but when they are loose, the surgeon should avoid extraction and consider the application of a miniplate, microplate, or bioabsorbable plate to the inferior border of the mandible.
9–11 years	During this time, the permanent teeth are in and the jaw is almost fully developed. Adult methods can be applied.

When faced with a condylar fracture, the management issues are controversial and there are several reasonable approaches. Many surgeons believe that the condylar fracture should be treated conservatively with intermaxillary fixation (Ivy loops or arch bars) for 2 weeks followed by elastic band exercises (see Chapter 19). Others believe that the condylar growth center must be repaired with open reduction and fixation (see Chapter 21). Still there is concern that surgical intervention causes further damage to the growth center.

In general open reduction and fixation can be considered for markedly displaced heads and necks of the condyle that do not reduce in 2 weeks, injury to the middle cranial fossa and/or external auditory canal and foreign bodies in the area of fracture.

Maxillary Fractures

B Many maxillary fractures are of the greenstick variety and can be treated successfully with analgesics and soft diet. For those fractures that are comminuted and/or displaced, open reduction and fixation with intermaxillary fixation may be necessary. Miniplate fixation with resorbable materials are placed deep to soft tissues (see Chapters 40 through 43).

Nasal Fracture

C Many nasal fractures in children are characterized by a splaying laterally of the nasal bones. Rapid healing mandates a closed reduction within several days of the injury and certainly before 1 week to 10 days after the injury. General anesthesia is the rule of thumb followed by application of a topical anesthetic and a nerve block (see Chapter 52). Subsequently each nasal bone is elevated laterally with a Boise elevator and then pinched toward the midline to provide a projected dorsum. Mobilization is obtained by internally placed antibiotic treated tampons for 2 days and an external cast for 5 days to prevent splaying.

Zygomatic and Orbital Fractures

Fractures in the periorbital area are treated as if the child were an adult. Double vision and/or enophthalmos or evidence of marked displacement of a wall or floor on CT Scan are indications for open reduction and repair with mesh or bone grafts (see Chapter 62). Displaced zygomatic fractures may require open reduction and fixation with miniplates again using resorbable materials applied to buttresses deep to the surface (see Chapter 57).

Naso-Orbital Fractures

Although rare, significant anteriorly to posteriorly directed forces can lead to displacement of the naso-orbital complex. In such cases displaced bone fragments need to be reduced either by elevation or by pulling the fragments into position with a towel clip

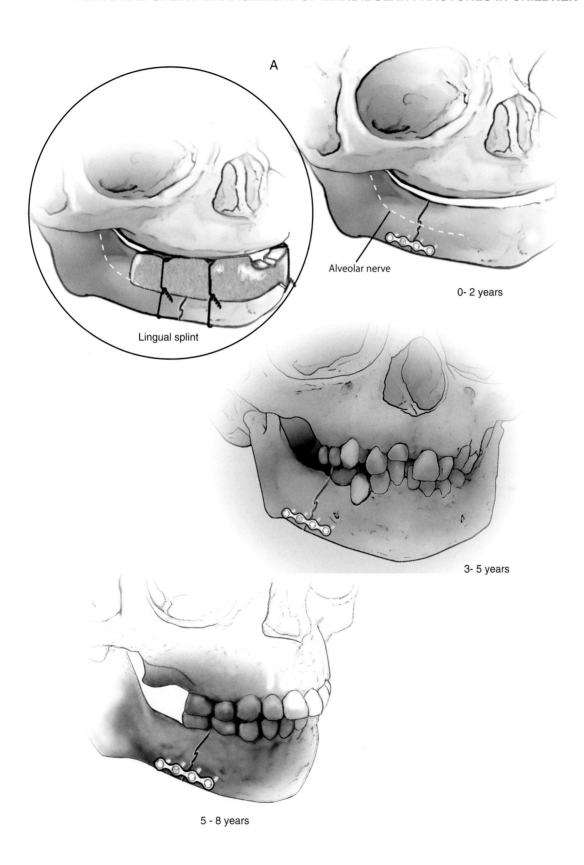

A

Alveolar nerve

Lingual splint

0- 2 years

3- 5 years

5 - 8 years

INTERMAXILLARY FIXATION MANAGEMENT OF MANDIBULAR FRACTURES IN CHILDREN

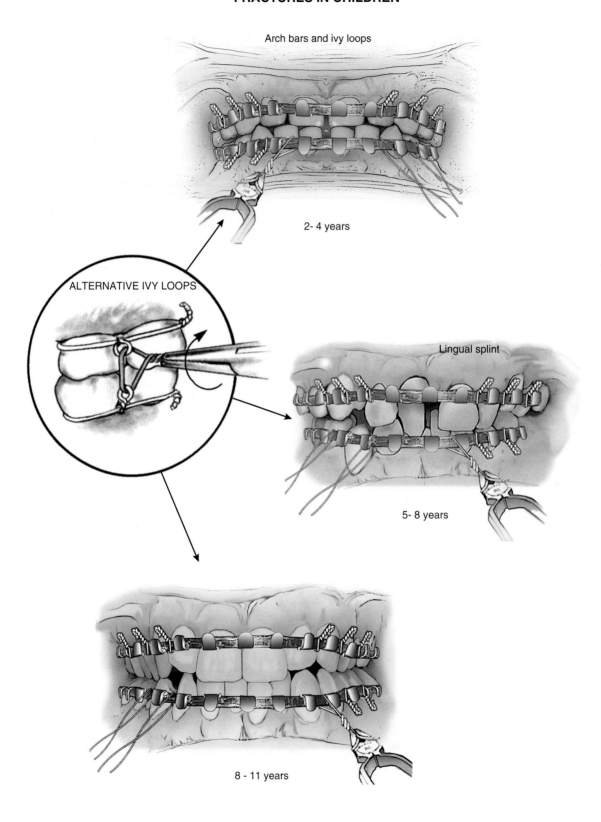

Arch bars and ivy loops

2- 4 years

ALTERNATIVE IVY LOOPS

Lingual splint

5- 8 years

8 - 11 years

MANAGEMENT OF MAXILLARY FRACTURES IN CHILDREN

B

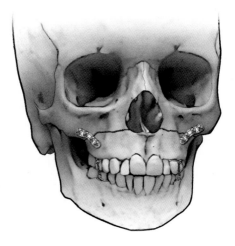

MANAGEMENT OF NASAL FRACTURES IN CHILDREN

C

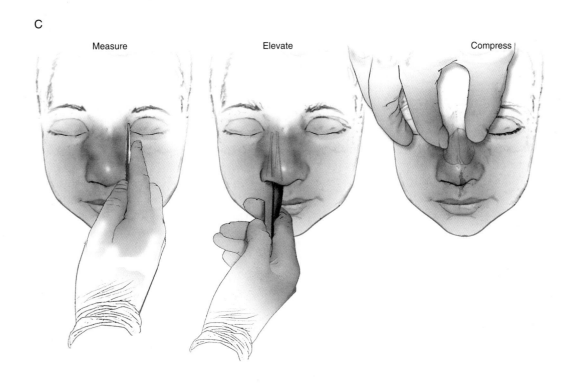

Measure   Elevate   Compress

(see Chapter 70). If the fracture is stable, plate fixation can be avoided. Repair of the medial canthal ligament (Chapters 67 through 69) will be necessary when there is comminution of medial wall of the orbit and/or lateral displacement of the eyelids but this is rare in children.

PITFALLS

1. Remember that the recovery in children from injury is rapid with a tendency to regenerate and reform normal architecture. This mandates conservative management with rare use of open reduction and fixation.

2. Avoid injury to growth centers that can lead to atrophy and dysfunction.

3. Avoid injury to developing teeth and extraction of deciduous teeth. Do not apply IMF to loose teeth and protect developing teeth and growth areas with monocortical screws and small (resorbable) plates.

4. Extended periods of immobilization of the jaws with intermaxillary fixation should be avoided as this may lead to ankylosis and long lasting trismus.

5. Titanium plates may restrict bone growth and probably should be substituted with resorbable plates when possible. Some surgeons recommend removal of titanium plates after a period of healing.

6. Greenstick fractures are usually stable and do not require fixation.

7. Nasal fractures should be treated within the first 5 to 7 days or else they may heal in malposition as a result of rapid healing.

8. Symptomatic blow-out fractures posterior to the equator of the globe must be recognized and repaired early to prevent enophthalmos and diplopia. Care should be taken to avoid injury to the optic nerve.

COMPLICATIONS

1. The atrophic mandible can be a complication of injury to the growth center of the condyle. Since open reduction and fixation can cause additional injury, the open approach should only be used when indicated. Should the mandible develop atrophy or malocclusion, the surgeon should consider orthodontia and/or orthoganthic surgery. Bone grafts and/or bone distraction methods may be necessary.

2. Hypoplasia of the maxilla can also occur as a result of injury to the growth centers in the septum and nasoethmoid complex. As in the mandibular deformity, sequela can be managed by orthodontia and/or orthognathic surgery (see Chapters 48 through 50).

3. Flattening or widening of the dorsum, saddle deformity, and hypoplasia of the nose can also occur following trauma. Most surgeons will wait until the child reaches maturity for correction but if the child has trouble breathing through the nose, surgery can be performed at an earlier time. The surgery is often a type of septorhinoplasty that will augment the nose with cartilage and/or bone.

4. Non union in the child is extremely rare. A moderate degree of malunion should be tolerated in as much as remodeling and reformation will occur. Conservative approaches are desirable.

ALTERNATIVE TECHNIQUE OF RESORBABLE PLATES (EPPLEY METHOD)

a–e Fractures of the mandible are usually exposed through an intraoral approach. Depending upon the age of the child and status of dentition, the reduction is accomplished by Ivy loops, arch bars, or by manual reduction of the fracture to approximate centric occlusion. The surgical exposure should show the lower margin of the mandible and avoid injury to the mental nerve. Following reduction a resorbable plate with at least two screw holes available on each side of the fracture is held in position. If the plate does not mold easily to the mandible then it should be warmed in a water bath or suitable heating media. Using short drill bits (usually under 5 mm in length), drill holes are placed in the outer cortex of the mandible. Drill holes are then tapped to cut screw threads. Resorbable screws of 4 to 5 mm are inserted to provide stability to the plate. Usually the plate will contour to the mandible without additional heating.

Monocortical screws usually will not strike a developing tooth bud and if placed inferiorly will often miss the area of developing teeth. The absorbable nature of the screws and plates will prevent migration into the bone tissues and moreover, there is less chance of restricting growth in the area of repair. Some of the more recent advances use sonic welding to obtain a more secure attachment.

These techniques can be applied to other fractures of the craniofacial skeleton. A prudent approach however is to apply these plates to areas which are covered abundantly with soft tissues since these plates can cause inflammation and reaction in that area. For zygomatic and maxillary fractures, the plates are optimally placed along the zygomaticomaxillary buttresses, avoiding plates in thin areas such as the nasal dorsum and orbital rims.

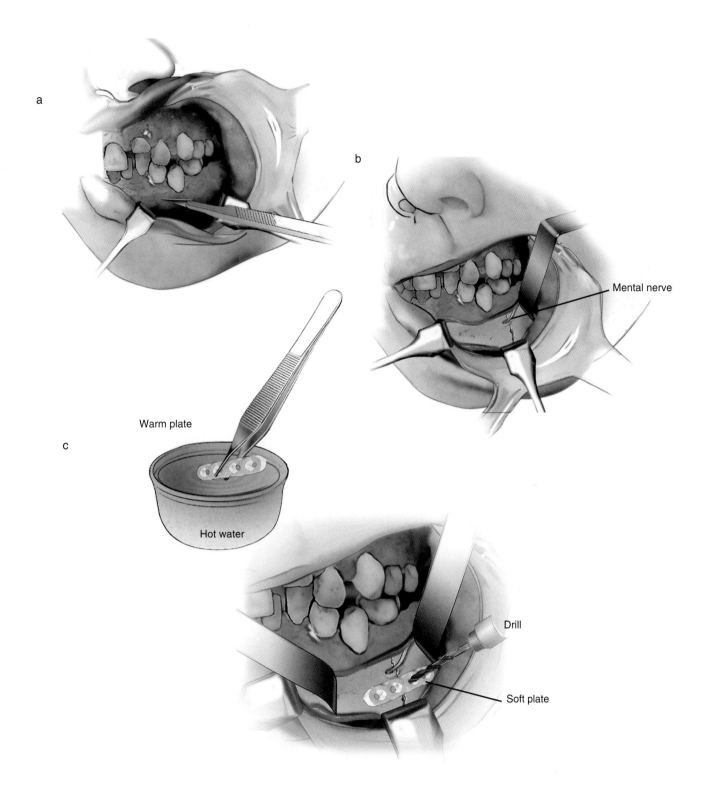

a

b

Mental nerve

c

Warm plate

Hot water

Drill

Soft plate

d

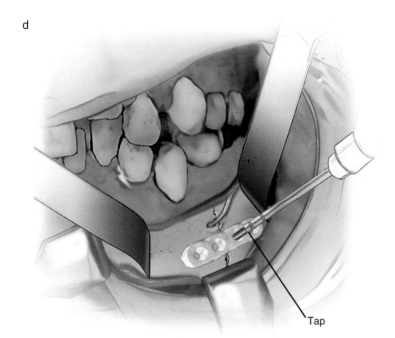

Tap

e

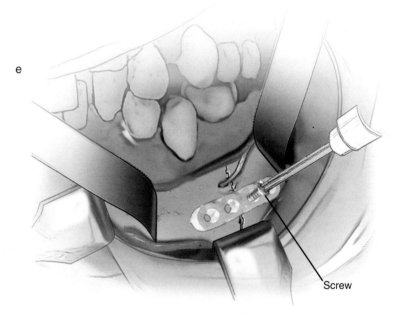

Screw

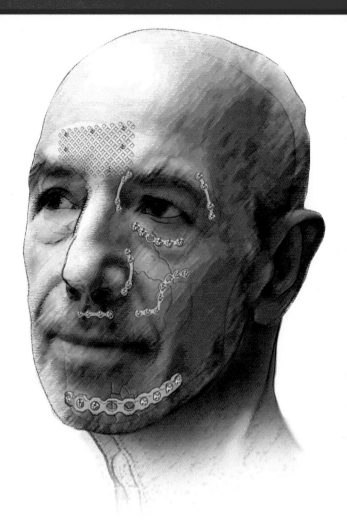

PART FIFTEEN

Complex Facial Fractures

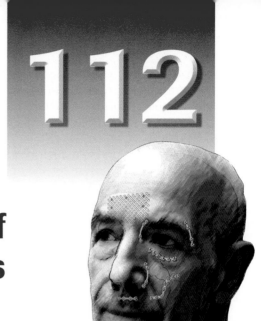

CHAPTER 112

Surgical Management of Complex Facial Fractures

INDICATIONS

Complex facial fractures, sometimes called pan facial fractures, require different considerations than those used in the isolated fracture. In these cases, the patient is often seriously injured and the reconstruction is similar to solving a puzzle although there are a variety of strategic approaches available to manage this challenging problem. Probably the most effective approach will be one based on time-tested principles that have been used traditionally in craniofacial surgery.

The patient's condition must first be stabilized before considering repair. As noted in Chapter 3, it is important to establish an airway, control bleeding, and restore circulation. A multidisciplinary approach is necessary to evaluate and treat any changes in neurological status, vascular supply, and vision. The craniofacial skeleton and soft tissues must be carefully evaluated by physical examination and appropriate imaging techniques (i.e., such as CT scans and MRIs). Preinjury photographs and dental studies are helpful.

The following principles are important to consider for the reconstruction:

1. The craniofacial repair should be built on a solid foundation using stable points of the skeleton to attach to adjacent unstable fractures.

2. The three dimensions of the craniofacial skeleton must be evaluated so that the height, length, and projection are returned to pre injury status. These objectives can be obtained by reducing and stabilizing selected beams and buttresses that constitute the facial skeleton.

3. The reconstruction should assure symmetry of the facial features.

4. Scars should be concealed as much as possible.

5. The reconstruction should improve and/or retain functions.

PROCEDURES

The strategic approach and reconstruction requires an appreciation of the type and degree of injury while establishing the goals and objectives of repair. The surgeon should be familiar with the normal anatomy and evaluate the craniofacial injuries using appropriate imaging studies and models. A tracheostomy should be considered at the start, since there will probably be a need for multiple procedures and repeated access to the airway; the tracheostomy will also provide for an improved exposure required for setting occlusion and reconstruction of the nasal passageways.

A *six step process* seems to be a rational approach.

A Step 1 requires planning of incisions for exposure and treatment of fractures. The entire face and portion of the head should be exposed and prepared

639

with a surgical scrub. Good lighting is important. There are many options for incisions that can provide exposure to the craniofacial skeleton but some are more concealed than others and should be first considered.

The coronal incision described in Chapter 43 provides excellent exposure for the upper portion of the craniofacial skeleton and for reduction and fixation at the zygomaticofrontal and nasomaxillary buttresses. It also provides exposure for the correction of the frontal bar, and with additional dissection, the zygomatic arch as it projects from the temporal suture line. Further dissection along the nasomaxillary buttress should also provide access to the medial wall of the orbit and medial canthal ligament. The transconjunctival incision (see Chapter 62) provides excellent exposure for the inferior orbital rim, floor of the orbit. When the incision is extended through lateral canthotomy, access is obtained for the lateral wall of the orbit and the zygomaticofrontal buttress. The maxillary degloving incision gives excellent exposure for the lower part of the nasomaxillary and zygomaticomaxillary buttresses as well as the lower maxillary alveolar arch (see Chapter 45). Intraoral exposures for the mandible as described in Chapters 25, 26, and 30 are also useful, but these concealed incisions may not give as good exposure as those from the external approach.

B Step 2 requires stabilization to the cranium or most stable superior structure(s) Using the cranium as a foundation, the adjacent displaced bone(s) can be attached to the stable cranial projection. From this point, additional buttresses and beams are reconstructed. The coronal incision will provide excellent exposure for correction of the zygomaticofrontal buttress as well as the upper part of the nasomaxillary buttress.

C The third step should be directed more toward the width and projection of the face. The zygomatic arches set these dimensions as well as the infraorbital rim and frontal bar beams. The zygomatic arches can be exposed through the coronal incision and stabilized at the zygomaticotemporal suture line. The frontal beam is repaired with a coronal exposure while the infraorbital rim is corrected through a transconjunctival approach.

D For step 4, attention is turned to the occlusal relationships. It is important to set the upper and lower jaws in occlusion as this will help in the relationships of the midface to the mandible.

E In step 5, the midface reconstruction is completed with attention to a correct positioning related to the nasomaxillary and zygomaticomaxillary buttresses. The palate, if split, can be stabilized. Usually these approaches can be accomplished through a degloving incision.

F For step 6, the mandibular reconstruction is completed with the application of plates to appropriate areas of fracture.

Other options for reconstruction are available. If the mandible is intact, it may be prudent to start the process with intermaxillary fixation using the mandible as a stable foundation. The reconstruction will then proceed upward to encompass the maxilla, nose, zygomatic/orbital area, and zygomatic arches.

Another option is to start at the zygomatic arches and achieve and secure accurate attachment to the zygomaticotemporal beams. This type of reconstruction concentrates more on the projection and width of the face. The reconstruction however requires significant exposure through the coronal approach.

Regardless of the strategy to reconstruct the craniofacial skeleton, it is essential that the surgeon reduce all fractures before stabilization. If this is not accomplished, it will be difficult, if not impossible, to fix the fractures in their anatomic position. Fixation most of the time will be accomplished by miniplates, rigid plates, and titanium mesh as described in earlier chapters. We prefer to keep the plating to a minimum and apply plates to only those beams/buttresses that are required for stability.

In proceeding with the reconstruction, functions must be addressed. The globe must be in the appropriate anatomic position and be able to move freely within the orbit. Correction of enophthalmos, hypothalamus, and diplopia are discussed in Chapters 55 through 65. Integrity of the medial canthal ligament must be restored to provide for normal collection and transport of tears (see Chapters 66 through 72). The nasal passageways must be kept patent by correct positioning of the nasal bones and septum. Occlusal relationships necessary for mastication must also be established during this reconstruction process.

Considering the complexity of the reconstruction, complications should be anticipated. Such deformities and/or dysfunctions should be evaluated in the immediate postoperative period and, if they are considered significant by the patient and/or surgeon, they should be corrected before there is a need for osteotomy or implants. Late correction of complications will require additional imaging and study models and a fresh strategic approach to correct the problems. These complications are discussed in detail in the earlier chapters of the book.

COMPLEX FACIAL FRACTURES

STEP 1: Conceal incisions

A

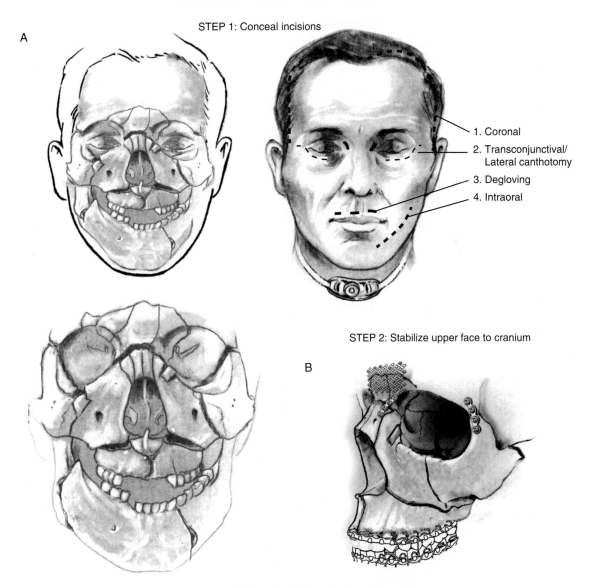

1. Coronal
2. Transconjunctival/
   Lateral canthotomy
3. Degloving
4. Intraoral

STEP 2: Stabilize upper face to cranium

B

STEP 3: Establish projection with repair
of horizontal beams

C

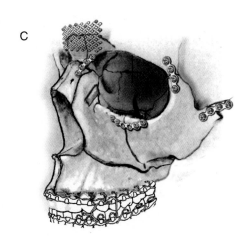

D

STEP 4: Stabilize occlusion

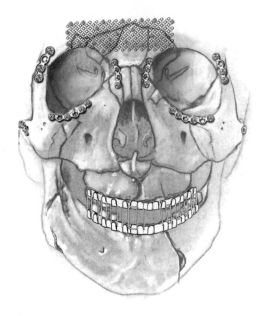

E

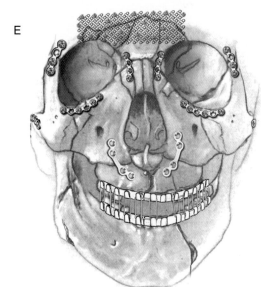

STEP 5: Stabilize buttresses and palate

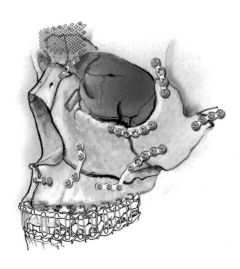

STEP 6: Repair mandible

F

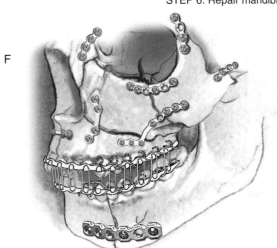

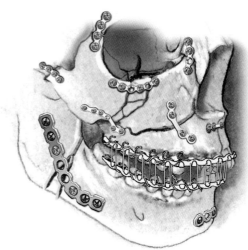

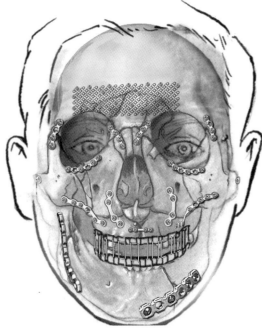

This atlas reflects the author's 40 years of experience in the treatment of craniomaxillofacial injuries. Textbooks and articles have provided much of the information that is used and sometimes modified for successful patient care. Below is a list of suggested readings that contain many of these excellent works.

GENERAL REFERENCES

American Colleges of Surgeons. Advanced Trauma Life Support Course (ATLS). 6th ed. 1997.

Andreason JO: Traumatic Injuries of the Teeth. 2nd ed. Philadelphia: WB Saunders, 1981.

Converse JM (ed): Reconstructive Plastic Surgery. vols 1–3. Philadelphia: WB Saunders, 1964.

Converse JM: Kazanjian and Converse's Surgical Treatment of Facial Injuries. vols 1 and 2. 3rd ed. Baltimore: Williams & Wilkins, 1974.

Cummings CW, Sessions DG, Weymuller EA Jr, Wood P: Atlas of Laryngeal Surgery. St Louis: CV Mosby, 1984.

Dingman RO, Natvig P: Surgery of Facial Fractures. 2nd ed. Philadelphia: WB Saunders, 1967.

Ellis E, Zide MF: Surgical Approach to the Facial Skeleton. 2nd ed. Baltimore: J Lippincott Williams and Wilkins, 2005.

Fonseca RJ, Walker RV, Betts NJ: Oral Maxillofacial Trauma. 3rd ed. Philadelphia: WB Saunders, 2004.

Habal MB, Ariyan S (eds): Facial Fractures. Philadelphia: BC Decker, 1989.

Haerle F, Champy M, Terry B (eds): Atlas of Craniomaxillofacial Osteosynthesis: Microplates, Miniplates and Screws. 2nd ed. Stuttgart, Germany: George Thieme Verag, 2009.

Jones N: Craniofacial trauma. New York: Oxford University Press, 1997.

Kellman RM (ed): Facial plating. Otolaryngol Clin North Am 20(3):1987.

Kellman RM, Marentette LJ: Atlas of Craniomaxillofacial Fixation. New York: Raven Press, 1995.

Killey HC: Fracture of the Middle Third of the Facial Skeleton. 2nd ed. Bristol, England: J Wright, 1971.

Manson PN (ed): Rigid fixation and bone grafts in craniofacial surgery. Clin Plastic Surg 16(1):1989.

Mathog RH (ed): Maxillofacial Trauma. Baltimore: Williams & Wilkins, 1984.

Mathog RH (ed): Symposium on maxillofacial trauma. Otolaryngol Clin North Am 9(2):1976.

Mathog RH, Crane LR, Nowak GS: Antimicrobial therapy following head and neck trauma. In Johnson JT (ed): Antibiotic therapy in head and neck surgery. New York: Morcal Deckker, 1987, pp 31–47.

Mustarde JC: Repair and Reconstruction of the Orbital Region. Baltimore: Williams & Wilkins, 1966.

Myers EN, Stool SE, Johnson JT (eds): Tracheotomy. New York: Churchill Livingstone, 1985.

Pham AM, Strong EB: Endoscopic management of facial fractures. Curr Opin Otolaryngol Head Neck Surg 14:234–241, 2006.

Prein J (ed): Manual of internal fixation in the craniofacial skeleton. Booth Springer-Verlog, 1998.

Rowe NL, Killey HC (eds): Fractures of the Facial Skeleton. 2nd ed. Edinburgh: E & S Livingstone, 1968.

Salyer KE: Techniques in Aesthetic Craniofacial Surgery. Philadelphia: JB Lippincott, 1989.

Schubert W, Jenabzadeh K: Endoscopic approach to maxillofacial trauma. J Craniofac Surg 20:154–156, 2009.

Schultz RC: Facial Injuries. 3rd ed. Chicago: Year Book Medical Publishers, 1988.

Smith B, Nesi F: Practical Techniques in Ophthalmic Plastic Surgery. St Louis: CV Mosby, 1981.

Spiessl B (ed): New Concepts in Maxillofacial Bone Surgery. Berlin: Springer-Verlag, 1976.

Spoor TC, Nesi FA (eds): Management of Ocular, Orbital, and Adnexal Trauma. New York: Raven Press, 1988.

Thaller S, McDonald WS: Facial Trauma. New York: Informa Healthcare, 2004.

Ward-Booth P, Eppley B, Schmelziesen R (eds): Maxillofacial Trauma and Esthetic Reconstruction. London: Churchill Livingston, 2003.

Wheeler RC: A Textbook of Dental Anatomy and Physiology. 4th ed. Philadelphia: WB Saunders, 1965.

Williams LI (ed): Rowe and Williams' Maxillofacial injuries. New York: Churchill Livingstone, 1994.

Yaremchuk MJ, Gruss JS, Manson PN: Rigid Fixation of the Craniomaxillofacial Skeleton. Boston: Butterworth-Heinemann, 1992.

SPECIFIC REFERENCES

Imaging

Barr RM, Gean AD, Le TH: Craniofacial trauma. In Brant WE, Helms CA (eds): Fundamentals of Diagnostic Radiology. 3rd ed. Philadelphia: Lippincott Williams & Wilkins, 2007, pp 55–85.

Curé JK: Head & Neck. In Jeffrey RB, Manaster BJ, Gurney JW, et al (eds): Diagnostic Imaging: Emergency. Salt Lake City, UT: Amirsys, 2007, pp I-1–I-59.

Harnsberger HR, Wiggins RH III, Hudgins PA, et al: Diagnosis Imaging: Head and Neck. Salt Lake City, UT: Amirsys, 2004.

Harris JH Jr, Castillo M, Smith MM: Face, including orbital soft tissues, and mandible. In Harris JH Jr, Harris WH (eds): The Radiology of Emergency Medicine. 4th ed. Philadelphia: Lippincott Williams & Wilkins, 2000, pp 40–135.

Hopper RA, Salemy S, Sze, RW: Diagnosis of Midface Fractures with CT: What the Surgeon Needs to Know. Radiographics 26:783–793, 2006.

Ouyang T, Branstetter BF: Advances in head and neck imagining: Oral maxillofac surg. Clin North Am 22:107–115, 2010.

Rhea JT, Novelline RA: How to simplify the CT diagnosis of Le Fort fractures: AJR Am J Roentgenol 184:1700–1705, 2005.

Sato Y: Head and Neck. In Erkonen WE, Smith WL (eds): Radiology 101. The Basics and Fundamentals of Imaging. 3rd ed. Philadelphia: Lippincott Williams & Wilkins, 2010, pp 311–321.

Scarfe WC: Imaging of maxilofacial trauma: Evolutions and emerging revelations. Oral Surg, Oral Med, Oral Pathol, Oral Radiol Endod 100(Suppl):75–96, 2005.

Zimmerman RD, Hertel KD: Spine. In Jeffrey RB, Manaster BJ, Gurney JW, et al (eds): Diagnostic Imaging: Emergency. Salt Lake City, UT: Amirsys, 2007, pp I-1–I-113.

Emergency Measures

CERVICAL SPINE INJURY AND AIRWAY EMERGENCIES

Atkin JP: Current utilization of cervical spine injury and emergency airway tracheotomy as a therapeutic measure: A review of the literature and an analysis of 526 cases. Laryngoscope 70:1672–1690, 1960.

Brantigan CO, Grow JB: Cricothyroidotomy: Elective use in respiratory problems requiring tracheotomy. J Thorac Cardiovasc Surg 71:72–80, 1976.

Committee on Trauma of the American College of Surgeons: Early Care of the Injured Patient. Philadelphia: WB Saunders, 1976.

Davidson JSD, Birdsell DC: Cervical spine injury of patients with facial skeletal trauma. J Trauma 29:1276–1278, 1989.

Elhai MM, Brar MS, Ahmed N, Howley DB, Nishtar S, Mahoney JL: Cervical spine injury in association with craniomaxillofacial injuries. Plast Reconstr Surg 121:201–208, 2008.

Glas WW, King OJ Jr, Lui A: Complications of tracheostomy. Arch Surg 85:56–63, 1962.

Haug RH, Wible RT, Likavec MJ, Conforti PJ: Cervical spine fractures in maxillofacial trauma. J Max Surg 49:725–729, 1991.

Herrin TJ, Brzustowitz R, Hendrickson M: Anesthetic management of neck trauma. South Med J 72:1102–1106, 1979.

Holmgren EP, Bagheri S, Dell RB, Bobek S, Dierks EJ: Utilization of tracheostomy in craniomaxillofacial trauma at a Level-1 Trauma Center. J Oral Maxillofac Surg 65:2005–2010, 2007.

Horton JM: Immediate care of head injuries. Anaesthesia 30:212–218, 1975.

Koopman CF, Feld RH, Coulthard SW: The effects of cricoid cartilage injury and antibiotics in cricothyroidotomy. Am J Otolaryngol 2:123–128, 1981.

Lewis VL, Manson PN, Morgan FG, et al: Facial injuries associated with cervical fractures: Recognition, patterns and management. J Trauma 25:90–93, 1985.

Mathog RH: Croup and laryngeal inflammation. Postgrad Med 52:106–110, 1972.

Mathog RH, Kenan PD, Hudson WR: Delayed massive hemorrhage following tracheostomy. Laryngoscope 81:107–119, 1971.

Meade JW: Tracheotomy: Its complications and their management. A study of 212 cases. N Engl J Med 265:519–523, 1961.

Melker JS, Gabrielli A: Melker cricothyroidectomy kit: An alternative to the surgical technique. Ann Otol Rhinol Laryngol 114:525–528, 2005.

Nelson TG: Tracheotomy: A clinical and experimental study. Am J Surg 23:660–694;750–783;941–981, 1957.

Ng M, Saadat D, Sinha UK: Managing emergency airway in LeFort Fractures. J Craniomaxillofac Trauma 4:38–43, 1998.

Oliver P, Richardson JR, Clubb RW, Flake CG: Tracheotomy in children. N Engl J Med 267:631–637, 1962.

Roberge RJ, Wears RC, Kelly M, et al: Selective application of cervical spine radiography in alert victims of blunt trauma: A prospective study. J Trauma 28:784–788, 1988.

Roccia F, Cassanino F, Boccaletti R, Stura G: Cervical spine fractures associated with mandibular trauma: 11 year review. J Craniofac Surg 18:1259–1263, 2007.

Ruskin JD, Tu HK: Integrated management of the maxillofacial trauma patient with multiple injuries. Oral Maxillofac Surg Clin North Am 2:15–27, 1990.

Schaefer SD, Bucholz RW, Jones RE, et al: "How I do it" head and neck: Treatment of transpharyngeal missile wounds to the cervical spine. Laryngoscope 91:146–148, 1981.

Schultz RC: Facial injuries from automobile accidents: A study of 400 consecutive cases. Plast Reconstr Surg 40:415–425, 1967.

Schultz RC, Oldham RJ: An overview of facial injuries. Surg Clin North Am 57:987–1010, 1977.

Smoot EC III, Jernigan JR, Kinsley E, Rey RM Jr: A survey of operative airway management practices for midface fractures. J Craniofac Surg 8:201–207, 1997.

Strate RG, Boies LR: The emergency management of trauma. Otolaryngol Clin North Am 9:315–329, 1976.

Thompson JN, Gibson B, Kohut R: Airway obstruction in Le Fort fractures. Laryngoscope 97:275–279, 1987.

Woo P, Kelly G, Kirschner P: Airway complications in the head injured. Laryngoscope 99:725–731, 1989.

Yarington CT, Frazer JP: Complications of tracheostomy. Arch Surg 91:652–655, 1968.

Epistaxis

Padua FGM, Voegels, RL: Several posterior epistaxis-endoscopy surgical anatomy. Laryngoscope 118:156–161, 2008.

Schwartzbauer HR, Shete M, Tarni TA: Endoscopic anatomy of the sphenopalatine and posterior nasal arteries: implications for the endoscopic management of epistaxis. Am J Rhinol 17:63–66, 2003.

Sharon AT: Endoscopic sphenopalatine artery ligation for refractory posterior epistaxis. Indian J Otolaryngol Head Neck Surg 37:215–217, 2005.

Siniluuto TM, Leinonen AS, Kartunnan AK: Embolization for management of posterior epistaxis. Arch Otolaryngol 119:837–841, 1993.

Soft Tissue Injury
PENETRATING WOUNDS AND VASCULAR INJURY

Azuaje RE, Jacobson LE, Glover J, Gomez GA, Rodman GH Jr, Broadie TA, Simons CJ, Bierke HS: Reliability of physical examination as a predictor of vascular injury after penetrating neck trauma. Am J Surg 69(9):804–807, 2003.

Beall AC Jr, Shirkey AL, DeBakey ME: Penetrating wounds of the carotid artery. J Trauma 3:276–287, 1963.

Bell RB, Osborn T, Dierks EJ, Potter BE, Long WB: Management of penetrating neck injuries-a new paradigm for civilian trauma. J Oral Maxillofac Surg 65:691–705, 2007

Brown MF, Graham JM, Feliciano DV, et al: Carotid artery injuries. Am J Surg 144:748–753, 1982.

Calcaterra TC, Hotz GP: Carotid artery injuries. Laryngoscope 82:321–329, 1972.

Campbell FC, Robbs JV: Penetrating injuries of the neck: A prospective study of 108 patients. Br J Surg 67:582–586, 1980.

Demetriades D, Asensio JA, Velmahos G, Thal E: Complex problems in penetrating neck trauma. Surg Clin North Am 76:661–683, 1996.

duToit DF, Strauss VC, Baszczyk M, deVilliers R, Warren BL: Endovascular treatment of penetrating thoracic outlet arterial injuries. Eur J Vasc Endovasc Surg 19:489–495, 2000.

Fackler ML: Physics of missile injury. In McSwain NE Jr, Kerstein MD (eds): Evaluation and Management of Trauma. East Norwalk: Appelton-Century-Crofts, 1987, pp 28–53.

Fanelli F, Salvatori FM, Ferrari R, Pacella S, Ross P, Passariello R: Stent repair of bilateral post traumatic dissection of internal carotid artery. J Endovasc 11:517–521, 2004.

Feliciano DV, Wald MJ Jr: Patterns of injury. In Moore E, Mattox KL, Feliciano DV (eds): Trauma. 2nd ed. East Norwalk: Appelton and Lang, 1991, pp 81–96.

Fitchett VH, Pomerantz M, Butsch DW, et al: Penetrating wounds of the neck: A military and civilian experience. Arch Surg 99:307–314, 1969.

Flint LM, Snyder WH, Perry MO, et al: Management of major vascular injuries in the base of the neck. Arch Surg 106:407–413, 1973.

Fry RE, Fry WJ: Extracranial carotid injury. Surgery 88:581–587, 1980.

Goldsmith MM, Postma DS, Jones FD: The surgical exposure of penetrating injuries to the carotid artery at the skull base. Otolaryngol Head Neck Surg 95:278–284, 1986.

Gracias VH, Reilly PM, Philpott J, Klein WP, Lee SY, Singer M, Schwab CW: Computed tomography in evaluation of penetrating neck trauma: A preliminary study. Arch Surg 136:1231–1235, 2001.

Harris JP, Anterasian G, Hoi SU, et al: Management of carotid artery transection resulting from a stab wound to the ear. Laryngoscope 95:782–785, 1985.

Holt GR: Wound ballistics of gunshot injuries to the head and neck. Arch Otolaryngol 109:313–318, 1983.

Jahrsdoerfer RA, Johns ME, Cantrell RW: Penetrating wounds of the head and neck. Arch Otolaryngol 105:721–725, 1979.

Jones RF, Terrell JC, Salyer KE: Penetrating wounds of the neck: An analysis of 274 cases. J Trauma 7:220–223, 1967.

Joo JY, Ahn JY, Chung SS, Chung YS, Kim SH, Yoon PN, Choi EN: Therapeutic endovascular treatments for traumatic carotid injuries. J Trauma 58:1159–1166, 2005.

Ledgerwood AM, Mullins RJ, Lucas CE: Primary repair vs. ligation for carotid artery injuries. Arch Surg 115:488–493, 1980.

Levine ZT, Wright DC, O'Malley S, Olan WS, Sekhar LN: Management of zone III missile injuries involving the carotid artery and cranial nerves. Skull Base Surg 10:17–27, 2000.

Liekweg WG, Greenfield LJ: Management of penetrating carotid arterial injury. Ann Surg 188:587–592, 1978.

Mahoney PF, Ryan J, Brooks, AJ, Schwab CW (eds): Ballastic trauma: A practical guide. 2nd ed. Leonard Chesier: Springer, 2004.

Mandavia DP, Qualls S, Rokos I: Emergency airway management in penetrating neck injury. Ann Emerg Med 35:221–225, 2000.

Mathog RH: Large facial wounds. In Gates GA (ed): Current Therapy in Otolaryngology—Head and Neck Surgery. Philadelphia: BC Decker, 1987, pp 73–77.

May M, Chadaratana P, West JW, Ogura JH: Penetrating neck wounds: Selective exploration. Laryngoscope 85:57–75, 1975.

May M, Tucker HM, Dillard BM: Penetrating wounds of the neck in civilians. Otolaryngol Clin North Am 9:361–391, 1976.

McConnell DD, Trunkey DD: Management of penetrating trauma to the neck. Adv Surg 27:97–127, 1994.

McNeil JD, Chiou AC, Gunlock MG, Grayson DE, Soares G, Hagino RT: Successful endovascular therapy of a penetrating zone III internal carotid injury. J Vasc Surg 36:187–190, 2002.

Munera F, Cohn S, Rivas LA: Penetrating injuries of the neck: Use of helicle computed tomographic angiography. J Trauma 58:413–418, 2005.

Munera F, Sota JA, Placio D, Velez SM, Medina E: Diagnosis of arterial injuries caused by penetrating trauma to the neck: Comparison of helicle CT angiography and conventional angiography. Radiology 216:356–362, 2000.

Munera F, Sota JA, Placio DM, Castaneda J, Morales C, Sanabria A, Gutierrez JE, Garcia G: Penetrating neck injuries: Helicle CT angiography for initial evaluation. Radiology 224:366–372, 2002.

Nanda A, Vannemreddy PS, Willis BK, Baskaya MK, Jawahar A: Management of carotid artery injuries: Louisiana State University Shreveport experience. Surg Neurol 59:184–190, 2003.

Navsaria P, Thoma M, Nicol A: Foley catheter balloon tamponade for life-threatening hemorrhage in penetrating neck trauma. World J Surg 30:1265–1268, 2006.

Nunez DB, Torres-Leon M, Munera F: Vascular injuries of the neck and thoracic inlet: Helical CT-angiographic correlation. Radiographics 24:1087–1098, 2004.

Padberg FT, Hobson RW, Yeager RH: Penetrating carotid arterial trauma. Am J Surg 50:277–282, 1984.

Pate JW, Casini M: Penetrating wounds of the neck: Explore or not? Am J Surg 10:38–43, 1980.

Pichtel WJ, Miller RH, Feliciano DV: Lateral mandibulotomy: A technique of exposure for penetrating injuries of the internal carotid artery at the base of the skull. Laryngoscope 94:1140–1144, 1984.

Pinto A, Brunese L, Scaglione M, Scuderi MG, Romano L: Gunshot wounds to the neck area: Balastic elements forensic issues. Semin Ultrasound CT MR 32:215–220, 2009.

Rao M, Bhatti FK, Gaudino J, et al: Penetrating injuries of the neck: Criteria for exploration. J Trauma 23:47–49, 1983.

Robbs JV, Baker LW, Human RR, et al: Cervicomediastinal arterial injuries. Arch Surg 116:663–667, 1981.

Samson D, Boone S: Extracranial-intracranial (EC-IC) arterial bypass: Past performance and current concepts. Neurosurgery 3:79–86, 1978.

Sriussadaporn S, Rattatlee P, Tharavej C, Sirichindakul B, Chiamanackthapong S: Selective management of penetrating neck injuries based on clinical presentations safe and practical. Int Surg 86:90–93, 2002.

Thompson EC, Porter JM, Fernandez LG: Penetrating neck trauma: An overview of management. J Oral Maxillofac Surg 60:918–923, 2002.

Tisherman SA, Bokhari F, Collier B, Ebert J, Holevar M, Cumming J, Kurek S, Leon S, Rhee P: Clinical practice guidelines: penetrating neck trauma. Chicago: Eastern Association for the Surgery of Trauma (EAST), 2008, p 52.

Unger SW, Tucker SW, Urdeza MH: Carotid arterial trauma. Surgery 87:477–483, 1980.

Yamada S, Kindt GW, Youmans JR: Carotid artery occlusion due to nonpenetrating injury. J Trauma 7:333–342, 1967.

Facial Nerve Injury

Baker DC, Conley J: Facial nerve grafting: A thirty year retrospective review. Clin Plast Surg 6:330–343, 1970.

Caboud HE: Epineural and perineural fascicular nerve repairs: A critical comparison. J Hand Surg 1:131–134, 1976.

Crumley RL: Interfascicular nerve repair: Is it applicable in facial nerve injuries? Arch Otolaryngol 106:313–316, 1980.

Fisch U: Facial nerve grafting. Otolaryngol Clin North Am 7:517–529, 1974.

Gullane PJ: Extratemporal facial rehabilitation. J Otolaryngol 8:477–486, 1979.

Hagan WE: Microneural techniques for nerve grafting. Laryngoscope 91:1759–1766, 1981.

Millesi H: Nerve grafting. Clin Plast Surg 11:105–113, 1984.

Millesi H: Technique of free nerve grafting in the face. In Rubin L (ed): Reanimation of the Paralyzed Face. St Louis: CV Mosby, 1977, pp 124–135.

Smith MFN, Goode RL: Eye protection in the paralyzed face. Laryngoscope 89:435–442, 1979.

Stroud WH, Yarbrough DR: Penetrating neck wounds. Am J Surg 140:323–326, 1980.

Szal G, Miller T: Surgical repair of facial nerve branches. Arch Otolaryngol 101:160–165, 1975.

Tucker H: The management of facial paralysis due to extracranial injuries. Laryngoscope 88:348–356, 1978.

Reconstruction

Baker SR: Local cutaneous flaps. Otolaryngol Clin North Am 27:139–159, 1994.

Baker SR (eds): Local flaps in facial reconstruction. St Louis: Mosby, 1995.

Baker SR: Regional flaps in facial reconstruction. Otolaryngol Clin North Am 23:925–946, 1990.

Borges A: Elective Incisions and Scar Revision. Boston: Little Brown and Company, 1973.

Brenner MJ, Perro CA: Recontouring, resurfacing and scar revision in skin cancer reconstruction. Facial Plast Surg Clin North Am 17:469–487, 2009.

Brown JB, Cannon B: Composite free grafts of skin and cartilage from the ear. Ann Surg 124:1101–1107, 1946.

Bukhari S, Khan I, Pasha B, Ahmed W: Management of facial gunshot wounds. J Coll Physicians Surg Pak 6:382–385, 2010.

Burget GC, Menick FJ: Aesthetic Reconstruction of the Nose. St Louis: Mosby-Year Book, 1996.

Burget GC, Menick FJ: Nasal reconstruction seeking a fourth dimension. Plast Reconstr Surg 78:145–157, 1986.

Burget GC, Menick FJ: Nasal support and lining: The marriage of beauty and blood supply. Plast Reconstr Surg 84:189–202, 1989.

Burget GC, Menick FJ: The subunit principal in nasal reconstruction. Plast Reconstr Surg 76:239–247, 1985.

Burget GC, Walton RL: Optimal use of microvascular free flaps, cartilage grafts, and a paramedian forehead flap for aesthetic reconstruction of the nose and adjacent facial units. Plast Reconstr Surg 120:1171–1207, 2007; discussion 1208–1216.

Danahey DG, Hilger PA: Reconstruction of large nasal defects. Otolaryngol Clin North Am 34:695–711, 2001.

Estlander JA: Eine methode aud der einen lippe substanzverluste der anderen zu erstegen. Arch Kiln Chir 14:622, 1872.

Fanelli F, Salvatori FM, Ferrari R, et al: Stent repair of bilateral post traumatic dissection of internal carotid artery. J Endovasc 11:517–521, 2004.

Futran ND: Maxillofacial trauma reconstruction. Facial Plast Surg Clin North Am 17:239–251, 2009.

Giberson WG, FreemanJL: Use of free auricular composite graft in nasal alar/vestibular reconstruction. J Otolaryngol 21:153–155, 1992.

Holt GR, Thomas JR (eds): Facial Scars: Incision, Revision and Camouflage. St. Louis: Mosby Inc., 1988.

Jackson I: Local Flaps in Head and Neck Reconstruction. St. Louis: CV Moseby Company, 1985.

Kountakis SE, Chamblee SA, Maillard AA, Stierberg CM: Animal bites to the head and neck. Ear Nose Throat J 77:216–220, 1998.

Kummoona R: Management of missile injuries of the facial skeleton; Primary, intermediate and secondary phases. J Craniofac Surg 21:976–981, 2010.

Mathog RH: Scar revision. Minn Med 57:31–36, 1974.

McCollough EG: Dermabrasion and Chemical Peel-a guide for Facial Plastic Surgeons. New York: Thieme Medical Publishers, 1988.

Menick FJ: A new modified method for nasal lining: The Menick technique for folded lining. J Surg Oncol 94:509–514, 2006.

Menick FJ: Nasal Reconstruction: Art and Practice. New York: Elsevier Publishing, 2008.

Monroy A, Behar P, Nagy M, Poje C, Pizzuto M, Brodsky L: Head and neck dog bites in children. Otolaryngol Head Neck Surg 140:354–357, 2009.

Mostafapour SP, Murakami, CS: Tissue expansion and serial excision in scar revision. Facial Plast Surg 17:245–252, 2001.

Patel BCK, Flaharty PM, Anderson RL: Reconstruction of the eyelids. In Baker SR, Swanson NA (eds): Local Flaps in Facial Reconstruction. St Louis: Mosby-Year Book Inc., 1995, pp 275–303.

Steinberg MJ, Herréra, AF: Management of parotid duct injuries. Oral Surg Oral Med Oral Pathol Oral Radiol Endod 99:136–141, 2005.

Thomas JR, Prendiville S: Update in scar revision. Facial Plast Surg Clin North Am 10:103–111, 2002.

Webster CC, Davidson JR, Smith RC: Broken line scar revision. Clin Plast Surg 4:263–274, 1977.

Webster CC, Smith RC: Scar revision and camouflaging. Otolaryngol Clin North Am 15:55–68, 1982.

Westine JG, Lopez, MA, Thomas JR: Scar revision. Facial Plast Surg Clin North Am 13:325–331, 2005.

Zitelli JA: The bilobed flap for nasal reconstruction. Arch Dermatol 125:957–959, 1989.

Mandible Fractures

Allgower M, Perren S, Pathew P: A new plate for internal fixation: The dynamic compression plate (DCP). Injury 2:40–47, 1970.

Barry CP, Kearns GJ: Superior border plating technique in the management of isolated mandibular angle fractures: A retrospective study of 50 consecutive patients. J Oral Maxillofac Surg 65:1544–1549, 2007.

Belvins C, Gores RJ: Fractures of the mandibular condylar process: Results of conservative treatment in 140 cases. J Oral Surg 19:393–407, 1961.

Bernstein L, McClurg FL: Mandibular fractures: A review of 156 consecutive cases. Laryngoscope 88:951–961, 1978.

Biller JA, Pletcher SD, Goldberg AN, Murr AH: Complications and the time to repair mandible fractures. Laryngoscope 115:769–772, 2005.

Blair VP: Operative treatment of ankylosis of the mandible. Trans South Surg Gynecol 26:435–465, 1913.

Boyne PJ, Upham C: The treatment of long standing bilateral fracture non- and malunion in atrophic edentulous mandibles. Int J Oral Surg 3:213–217, 1974.

Braham RL, Roberts MW, Morris ME: Management of dental trauma in children and adolescents. J Trauma 17:857–865, 1977.

Brown AE, Obeid G: A simplified method for the internal fixation of fractures of the mandibular condyle. Br J Oral Maxillofac Surg 22:145–150, 1984.

Bruce RH, Strachan DS: Fractures of the edentulous mandible: The chalmers J Lyons academy study. J Oral Surg 34:973–979, 1976.

Calhoun KH, Spencer L, Clark WD, et al: Surgical care of submental gunshot wounds. Arch Otolaryngol 114:513–519, 1988.

Cameron JR: Complications in the treatment of fractures. J Oral Surg 23:14–16, 1965.

Cascone P, Spallacia F, Fatone FMJ, Rivarol A, Saltarel A, Iannetti G: Rigid versus semi-rigid fixation for condylar fractures: Experience with the external fixation system. J Oral Maxillofac Surg 66:265–271, 2008.

Champy M, Lodde JP, Schmitt R, et al: Mandibular osteosynthesis by miniature screwed plates via a buccal approach. J Maxillofac Surg 6:14–21, 1978.

Cillo JE, Ellis E III: Treatment of patients with double unilateral fractures of the mandible. J Oral Maxillofac Surg 65:1461–1469, 2007.

Coletti DP, Salama H, Caccamesi JF: Application of intermaxillary fixation screws in maxillofacial trauma. J Oral Maxillofac Trauma 65:1746–1750, 2007.

Converse JM: Surgical release of bilateral intractible temporomandibular ankylosis. Plast Reconstr Surg 64:404–407, 1979.

Czerwinski M, Parker WL, Correa JA, Williams HB: Effect of treatment delay on mandibular fracture infection rate. Plast Reconstr Surg 122:881–885, 2008.

Danda AK, Muthusekhar MR, Narayanan V, Barg MF, Siddareddi A: Open versus closed treatment of unilateral subcondylar and condylar neck fractures: A prospective, randomized clinical study. J Oral Maxillofac Surg 68:1238–1241, 2010.

Davis WH, Delo RI, Weiner JR, Terry B: Transoral bone graft for atrophy of the mandible. Oral Surg 28:760–765, 1970.

Dierks E: Transoral approach to fractures of the mandible. Laryngoscope 97:4–6, 1987.

Dingman RO, Grabb WC: Intra-articular temporomandibular joint arthroplasty. Plast Reconstr Surg 38:179–185, 1966.

Dingman RO, Grabb WC: Reconstruction of both mandibular condyles with metatarsal bone grafts. Plast Reconstr Surg 34:441–451, 1964.

Doctor VS, Farwell DG: Gunshot wounds to the head and neck. Curr Opin Otolaryngol Head Neck Surg 15:213–218, 2007.

Ducic Y: Endoscopic treatment of subcondylar fractures. Laryngoscope 118:1164–1167, 2008.

Ellis E III: Method to determine when open treatment of condylar process fractures is not necessary. J Maxillofac Surg 67:1685–1690, 2009.

Ellis E III, Price C: Treatment protocol for fractures of the atrophic mandible. J Oral Maxillofac Surg 66:421–435, 2008.

Ellis E III, Muniz O, Anand K: Treatment considerations for comminuted mandible fractures. J Oral Maxillofac Surg 161:861–870, 2003.

Fernandez JA, Mathog RH: Open treatment of condylar fractures with biphase technique. Arch Otolaryngol 113:262–266, 1987.

Furr AN, Schweinfurth JN, May WL: Factors associated with long-term complications after repair of mandibular fractures. Laryngoscope 116:427–430, 2006.

Futran ND: Maxillofacial trauma reconstruction. Facial Plast Surg Clin North Am 17:239–251, 2009.

Gear AJ, Apasova E, Schmitz JP, Schubert W: Treatment modalities for mandibular angle fractures. J Oral Maxillofac Surg 63:655–663, 2005.

Georgiade NG, Masters FW, Metzger JT, Pickrell KL: Fractures of the mandible and maxilla in children. J Pediatr 42:440–449, 1953.

Georgiade NG, Pickrell K, Douglas W, Altany F: External pinning of displaced condylar fractures. Plast Reconstr Surg 18:377–383, 1956.

Gerbino G, Boffano P, Tosco P, Berrone S: Long-term clinical and radiological outcomes for surgical treatment of mandibular condylar fractures. J Oral Maxillofac Surg 67:109–1141, 2009.

Laurentjoye M, Majoufre-Lefebre CM, Siberchicot F, Ricard AS: Result of maxillomandibular fixation using intraoral cortical bone screws for condylar fractures of the mandible. J Oral Maxillofac Surg 67:767–770, 2009.

Li Z, Zhang W, Li Z-B, Li J-R: Abnormal union of mandibular fractures. A review of 84 cases. J Oral Maxillofac Surg 64:1225–1231, 2006.

Lieger O, Zix J, Kruse A, Iizuka T: Dental injuries in association with facial fractures. J Oral Maxillofac Surg 67:1680–1684, 2009.

Loveless TP, Bjornland T, Dodson T, Keith DA: Efficacy of temporomandibular joint ankylosis surgical treatment. J Oral Maxillofac Surg 68:1266–1282, 2010.

Madsen MJ, Haug RH, Christensen BS, Aldridge E: Management of atrophic mandibular fractures. Oral Maxillofac Surg Clin North Am 21:175–183, 2009.

Mary RE, Cillo JE, Broumand V, Illoa, JJ: Outcome analysis of the mandibular condyle replacements in tumor and trauma reconstruction: A prospective analysis of 131 cases with long-term follow-up. J Oral Maxillofac Surg 66:2515–2523, 2008.

Mehra P, Murad H: Internal fixation of mandibular angle fractures: A comparison of 2 techniques. J Oral Maxillofac Surg 66:2254–2260, 2008.

Mehra P, Van Heukelom EV, Cottrell DA: Rigid internal fixation of infected mandibular fractures. J Oral Maxillofac Surg 66:1046–1051, 2009.

Schneider M, Erasmus F, Gerlach KL, Kuhlich E, Loukota RA, Rasse M, Schubert J, Terbeyden H, Eckelt U: Open reduction and internal fixation versus closed treatment and mandibulomaxillary fixation of fractures of the mandibular condylar process: A randomized prospective multi-center study with special evaluation of fracture level. J Oral Maxillofac Surg 66:2537–2544, 2008.

Singh V, Bhagol A, Goel M, Kumar I, Verma A: Outcomes of open versus closed treatment of mandibular subcondylar subfractures: A prospective randomized study. J Oral Maxillofac Surg 68:1304–1309, 2010.

Suhhashra K: A study on the impact of mandibular third molars on angle fractures. J Maxillofac Surg 67:968–972, 2009.

Tiwana PS, Abraham MS, Kushner GM, Alpert B: Management of atrophic edentulous mandibular fractures. The case for primary reconstruction with immediate bone grafting. J Oral Maxillofac Surg 67:882–887, 2009.

Urken, ML, Sullivan MJ, Biller, HF: Atlas of Regional and Free Flaps for Head and Neck Reconstruction. 1st ed. New York: Raven Press, 1995.

Wittwer G, Adeyemo WL, Turbani D, Ploder O: Treatment of atrophic mandibular fractures based on the degree of atrophy-experience with different plating systems: A retrospective study. J Oral Maxillofac Surg 64:230–234, 2006.

Yilmaz M, Vayvada M, Menderes A, Demirdover C, Kizitkaya A: A comparison of vascularized fibular flap and iliac crest flap for mandibular reconstruction. J Craniofac Surg 19:54–61, 2008.

Maxillary Fractures

Antoni AA, Vandemark TB, Weinberg S, Schofield L: Surgical treatment of longstanding malunited horizontal fractures of the maxilla. Can Dent Assoc J 31:22–25, 1965.

Arden RL, Mathog RH: Maxillary fractures. In Paparella MM, Shumrick DA, Gluckman JL, Myerhoff WL (eds): Otolaryngology. 3rd ed. Philadelphia: WB Saunders, 1991, pp 2927–2938.

Bell RB, Kindsfater CS: The use of biodegradable plates and screws to stabilize facial fractures. J Oral Maxillofac Surg 64:31–39, 2006.

Chen C-H, Wang TY, Tsay P-K, Lai J-B, Chen C-T, Liao H-T, Lin C-H, Chen Y-R: A 162 case review of palatal fractures: Management strategy from a 10 year experience. Plast Reconstr Surg 121:2065–2073, 2008.

Conway H, Smith JW, Behrman JJ: Another method of bringing the midface forward. Plast Reconstr Surg 46:325–331, 1970.

Ellis E III: Passive repositioning of maxillary fractures: Occasional impossibility without osteotomy. J Oral Maxillofac Surg 62:1477–1485, 2004.

Eppley BL: Use of absorbable fixation technique for maxillary fractures. J Craniofac Surg 9:317–321, 1998.

Furnas DW: Transverse maxillary osteotomy for malunion of maxillary fractures. Plast Reconstr Surg 42:378–383, 1968.

Georgiade N, Nash T: An external cranial fixation apparatus for severe maxillofacial injuries. Plast Reconstr Surg 38:142–146, 1966.

Gruss JS, MacKinnon SE: Complex maxillary fractures: Role of buttress reconstruction and immediate bone grafts. Plast Reconstr Surg 78:9–22, 1986.

Gruss JS, MacKinnon SE, Kassel EE, Cooper PW: Role of primary bone grafting in complex craniomaxillofacial trauma. Plast Reconstr Surg 75:17–24, 1983.

He D, Zhang W, Ellis E III: Pan facial fractures: Analysis of 33 cases treated late. J Oral Maxillofac Surg 65:2459–2465, 2007.

Hendrickson M, Clark N, Manson PN, Yaremchuk M, Robertson B, Slezak KS, Crawley N, Vander Kolk C: Palatal fractures: Classification, patterns and treatment with rigid internal fixation. Plast Reconstr Surg 101:319–332, 1998.

Hillstrom RP, Mathog RH, Moore GK: Medial maxillary fractures. Otolaryngol Head Neck Surg 104:270–275, 1991.

Jackson IT, Somers PC, Kjar JG: The use of champy miniplates for osteosynthesis in craniofacial deformities and trauma. Plast Reconstr Surg 77:729–736, 1986.

Kellman RM, Schilli W: Plate fixation of the mid and upper face. Otolaryngol Clin North Am 20:559–572, 1987.

Le Fort R: Experimental study of fractures of the upper jaw. Rev Chir de Paris 23:208–217;360–379, 1901. (Reprinted in Plast Reconstr Surg 50:497–506, 1972.)

Lewis JES, Losken HW: LeFort III osteotomy to correct dish face deformity resulting from trauma. S Afr Med J 49:1915–1920, 1975.

Manson PN, Crawley WA, Yaremchuk MJ, et al: Midfacial fractures: Advantages of extended open reduction and immediate bone grafting. Plast Reconstr Surg 76:1–10, 1985.

Manson PN, Hoopes JE, Su CT: Structural pillars of the facial skeleton: An approach to the management of LeFort fractures. Plast Reconstr Surg 66:54–61, 1980.

Manson PN, Shack RB, Leonard LG, et al: Sagittal fractures of the maxilla and palate. Plast Reconstr Surg 72:484–488, 1983.

Mathog RH, Crane LR, Nowak GS: Antimicrobial therapy following head and neck trauma. In Johnson JT (ed): Antibiotic Therapy in Head and Neck Surgery. New York: Marcel Dekker, 1987, pp 31–49.

Mathog RH, Leonard M, Bevis R: Surgical correction of maxillary hypoplasia. Arch Otolaryngol 105:399–403, 1979.

Mathog RH, Rosenberg Z: Complications in the treatment of facial fractures. Otolaryngol Clin North Am 9:533–553, 1976.

May M, Phipatanakul P: Fracture of the medial aspect of the maxilla. Arch Otolaryngol 97:286–287, 1973.

Mixter RC, Feldman PD: Stabilization of the midface with a cranium-to-alveolus bone graft. Plast Reconstr Surg 83:348–355, 1989.

Nahum AM: The biomechanics of maxillofacial trauma. Clin Plast Surg 2:59–64, 1978.

Obwegeser HL: Surgical correction of small or retrodisplaced maxillae. Plast Reconstr Surg 43:351–365, 1969.

Schultz RC, Carbonell AM: Midfacial fractures from vehicular accidents. Clin Plast Surg 2:107–130, 1975.

Sofferman RA, Danielson PA, Quatela V, et al: Retrospective analysis of surgically treated LeFort fractures. Arch Otolaryngol 109:446–448, 1983.

Stanley RB: Reconstruction of the midface vertical dimension following LeFort fractures. Arch Otolaryngol 110:571–575, 1984.

Stanley RB, Funk GF: Rigid internal fixation for fractures involving tooth-bearing maxillary segments. Arch Otolaryngol 114:1295–1299, 1988.

Stanley RB, Nowak GM: Midfacial fractures. Importance of angle of impact to horizontal craniofacial buttresses. Otolaryngol Head Neck Surg 93:186–191, 1985.

Tessier P: Total osteotomy of the middle third of the face for faciostenosis or for sequela of LeFort III fractures. Plast Reconstr Surg 48:533–541, 1971.

Zachariades N, Vairaktaris E, Papavassiliou D, et al: Traumatic LeFort III osteotomy. Br J Oral Maxillofac Surg 24(1):69–71, 1986.

Nasal Fractures

Beekhuis GJ: Nasal fractures. Trans Am Acad Ophthalmol Otolaryngol 74:1058–1059, 1970.

Clark WD: Nasal and nasal septal fractures. Ear Nose Throat J 62:25–32, 1983.

Clark GM, Wallace CS: Analysis of nasal support. Arch Otolaryngol 92:118–123, 1970.

Courtiss EH: Septorhinoplasty of the traumatically deformed nose. Ann Plast Surg 1:443–449, 1978.

Farrior RT, Connolly ME: Septorhinoplasty in children. Otolaryngol Clin North Am 3:345–364, 1970.

Farrior RT: Corrective and reconstructive surgery of the external nose. In Naumann HH (ed): Head and Neck Surgery. Stuttgart; Georg Thieme, 1980, pp 173–277.

Farrior RT: Modifications in rhinoplasty: Where and when. Trans Am Acad Ophthalmol Otolaryngol 78:341–348, 1974.

Farrior RT: The osteotomy in rhinoplasty. Laryngoscope 88:1449–1459, 1978.

Fattahi T, Steinberg B, Ferrandes R, Mohan M, Reitter E: Repair of nasal complex fractures and the need for secondary septorhinoplasty. J Oral Maxillofac Surg 64:1785–1789, 2006.

Fry H: Nasal skeletal trauma and the interlocked stresses of the nasal septal cartilage. Br J Plast Surg 20:146–158, 1967.

Goldman IB: When is rhinoplasty indicated for a correction of recent nasal fractures? Laryngoscope 74:689–700, 1964.

Harrison DH: Nasal injuries: Their pathogenesis and treatment. Br J Plast Surg 32:57–64, 1979.

Higuera S, Lee E, Cole P, Hollier LH, Stal S: Nasal trauma and the deviated nose. Plast Reconstr Surg 120(Suppl):64–75, 2007.

Holt GR: Immediate open reduction of nasal septal injuries. Ear Nose Throat J 57:345–354, 1978.

Kane AP, Kane LA: Open reduction of nasal fractures. J Otolaryngol 7:183–186, 1978.

Mackay IS: The deviated nose. Plast Reconstr Surg 3:253–265, 1986.

Marshall DR, Slattery PG: Intracranial complications of rhinoplasty. Br J Plast Surg 36:342–344, 1983.

Mathog RH: Management of acute nasal fractures. In Cummings GW, Fredrickson JM, Harkin LA, et al (eds): Otolaryngology—Head and Neck Surgery. St Louis: CV Mosby, 1986, pp 611–624.

Mondin V, Rinaldo A, Ferlito A: Management of nasal bone fractures. Am J Otolaryngol 26:181–188, 2005.

Murray JAM, Maran AGD: The treatment of nasal injuries by manipulation. J Laryngol Otolaryngol 94:1405–1410, 1980.

Murray JAM, Maran AGD, MacKenzie IJ: Open vs closed reduction of the fractured nose. Arch Otolaryngol 110:797–802, 1984.

Schultz RC: The management of common facial fractures. Surg Clin North Am 53:3–32, 1973.

Schultz RC, deVillers YT: Nasal fractures. J Trauma 15:319–327, 1974.

Smith B: Reduction of nasal orbital fractures and simultaneous dacryocystorhinostomy. Trans Am Acad Ophthalmol Otolaryngol 82:527–530, 1976.

Stranc MF, Robertson GA: A classification of injuries of the nasal skeleton. Ann Plast Surg 2:468–474, 1979.

Zygoma Fractures

Antonyshyn O, Gruss JS, Kassel EE: Blow-in fractures of the orbit. Plast Reconstr Surg 84:10–20, 1989.

Briggs PC, Heckler FR: Lacrimal gland involvement in zygomaticofrontal fracture site. Plast Reconstr Surg 80:682–685, 1987.

Carr R, Mathog RHM: Early and delayed repair of orbitozygomatic fractures. J Oral Maxillofac Surg 55:253–258, 1997.

Crumley RL, Leibsohn J, Krause CJ, Burton TC: Fractures of the orbital floor. Laryngoscope 87:934–947, 1977.

Czerwinski M, Martin M, Lee C: Quantitative comparison of open reduction and internal fixation vs. the Gilles method in the treatment of orbitozygomatic complex fractures. Plast Reconstr Surg 115:1948–1954, 2005.

Dingman RO, Natvig P: Surgery of facial fractures. Philadelphia: WB Saunders, 1964, pp 211–245.

Eisele DW, Duckert LF: Single-point stabilization of zygomatic fractures with the minicompression plate. Arch Otolaryngol 113:267–270, 1987.

Ellis E, El-Attar A, Moos KF: Analysis of 2,067 cases of zygomatico-orbital fracture. Oral Maxillofac Surg 43:417–428, 1985.

Fugaça WC, Fereirra MC, Dellon AL: Infraorbital nerve injury associated with zygoma fracture: Documentation and neurosensory testing. Plast Reconstr Surg 113:834–838, 2004.

Gillies MD, Kelner TP, Stone D: Fractures of the malar-zygomatic compound. Br J Plast Surg 14:651–675, 1927.

Gordon S, McCrae II: Monocular blindness as a complication of the treatment of a malar fracture. Plast Reconstr Surg 6:228–232, 1950.

Hinderer UT: Malar implants for improvement of the facial appearance. Plast Reconstr Surg 56:157–165, 1975.

Holmes KD, Matthews BL: Three point alignment of zygoma fractures with miniplate fixation. Arch Otolaryngol Head Neck Surg 115:961–963, 1989.

Jamal BT, Pfahler SM, Lane KA, BIlyk JR, Pribitken EA, Diecidue RJ, Taub DI: Ophthalmalic injuries in patients with zygomaticomaxillary complex fractures requiring surgical repair. J Oral Maxillofac Surg 67:986–989, 2009.

Karlan MS, Cassisi NJ: Fractures of the zygoma. Arch Otolaryngol 105:320–327, 1979.

Karlan M, Skobel BS: Reconstruction for malar asymmetry. Arch Otolaryngol 106:20–24, 1980.

Kazanjian ES, Converse JM: Surgical Treatment of Facial Injuries. 3rd ed. Baltimore: Williams & Wilkins, 1974, pp 287–306.

Knight JS, North JF: The classification of malar fractures: An analysis of displacement as a guide to treatment. Br J Plast Surg 13:325–332, 1961.

Lederman IR: Loss of vision associated with surgical treatment of zygomatico-orbital floor fracture. Plast Reconstr Surg 68:94–99, 1981.

Lund K: Fractures of the zygoma: A follow-up study of 62 patients. J Oral Surg 29:557–560, 1971.

Mathog RH: Reconstruction of the orbit following trauma. Otolaryngol Clin North Am 16:585–607, 1983.

Mathog RH, Rosenberg Z: Complications in the treatment of facial fractures. Otolaryngol Clin North Am 9:547–550, 1976.

Mustarde JC: The role of Lockwood's suspensory ligament in preventing downward displacement of the eye. Br J Plast Surg 21:73–81, 1968.

Nordgaard JO: Persistent sensory disturbances and diplopia following fractures of the zygoma. Arch Otolaryngol 102:80–82, 1976.

Rinehart GG, Marsh JL, Hemmer KM, Bresina S: Internal fixation of malar fractures: An experimental biophysical study. Plast Reconstr Surg 84:21–25, 1989.

Rohrich RJ, Watamull D: Comparison of rigid plates vs. wire fixation in management of zygomatic fractures: A long-term follow up clinical study. Plast Reconstr Surg 96:570–575, 1995.

Rowe NL, Killey HC: Fractures of the Facial Skeleton. Baltimore: Williams & Wilkins, 1986, pp 276–344.

Scrimshaw GC: Malar-orbital-zygomatic fracture causing fracture of underlying coronoid process. J Trauma 18:367–368, 1978.

Stanley RB, Mathog RH: Evaluation and correction of combined orbital trauma syndrome. Laryngoscope 93:856–865, 1983.

Stanley RB, Mathog RH: Late reconstruction of the orbit after trauma to the inferior and lateral walls. In Ward PH, Berman WC (eds): Plastic and Reconstructive Surgery: Proceedings of the Fourth International Symposium. St Louis: CV Mosby, 1984.

Tahernia A, Erdmann D, Follmar K, Mukundan S, Grimes J, Marcus J: Clinical implications of orbital volume changes in the management of isolated and zygomaticomaxillary complex-associated orbital floor injuries. Plast Reconstr Surg 123:968–975, 2009.

Whitaker LA: Aesthetic augmentation of the malar-midface structures. Plast Reconstr Surg 80:337–346, 1987.

Vrieris JP, VanderGlas HW, Bosman F, Koole R, Moos KF: Information on infraorbital nerve damage from multitesting of sensory function. Int J Oral Maxillofac Surg 27:20–26, 1998.

Yamamoto K, Murakami K, Sugiura T, Fujmoto M, Inoue M, Kawakami M, Ohgi K, Kirita T: Clinical analysis of isolated zygomatic arch fractures. J Oral Maxillofac Surg 65:457–461, 2007.

Yanigasawa E: Symposium on maxillofacial trauma. III: Pitfalls in the management of zygomatic fractures. Laryngoscope 88:527–546, 1973.

Yaremchuk MJ: Orbital deformity after craniofacial fracture repair: Avoidance and treatment. J Craniomaxillofac Trauma 5:7–16, 1999.

Orbital Wall Fractures

Antonyshyn O, Gruss JS, Galbraith DJ, Hurwitz JJ: Complex orbital fractures: A critical analysis of immediate bone graft reconstruction. Ann Plast Surg 22:220–235, 1989.

Bite V, Jackson IT, Forbes GS, Gehring DG: Orbital volume measurements in enophthalmos using three-dimensional CT imaging. Plast Reconstr Surg 75:502–507, 1985.

Burres S, Cohn AM, Mathog RH: Repair of orbital blow-out fractures with Marlex mesh and Gelfilm. Laryngoscope 91:1881–1886, 1981.

Converse JM: Correction of enophthalmos by disentrapment of an orbital blowout fracture. Plast Reconstr Surg 62:788–789, 1978.

Converse JM, Smith B: Enophthalmos and diplopia in fractures of the orbital floor. Br J Plast Surg 9:265–274, 1975.

Converse JM, Smith B: Reconstruction of the floor of the orbit by bone grafts. Arch Ophthalmol 44:1–21, 1950.

Converse JM, Wood-Smith D: Orbital and naso-orbital fractures. In Converse JM (ed): Reconstructive Plastic Surgery, vol 2. Philadelphia: WB Saunders, 1977, pp 740–776.

Converse JM, Cole G, Smith B: Late treatment of blowout fractures of the orbit. Plast Reconstr Surg 28:183–190, 1961.

Converse JM, Smith B, Obear M: Orbital blowout fractures: A ten year survey. Plast Reconstr Surg 39:20–26, 1967.

Converse JM, Smith B, Wood-Smith D: Deformities of the midface resulting from malunited orbital and naso-orbital fractures. Clin Plast Surg 2:107–130, 1975.

Converse JM, Smith B, Wood-Smith D: Malunited fractures of the orbit. In Converse JM (ed): Reconstructive Plastic Surgery, vol 2. Philadelphia: WB Saunders, 1977, pp 989–1033.

Converse JM, Firmin T, Wood-Smith D, Friedland JA: The conjunctival approach in orbital fractures. Plast Reconstr Surg 52:656–657, 1973.

Crumley RL, Leibsohn J, Krause CJ, Burton TC: Fractures of the orbital floor. Laryngoscope 97:934–947, 1977.

Dulley B, Fells P: Long-term follow-up of orbital blow-out fractures with and without contrast surgery. Mod Probl Ophthalmol 14:467–470, 1975.

Ellis E, Tan Y: Assessment of internal orbital reconstruction for pure blowout fractures: Cranial bone grafts versus titanium mesh. J Oral Maxillofac Surg 61:442–453, 2003.

Emery JM, Von Noorden GK, Schlernitzauer DA: Orbital floor fractures: Long-term follow-up of cases with and without surgical repair. Trans Am Acad Ophthalmol Otolaryngol 75:802–812, 1971.

Fan X, Li J, Zhu J, Li H, Zhang D: Computer-associated orbital volume measurements in the surgical correction of late enophthalmos caused by blow out fracture. Ophthal Plast Reconstr Surg 19:207–211, 2003.

Fujino T: Experimental "blowout" fracture of the orbit. Plast Reconstr Surg 54:81–82, 1974.

Fujino T, Makino K: Entrapment mechanism and ocular injury in orbital blowout fracture. Plast Reconstr Surg 65:571–574, 1980.

Graham SM, Thomas RD, Carter AD, Nerad J: The Transcaruncular approach to the medial orbital wall. Laryngoscope 112:986–989, 2002.

He D, Blomquist PH, Ellis E III: Association between ocular injuries and internal orbital fractures. J Oral Maxillofac Surg 67:713–720, 2007.

Heckler FR, Songcharoen S, Sultani FA: Subciliary incision and skin-muscle flap for orbital fractures. Ann Plast Surg 10:309–313, 1983.

Ioannides C, Treffers W, Rutten M, Neverraz P: Occular injuries associated with fractures involving the orbit. J Craniomaxillofac Surg 16:157–159, 1988.

Jabaley ME, Lerman M, Sanders HJ: Ocular injuries in orbital fractures: A review of 119 cases. Plast Reconstr Surg 56:410–418, 1975.

Jones DEP, Evans JNG: "Blowout" fractures of the orbit: An investigation into their anatomical basis. J Laryngol Otol 81:1109–1120, 1967.

Kawamoto HK: Late posttraumatic enophthalmos: A correctable deformity? Plast Reconstr Surg 69:423–432, 1982.

Kersten RC: Blowout fracture of the orbital floor with entrapment caused by isolated trauma to the orbital rim. Am J Ophthalmol 103:215–219, 1987.

Kokemueller H, Zizelmann C, Tavassel F, Puling T, Gellrich N-C: A comprehensive approach to objective quantification of orbital dimensions. J Oral Maxillofac Surg 66:401–407, 2008.

Kolk A, Pautke C, Schott V, Ventrella E, Weiner E, Ploder O, Horch HH, Neff H: Secondary post-traumatic enophthalmos high-resolution magnetic resonance imaging compared with multi-slice computed tomography in post-operative orbital volume measurements. J Maxillofac Surg 65:1926–1934, 2007.

Kontio RK, Laine P, Salo H, Paukku P, Lindqvist C, Suuronen R: Reconstruction of internal orbital wall fracture with iliac crest free bone graft: Clinical, computed tomography in magnetic resonance imaging follow-up study. Plast Reconstr Surg 118:1365–1374, 2006.

Koornneef L: Current concepts on the management of orbital blow-out fractures. Ann Plast Surg 9:185–200, 1982.

Lang W: Traumatic enophthalmos with retention of perfect acuity of vision. Eye 9:44–45, 1889.

Maisel RH, Acomb TE, Cantrell RW: Medial orbital blow-out fracture: A case report. Laryngoscope 85:1211–1215, 1975.

Malauskas AT, Fueges GF: Serious ocular complications associated with blowout fractures of the orbit. Am J Ophthalmol 62:670–672, 1966.

Maniglia AJ: Conjunctival approach to the orbit for repair of blowout fracture. Laryngoscope 90:1564–1568, 1980.

Manson PN: Pure orbital blowout fracture. New concepts and importance of the medial orbital blowout fracture. Plastic Reconstr Surg 104:878–882, 1999.

Manson PN, Clifford CM, Su CT, et al: Mechanisms of global support and posttraumatic enophthalmos: I. The anatomy of the ligament sling and its relation to intramuscular cone orbital fat. Plast Reconstr Surg 77:193–202, 1986.

Manson PN, Grivas A, Rosenbaum A, et al: Studies on enophthalmos II: The measurement of orbital injuries and their treatment by quantitative computed tomography. Plast Reconstr Surg 77:203–214, 1986.

Mathog RH: Maxillofacial orbital blowout fractures. In Pillsbury HC, Goldsmith MM (eds): Operative Challenges in Otolaryngology—Head and Neck Surgery. Chicago: Year Book Medical Publishers, 1991, pp 471–496.

Mathog RH: Reconstruction of the orbit following trauma. Otolaryngol Clin North Am 16:585–607, 1983.

Mathog RH, Rosenberg Z: Complications in the treatment of facial fractures. Otolaryngol Clin North Am 9:533–553, 1974.

Mathog RH, Archer KF, Nesi FA: Posttraumatic enophthalmos and diplopia. Otolaryngol Head Neck Surg 94:69–77, 1986.

Miller GR: Blindness developing a few days after a midface fracture. Plast Reconstr Surg 42:384–385, 1968.

Nesi F, LiVecchi F, Mathog RH: Orbital blowout fractures. In Mathog RH (ed): Maxillofac Trauma. Baltimore: Williams & Wilkins, 1983, pp 318–320.

Nicholson DH, Guzak ST: Visual loss complicating repair of orbital fractures. Arch Ophthalmol 86:370–375, 1971.

Nishiike S, Nagai M, Nakagawa A, Konishi M, Kato T, Sakata Y, Yasakura T, Harada T: Endoscopic transantral orbital floor repair with antral bone grafts. Arch Otolaryngol Head Neck Surg 131:911–915, 2005.

Panje WR, Gross CE, Anderson RL: Sudden blindness following trauma. Otolaryngol Head Neck Surg 87:941–948, 1981.

Parkin JL, Stevens MH, Stringham JC: Absorbable gelatin film versus silicone rubber sheeting in orbital fracture treatment. Laryngoscope 97:1–3, 1987.

Parsons GS, Mathog RH: Orbital wall and volume relationships. Arch Otolaryngol 114:743–747, 1988.

Pearl RM: Surgical management of volumetric changes in the bony orbit. Ann Plast Surg 19:349–358, 1987.

Pearl RM, Vistnes LM: Orbital blowout fractures: An approach to management. Ann Plast Surg 1:267–270, 1978.

Pfeiffer RL: Traumatic enophthalmos. Arch Ophthalmol 30:718–726, 1943.

Pham AM, Strong EB: Endoscopic management of facial fractures. Curr Opin Otolaryngol Head Neck Surg 14:234–241, 2006.

Polley JW, Ringler SL: The use of Teflon in orbital floor reconstruction following blunt facial trauma: A 20 year experience. Plast Reconstr Surg 79:39–43, 1987.

Potter JK, Ellis E III: Biomaterials for reconstruction of the internal orbit. J Oral Maxillofac Surg 62:1280–1297, 2004.

Putterman AM: Late management of blowout fractures of the orbital floor. Trans Am Acad Otol 83:650–659, 1977.

Putterman AM, Stevens T, Urist M: Nonsurgical management of blowout fractures of the orbital floor. Am J Ophthalmol 77:232–238, 1974.

Putterman AM, Urist MJ: Treatment of enophthalmic narrow palpebral fissure after blowout fracture. Ophthalmic Surg 6:45–49, 1975.

Raflo GT: Blow-in and blow-out fractures of the orbit: Clinical correlations and proposed mechanisms. Ophthalmic Surg 15:114–119, 1984.

Rauch SD: Medial orbital blow-out fracture with entrapment. Arch Otolaryngol 111:53–55, 1985.

Siddique SA, Mathog RH: A comparison of parietal and iliac bone grafts for orbit reconstruction. J Oral Maxillofac Surg 60:44–50, 2002.

Smith B, Lisman RD, Simonton J, DellaRocca R: Volkmann's contracture of the extraocular muscles following blowout fracture. Plast Reconstr Surg 74:200–214, 1984.

Smith B, Regan WF: Blowout fractures of the orbit: Mechanism and correction of inferior orbital fracture. Am J Ophthalmol 44:733–739, 1957.

Smith B, Taiara C: Correction of enophthalmos and deep supratarsal sulcus by posterior subperiosteal glass bead implantation. Br J Ophthalmol 57:741–746, 1974.

Stanley RB, Mathog RH: Evaluation and correction of combined orbital trauma syndrome. Laryngoscope 93:856–865, 1983.

Stasior OG, Roen JL: Traumatic enophthalmos. Ophthalmol 89:1267–1273, 1982.

Sullivan WG, Smith AA: The split calvarial graft donor site in the elderly: A study in cadavers. Plast Reconstr Surg 84:29–31, 1988.

Tessier P: The conjunctival approach to the orbital floor and maxilla in congenital malformation and trauma. J Maxillofac Surg 1:3–8, 1973.

Thering HR, Bogart JN: Blowout fracture of the medial orbital wall with entrapment of the medial rectus muscle. Plast Reconstr Surg 63:848–852, 1979.

Tse R, Allen L, Matic D: The white-eyed medial blowout fracture. Plast Reconstr Surg 119:277–286, 2007.

Villarreal PM, Monje F, Morillo AJ, Junguera LM, Gonzalez C, Barbon JJ: Porous polyethylene implants in orbital floor reconstruction. Plast Reconstr Surg 109:877–885, 2002.

Wolfe SA: Application of craniofacial surgical precepts in orbital reconstruction following trauma and tumour removal. J Maxillofac Surg 10:212–223, 1982.

Wolfe SA: Surgical treatment of exophthalmos and enophthalmos. Ann Ophthalmol 13:995–1002, 1981.

Yano H, Nakano M, Anraku K, Suzuki Y, Ishida H, Murakami R, Hirano A: A consecutive case review of orbital blowout fractures and recommendations for comprehensive management. Plast Reconstr Surg. 124:602–11, 2009.

Naso-Orbital Fractures

Arden R, Mathog RH, Nesi FA: Flap reconstruction techniques in conjunctivorhinostomy. Otolaryngol Head Neck Surg 102(2):150–155, 1990.

Balle VH, Andersen R, Sum C: Incidence of lacrimal obstruction following trauma to the facial skeleton. Ear Nose Throat J 67:66–70, 1988.

Beyer CK, Fabian RL, Smith B: Naso-orbital fractures: Complications and treatment. Ophthalmology 89:456–463, 1982.

Beyer CK, Smith B: Naso-orbital fractures, complications and treatment. Ophthalmologica 163:418–427, 1972.

Busse H: The Kaleff-Hollwich technique and results of external-dacryocysto-rhinostomy operation. J Maxillofac Surg 7:135–141, 1979.

Converse JM, Hogan MV: Open sky approach for reduction of naso-orbital fractures. Plast Reconstr Surg 46:396–398, 1970.

Converse JM, Smith B: Canthoplasty and dacryocystorhinostomy in malunited fractures of the medial wall of the orbit. Am J Ophthalmol 35:1103–1114, 1952.

Converse JM, Smith B: Nasoorbital fractures and traumatic deformities of the medial canthus. Plast Reconstr Surg 38:147–162, 1966.

Converse JM, Smith B, Wood-Smith D: Deformities of the midface resulting from malunited orbital and naso-orbital fractures. Clin Plast Surg 2:107–130, 1975.

DeSouza C, Nissan J: Experience with endoscopic dacryocystorhinostomy using four methods. Otolaryngol Head Neck Surg 142:389–393, 2010.

Dingman RO, Grabb WC, Oneal RM: Management of injuries of the naso-orbital complex. Arch Surg 98:566–571, 1969.

Duvall AJ, Banovetz JD: Nasoethmoid fractures. Otolaryngol Clin North Am 9:507–515, 1976.

Freihoffer HPM: Experience with transnasal canthopexy. J Maxillofac Surg 8:119–124, 1980.

Freihoffer HPM: Inner intercanthal and interorbital distances. J Maxillofac Surg 8:324–326, 1980.

Furnas DW: The pulley canthoplasty for residual telecanthus after hypertelorism repair or facial trauma. Ann Plast Surg 5:85–94, 1979.

Furnas DW, Bircoll MJ: Eyelid traction test to determine if the medial canthal ligament is detached. Plast Reconstr Surg 52:315–317, 1973.

Gruss JS: Nasoethmoid-orbital fractures. Classification and role of primary bone grafting. Plast Reconstr Surg 75:303–317, 1985.

Gruss JS, Hurwitz JJ, Nik NA, Kassel EE: The pattern and incidence of nasolacrimal injury in naso-orbital-ethmoid fractures: The role of delayed assessment and dacryocystorhinostomy. Br J Plast Surg 38:116–121, 1985.

Hanna DC, Clairmont AA: Nasolacrimal duct reconstruction with a vein graft: A non-invasive technique. Plast Reconstr Surg 62:85–88, 1978.

Herford AS, Ying T, Brown V: Outcomes of severely comminuted (Type III) nasorbitoethmoid fractures. J Oral Maxillofac Surg 63:1266–1277, 2005.

Jones LT: The cure of epiphora due to canalicular disorders: Trauma and surgical failure on the lacrimal passages. Trans Am Acad Ophthalmol Otol 66:506–524, 1962.

Lauer G, Pinzer T: Transcaruncular sutures: A modification of medial canthopexy. J Oral Maxillofac Surg 66:2178–2184, 2008.

Macomber WB, Wang MKH, Linton PC: A technique of canthal ligament reconstruction. Plast Reconstr Surg 33:253–257, 1964.

Marsh JL: Blepharo-canthal deformities in patients following craniofacial surgery. Plast Reconstr Surg 61:842–853, 1978.

Mathog RH: Reconstruction of the orbit following trauma. Otolaryngol Clin North Am 16:585–607, 1983.

Mathog RH: Traumatic telecanthus. In Mathog RH (ed): Textbook of Maxillofacial Trauma. Baltimore: Williams & Wilkins, 1983, pp 303–318.

Mathog RH, Bauer W: Post-traumatic pseudohypertelorism (telecanthus). Arch Otolaryngol 105:81–85, 1979.

Mathog RH, Rosenberg Z: Complications in the treatment of facial fractures. Otolaryngol Clin North Am 9:547–550, 1976.

Melson R: Dacryocystorhinostomy. In Kennedy DW, Bolger WE, Zinreich JJ (eds): Diseases of the Sinus, Diagnosis and Management. Hamilton: Decker, 2001, pp 317–324.

Mishra P, Sonkhya N: Endoscopic transnasal dacryocystorhinostomy with nasal mucosal and posterior lacrimal sac flap. J Laryngol Otolaryngol 123:320–326, 2009.

Mustarde JC: Epicanthus and telecanthus. Br J Plast Surg 16:345–356, 1963.

Papadopoulos H, Salib NK: Management of nasal-orbital-ethmoidal fractures. Oral Maxillofac Surg Clin North Am 21:221–225, 2009.

Ramselaar JM, Van der Meulen JC, Bloem JJ: Naso-orbital fractures. Mod Probl Ophthalmol 14:107–110, 1975.

Rice DH: Endoscopic intranasal dacryocystorhinostomy: A cadaver study. Am J Rhinol 2:127–128, 1988.

Sargent LA: Nasoethmoid orbital fractures: Diagnosis and Treatment. Plast Reconstr Surg 120 (Suppl):16–31, 2007.

Smith B: Reduction of nasal orbital fractures and simultaneous dacryocystorhinostomy. Trans Am Acad Ophthalmol Otol 82:525–530, 1976.

Smith B, Beyer CK: Medial canthoplasty. Arch Ophthalmol 82:344–348, 1969.

Spinelli HM, Shapiro MD, Wei LL, Elahi E, Hirmand H: The role of lacrimal intubation in the management of facial trauma and tumor resection. Plastic Reconstr Surg 115:1871–1876, 2005.

Stranc MF: Primary treatment of nasoethmoid injuries with increased intercanthal distance. Br J Plast Surg 23:8–25, 1970.

Stranc MF: The pattern of lacrimal injuries in nasoethmoid fractures. Br J Plast Surg 23:335–346, 1970.

Tessier P: Experiences in the treatment of orbital hypertelorism. Plast Reconstr Surg 53:1–18, 1974.

Whitaker LA, Katowitz JA, Jacobs WE: Ocular adnexal problems in craniofacial deformities. J Maxillofac Surg 7:55–60, 1979.

Whitaker LA, Schaffer DB: Severe traumatic oculo-orbital displacement: Diagnosis and secondary treatment. Plast Reconstr Surg 59:352–359, 1977.

Frontal Sinus Fractures

Arden RL, Mathog RH, Thomas LM: Temporalis muscle-galea flap in craniofacial reconstruction. Laryngoscope 97:1336–1342, 1987.

Bell RB, Dierks EJ, Brar P, Potter JK, Potter BE: A protocol for the management of frontal sinus fractures emphasizing preservation. J Maxillofac Surg 65:825–834, 2007.

Bloem JJ, van der Meulen JC, Ramselaar JM: Orbital roof fractures. Mod Probl Ophthalmol 14:510–512, 1975.

Bordley JE, Bischofberger W: Osteomyelitis of the frontal bone. Laryngoscope 77:1234–1244, 1967.

Cabbage EB, Shively RS, Malik P: Cranioplasty for traumatic deformities of the frontoorbital area. Ann Plast Surg 13:175–184, 1984.

Calcaterra TC: Extracranial surgical repair of cerebrospinal fluid rhinorrhea. Ann Otol Rhinol Laryngol 87:108–116, 1980.

Capanna AH: A new method of cranioplasty. Surg Neurol 14:385–386, 1980.

Chen K-T, Chen C-T, Mardini S, Tsay PK, Chen Y-R: Frontal sinus fracture: A treatment algorthim and assessment of outcomes based on 78 clinical cases. Plast Reconstr Surg 118:457–468, 2006.

Curtin H, Wolfe D, Schramm V: Orbital roof blowout fractures. AJR Am J Roentgenol 139:969–972, 1982.

Donald PJ: Frontal sinus ablation by cranialization. Arch Otolaryngol 108:142–146, 1982.

Donald PJ, Bernstein L: Compound frontal sinus injuries with intracranial penetration. Laryngoscope 88:225–232, 1978.

Donald PJ, Ettin M: The safety of frontal sinus obliteration when sinus walls are missing. Laryngoscope 96:190–193, 1986.

Donath A, Sindwani R: Frontal sinus cranialization using the pericranial flap: An additional layer of Protection. Laryngoscope 116:1585–1588, 2006.

Fattahi T, Johnson C, Steinberg B: Comparison of two preferred methods used for frontal sinus obliteration. J Oral Maxillofac Surg 63:487–491, 2005.

Flanagan JC, McLachlan DL, Shannon GM: Orbital roof fractures. Neurologic and neurosurgical considerations. Am Acad Ophthalmol 87:325–339, 1980.

Gerbino C, Roccia F, Benech A, Calderelli C: Analysis of 158 frontal sinus fractures: Current surgical management and complications. J Craniomaxillofac Trauma 28:133–140, 2000.

Gossman D, Archer SA, Arosarena O: Management of frontal sinus fractures: A review of 96 cases. Laryngoscope 116:1357–1362, 2006.

Gruss JS: Fronto-naso-orbital trauma. Clin Plast Surg 9:577–589, 1982.

Heller EM, Jacobs JB, Holliday RH: Evaluation of the frontonasal duct in frontal sinus fractures. Head Neck 11:46–50, 1989.

Herford AS, Ying T, Brown B: Outcomes of severely comminuted (Type III) nasorbital ethmoid fractures. J Oral Maxillary Surg 63:1266–1277, 2005.

Horowitz JH, Persing JA, Winn HR, Edgerton MT: The late treatment of vertical orbital dystopia resulting from orbital roof fracture. Ann Plast Surg 13:519–524, 1984.

Hybels RL: Posterior table fractures of the frontal sinus II: Clinical aspects. Laryngoscope 87:1740–1745, 1977.

Hybels RL, Newman MH: Posterior table fractures of the frontal sinus 1: An experimental study. Laryngoscope 87:171–179, 1977.

Ioannides C, Freihofer HPM, Bruaset I: Trauma of the upper third of the face: Management and follow-up. J Maxillofac Surg 12:255–261, 1984.

Jackson IT, Adham MN, Marsh WR: Use of the galeal frontalis myofascial flap in craniofacial surgery. Plast Reconstr Surg 77:905–910, 1986.

Kennedy DW: Functional endoscopic sinus surgery techniques. Arch Otolaryngol 111:643–649, 1988.

Lakani RS, Shibuya TY, Mathog RH, Marks SC, Burgio DL, Yoo GH: Titanium mesh repair of the severely comminuted frontal sinus fracture. Arch Otolaryngol Head Neck Surg 127:665–669, 2001.

Larrabee WF, Travis LW, Tabb HG: Frontal sinus fracture—their suppurative complications and surgical management. Laryngoscope 90:1810–1813, 1980.

Levine SB, Rowe LD, Keane WM, Atkins JP: Evaluation and treatment of frontal sinus fractures. Otolaryngol Head Neck Surg 95:19–22, 1986.

Lynch RC: The technique of a radical frontal sinus operation which has given me the best results. Laryngoscope 31:1–5, 1921.

Manson PN, Crawley WA, Hoopes JE: Frontal cranioplasty: Risk factors and choice of cranial vault reconstruction material. Plast Reconstr Surg 77:888–898, 1986.

Mathog RH: Frontoethmoid fractures. In Gates GA (ed): Current Therapy in Otolaryngology—Head and Neck Surgery. Philadelphia: BC Decker, 1984–1985, pp 100–104.

Mathog RH, Crane LR, Nowak GS: Antimicrobial therapy following head and neck trauma. In Johnson JT (ed): Antibiotic Therapy in Head and Neck Surgery. New York: Marcel Dekker, 1987, pp 31–47.

Maves MD, Matt BH: Calvarial bone grafting of facial defects. Otolaryngol Head Neck Surg 95:464–470, 1986.

May M, Ogura JH, Schramm V: Nasofrontal duct in frontal sinus fractures. Arch Otolaryngol 92:534–538, 1970.

McClurg FL, Swanson PJ: An orbital roof fracture causing diplopia. Arch Otolaryngol 102:497–498, 1976.

McLachlan DL, Flanagan JC, Shannon GM: Complications of orbital roof fractures. Am Acad Ophthalmol 89:1274–1278, 1982.

Messerklinger N: On the drainage of the normal frontal sinus of man. Acta Otolaryngol 63:176–181, 1967.

Messinger A, Radkowski MA, Greenwald MJ, Pensler JM: Orbital root fractures in the pediatric population. Plast Reconstr Surg 84:213–216, 1984.

Newman MH, Travis LW: Frontal sinus fractures. Laryngoscope 83:1281–1291, 1973.

Ousterhout DK, Tessier P: Closure of large cribriform defects with a forehead flap. J Maxillofac Surg 9:7–9, 1981.

Panje WR, Gross CE, Anderson RL: Sudden blindness following trauma. Otolaryngol Head Neck Surg 87:941–948, 1981.

Pfaltz CR: The indications of infraorbital nerve decompression. ORL J Otorhinolaryngol Relat Spec 35:214–216, 1973.

Pollack K, Payne EE: Fractures of the frontal sinus. Otolaryngol Clin North Am 9:517–522, 1976.

Potter JA, Siddoway JR, Mathog RH: Injury to the orbital plate of the frontal bone. Head Neck Surg 10:78–84, 1987.

Prendergast ML, Wildes TO: Evaluation of the orbital floor in zygoma fractures. Arch Otolaryngol Head Neck Surg 114:446–450, 1988.

Prolo DJ, Oklund SA: Composite autogeneic human cranioplasty: Frozen skull supplemented with fresh iliac corticocancellous bone. Neurosurgery 15:846–851, 1984.

Psillakis JM, Nocchi LB, Zanini SA: Repair of large defect of frontal bone with free graft and outer table of parietal bones. Plast Reconstr Surg 64:827–830, 1979.

Raveh J, Vuillemen T: Subcranial management of 395 combined frontobasal-midface fractures. Arch Otolaryngol Head Neck Surg 114:1114–1122, 1988.

Rice DH: Management of frontal sinus fractures. Curr Opin Otolaryngol Head Neck Surg 12:46–48, 2004.

Rodriquez ED, Stanwix MG, Nan A, St. Hilaire H, Simmons O, Christy MR, Grant MP, Manson PN: Twenty-six-year experience treating frontal sinus fractures: A novel algorithm based on anatomical fracture, pattern and failure of conventional techniques. Plast Reconstruc Surg 122:1850–1866, 2008.

Sataloff RT, Sariego J, Myers DF, Richter HJ: Surgical management of the frontal sinus. Neurosurgery 15:593–596, 1984.

Schenck NL: Frontal sinus disease III: Experimental and clinical factors in failure of the frontal osteoplastic operation. Laryngoscope 85:76–92, 1975.

Schenck NL, Rauchbach E, Ogura JE: Frontal sinus disease II development of the frontal sinus model: Occlusion of the nasofrontal duct. Laryngoscope 84:1233–1247, 1974.

Schultz RC: Frontal sinus and supraorbital fractures from vehicle accidents. Clin Plast Surg 2:93–106, 1975.

Schultz RC: Supraorbital and glabellar fractures. Plast Reconstr Surg 45:227–233, 1980.

Shockley WW, Stucker FJ, Gage-White L, Anthony SO: Frontal sinus fractures: Some problems and some solutions. Laryngoscope 98:18–22, 1988.

Smith TL, Han JK, Loehre JA, Rhee JS: Endoscopic management of the frontal sinus recess and frontal sinus fractures: A shift in paradigm? Laryngoscope 112:784–790, 2002.

Stanley RB, Becker TS: Injuries of the nasofrontal orifices in frontal sinus fractures. Laryngoscope 97:728–731, 1987.

Stanley RB, Schwartz MS: Immediate reconstruction of contaminated central craniofacial injuries with free autogenous grafts. Laryngoscope 99:1011–1015, 1989.

Strong EB, Buchalter GM, Moulthrop TH: Endoscopic repair of isolated anterior table frontal sinus fractures. Arch Facial Plast Surg 5:514–521, 2003.

Tiwari P, Higuera S, Thornton J, Hollier LH: The management of frontal sinus fractures. J Oral Maxillofac Surg 63:1354–1360, 2005.

Van Gool A: Preformed polymethylmethacrylate cranioplasties. J Maxillofac Surg 13:2–8, 1988.

Wallis A, Donald PJ: Frontal sinus fractures: A review of 72 cases. Laryngoscope 98:593–598, 1988.

Waring GO, Flanagan JC: Pneumocephalus. A sign of intracranial involvement in orbital fracture. Arch Ophthalmol 93:847–850, 1975.

Williamson LK, Miller RH, Sessions RB: Treatment of nasofrontal ethmoidal complex fractures. Otolaryngol Head Neck Surg 89:587–593, 1981.

Wilson BC, Davidson B, Corey JP, Haydon RC: Comparison of complications following frontal sinus fractures managed with exploration with or without obliteration over 10 years. Laryngoscope 98:516–520, 1988.

Wolfe SA: The utility of pericranial flaps. Ann Plast Surg 1:146–153, 1978.

Wolfe SA, Johnson P: Frontal sinus injuries: Primary care and management of late complications. Plast Reconstr Surg 82:781–789, 1988.

Sphenoid Fractures

Anderson RL, Panje WR, Gross CE: Optic nerve blindness following blunt forehead trauma. Ophthalmology 89:445–455, 1982.

Cook MW, Levin LA, Joseph MP, Pinczower EF: Traumatic optic neuropathy. A meta-analysis. Arch Otolaryngol Head Neck Surg 122:389–392, 1996.

Fukado Y: Results in 400 cases of surgical decompression of the optic nerve. Mod Probl Ophthalmol 14:474–481, 1975.

Funk GF, Stanley RB, Becker TS: Reversible visual loss due to impacted lateral orbital wall fractures. Head Neck Surg 11:295–300, 1989.

Ghobrial W, Amstatz S, Mathog RH: Fractures of the sphenoid bone. Head Neck Surg 8:447–455, 1986.

Habal MB, Maniscalco JE: Surgical relations of the orbit and optic nerve: An anatomical study under magnification. Ann Plast Surg 4:265–275, 1979.

Holt RG, Holt JE: Incidence of eye injuries in facial fractures: An analysis of 727 cases. Otolaryngol Head Neck Surg 91:276–279, 1983.

Jabaley ME, Lerman M, Sanders HJ: Ocular injuries in orbital fractures. Plast Reconstr Surg 56:410–418, 1975.

Kennerdell JS, Amsbaugh GH, Myers EN: Transantralethmoidal decompression of optic canal fracture. Arch Ophthalmol 94:1040–1043, 1976.

Ketchum LD, Ferris B, Masters FW: Blindness without direct injury to the globe—a complication of facial fractures. Plast Reconstr Surg 58(2):187–191, 1976.

Kountakis SE, Maillard AA, El-Hanazi SM, Longhini L, Urso RG: Endoscopic optic nerve decompression with traumatic blindness. Otolaryngol Head Neck Surg 123:34–37, 2000.

Krausen AS, Ogura JH, Burde RM, Ostrow DE: Emergency orbital decompression: A reprieve from blindness. Otolaryngol Head Neck Surg 89:252–256, 1981.

Li HB, Shi JB, Cheng L, Yun O, Xu G: Salvage optic nerve decompression for traumatic blindness under nasal endoscopy: Risk and Benefit Analysis. Clin Otolaryngol 34:347–351, 2007.

Li KK, Teknos TN, Lai A, Laurtano A, Joseph MP: Traumatic optic neuropathy: Result in 45 consecutive surgical treated patients. Otolaryngol Head Neck Surg 120:5–11, 1999.

Lipkin AT, Woodson GE, Miller RH: Visual loss due to orbital fracture. Arch Otolaryngol 113:81–83, 1987.

Manfredi SJ, Rajii MR, Sprinkle PM, et al: Computerized tomographic scan findings in facial fractures associated with blindness. Plast Reconstr Surg 68:479–489, 1981.

Niho S, Niho M, Niho K: Decompression of the optic canal by the transethmoidal route and decompression of the superior orbital fissure. Can J Ophthalmol 5:22–40, 1970.

Niho S, Yasuda K, Sato T, et al: Decompression of the optic canal by the transethmoidal route. Am J Ophthalmol 51:659–665, 1961.

Osguthorpe JD, Sofferman RA: Optic nerve decompression. Otolaryngol Clin North Am 21:155–169, 1988.

Panje WR, Gross CE, Anderson RL: Sudden blindness following trauma. Otolaryngol Head Neck Surg 89:941–948, 1981.

Rajiniganth MG, Gupta AK, Gupta A, Bapuraj JR: Traumatic optic neuropathy: Visual outcome following combined therapy protocol. Arch Otolaryngol Head Neck Surg 129:1203–1206, 2003.

Ramsay JH: Optic nerve injury in fracture of the canal. Br J Ophthalmol 63:607–610, 1979.

Raveh J, Vuillemin T: Subcranial management of 395 combined frontobasal-midface fractures. Arch Otolaryngol Head Neck Surg 114:1114–1122, 1988.

Resneck JD, Lederman IR: Traumatic chiasmal syndrome associated with pneumocephalus and sellar fracture. Am J Ophthalmol 92:233–237, 1987.

Sherman R, Gottlieb LJ: Carotid-cavernous sinus fistula complicating a complex shotgun facial injury. Ann Plast Surg 21:251–256, 1988.

Shoji N, Kazuhide Y, Yikasi S, et al: Decompression of the optic canal by the transethmoidal route. Am J Ophthalmol 51:659–665, 1961.

Sofferman RA: Sphenoethmoid approach to the optic nerve. Laryngoscope 91:184–196, 1981.

Spoor TC, Mathog RH: Restoration of vision after optic nerve decompression. Arch Ophthalmol 104:804–805, 1986.

Stanley RB: The temporal approach to impacted lateral orbital wall fractures. Arch Otolaryngol Head Neck Surg 114:550–553, 1988.

Unger JD, Unger GF: Fractures of the pterygoid process accompanying severe facial bone injury. Radiology 98:311–316, 1971.

Walsh FB: Pathological clinical correlations 1: Indirect trauma to the optic nerves and chiasm. Invest Ophthalmol 5:433–449, 1966.

Weymuller EA: Blindness and LeFort III fractures. Ann Otol Rhinol Laryngol 93:2–5, 1984.

Yoshinao F: Results in 350 cases of surgical decompression of the optic nerve. Trans Fourth Asia-Pacific Congress Ophthalmol 4:96–99, 1972.

Ethmoid Fractures

Arness JS: Nasoethmoid orbital fractures: Classification and role of primary bone grafting. Plast Reconstr Surg 75:303–317, 1985.

Barrs DM, Kern EB: Use of intranasal pledgets for localization of cerebrospinal fluid rhinorrhea (notes in technique). Rhinology 17:227–230, 1979.

Brandt F, Nahser HC, Hartjes H, Kunitsch G: The value of metrizamide CT cisternography in the diagnosis of CSF fistulae. Acta Neurochir 69:37–42, 1983.

Calcaterra TC: Extracranial surgical repair of cerebrospinal fluid rhinorrhea. Ann Otol Rhinol Laryngol 89:108–116, 1980.

Chiro GD, Ommaya AK, Ashburn WL, Briner WH: Isotope cisternography in the diagnosis and follow-up of cerebrospinal fluid rhinorrhea. J Neurosurg 28:522–529, 1960.

Chow JM, Goodman D, Mafee MF: Evaluation of CSF rhinorrhea by computerized tomography with metrizamide. Otolaryngol Head Neck Surg 100:99–100, 1989.

Dukert LG, Mathog RH: Diagnosis in persistent cerebrospinal fluid fistulas. Laryngoscope 87:18–25, 1977.

Gruss JS: Nasoethmoid-orbital fractures: Classification and role of primary bone grafting. Plast Reconstr Surg 75:303–317, 1988.

Hanley J, Bales J, Byrd B: Recurrent meningococcal meningitis with occult CSF leak. Arch Intern Med 139:702–703, 1979.

Kirchner FR, Proud GO: Method for identification and localization of cerebrospinal fluid rhinorrhea and otorrhea. Laryngoscope 70:921–930, 1960.

Klatersky J, Sadeghi M, Brihaye J: Antimicrobial prophylaxis in patients with rhinorrhea or otorrhea: A double blind study. Surg Neurol 6:111–114, 1976.

Mahaley MS, Odom GL: Complication following intrathecal injection of fluorescein. J Neurosurg 25:298–299, 1966.

Markham JW: Clinical features of pneumocephalus based upon a survey of 284 cases with report of 11 additional cases. Acta Neurol 15:1–78, 1967.

Mathog RH: Frontoethmoid fractures. In Gates G (ed): Current Therapy in Otolaryngology—Head and Neck Surgery. Philadelphia: BC Decker, 1984, pp 100–104.

May M: Nasal frontal ethmoidal injuries. Laryngoscope 87:948–953, 1977.

McCabe BF: The osteomucoperiosteal flap in repair of cerebrospinal fluid rhinorrhea. Laryngoscope 86:537–539, 1976.

Moseley JI, Carton CA, Stern WE: Spectrum of complications in the use of intrathecal fluorescein. J Neurosurg 48:765–767, 1978.

North JB: The importance of intracranial air. Br J Surg 58:826–829, 1971.

Ramsden RT, Block T: Traumatic pneumocephalus. J Laryngol Otol 90:345–355, 1990.

Schaefer SD, Diehl JT, Briggs WH: The diagnosis of CSF rhinorrhea by metrizamide CT scanning. Laryngoscope 90:871–875, 1980.

Schnabel C, DiMartino E, Gilsbach JM, Riediger D, Gressnen AM, Kunz D: Comparison of beta 2-transferrin and beta–trace protein for detection of cerebrospinal fluid in nasal and ear fluids. Clin Chem 56:61–63, 2004.

Shetty PG, Shroff M, Sahani DV, Kirtane MV: Evaluation of high-resolution CT and MR cistenography in the diagnosis of cerebrospinal fluid fistula. Am J Neuroradiol 19:633–639, 1998.

Shibuya TY, Carron MA, Doerr T, Stachler R, Zormier M, Mathog RH, McLaren TL, Li K-T: Facial Fracture repair in the traumatic brain injury patient. J Maxillofac Surg 65:1693–1699, 2007.

Stammberger H: Endoscopic endonasal surgery-concepts and treatment of recurring rhinosinusitis Part 1 anatomic and pathophysiologic correlations. Otolaryngol Head Neck Surg 94:143–147, 1986.

Stankiewicz JA, Welch KC: A contemporary view of endoscopic sinus surgery: Techniques, tools and outcomes. Laryngoscope 119:2258–2268, 2009.

Waring GO, Flanagan JC: Pneumocephalus—a sign of intracranial involvement in orbital fracture. Arch Ophthalmol 93:847–850, 1975.

Yokoyama K, Hasegawa M, Shiba K, et al: Diagnosis of CSF rhinorrhea: Detection of tau-transferrin in nasal discharge. Otolaryngol Head Neck Surg 98:328–332, 1988.

Zuckerman JD, Delgaudio JM. Utility of preoperative high resolution CT and intraoperative image guidance in identification of cerebral spinal fluid leaks for endoscopic repair. Am J Rhinol 22:151–154, 2008.

Temporal Bone Fractures

Alford BR, Weber SC, Sessions RB: Neurodiagnostic studies in facial paralysis. Ann Otol 79:227–233, 1970.

Barber HO: Dizziness and head injury. Canad Med Assoc J 92:974–978, 1965.

Barber HO: Head injury. Audiological and vestibular findings. Ann Otol 78:239–252, 1969.

Barber HO: Positional nystagmus, especially after head injury. Laryngoscope 4:891–944, 1964.

Bellucci RJ: Traumatic injuries of the middle ear. Otolaryngol Clin North Am 16:633–650, 1983.

Benitez JT, Bouchard KR, Lane R, Szopo D: Pathology of deafness and dysequilibrium in head injury: A human temporal bone study. Am J Otol 1:163–167, 1980.

Bergemalm P-O: Progressive hearing loss after closed head injury: A predictable outcome? Acta Otolaryngol 123:836–845, 2003.

Brodie HA, Thompson TC: Management of complications from 820 temporal bone fractures. Am J Otol 18:188–197, 1997.

Camilleri AE, Toner JG, Howarth KL, Hampton S, Ramsden RT: Cochlear implantation following temporal bone fracture. J Laryngol Otol 113:454–457, 1999.

Cannon CR, Jahrsdoerfer R: Temporal bone fractures. Arch Otolaryngol 109:285–288, 1983.

Chalat NT: Middle ear effects of trauma. Laryngoscope 81:1286–1303, 1971.

Chang CY, Cass SP: Management of facial nerve injury due to temporal bone trauma. Am J Otol 20:96–114, 1999.

Coker NJ, Kendall KH, Jenkins HA, Alford BR: Traumatic intratemporal facial nerve injury: Management rationale for preservation of function. Otolaryngol Head Neck Surg 97:262–269, 1987.

Dahiya R, Keller JD, Litofsky NS, Bankey PE, Bonassar LJ, Megerian CA: Temporal Bone fractures: Otic capsule sparing versus otic capsule violating clinical and radiographic considerations. J Trauma 47:1079–1083, 1999.

Darrouzet V, Duclos JY, Liquoro D, Trulhe Y, DeBontils C, Bobean JP: Management of facial paralysis resulting from temporal bone fractures: Our experience in 115 cases. Otolaryngol Head Neck Surg 125:77–84, 2001.

Dawkes DK: Ossicular fixation. J Laryngol Otol 94:573–593, 1980.

Derlacki EL: Office closure of central tympanic membrane perforations: A quarter century of experience. Trans Am Acad Ophthalmol Otol 77:53–66, 1973.

Dommerby H, Tos M: Sensorineural hearing loss in post-traumatic incus dislocation. Arch Otolaryngol 109:257–261, 1983.

Eby TL, Pollak A, Fisch U: Histopathology of the facial nerve after longitudinal temporal bone fracture. Laryngoscope 98:717–720, 1988.

Emmett JR, Shea JJ: Traumatic perilymph fistula. Laryngoscope 90:1513–1520, 1980.

Fisch U: Facial paralysis in fractures of the petrous bone. Laryngoscope 84:2141–2154, 1974.

Fisch U: Management of intratemporal facial nerve injuries. J Laryngol Otol 94:129–134, 1980.

Fisch U: Prognostic value of electrical tests in acute facial paralysis. Am J Otol 5:494–498, 1984.

Fredrickson JM, Griffith HW: Transverse fracture of the temporal bone. Arch Otolaryngol 78:54–68, 1963.

Freeman J: Temporal bone fractures and cholesteatoma. Ann Otol Rhinol Laryngol 92:558–560, 1983.

Ghorayeb BY, Yeakley JW, Hall JW, Jones BE: Unusual complications of temporal bone fractures. Arch Otolaryngol Head Neck Surg 113:749–753, 1987.

Goodhill V, Harris I, Brockman SJ, Hantz O: Sudden deafness and labyrinthine window ruptures. Ann Otol 82:2–12, 1973.

Goodwin WS Jr: Temporal bone fractures. Otolaryngol Clin North Am 16:651–659, 1983.

Graham MD: Surgical exposure of the facial nerve. Otolaryngol Clin North Am 7:437–456, 1974.

Grant JR, Arganbirght J, Friedland DR: Outcomes for conservative management of traumatic conductive hearing loss. Otol Neurotol 29:344–349, 2008.

Griffin WL: A retrospective study of traumatic tympanic membrane perforations in a clinical practice. Laryngoscope 89:261–282, 1979.

Griffiths MV: The incidence of auditory and vestibular concussion following minor head injury. J Laryngol Otol 93:253–265, 1979.

Gros JC: The ear in skull trauma. South Med J 60:705–711, 1967.

Hasso AN, Ledington JA: Traumatic injuries of the temporal bone. Otolaryngol Clin North Am 21:295–316, 1988.

Heid L, Claussen C-F, Kersebaum M, Nagy E, Bencze G, Bencsik B: Vertigo, dizziness, and tinnitus after otobasal fractures. Int Tinnitus J 10:94–100, 2004.

Hicks GW, Wright JW Jr, Wright JW: Cerebrospinal fluid otorrhea. Laryngoscope 90(suppl 25):1–25, 1980.

Hough JVD: Restoration of hearing loss after head trauma. Ann Otol 78:210–226, 1969.

Hough JVD, Stuart WD: Middle ear injuries in skull trauma. Laryngoscope 78:899–937, 1968.

Ishman SL, Friedland DR: Temporal bone fractures: Traditional classification and clinical relevance. Laryngoscope 114:1734–1741, 2004.

Johnson F, Semaan MT, Megerian CA: Temporal bone fracture: Evaluation and management in the modern era. Otolaryngol Clin North Am 41:597–618, 2008.

Kamerer DB: Intratemporal facial nerve injuries. Otolaryngol Head Neck Surg 90:612–615, 1982.

Kettel K: Peripheral facial palsy in fractures of the temporal bone. Arch Otolaryngol 51:25–41, 1950.

Lambert PR, Brackman DE: Facial paralysis in longitudinal temporal bone fractures: A review of 26 cases. Laryngoscope 94:1022–1026, 1984.

Laumans EPJ, Yongkees LBW: On the prognosis of peripheral facial paralysis of endotemporal origin. Ann Otol Rhinol Laryngol 72:622–636, 894–899, 1963.

Little SC, Kesser BW: Radiographic classification of temporal bone fractures: Clinical predictability using a new system. Arch Otolaryngol Head Neck Surg 132:1300–1304, 2006.

Lyos AT, March MA, Jenkins HA, Coker, NJ: Progressive hearing loss after transverse temporal bone fracture. Arch Otolaryngol Head Neck Surg 121:795–799, 1995.

Mcfeely WJ, Bojrab DI, Davis KG, Hegyi DF: Otologic injuries caused by airbag deployment. Otolaryngol Head Neck Surg 121:367, 1999.

Nosan D, Benecke JE, Murr AH: Current perspectice on temporal bone trauma. Otolaryngol Head Neck Surg 117:67–71, 1997.

Pennington CL: Incus transposition techniques. Ann Otol Rhinol Laryngol 82:518–531, 1973.

Podoshin L, Fradis M: Hearing loss after head injury. Arch Otolaryngol 101:15–18, 1975.

Pulec JL: Total facial nerve exposure. Arch Otolaryngol 89:179–183, 1969.

Quaranta A, Campobasso G, Piazza F, Quaranta N, Salonna I: Facial nerve paralysis in temporal bone fractures: Outcomes after late decompression surgery. Acta Otolaryngol 121:652–655, 2001.

Savva A, Taylor MJ, Beatty CW: Management of cerebrospinal fluid leaks involving the temporal bone: Report on 92 patients. Laryngoscope 113:50–56, 2003.

Schuknecht HF: Mechanism of inner ear injury from blows to the head. Ann Otol 78:253–262, 1969.

Schuknecht HF, Davison RC: Deafness and vertigo from head injury. Arch Otolaryngol 63:513–528, 1956.

Shea JJ, Emmett JR: Traumatic perilymph fistula. Laryngoscope 90:1513–1520, 1980.

Strom M: Trauma of the middle ear. Adv Otorhinolaryngol 35:1–254, 1986.

Tos M: Prognosis of hearing loss in temporal bone fractures. J Laryngol Otol 85:1147–1159, 1979.

Travis LW, Stalnaker RL, Melvin JW: Impact trauma of the human temporal bone. J Tauma 17:761–766, 1977.

Ulug T, Ulubil SA: Contralateral labyrinthine concussion in temporal bone fractures. J Otolaryngol 35:380–383, 2006.

Wennmo C, Svennson C: Temporal bone fractures-vestibular and other related ear sequel. Acta Otolaryngol (Suppl) 468:379–383, 1989.

Yanagihara N: Transmastoid decompression of the facial nerve in the temporal bone fracture. Otolaryngol Head Neck Surg 90:616–621, 1982.

Ylikosky J, Sanna M: Vestibular neurectomy for dizziness after head trauma. ORL J Otorhinolaryngol Relat Spec 45:216–225, 1983.

Laryngeal Injuries

Alonso WA, Pratt LL, Zollinger WK: Complications of laryngotracheal disruption. Laryngoscope 84:1276–1290, 1974.

Bogdasarian RS, Olson NR: Posterior glottic laryngeal stenosis. Otolaryngol Head Neck Surg 88:765–772, 1980.

Bryce DP: Subglottic stenosis. Laryngoscope 89:320–324, 1979.

Bryce DP: The surgical management of laryngotracheal injury. J Laryngol Otol 86:547–587, 1972.

Chandler JR: Avulsion of the larynx and pharynx as the result of a water ski rope injury. Arch Otolaryngol 96:365–367, 1972.

Cummings CW, Sessions DG, Weymuller EA Jr, Wood P: Atlas of Laryngeal Surgery. St. Louis: CV Mosby, 1984, pp 43–190.

Dedo HH, Rowe LP: Laryngeal reconstruction in acute and chronic injuries. Otolaryngol Clin North Am 16:373–388, 1983.

Dedo HH, Sooy FA: Surgical repair of late glottic stenosis. Ann Otol 77:435–441, 1968.

deMello-Filho FV, Carrau RL: The management of laryngeal fractures using internal fixation. Laryngoscope 110:2143–2146, 2000.

Fearon B, Cotton R: Surgical correction of subglottic stenosis of the larynx. Ann Otol 81:508–513, 1972.

Finnegan DA, Wong ML, Kashima HK: Hyoid autograft repair of chronic subglottic stenosis. Ann Otol Rhinol Laryngol 84:643–649, 1975.

Geffin B, Grillo HC, Cooper JC, Pontoppidant L: Stenosis following tracheostomy for respiratory care. JAMA 216:1984–1988, 1971.

Grillo HC: Circumferential resection and reconstruction of the mediastinal and cervical trachea. Ann Surg 162:374–388, 1965.

Grillo HC: Management of cervical mediastinal lesions of the trachea. JAMA 197:1085–1090, 1966.

Gussack GS, Jurkovich GJ, Luterman A: Laryngotracheal trauma: A protocol approach to a rare injury. Laryngoscope 96:660–665, 1986.

Harris HH, Ainsworth JZ: Immediate management of laryngeal and tracheal injuries. Laryngoscope 75:1103–1115, 1965.

Hwang SY, Yeak SC: Management dilemmas in laryngeal trauma. J Laryngol Otol 118:325–328, 2004.

Isshiki N: Vocal mechanics as the basis of phonosurgery. Laryngoscope 108:1761–1766, 1998.

Kennedy TL: Epiglottic reconstruction of laryngeal stenosis secondary to cricothyroidostomy. Laryngoscope 90:1130–1134, 1980.

Kuttenberger JJ, Hardt N, Schlegel C: Diagnosis and initial management of laryngotracheal injuries associated with facial fractures. J Craniomaxillofac 32:80–84, 2004.

LeJeune FE: Laryngotracheal separation. Laryngoscope 88:1956–1962, 1976.

Lewy RB: Experience with vocal cord injection. Ann Otol 85:440–450, 1976.

McNaught RC: Surgical correction of anterior web of the larynx. Laryngoscope 60:264–272, 1950.

Montgomery WW: Surgery of the Upper Respiratory System. 1st ed. Philadelphia: Lea & Febiger, 1973, pp 315–372.

Montgomery WW: The surgical management of supraglottic and subglottic stenosis. Ann Otol Rhinol Laryngol 77:534–546, 1968.

Montgomery WW, Blaugrund SM, Varvares MA: Thryoplasty: A new approach. Ann Otol Rhinol Laryngol 102:571–579, 1993.

Montgomery WW, Gamble JE: Anterior glottic stenosis. Arch Otolaryngol 92:560–567, 1970.

Myer CM, Orobello P, Cotton RT, Bratcher GO: Blunt laryngeal trauma in children. Laryngoscope 97:1043–1048, 1987.

Netterville JL, Stone RE, Luken ES, Civantos FJ, Ossoff RH: Silastic medialization and arytenoid adduction: The vanderbilt experience: A review of the phonosurgical procedures. Ann Otol Rhinol Laryngol 102:413–424, 1993.

Newman MH, Work WP: Arytenoidectomy revisited. Laryngoscope 86:840–849, 1976.

Ogura JH, Biller HF: Reconstruction of the larynx following blunt trauma. Ann Otol Rhinol Laryngol 80:492–506, 1971.

Ogura JH, Powers WE: Functional restitution of traumatic stenosis of the larynx and pharynx. Laryngoscope 74:1081–1110, 1964.

Olson NR: Laryngeal suspension and epiglottic flap in laryngotracheal trauma. Ann Otol Rhinol Laryngol 85:533–538, 1976.

Olson NR: Surgical treatment of acute blunt laryngeal injuries. Ann Otol Rhinol Laryngol 87:716–721, 1978.

Olson NR: Wound healing by primary intention in the larynx. Otolaryngol Clin North Am 12:735–740, 1977.

Olson NR, Miles WK: Treatment of acute blunt laryngeal injuries. Ann Otol Rhinol Laryngol 80:704–710, 1971.

Pennington CL: External trauma of the larynx and trachea. Ann Otol Rhinol Laryngol 81:546–554, 1972.

Pennington CL: Glottic and supraglottic laryngeal injury and stenosis from external trauma. Laryngoscope 77:317–345, 1964.

Potter CR, Sessions DG, Ogura JH: Blunt laryngotracheal trauma. Otolaryngol 86:909–923, 1978.

Quick CA, Merwin GE: Arytenoid dislocation. Arch Otolaryngol 104:267–270, 1978.

Rethi A: An operation for cicatricial stenosis of the larynx. J Otolaryngol 72:283–293, 1956.

Schaefer SD: The acute management of external laryngeal trauma: A 27 year experience. Arch Otolaryngol Head Neck Surg 118:598–604, 1992.

Schaefer SD, Close LG: Acute management of laryngeal trauma: Update. Ann Otol Rhinol Laryngol 98:98–104, 1989.

Schaefer SD, Close LG, Brown OE: Mobilization of the fixed arytenoid in the stenotic posterior laryngeal commissure. Laryngoscope 96:656–659, 1986.

Schuller DE, Parrish RT: Reconstruction of the larynx and trachea. Arch Otolaryngol Head Neck Surg 114:211–219, 1988.

Stanley RB, Coleman WF: Unilateral degloving injuries of the arytenoid cartilage. Arch Otolaryngol Head Neck Surg 112:516–518, 1986.

Stanley RB, Cooper DS, Florman SH: Phonatory effects of thyroid cartilage fractures. Ann Otol Rhinol Laryngol 96:493–496, 1987.

Thawley SE, Ogura JE: Use of the hyoid graft for treatment of laryngotracheal stenosis. Laryngoscope 91:226–232, 1981.

Trone TH, Schaefer SD: Blunt and penetrating laryngeal trauma: A 13 year review. Otolaryngol Head Neck Surg 88:257–261, 1980.

Tucker HM: Human laryngeal reinnervation: Long-term experience with the nerve-muscle pedicle technique. Laryngoscope 88:598–604, 1978.

Tucker HM, Wood BJ, Levine H, Katz R: Glottic reconstruction after near total laryngectomy. Laryngoscope 89:609–617, 1979.

Verschueren DS, Bell RB, Bagheri SC, Dierks EJ, Potter BE: Management of Laryngo-tracheal injuries associated with craniomaxillofacial trauma. J Oral Maxillofac Surg 64:203–214, 2006.

Ward RH, Canalis R, Fee W, Smith G: Composite hyoid sternohyoid muscle grafts in humans. Arch Otolaryngol 103:531–534, 1977.

Pediatric Fractures

Bos, Rudolf RM: Treatment of pediatric facial fractures: The case for metallic fixation. J Oral Maxillofac Surg 63:382–384, 2005.

Drumholler FH: Nasal fractures in children. Postgrad Med 48:123–127, 1970.

Eggensperger Wymann MN, Hölzie A, Zachariou Z, Iizuka T: Pediatric craniofacial trauma. J Oral Maxillofac Surg 66:58–64, 2008.

Eppley BL: Use of absorbable plates and screws in pediatric facial fractures. J Oral Maxillofac Surg. 63:385–391, 2005.

Eppley BL, Sadove AM, Havlik RJ: Resorbable plate fixation in pediatric craniofacial surgery. Plast Reconstr Surg 100:1–7, 1997.

Ferreira P, Amarante J, Silva P, Rodrigues J, Choupina M, Silva A, Barbosa R, Cardoso M, Reis J: Retrospective study of 1251 maxillofacial fractures in children and adolescents. Plast Reconstr Surg 115:1500–1508, 2005.

Gerbino G, Roccia F, Bianchi, FA, Zavattero E: Surgical management of orbital trap-door fracture in pediatric population. J Oral Maxillofac Surg 68:1310–1316, 2010.

Goode RL, Spooner TR: Management of nasal fractures in children: A review of current practices. Clin Pediatr 11:526–529, 1972.

Hatef DA, Cole PD, Hollier LH: Contemporary management of pediatric facial trauma. Curr Opin Otolaryngol Head Neck Surg 17:308–314, 2009.

Hatton MP, Watkins LM, Rubin PA: Orbital fractures in children. Ophthalmol Plast Reconstr Surg 117:174–179, 2001.

Holland AJ, Broome C, Steinberg A, Cass DT: Facial fractures in children. Pediatr Emerg Care 17:157–160, 2001.

Imola MJ, Hamlar DO, Shao W, Choudhury K, Tatum S: Resorbable plate fixation in pediatric craniofacial surgery: Long term outcome. Arch Facial Plast Surg 3:79–90, 2001.

James D: Maxillofacial injuries in children in Rowe and Williams' Maxillofacial Injuries. William JL (ed): London: Churchill Livingstone, 1994, pp 387–403; 448–456.

Kaban LB, Mulliken JB, Murry JE: Facial fractures in children: An analysis of 122 fractures I 109 patients. Plast Reconstr Surg 9:15–20, 1977.

Koltai PJ, Rabkin D: Management of facial trauma in children. Pediatr Clin North Am 43:1253–1275, 1996.

Kwon J, Moon J, Kwon M, Cho J: The differences of blowout fracture of the inferior orbital wall between children and adults. Arch Otolaryngol Head and Neck Surg 131:723–727, 2005.

Losee J, Afifi A, Jiang S, Smith D, Chao M, Vecchione L, Hertle R, Davis J, Naran S, Hughes J, Paviglianiti J, Deleyiannis F: Pediatric orbital fractures: Classification, management, and early follow-up. Plast Reconstr Surg 122(3):886–897, 2008.

McCoy F, Chandler RA, Crow ML: Facial fractures in children. Plast Reconstr Surg 37:209–215, 1966.

McGraw BL, Cole RR: Pediatric maxillofacial trauma: Age-related variables in injury. Arch Otolaryngol 116:41–45, 1999.

Messinger A, Radkowski MA, Greenwald MJ, Penslow JM: Orbital roof fractures in the pediatric population. Plast Reconstr Surg 84:213–216, 1989.

Morales JL, Skowronski PD, Thaller SR: Management of pediatric maxillary fractures. J Craniofac Surg 21:1226–1233, 2010.

Moran WB: Nasal trauma in children. Otolarygol Clin North Am 10:95–101, 1977.

Olsen KD, Carpenter RJ, Kern EB: Nasal septal injury in children. Arch Otolargol 106:317–320, 1980.

Posnick JC, Wells M, Pron GE: Pediatric facial fractures: Evolving patterns of treatment. J Oral Maxillofac Surg 51(8):836–844, 1993.

Rowe NL: Fracture of the jaws in children. J Oral Surg 27:497–507, 1969.

Stucker FJ, Bryarly RC, Shockley MW: Management of nasal trauma in children. Arch Otolaryngol 110:190–192, 1984.

Suei Y, Mallick P, Nagasaki T, Taguchi A, Fujita M, Tanimoto K: Radiographic evaluation of the fate of developing tooth buds on the fracture line of Mandibular fractures. J Oral Maxillofac Surg 64:94–99, 2006.

Zimmermann CE, Troulis MJ, Kaban LB: Pediatric facial fractures: Recent advances in prevention, diagnosis and management. Int J Oral Maxillofac Surg 35:2–13, 2006.

Nonunion, after palatal split, 276
  of condylar fracture, 128, 131, 145
  of mandible. See *Mandible nonunion*
  of mandibular body fracture, 169
  of maxilla, 255, 262–263
Nose. See *Nasal entries*
Nose injury, 65, 307, 406
Nosebleeds, 52, 330, 503
Nutation, *66, 67*
Nylon suture, 105, 110, 167, 204, 211, 221,
          258, 331, 346, 350, 375, 376, 381, 388,
          391, 404, 406, 417, 421, 429, 431, 433,
          444, 452, 462, 471, 476, 526, 562, 576,
          584, 595, 597, 604, 613, 616, 1020

O

Obstruction, postoperative, tracheostomy
          and, 16, 48
Onlay graft technique, for malunited
          zygoma fractures, 357, 358, *359,*
          360, 361
  for mandible malunion, 225–228, *227*
  for upper lip retrusion or accentuation of
          nasolabial fold, 289
Open fracture, of mandible, 115
Open rhinoplasty, for nasal deformity after
          trauma, 330–331, *332*
Open sky incision, 444
Optic nerve damage, 499
Optic nerve decompression, 499, 500, *501,*
          502, 503, 504, *505, 506,* 507, 508, *509*
Optic nerve, localization of, 500, 502
Oral airway, 27, *28–29*
Orbicularis oculi, 399
Orbit, anatomic relationships of, 399, 400,
          401, 402
  roof of, fractures of, 478
Orbital deformity and dysfunction, from
          wire fixation of zygoma fracture,
          349–350
Orbital fat herniation, 375
Orbital floor and rim osteotomy, 287, *300*
Orbital floor fractures, polyethylene mesh
          repair of, indications for, 372, 375
Orbital reconstruction, cranial grafts for, 390,
          391, *392*
  for combined orbital trauma syndrome,
          394–395, *396*
  iliac crest grafts for
    complications of, 214
    indications for, 210
    pitfalls of, 214
    procedure for, 210–211, *212–213,* 214
  osteotomy for, 391, *392, 393*
Orbital wall fractures, blow-out type of,
          Caldwell-Luc approach for, 377,
          378, 379
  classification of, 367, *368, 369*
  contraindications to repair of, 375
  medial area, polyethylene mesh repair of,
          380, 381, *382, 383*
  parietal cortex grafts for, *374,* 377
  pathophysiology of, 367, *368, 369*
  polyethylene mesh repair of
    pitfalls of, 375
  polyethylene mesh repair of
    complications of, 375–376
    procedure for, 372, *373–374,* 375
    titanium mesh repair of, 371, *374,* 376
  timing of repair of, 375
Oropharyngeal intubation, 33, *34,* 35
Orotracheal intubation
  pitfalls of, 38

  procedure for, 36, *37, 38*
Orthodontic bracket technique, for tooth
          injuries, 189, *190,* 191, *192,*
          193, 194
Ossicular chain, damage of, 514
  repair of, 448, 450, *449*
Osteointegrated implant, *223*
Osteomyelitis, at mandibular body fracture
          site, 167, 169
Osteoplastic flap, coronal, for inferior wall
          fracture of frontal sinus, 465, 466,
          467, 468
Osteoradionecrosis, 221
Osteotomy, for zygoma fracture malunion,
          353, 354, *355, 356*
  for mandible malunion, 226, 227
  for orbital reconstruction, 391, *392*
Oxymetazoline, 33, 52, 53, 56, 311, 491,
          503, 518

P

Palatal osteotomy, *295, 300*
Palatal split, arch bar fixation of
  indications for
    pitfalls of, 276
    procedure for, 275–276, *277*
  miniplate fixation of, 275, 276, *277,* 278
  reduction and fixation of, with prosthesis
          and screws, 279, *280,* 281
Palatal split, arch bar fixation of, indications
          for, 275
Panorex (orthopanthogram), 3, 6, *7*
Papillary dermis, 59, *60,* 61, *62,* 93
Parasymphyseal fractures, 116, *118*
  closed reduction of, in children, 181, *182,*
          183, 184
  external pin fixation of, 177, *178, 179, 180*
  interosseous wiring and intermaxillary
          fixation for, indications for, 177
    procedure for, 177, *178,* 179
    using rigid internal plate fixation, *178,*
          179, 180
  open reduction of, with interosseous
          wiring and intermaxillary fixation,
          177, *178,* 179, 185, *186, 187*
  rigid internal plate fixation of, 177, *178,*
          179, 180, 185
  splint fabrication on patient's dental arch
          in, 181, *182, 183, 184*
Parietal cortex grafts, for Le Fort II fracture
          repair, 255, *256*
  for orbital wall fracture repair, *374, 376*
Parotid duct injury, open repair of, 110,
          111, 112
Parotitis, 112
Pasteurella, 79
Pectoralis major flap, 64
Penetrating injury, 31, 65–78
Perilymph fistula, 543, *544*
Perineal artery, 102
Periodontal infection, 199
Periosteal elevation, for tooth extraction,
          197, *198,* 199
Pharyngeal intubation, 33, *34,* 35
Pharyngotomy, anterior, with partial supra-
          glottic resection, 575, 576, *577, 578,*
          579, *580, 581*
Pharynx, bleeding from, 53
Phrenic nerve, *69, 74, 76*
Plate bender, 20, *22*
Plate cutter, *15,* 20, 23
Plate exposure, postoperative, from miniplate
          fixation of Le Fort II fractures, 255

Plate fixation, of anterior wall frontal sinus
          fractures, 443, 444, *445,* 446, *447,*
          448, 449
Plate holder, 20, *23,* 157, 167
Plating, 3–24, 146, 153, 155–163, 241, *254,*
          258, 262, *352,* 353, 443–450, 452, *457,*
          477, 564, 629, 640
Pledgets (nasal), 52, 53, 270, 273, 311, 312,
          420, 424, 470, 490–494, *495,* 503, 508,
          522, 606, 607
Pneumothorax, 30, 31, *32,* 46, 48, 67, 70
Pneumothorax, after tracheostomy, 48
Poly-L-lactic acid, 14
Polyethylene mesh repair, of orbital wall
          fractures, *372, 373, 374,* 375
  complications of, 175–176
  pitfalls of, 375
Posterior nasal artery, 56
Posterior tibial artery, 216, *217,* 218, 221
Postintubation care, 38
Postoperative depression, from wire fixation
          of malar fracture, 349
Preauricular incision, 107, *109*
Precession, *66, 67*
Prolene suture, 80, 84, 89, 579
Prosthetic stabilization, of palatal split
  complications of, 281
  pitfalls of, 279
  procedure for, 279, *280*
Pseudoarthrosis, of condylar fracture, 131
Pterygoid plate displacement, 487
Pterygomaxillary buttress, 239
Pterygomaxillary osteotomy, *286,* 291,
          295, 300
PTFE graft, 77
Pulse Doppler thrombosis, 221

R

Rabies, 79, 89
Ramus fractures
  ascending, closed and open treatment of,
          153, *154*
    pitfalls of, 153
  closed and open treatment of, indications
          for, 153
Reankylosis, 233
Reconstruction plate, 14, 16, *17,* 157, 163,
          167, 170–176, 203–215, 218, 220,
          222, 226
Recurrent laryngeal nerve, neurorrhaphy
          of, 590
Recurrent laryngeal nerve, neurorrhaphy of
  paralysis of, from subglottic stenosis
          repair, 613
Regurgitation of stomach contents, tracheal
          intubation and, 36
Reidel procedure, 458
Reiger flap (dorsal nasal), 84, *86*
Residual contour defects, after Le Fort II
          osteotomy, 294
Resorbable plates-absorbable, 14, 16, 24, 246,
          252, 255, 270, 562, 564, 584, 629–636
Resorption, of bone graft, 211
Respiratory difficulty, cricothyrotomy for,
          41, *42*
Resuscitation, 30, 67, 70
Reticular dermis, 59, 60, 62
Retinal tear, 375
Rhomboid flap, 80, *82,* 89
Rib graft technique, for malunion of zygoma
          fractures, 358, *360*
  for temporomandibular ankylosis, 230,
          231–232, 233